Human
Embryology

Human Embryology

THIRD EDITION

William J. Larsen, Ph.D.

Professor, Department of Cell Biology, Neurobiology and Anatomy
Faculty Member, Developmental Biology Graduate Program
University of Cincinnati College of Medicine
Research Faculty, Perinatal Research Institute
Children's Hospital and University of Cincinnati College of Medicine
Cincinnati, Ohio

This Edition Specially Edited By

Lawrence S. Sherman, Ph.D.

Assistant Professor, Department of Cell Biology, Neurobiology and Anatomy
University of Cincinnati College of Medicine
Vontz Center for Molecular Studies
Cincinnati, Ohio

S. Steven Potter, Ph.D.

Professor of Pediatrics, Division of Developmental Biology
The Children's Hospital Research Foundation
Children's Hospital
Cincinnati, Ohio

William J. Scott, Ph.D.

Professor of Pediatrics, Division of Developmental Biology
The Children's Hospital Research Foundation
Children's Hospital
Cincinnati, Ohio

TM

CHURCHILL LIVINGSTONE
An Imprint of Elsevier

CHURCHILL LIVINGSTONE
An Imprint of Elsevier

The Curtis Center
Independence Square West
Philadelphia, Pennsylvania 19106

Library of Congress Cataloging-in-Publication Data

Larsen, William J.   (William James)
    Human embryology / William J. Larsen.—3rd ed.

        p.   ;   cm.

    Includes bibliographical references and index.

    ISBN 0–443–06583–7

    1. Embryology, Human.
        [DNLM: 1.   Embryology.   QS 604 L334h 2001]   I. Title.

QM601   L37   2001

612.6'4—dc21   2001017467

Acquisitions Editor: William Schmitt
Developmental Editor: David Orzechowski
Manuscript Editor: Mary Reinwald
Production Manager: Frank Polizzano
Illustration Specialist: Peg Shaw
Book Designer: Marie Gardocky-Clifton

HUMAN EMBRYOLOGY   ISBN 0-443-06583-7

Permissions may be sought directly from Elsevier's Health Sciences Rights Department in Philadelphia, USA: phone: (+1)215-238-7869, fax: (+1)215-238-2239, email: healthpermissions@elsevier.com. You may also complete your request on-line via the Elsevier Science homepage (http://www.elsevier.com), by selecting 'Customer Support' and then 'Obtaining Permissions'.

CHURCHILL LIVINGSTONE and the Sail Boat Design are trademarks of Elsevier.

Printed in China

Last digit is the print number: 9   8   7   6   5   4

William J. Larsen, Ph.D.
1942–2000
Developmental biology research scientist and teacher par excellence,
author of *Human Embryology* and *Human Anatomy* (in press),
furniture builder, lover of the Southwest, superlative storyteller and
humorist, gourmet cook, thoughtful advisor,
exciting and generous personality—a truly unique and exceptional
human being.

Preface to the Third Edition

The completion of the human genome project was indeed an amazing milestone for research in human genetics. This work is generating—and will undoubtedly continue to generate—an incredible new surge of experimental studies, with exciting prospects for applying the knowledge of human genetics to human embryology and medical clinical practice. The National Board of Medical Examiners has, in fact, recognized the growing importance of this area of medical education and has created both an Embryology and a Developmental Biology and Human Genetics Task Force. Dr. Larsen was invited to participate in both. (After he served on these task forces, he joined the Anatomy Test Committee.)

A short time ago, I received a concrete example of the relevance of human embryology to the practice of medicine: A physician wrote to Dr. Larsen requesting his collaboration on a chapter of a book for pediatric physicians. The goal of the chapter would be to present the ways in which knowledge of the embryology of congenital heart defects informs clinical practice for pediatric anesthesiology. It is with great sorrow, however, that I must announce that William Larsen died suddenly in January of 2000 and therefore was not able to participate personally in this project. He would have been delighted by this evidence of a real and direct use of embryologic knowledge for diagnosing and treating patients—a trend that will undoubtedly grow exponentially in the coming years.

Dr. Larsen had the work for this edition well under way before he died. He had completed several of the experimental and clinical section updates, selected current research, and outlined areas to be revised for all other chapters. Three colleagues in the area of developmental research, who had contributed to and reviewed previous editions, graciously agreed to take on the task of completing this revision. They are Doctors Lawrence S. Sherman, S. Steven Potter, and William J. Scott. These three individuals reviewed vast amounts of current published research articles and conferred with, or elicited the help of, other clinical and research colleagues to update both the experimental and clinical sections of each chapter—exactly as Bill had done in previous editions. Descriptive embryology sections of the book were also updated where necessary, and over 40 figures were enhanced. I am incredibly grateful to them for taking on this task. Their commitment, time, and expertise, as well as their good humor and positive interactions, have made a difficult job much more enjoyable. Together, they have produced a book current in every respect.

The Human Embryology website has also been updated with the addition of a number of new animations and will be kept current by Bill's son, Eric Larsen, who originally created the website and the animations.

I have lost the love of my life, my inspiration and supporter, the marvelous father of our children, and my closest friend. The world has lost a person with a great zest for life, a superlative storyteller, and a caring, generous person. His gift to embryology and medical education was his ability to see the whole picture and synthesize it for others—a gift that makes this book unique among embryology textbooks. His vision is reflected in the structure of this book in which classical embryology has been combined with a brief overview of exciting new research. This provides beginning medical students with the tools to understand research discoveries that will forever change the future of their medical careers. I am happy that this book, which reflects Bill's greatest professional passions—his excitement about embryology and his devotion to the art of teaching—so excellently carries on his spirit.

Human Embryology **Third Edition Editors**
Lawrence S. Sherman, Ph.D., Assistant Professor—Graduate Programs in Neuroscience, Molecular and Developmental Biology, Cell and Molecular Biology, and Physician Scientist Training Program. His research area is development of the

peripheral nervous system, with a focus on how processes that occur during development are recapitulated after nerve injury and in nervous system cancers.

S. Steven Potter, Ph.D., Professor of Pediatrics in the Division of Developmental Biology. He is studying the roles of homeobox genes in limb, urogenital, and central nervous system development, with a special focus on left-right axis determination.

William J. Scott, Ph.D., Professor of Pediatrics, codirected (with William Larsen) a graduate level course for students of Developmental Biology research and genetic counseling. His research interests are in teratology, especially drug-induced congenital malformations of the limbs.

The following people reviewed and offered suggestions on various sections of the text for this edition: Jeffrey Whitsett, Larry Patterson, Richard Miller, Robert Gendron, and Robert Arceci. I am grateful to all of them.

I am also indebted to Marianne Bronner-Fraser, George Daston, David Repaske, Sheila Bell, Cliff Tabin, Andrew McMahon, Dorothy Supp, Jay Hoying, Peter Stambrook, Gail Benson, Tom Doetschman, Stephen D. Smith, Richard Maas, R. A. Conlon, Mario Cappechi, Susan Wert, Kathryn Yutzey, Melissa Colbert, Margaret Kirby, Bjorn Olsen, Thomas Reid, George Nikas, Tariq Siddiqui, K. Lawson, Jonathan Cooke, J. E. Cook, Lee Niswander, Raymond Gasser, C. R. Ball, Donald R. Cahill, Lewis Williams, Y. Fukui, Stephan Carmichael, Ann Hirschfield, David Chan, Martin J. Coh, R. Hunt, C. Ward Kirscher, Stefan Mundlos, Herbert Steinbeisser, Richard Brand, Robb Krumlauf, Claire Shreiner, Igor Dawid, Michael Gershon, Bruce Carlson, Colin Wendell-Smith, Jean Marx, M. Bruecker, John Saunders, Cynthia Loomis, John Fallon, and E. L. Cardell. Without their insights and suggestions, this book would not have been possible.

JUDITH I. LARSEN

Preface to the Second Edition

The revolution in mammalian and human embryology described in the preface to the first edition of *Human Embryology* has continued and accelerated. It has been just ten years since *Hox* genes were discovered in mammals; by the time the first edition of this book was written, only a few other regulatory genes inherited from our evolutionary ancestors had been described. Nevertheless, it seemed likely that these initial discoveries held fundamental significance for our understanding of human development. Research carried out in the last few years has clearly demonstrated the authenticity of this hope. The number and functions of developmental regulatory genes in mammals, including humans, have expanded exponentially. Indeed, it appears that many ancestral gene cascades have been co-opted for the regulation of unique vertebrate or mammalian developmental processes that do not even occur in lower organisms.

These new findings are exciting in their own right, but the significance of the new molecular discoveries to congenital disease and clinical practice attests to their practical value as well. This is illustrated by the movement of several discussions in the Experimental Principles sections of the first edition to Clinical Applications sections of the second. In most cases, this has occurred as a consequence of mapping and/or cloning of the human homolog of specific regulatory genes or discovery that their disruption results in human congenital disease. A few of the many examples include *PAX3* (Hirschsprung's disease), surfactant B (surfactant B deficiency), *HOXD13* (syndactyly), and *SHH* (limb and craniofacial malformations). Identification of genes that underlie many other human congenital malformations are also on the horizon, including genes that underlie situs defects and Down syndrome. In addition, it is now known that several human regulatory genes or related genes also function as tumor suppressor genes. Indeed, disruptions of some of these genes are among the most common causes of significant human cancers. While this information is particularly relevant to diagnosis, it is likely that effective therapies will also evolve more rapidly once the genetic and mechanistic bases of specific congenital disease are understood. Finally, advances in techniques such as spectral karyotyping, Southern blotting, and RT-PCR have also improved the efficiency and accuracy of clinical screening and diagnoses. This second edition, therefore, has attempted to update many of these new advances, although the rapidity and volume of change and limitations of space have forced the need to be selective.

The study of human embryology continues to provide a useful basis for the understanding of definitive human anatomy; to this end, several revisions to figures and new scanning electron micrographs have also been included in this second edition. Perhaps the most important didactic improvements of this edition to the teaching of descriptive embryology and anatomy, however, are numerous animations and interactive testing exercises that can be found on the new World Wide Web site for *Human Embryology* (http://www.med.uc.edu/embryology). The web site will also be useful to those who wish to keep abreast of new information as it unfolds between the second and third editions and for those who wish to comment or provide suggestions for improvements.

I owe a debt of sincere gratitude to the many colleagues who graciously contributed figures or who read, critiqued, or made suggestions for the second edition. They include George Daston, David Repaske, William J. Scott, Sheila Bell, Cliff Tabin, Andrew McMahon, Larry Sherman, Steve Potter, Dorothy Supp, Jay Hoying, Robert Gendron, Peter Stambrook, Gail Benson, Tom Doetschman, Stephen D. Smith, Richard Maas, R. A. Conlon, Mario Cappechi, Susan Wert, Kathryn Yutzey, Melissa Colbert, Margaret Kirby, Bjorn Olsen, Thomas Reid, George Nikas, Tariq Siddiqui, K. Lawson, Jonathan Cooke, J. E. Cook, Lee Niswander, Raymond Gasser, C. R. Ball, Donald R.

Cahill, Lewis Williams, Y. Kukui, Stephen Carmichael, Ann Hirschfield, David Chan, Martin J. Cohn, R. Hunt, C. Ward Kischer, Stefan Mundlos, Herbert Steinbeisser, Richard Brand, Robb Krumlauf, Robert Arceci, Igor Dawid, Michael Gershon, Bruce Carlson, Colin Wendell-Smith, Jean Marx, M. Brueckner, John Saunders, Cynthia Loomis, John Fallon, and E. L. Cardell.

WILLIAM J. LARSEN, PH.D.

Preface to the First Edition

A torrent of new findings and techniques has revolutionized embryology. As a result, this discipline is relevant not only to understanding adult structure but also, increasingly, to a physician's direct practice. I have written *Human Embryology* to meet the needs of first-year medical students in gross anatomy and neuroanatomy courses and to offer them a glimpse of some of the exciting applications that are currently in use or on the horizon. This text is used at the University of Cincinnati in conjunction with the twelve embryology lectures given in the gross anatomy course. It will also interest other readers, including premedical undergraduates, graduate students in developmental biology programs, nursing students, and allied health students in disciplines such as the burgeoning field of genetic counseling.

I researched this book intensively in an attempt to make it wholly up-to-date. In the course of that process, I learned a great deal that has renewed my own fascination with embryology, including the truth behind a number of venerable chestnuts that have been passed down in generations of embryology texts. It is my hope that the students who read this text will be as enthralled by modern embryology as I am.

This text uses a modular design that allows students to review the material in several ways and that will let instructors tailor the book to their specific needs. The first six chapters describe gametogenesis, fertilization, and the initial weeks of development; Chapters 7 to 14 deal with the individual organ systems; and the last chapter covers aspects of fetal development. Each chapter opens with a summary that gives a condensed version of the material in the chapter. In accordance with a frequent demand of my students, these summaries are supplemented by full-page timeline illustrations that graphically display the timing of the events described. The main portion of each chapter is devoted to a concise descriptive embryology of its subject. Other topics, such as theoretical discussions and description of congenital anomalies, are segregated in special Clinical Applications and Experimental Principles sections, where they will not clutter the essential story. I have worked hard to make the descriptions of morphogenetic processes complete as well as concise, because I know from experience that gaps in the explanation make these processes difficult to visualize and, hence, to remember. The text headings are written in sentence style so as to encapsulate the main points of the chapter.

Good three-dimensional illustrations are obviously central to an embryology text. Once a chapter has been mastered, the reader ought to be able to review it by thumbing through the pictures and skimming the captions. Within the limits of space and expense, I have tried to illustrate enough critical stages of each process to obviate "leaps of faith." In the interests of clarity, I have converted all length, somite number, and stage designations to approximate gestation time in days and weeks. However, a complete table relating Carnegie stages, embryo length in millimeters, and numbers of somites is provided on pages xv and xvi. Structures are usually shown in their real context in the embryo, rather than left to float on the page, and color is used abundantly to indicate the derivation of structures and tissues. Where possible, I have included scanning electron micrographs to show how the structures in question actually look.

Although the Clinical Applications and Experimental principles sections relate to the descriptive text, they are free-standing and can be assigned or omitted at will. Topics such as multifactorial inheritance, sensitive periods, teratogenicity, and prenatal diagnosis, as well as a selection of congenital abnormalities, are covered in the Clinical Applications sections. These sections will sharpen the interest of first-year students by showing the relation of embryology to clinical practice. Some of them will also prove useful in later training. A student studying Hirschsprung's disease in a second-year pathology course, for example, can refer to the section on the pathogenesis of the underlying parasympathetic anomaly, and a student on a third-year clinical rotation can review the common cardiac anomalies.

Even a cursory reading of the short Experimental Principles sections will show how the information in the description embryology sections was obtained and will give a glimpse of the frontiers of diagnosis, therapy, and research. Some of these sections are essential to a first-year student, but others are of fundamental utility, such as the discussion of induction in Chapter 4 and the section on the pathogenetic bases of cardiac anomalies in Chapter 7. These sections may also be used to support the multidisciplinary approaches currently employed in some schools.

The past decade has witnessed a revolution in the diagnosis and treatment of congenital diseases. Many diseases can be identified in utero, and fetal operations may soon be routine. However, the revolution is only beginning: The studies now being carried out on novel molecular techniques, such as gene therapy, are thrusting us abruptly into a new age of prenatal medicine. Techniques to cure such diseases as congenital immunodeficiency syndromes and cystic fibrosis are being tested in animal models, for example. Because of this prospect of therapeutic payoff, the molecular basis of development has become a highly funded topic in medical research. Here in the United States, the number of grant applications submitted to the Molecular Genetics section of the National Institute of Child Health and Human Development is increasing at an unprecedented rate. It will not be possible to develop appropriate applications for these new molecular techniques, however, without input from classical experimental and descriptive embryologic research. That task of integration and application—as well as the daunting social and ethical challenges that the new prenatal and genetic techniques will bring in their train—will fall largely to the students who are now studying medicine, nursing, developmental and molecular biology, and genetic counseling.

WILLIAM J. LARSEN, PH.D.

Now the Mother Earth
and the Father Sky
Meeting, joining one another,
Helpmates ever, they

All is beautiful
All is beautiful
All is beautiful, indeed

And the white corn
And the yellow corn
Meeting, joining one another
Helpmates ever, they

All is beautiful
All is beautiful
All is beautiful, indeed

(From Song of the Earth [Navajo], George W. Cronin [ed]: Songs of the Southwest. In: American Indian Poetry: Anthology of Songs and Chants. Liveright, New York, 1934, with permission.)

Contents

Correlation of Timing Systems Used For Human Embryos (Weeks 1 Through 8)

Week	Day	Length (mm)[a]	Number of Somites	Carnegie Stage	Features (chapters in which features are discussed)[b]
1	1	0.1–0.15	—	1	Fertilization (1)
	1.5–3	0.1–0.2	—	2	First cleavage divisions occur (2–16 cells) (1)
	4	0.1–0.2	—	3	Blastocyst is free in uterus (1)
	5–6	0.1–0.2	—	4	Blastocyst hatches and begins implanting (1, 2)
2	7–12	0.1–0.2	—	5	Blastocyst fully implanted (1, 2)
	13	0.2	—	6	Primary stem villi appear (2); primitive streak develops (3)
3	16	0.4	—	7	Gastrulation commences; notochordal process forms (3)
	18	1–1.5	—	8	Primitive pit forms (3); neural plate and neural groove appear (3, 4)
	20	1.5–2.5	1–3	9	Caudal eminence and first somites form (3); neuromeres appear in presumptive brain vesicles (4, 13); primitive heart tube is forming (7); vasculature begins to develop in embryonic disc (8)
4	22	2–3.5	4–12	10	Neural folds begin to fuse; cranial end of embryo undergoes rapid flexion (4, 13); pulmonary primordium appears (6); myocardium forms and heart begins to pump (7); hepatic plate appears (9); first two pharyngeal arches and optic sulci begin to form (12)
	24	2.5–4.5	13–20	11	Primordial germ cells begin to migrate from wall of yolk sac (1); cranial neuropore closes (4); buccopharyngeal membrane ruptures (12); optic vesicles develop (12); optic pit begins to form
	26	3–5	21–29	12	Caudal neuropore closes (4); cystic diverticulum and dorsal pancreatic bud appear (9); urorectal septum begins to form (9, 10); upper limb buds appear (11); pharyngeal arches 3 and 4 form (12)
	28	4–6	30+	13	Dorsal and ventral columns begin to differentiate in mantle layer of spinal cord and brain stem (4, 13); septum primum begins to form in heart (7); spleen appears (9); ureteric buds appear (10); lower limb buds appear (11); otic vesicle and lens placode appear (12); motor nuclei of cranial nerves appear (13)
5	32	5–7	—	14	Spinal nerves begin to sprout (5); semilunar valves begin to form in heart (7); lymphatics and coronary vessels appear (8); greater and lesser stomach curvatures and primary intestinal loop form (9); metanephros begins to develop (10); lens pit invaginates into optic cup; endolymphatic appendage appears (12); secondary brain vesicles begin to form; cerebral hemispheres become visible (13)
	33	7–9	—	15	Atrioventricular valves and definitive pericardial cavity begin to form (7); cloacal folds and genital tubercle appear (10); hand plate develops (11); lens vesicle forms and invagination of nasal pit creates medial and lateral nasal processes (12); sensory and parasympathetic cranial nerve ganglia begin to form; primary olfactory neurons send axons into telencephalon (13)

Correlation of Timing Systems Used For Human Embryos (Weeks 1 Through 8)

Week	Day	Length (mm)[a]	Number of Somites	Carnegie Stage	Features (chapters in which features are discussed)[b]
6	37	8–11	—	16	Muscular ventricular septum begins to form (7); gut tube lumen becomes occluded (9); major calyces of kidney begin to form and kidneys begin to ascend; genital ridges appear (10); foot plate forms on lower limb bud (11); pigment appears in retina; auricular hillocks develop (12)
	41	11–14	—	17	Bronchopulmonary segment primordia appear (6); septum intermedium of heart is complete (7); subcardinal vein system forms (8); minor calyces of kidney are forming (10); finger rays are distinct (11); nasolacrimal groove forms (12); cerebellum begins to form (13); melanocytes enter epidermis; dental laminae form (14)
7	44	13–17	—	18	Skeletal ossification begins (4, 11); Sertoli cells begin to differentiate in the male gonad (10); elbows and toe rays appear (11); intermaxillary process and eyelids form in face (12); thalami of diencephalon expand (13); nipples and first hair follicles appear (14)
	47	16–18	—	19	Septum primum fuses with septum intermedium in heart (7); urogenital membrane ruptures (10); trunk elongates and straightens (15)
8	50	18–22	—	20	Primary intestinal loop completes initial counterclockwise rotation (9); in males, paramesonephric ducts begin to regress and vasa deferentia begin to form (10); upper limbs bend at elbows (11)
	52	22–24	—	21	Pericardioperitoneal canals close (6); hands and feet approach each other at the midline (11)
	54	23–28	—	22	Eyelids and auricles are more developed (12)
	56	27–31	—	23	Chorionic cavity is obliterated by the growth of the amniotic sac (6); definitive superior vena cava and major branches of the aortic arch are established (8); lumen of gut tube is almost completely recanalized (9); primary teeth are at cap stage (14)

[a]Length is the greatest length of embryo.

[b]Timing of some events will differ slightly in some embryos.

(Columns 1 through 5 from O'Rahilly R, Müller F. 1987. Developmental Stages in Human Embryos. Carnegie Institute, Washington, D.C., Publ. No. 637, with permission.)

Gametogenesis, Fertilization, and the First Week

Summary

The discussion of human embryology could be initiated at any of several points in the human reproductive cycle. In this text, we begin our description of the developing human with the formation and differentiation of the male and female sex cells or **gametes**, which will unite at fertilization to initiate the embryonic development of a new individual. The cell line that leads to the gametes, called the **germ line**, arises within the primary ectoderm and then becomes distinct during the fourth week of embryonic development, as cells called **primordial germ cells** differentiate within the wall of the yolk sac. These cells then actively migrate to the posterior body wall of the embryo, where they populate the developing gonads and differentiate into the gamete precursor cells called **spermatogonia** in the male and **oogonia** in the female. Like the normal somatic cells of the body, the spermatogonia and oogonia are **diploid**; that is, they contain a complement of 23 pairs of chromosomes (a total of 46 chromosomes). When these cells produce gametes by the process of **gametogenesis** (called **spermatogenesis** in the male and **oogenesis** in the female), they undergo **meiosis**, a sequence of two specialized cell divisions by which the number of chromosomes in the gametes is halved. The gametes thus contain 23 chromosomes (one of each pair) and are said to be **haploid**. The developing gametes also undergo cytoplasmic modifications, resulting in the production of mature **spermatozoa** in the male and **definitive oocytes** in the female.

In the male, formation of spermatogonia and spermatogenesis take place in the seminiferous tubules of the testes and do not occur until puberty. In the female, in contrast, all the primary oocytes that the individual will ever possess are produced during fetal life. Between the third and fifth months of fetal life, the oogonia commence the first meiotic division but then immediately enter a state of meiotic arrest that persists until after puberty. After puberty, a few oocytes and their enclosing follicles resume development each month in response to the production of pituitary gonadotropic hormones. Only one of these follicles matures fully and undergoes **ovulation** to release the enclosed oocyte, and the oocyte completes meiosis only if it is fertilized by a spermatozoon. Fertilization takes place in the oviduct. After the oocyte finishes meiosis, the paternal and maternal chromosomes come together,

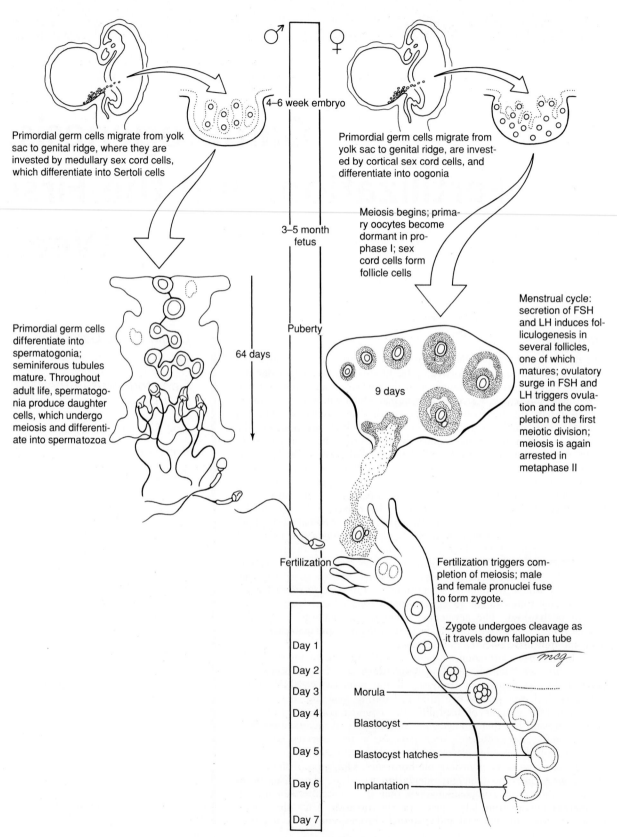

4–6 week embryo

Primordial germ cells migrate from yolk sac to genital ridge, where they are invested by medullary sex cord cells, which differentiate into Sertoli cells

Primordial germ cells migrate from yolk sac to genital ridge, are invested by cortical sex cord cells, and differentiate into oogonia

3–5 month fetus

Meiosis begins; primary oocytes become dormant in prophase I; sex cord cells form follicle cells

Puberty

64 days

Primordial germ cells differentiate into spermatogonia; seminiferous tubules mature. Throughout adult life, spermatogonia produce daughter cells, which undergo meiosis and differentiate into spermatozoa

9 days

Menstrual cycle: secretion of FSH and LH induces folliculogenesis in several follicles, one of which matures; ovulatory surge in FSH and LH triggers ovulation and the completion of the first meiotic division; meiosis is again arrested in metaphase II

Fertilization

Fertilization triggers completion of meiosis; male and female pronuclei fuse to form zygote.

Zygote undergoes cleavage as it travels down fallopian tube

Day 1
Day 2
Day 3   Morula
Day 4
        Blastocyst
Day 5   Blastocyst hatches
Day 6   Implantation
Day 7

Timeline. Gametogenesis and the first week of development.

resulting in the formation of a **zygote** containing a single diploid nucleus. Embryonic development is considered to begin at this point.

The newly formed embryo undergoes a series of cell divisions called **cleavage** as it travels down the oviduct toward the uterus. The cleavage divisions subdivide the zygote first into two cells, then into four, then into eight, and so on. These daughter cells do not grow between divisions, so the entire embryo remains the same size. Starting at the 8- to 16-cell stage, the cleaving embryo differentiates into two groups of cells: a peripheral **outer cell mass** and a central **inner cell mass.** The outer cell mass, also called the **trophoblast,** is the main source of the placenta and associated membranes, whereas the inner cell mass, also called the **embryoblast,** gives rise to the embryo proper and the amnion. By the 30-cell stage, the embryo, now called a **morula,** begins to form a fluid-filled central cavity, the **blastocyst cavity.** By the fifth to sixth day of development, the embryo is a hollow ball of about 100 cells called a **blastocyst.** At this point, it enters the uterine cavity and begins to implant into the endometrial lining of the uterine wall.

THE GERM CELLS ARISE WITHIN THE EMBRYO PROPER

The Primordial Germ Cells Originate Within the Primary Ectoderm of the Embryo and Then Migrate Into the Yolk Sac

Cells that give rise to the **gametes** in both male and female mammals (including humans) originate within the primary ectoderm of the embryo during the second week of development (see Ch. 3). They then detach from the ectoderm and migrate by ameboid movement into an extraembryonic structure called the **yolk sac.** At first, they may be distinguished within a mass of extraembryonic mesoderm at the caudal end of the embryo, and then within the endoderm of the yolk sac wall (Fig. 1–1*A*). These cells are called the **primordial germ cells,** and their lineage constitutes the **germ line.** Primordial germ cells can easily be recog-

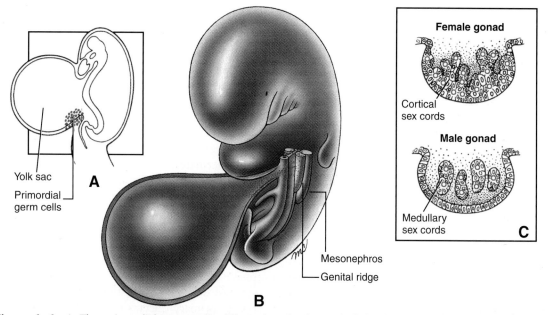

Figure 1–1. *A,* The primordial germ cells differentiate in the endodermal layer of the yolk sac at 4 to 6 weeks of development and migrate to the dorsal body wall. *B,* Between 6 and 12 weeks, the primordial germ cells induce formation of the genital ridges. *C,* Sex cord cells differentiate and invest the primordial germ cells. In females, the sex cords of the cortical region survive and become the ovarian follicle cells; in males, the medullary sex cords survive and become the Sertoli cells of the seminiferous tubules.

nized during their migration because of their distinctive pale cytoplasm and ovoid shape and because they specifically stain intensely with reagents that localize the enzyme alkaline phosphatase.

During the Fourth Week, the Primordial Germ Cells Migrate Back Into the Posterior Body Wall of the Embryo

Between 4 and 6 weeks, the primordial germ cells migrate by ameboid movement from the yolk sac to the wall of the gut tube and from the gut tube via the mesentery to the dorsal body wall (see Fig. 1–1B). In the dorsal body wall, these cells come to rest on either side of the midline in the loose mesenchymal tissue just deep to the membranous lining of the coelomic cavity. Most of the primordial germ cells populate the region of the body wall adjacent to the 10th thoracic vertebral level that will form the gonads (see Ch. 10). The primordial germ cells continue to multiply by mitosis during their migration. A few cells may become stranded along the route of migration or at inappropriate sites in the dorsal body wall. Occasionally, stray germ cells of this type may give rise to a type of tumor called a **teratoma** (see Experimental Principles Section later).

The Germ Cells Induce the Formation of the Gonads in the Dorsal Body Wall

The differentiation of the gonads is described in detail in Chapter 10. When the germ cells arrive in the presumptive gonad region, they stimulate cells of the adjacent coelomic epithelium and mesonephros (embryonic kidney) to proliferate and form compact strands of tissue called **primitive sex cords** (see Fig. 1–1C; see also Fig. 10–14). The proliferating sex cords create a swelling just medial to each mesonephros on either side of the vertebral column. These swellings, the **genital ridges,** represent the primordial gonads. The sex cords invest the primordial germ cells and give rise to the tissues that will nourish and regulate the development of the maturing sex cells—the **ovarian follicles** in the female and the **Sertoli cells** of the **germinal epithelium (seminiferous epithelium)** of the **seminiferous tubules** in the male (see Fig. 1–1C). The sex cords are essential to germ cell development: Germ cells that are not invested by sex cord cells either degenerate or first initiate premature meiosis and then degenerate. Conversely, if the germ cells do not arrive in the presumptive gonadal region, gonadal development is disrupted.

GAMETOGENESIS IS THE PROCESS OF MEIOSIS AND CYTODIFFERENTIATION THAT CONVERTS GERM CELLS INTO MATURE MALE AND FEMALE GAMETES

The Timing of Gametogenesis Is Different in Males and Females

In both males and females, the primordial germ cells undergo further mitotic divisions within the gonads and then commence **gametogenesis,** the process that converts them to mature male and female gametes (**spermatozoa** and **definitive oocytes,** respectively). The timing of these processes differs in the two sexes, however (see timeline and Fig. 1–3). In males, the primordial germ cells remain dormant from the sixth week of embryonic development until puberty. At puberty, the seminiferous tubules mature and the germ cells differentiate into spermatogonia. Successive waves of spermatogonia undergo meiosis (the process by which the number of chromosomes in the sex cells is halved; see the following section) and mature into spermatozoa. Spermatozoa are produced continuously from puberty until death.

In females, by contrast, the primordial germ cells undergo a few more mitotic divisions after they are invested by the sex cord cells, differentiate into oogonia, and then all begin meiosis by the fifth month of fetal development. During an early phase of meiosis, however, all the sex cells enter a state of dormancy, and they remain in meiotic arrest as primary oocytes until sexual maturity. Starting at puberty, a few ovarian follicles each month resume development in response to the monthly surge of pituitary gonadotropic hormones. However, usually only one primary oocyte matures into a secondary oocyte and is ovulated each month. This oocyte enters a second phase of meiotic arrest and does not actually complete meiosis unless it is fertilized. These monthly cycles continue until menopause at approximately 50 years of age.

The process of gametogenesis in the male and female (called **spermatogenesis** and **oogenesis,** respectively) are discussed in detail later in this chapter.

Meiosis Halves the Number of Chromosomes and DNA Strands in the Sex Cells

Although the timing of meiosis is very different in the male and female, the basic chromosomal events of the process are the same in the two sexes (Fig. 1–2). Like all normal somatic (non-germ) cells, the primordial germ cells contain 23 pairs of chromosomes, or a total of 46. One chromosome of each pair is obtained from the maternal gamete and the other from the paternal gamete (see later). These chromosomes contain the **deoxyribonucleic acid (DNA)** that encodes virtually all the information required for the development and functioning of the organism. Of the total complement of 46 chromosomes, 22 pairs consist of matching, homologous chromosomes called **autosomes.** The remaining two chromosomes are called the **sex chromosomes** because they determine the sex of the individual. There are two kinds of sex chromosome, X and Y. Individuals with one X chromosome and one Y chromosome (XY) are genetically male; individuals with two X chromosomes (XX) are genetically female. Nonetheless, one of the X chromosomes in the female genome is randomly inactivated, leaving only one active X chromosome in each cell (see discussion of X-inactivation in Ch. 2). In addition, the mechanisms underlying sex determination are discussed in detail in Chapter 10.

Two designations that are often confused are the **ploidy** of a cell and its **N number.** *Ploidy* refers to the number of copies of each *chromosome* present in a cell nucleus, whereas the *N number* refers to the number of copies of each unique double-stranded *DNA molecule* in the nucleus. Each chromosome contains one or two molecules of DNA at different stages of the cell cycle (whether mitotic or meiotic), so the ploidy and N number

of a cell do not always coincide. Somatic cells and primordial germ cells have two copies of each kind of chromosome and hence are called **diploid.** Mature gametes, in contrast, have just one copy of each kind of chromosome and are called **haploid.** Haploid gametes with one DNA molecule per chromosome are said to be **1N.** In some stages of the cell cycle, diploid cells also have one DNA molecule per chromosome and hence are **2N.** During the earlier phases of meiosis or mitosis, however, each chromosome of a diploid cell has two molecules of DNA, and so the cell is **4N.**

Meiosis is a specialized process of cell division that occurs only in the germ line. Figure 1–2 compares the processes of mitosis and meiosis. In **mitosis** (normal cell division), a diploid, 2N cell undergoes a single division to yield two diploid, 2N daughter cells. In meiosis, a diploid germ cell undergoes two successive, qualitatively different nuclear and cell divisions to yield four haploid, 1N offspring. In males, the cell divisions of meiosis are equal and yield four identical spermatozoa. In females, however, the meiotic cell divisions are dramatically unequal and yield a single, massive, haploid definitive oocyte and three minute, non-functional, haploid **polar bodies.**

Occasionally, an error during meiosis yields a gamete with an abnormal number of somatic or sex chromosomes. Some of these chromosomal anomalies and their effects on embryonic development are discussed in the Clinical Applications section at the end of this chapter.

The First Meiotic Division Involves DNA Replication and Recombination and Yields Two Haploid, 2N Daughter Cells. The steps of meiosis are illustrated in Figure 1–2 and summarized in Table 1–1. The preliminary step in meiosis, as in mitosis, is the replication of each chromosomal DNA molecule; thus, the diploid cell is converted from 2N to 4N. This event marks the beginning of gametogenesis. In the female, the oogonium is now called a **primary oocyte,** and in the male, the spermatogonium is now called a **primary spermatocyte** (Fig. 1–3). Once the DNA replicates, each chromosome consists of two parallel strands or **chromatids** joined together at a structure called the **centromere.** Each chromatid contains a single DNA molecule.

In the next step, called **prophase,** the chromosomes condense into compact, double-stranded

Mitosis

Diploid, 2N

Preparatory phase: DNA doubles

Diploid, 4N

Prophase: chromosomes condense

Metaphase: chromosomes line up on
mitotic spindle; centromeres replicate

Anaphase: single-stranded
chromosomes pull apart

Cell divides; each daughter cell
contains two chromosomes of each type

Diploid, 2N

A

Meiosis

Diploid, 2N
    Chromosomes each
contain one chromatid

Preparatory phase: DNA doubles

Diploid, 4N
    Chromosomes each
contain two chromatids

Prophase I: chromosomes condense

Chiasmata form; crossing over can occur

Metaphase I—anaphase I: double-stranded
chromosomes pull apart

Telophase I: cell division

Haploid, 2N

Anaphase II: centromeres replicate and each
double-stranded chromosome pulls apart to form
two single-stranded chromosomes

Cell division yields four gametes

Haploid, 1N

B

Figure 1–2. *A,* Mitosis. *B,* Meiosis. See Table 1–1 for a description of the stages.

Table 1–1
The Events During Mitotic and Meiotic Cell Divisions in the Germ Line

STAGE	EVENTS	NAME OF CELL	CONDITION OF GENOME
Resting interval between mitotic cell divisions	Normal cellular metabolism occurs.	♀ Oogonium ♂ Spermatogonium	Diploid, 2N
Mitosis			
Preparatory phase	DNA replication yields double-stranded chromosomes.	♀ Oogonium ♂ Spermatogonium	Diploid, 4N
Prophase	The double-stranded chromosomes condense.		
Metaphase	The chromosomes align along the equator. The centromeres replicate.		
Anaphase and telophase	Each double-stranded chromosome splits into two single-stranded chromosomes, one of which is distributed to each daughter nucleus.		
Cytokinesis	The cell divides.	♀ Oogonium ♂ Spermatogonium	Diploid, 2N
Meiosis I			
Preparatory phase	DNA replication yields double-stranded chromosomes.	♀ Primary oocyte ♂ Primary spermatocyte	Diploid, 4N
Prophase	The double-stranded chromosomes condense. The two chromosomes of each homologous pair then pair up at the centromeres to form a four-limbed chiasma structure. Recombination by crossing over may occur.		
Metaphase	The chromosomes align along the equator. *The centromeres do not replicate.*		
Anaphase and telophase	One double-stranded chromosome of each homologous pair is distributed to each daughter cell.		
Cytokinesis	The cell divides.	♀ One secondary oocyte and the first polar body ♂ Two secondary spermatocytes	Haploid, 2N
Meiosis II			
Prophase	*No DNA replication takes place during the second meiotic division.* The double-stranded chromosomes condense.		
Metaphase	The chromosomes align along the equator. The centromeres replicate.		
Anaphase and telophase	Each chromosome splits into two single-stranded chromosomes, one of which is distributed to each daughter nucleus.		
Cytokinesis	The cell divides.	♀ One definitive oocyte and three polar bodies ♂ Four spermatids	Haploid, 1N

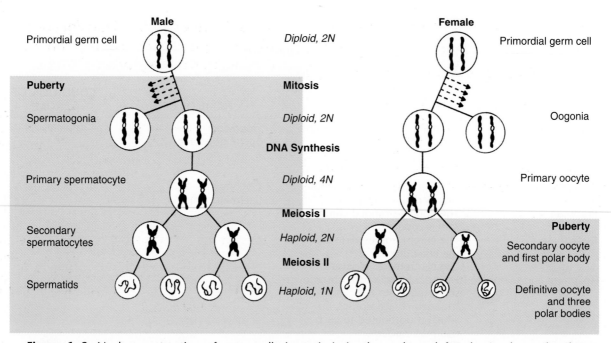

Figure 1–3. Nuclear maturation of germ cells in meiosis in the male and female. In the male, the primordial germ cells remain dormant until puberty, when they differentiate into spermatogonia and commence mitosis. Throughout adulthood, the spermatogonia produce primary spermatocytes, which undergo meiosis and spermatogenesis. Each primary spermatocyte yields four spermatozoa. In the female, the primordial germ cells differentiate into oogonia, which undergo mitosis and then commence meiosis as primary oocytes during fetal life. The primary oocytes remain arrested in prophase I until stimulated to resume meiosis during a menstrual cycle. Each primary oocyte yields one definitive oocyte and three polar bodies.

structures. During the late stages of prophase, the double-stranded chromosomes of each homologous pair match up, centromere to centromere, to form a joint structure called a **chiasma.** Chiasma formation makes it possible for the two homologous chromosomes to exchange large segments of DNA by a process called **crossing over.** The resulting **recombination** of the genetic material on homologous maternal and paternal chromosomes is largely random and, therefore, increases the genetic variability of the future gametes. As mentioned earlier, the primary oocyte enters a phase of meiotic arrest during the first meiotic prophase.

During **metaphase,** the four-stranded chiasma structures are organized on the equator of a spindle apparatus similar to the one that forms during mitosis, and during **anaphase,** one double-stranded chromosome of each homologous pair is distributed to each of the two daughter nuclei. During the first meiotic division, the centromeres of the chromosomes do not replicate, and, there-

fore, the two chromatids of each chromosome remain together. The resulting daughter nuclei thus are haploid but 2N: they contain the same amount of DNA as the parent germ cell but half as many chromosomes. After the daughter nuclei form, the cell itself divides (undergoes **cytokinesis**). The first meiotic cell division produces two **secondary spermatocytes** in the male and a **secondary oocyte** and a **first polar body** in the female (see Fig. 1–3).

In the Second Meiotic Division, the Double-Stranded Chromosomes Divide, Yielding Four Haploid, 1N Daughter Cells. No DNA replication occurs during the second meiotic division. The 23 double-stranded chromosomes condense during the second meiotic prophase and line up during the second meiotic metaphase. The chromosomal centromeres then replicate, and during anaphase, the double-stranded chromosomes pull apart into two single-stranded chromosomes, one of which is distributed to each of the daughter nuclei. In males, the second meiotic cell division produces two **definitive spermatocytes or spermatids** (i.e., a total of four from each germ cell entering meiosis). In the female, the second meiotic cell division, like the first, is radically unequal, producing a large **definitive oocyte** and another diminutive polar body. The first polar body may simultaneously undergo a second meiotic division to produce a third polar body (see Fig. 1–3).

In the female, the oocyte enters a second phase of meiotic arrest during the second meiotic metaphase before the replication of the centromeres. Meiosis does not resume unless the cell is fertilized.

SPERMATOGENESIS BEGINS AT PUBERTY AND CONTINUES THROUGHOUT ADULT LIFE

Now that meiosis has been described, it is possible to investigate and compare the specific processes of spermatogenesis and oogenesis. At puberty, the testes begin to secrete greatly increased amounts of the steroid hormone **testosterone.** This hormone has a multitude of effects. In addition to stimulating the development of many secondary sex characteristics, it triggers the growth of the testes, the maturation of the seminiferous tubules, and the commencement of spermatogenesis.

Under the influence of testosterone, the Sertoli cells differentiate into a system of seminiferous tubules. The dormant primordial germ cells resume development, divide several times by mitosis, and then differentiate into spermatogonia. These spermatogonia are located immediately under the basement membrane surrounding the seminiferous tubules, where they occupy pockets between the Sertoli cells (Fig. 1–4A). Each spermatogonium is connected to the adjacent Sertoli cells by specialized membrane junctions. In addition, all the Sertoli cells are joined to each other by dense bands of intercellular membrane junctions that completely surround each Sertoli cell and thus isolate the trapped spermatogonia from the tubule lumen.

Male Germ Cells Are Translocated to the Seminiferous Tubule Lumen During Spermatogenesis

The cells that will undergo spermatogenesis arise by mitosis from the spermatogonia. These cells are gradually translocated between the Sertoli cells from the basal to the luminal side of the seminiferous epithelium while spermatogenesis takes place (see Fig. 1–4A). During this migratory phase, the recruited primary spermatocytes pass without interruption through both meiotic divisions, producing first two secondary spermatocytes and then four spermatids. The spermatids undergo the dramatic changes that convert them into mature sperm while they complete their migration to the lumen. This process of sperm cell differentiation is called **spermiogenesis.**

The Sertoli Cells Are Also Instrumental in Spermiogenesis

The Sertoli cells participate intimately in the differentiation of the gametes. Maturing spermatocytes and spermatids are connected to the surrounding Sertoli cells not only by tight junctions and gap junctions but also by unique cytoplasmic processes called **tubulobulbar complexes** that extend into the Sertoli cells. The cytoplasm of the developing gametes shrinks dramatically during spermiogenesis; these tubulobulbar complexes are thought to provide a mechanism by which the excess cytoplasm is transferred to the Sertoli cells. As cytoplasm is removed, the spermatids undergo the dramatic changes in shape and internal organization that transform them into spermatozoa. Finally, the last connections with the Sertoli cells break, releasing the spermatozoa into the tubule lumen. This final step is called **spermiation.**

As shown in Figure 1–4B, a spermatozoon consists of a **head,** a **midpiece,** and a very long **tail.** The head contains the condensed nucleus and is capped by an apical vesicle filled with hydrolytic enzymes. This vesicle, the **acrosome,** plays an essential role in fertilization (see later). The midpiece contains large, helical mitochondria and generates the power for swimming. The tail contains the microtubules that form part of the propulsion system of the spermatozoon.

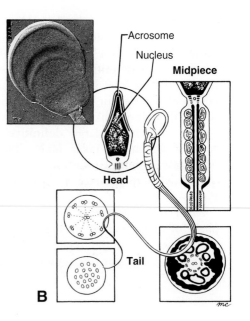

Figure 1–4. *A,* A schematic section through the seminiferous tubule wall. The spermatogonium just under the outer surface of the tubule wall (basal side) undergoes mitosis to produce daughter cells, which may either continue to divide by mitosis (thus renewing the spermatogonial stem cell population) or commence meiosis as primary spermatocytes. As spermatogenesis and spermiogenesis occur, the differentiating cell is translocated between adjacent Sertoli cells to the tubule lumen. The daughter spermatocytes and spermatids remain linked by cytoplasmic bridges. The entire clone of spermatogonia derived from each primordial germ cell is linked by cytoplasmic bridges. *B,* Structure of the mature spermatozoon. The head contains the nucleus capped by the acrosome; the midpiece contains coiled mitochondria; the tail contains propulsive microtubules. The inset micrograph shows a piece of a human sperm. (*B,* Photo courtesy of Dr. Daniel S. Friend.)

Errors in spermatogenesis or spermiogenesis are not at all uncommon. Examination of a sperm sample will reveal spermatozoa with abnormalities such as small, narrow, or piriform (pear-shaped) heads, double or triple heads, acrosomal defects, and double tails.

Continual Waves of Spermatogenesis Occur Throughout the Seminiferous Epithelium

Spermatogenesis takes place continuously from puberty to death. Gametes are produced in synchronous waves in each local area of the germinal epithelium, although the process is not synchronized throughout the seminiferous tubules. In many different mammals, the clone of spermatogonia derived from each spermatogonial stem cell populates a local area of the seminiferous tubules and displays synchronous spermatogenesis. That may be the case in humans as well. About four waves of synchronously differentiating cells can be observed in a given region of the human tubule epithelium at any time. Ultrastructural studies provide some evidence that these waves of differentiating cells remain synchronized because of incomplete cytokinesis throughout the series of mitotic and meiotic divisions between the division of a spermatogonium and the formation of spermatids. Instead of fully separating, the daughter cells produced by these divisions remain connected by slender cytoplasmic bridges that could allow passage of small signal molecules or metabolites (see Fig. 1–4A).

In the human male, each cycle of spermatogenesis takes about 64 days. Spermatogonial mitosis occupies about 16 days, the first meiotic division takes about 8 days, the second meiotic division takes about 16 days, and spermiogenesis requires about 24 days.

Spermatozoa Undergo a Terminal Step of Functional Maturation Called Capacitation

During its journey from the seminiferous tubules to the ampulla of the oviduct, a sperm cell undergoes a process of functional maturation that prepares it to fertilize an oocyte. Sperm produced in the seminiferous tubules are stored in the lower part of the **epididymis**, a special coiled duct connected to the **vas deferens** near its origin in the testis. During ejaculation, the sperm are propelled through the vas deferens and urethra and are mixed with nourishing secretions from the **seminal vesicles, prostate,** and **bulbourethral glands** (see Ch. 10 for further discussion of these structures). As many as 200 million spermatozoa may be deposited in the vagina by a single ejaculation, but only a few hundred succeed in navigating through the cervix, uterus, and oviduct and into their expanded ampullar region. In the **ampulla,** sperm survive and retain their capacity to fertilize an oocyte for 1 to 3 days.

Capacitation is defined as the final step of sperm maturation, consisting primarily of changes in the acrosome that prepare it to release the enzymes required to penetrate the zona pellucida, a shell of glycoprotein surrounding the oocyte (see later). Capacitation is thought to take place within the female genital tract and to require contact with the secretions of the oviduct. Spermatozoa used in in vitro fertilization procedures are artificially capacitated. Spermatozoa with defective acrosomes may be injected directly into oocytes to assist reproduction in humans (see Clinical Applications later).

OOGENESIS IS DISCONTINUOUS AND BEGINS DURING FETAL LIFE

The Total Number of Primary Oocytes Is Produced in the Ovaries by 5 Months of Fetal Life

As mentioned earlier, the female germ cells undergo a series of mitotic divisions after they are invested by the sex cord cells and then differentiate into oogonia (see Fig. 1–3). By 12 weeks of development, a proportion of the several million oogonia in the genital ridges enters the first meiotic prophase and then almost immediately becomes dormant. The nucleus of these dormant primary oocytes, containing the partially condensed prophase chromosomes, becomes very large and watery and is referred to as a **germinal vesicle.** The germinal vesicle is thought to protect the DNA during the long period of meiotic arrest.

Each primary oocyte becomes tightly enclosed by a single-layered, squamous capsule of epithelial **follicle cells** derived from the sex cord cells. This capsule and its enclosed primary oocyte constitute a **primordial follicle.** By 5 months, the number of primordial follicles in the ovaries peaks at about 7 million. Most of these follicles subsequently degenerate. By birth only 700,000 to 2 million remain, and by puberty, only about 400,000.

The Hormones of the Female Cycle Control Folliculogenesis, Ovulation, and the Condition of the Uterus

After a girl reaches menarche (female puberty), monthly cycles in the secretion of hypothalamic, pituitary, and ovarian hormones control a **menstrual cycle,** which has the purpose of producing each month a single female gamete and a uterus in a condition to receive a fertilized embryo. This cycle consists of the monthly maturation of (usually) a single oocyte and its enclosing follicle, the concurrent proliferation of the uterine endometrium, the process of ovulation by which the oocyte is released, the continued development of the follicle into an endocrine corpus luteum, and, finally—unless a fertilized ovum implants in the uterus and begins to develop—the sloughing of the uterine endometrium and the involution of the corpus luteum. This entire cycle takes about 28 days.

The menstrual cycle is considered to begin with **menstruation** (also called the **menses**), the shedding of the degenerated uterine endometrium from the previous cycle. On about the fifth day of the cycle (the fifth day after the beginning of menstruation), an increase in secretion by the hypothalamus of the brain of a small peptide hormone, **gonadotropin-releasing hormone (GnRH),** stimulates the pituitary gland to increase its secretion of two **gonadotropic hormones (gonadotropins): follicle-stimulating hormone (FSH)** and **luteinizing hormone (LH)** (Fig. 1–5). Increased secretion of GnRH by the hypothalamus is also the event that initiates the first menstrual cycle at menarche. The rising levels of pituitary gonadotropins regulate later phases of **folliculogenesis** in the ovary and the **proliferative phase** in the uterine endometrium.

About 5 to 12 Primary Follicles Resume Development Each Month

Before a particular cycle and independent of pituitary gonadotropins, the cells of the single-layered follicular epithelium of a small group of primordial follicles thicken from squamous to cuboidal (Fig. 1–6A), These follicles are now called **primary follicles.** The follicle cells and the oocyte jointly secrete a thin layer of acellular material, composed of only a few types of glycoprotein, onto the surface of the oocyte. Although this layer, the **zona pellucida,** appears to form a complete physical barrier between the follicle cells and the oocyte (Figs. 1–6B and 1–7A), actually it is penetrated by thin extensions of the follicle cells that are connected to the oocyte cell membrane by gap junctions and intermediate cell junctions (see Fig. 1–7B). These extensions and their membrane junctions remain intact until just before ovulation and probably convey both developmental signals and metabolic support to the oocyte. The epithelium of 5 to 12 of these primary follicles then proliferates to form a multilayered capsule around the oocyte (see Figs. 1–5 and 1–6). They are now called **growing follicles.** At this point, some of the growing follicles cease to develop and eventually degenerate, whereas a few continue to enlarge in response to rising levels of FSH, mainly by taking up fluid and developing a central fluid-filled cavity called the **antrum.** These follicles are called **antral** or **vesicular follicles.** At the same time, the connective tissue of the ovarian stroma surrounding each of these follicles differentiates into two layers, an inner layer called the **theca interna** and an outer layer called the **theca externa.** These two layers become vascularized, in contrast to the follicle cells, which do not.

A Single Follicle Becomes Dominant and the Rest Degenerate

Eventually, one of the growing follicles gains primacy and continues to enlarge by absorbing fluid,

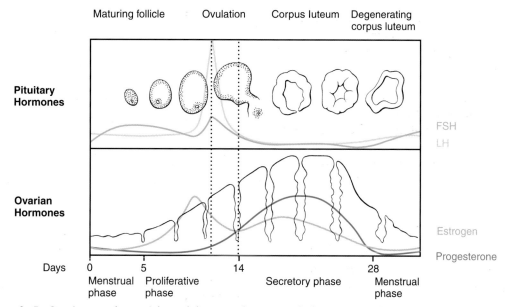

Figure 1–5. Ovarian, endometrial, and hormonal events of the menstrual cycle. The pituitary follicle-stimulating hormone (FSH) and luteinizing hormone (LH) directly control the ovarian cycle and also control the production of estrogens and progesterone by the responding follicles and corpus luteum of the ovary. These ovarian hormones in turn control the cycle of the uterine endometrium.

whereas the remainder of the follicles recruited during the cycle degenerate (undergo **atresia**). The oocyte, surrounded by a small mass of follicle cells called the **cumulus oophorus,** increasingly projects into the expanding antrum but remains connected to the layer of follicle cells that lines the antral cavity and underlies the basement membrane of the follicle. This layer is called the **membrana granulosa.** The large, swollen follicle is now called a **mature vesicular follicle** or **mature graafian follicle** (see Fig. 1–6). At this point, the oocyte still has not resumed meiosis.

Various Theories Have Been Proposed for the Mechanism That Selectively Stimulates Folliculogenesis in a Few Follicles

The reason why only 5 to 12 primordial follicles commence folliculogenesis each month, and why, of this group, all but one eventually degenerate is not well understood. One theory suggests that follicles become progressively more sensitive to the stimulating effects of FSH as they advance in de-

velopment. Follicles that are slightly more advanced simply on a random basis would, therefore, respond more acutely to FSH and would be favored. Another theory proposes that the selection process is regulated by a complex system of feedback between the pituitary and ovarian hormones and growth factors.

The Resumption of Meiosis and Ovulation Are Stimulated by an Ovulatory Surge in the Levels of FSH and LH

On about day 13 or 14 of the menstrual cycle (at the end of the proliferative phase of the uterine endometrium), the levels of FSH and LH suddenly rise very sharply (see Fig. 1–5). This **ovulatory surge** in the pituitary gonadotropins stimulates the primary oocyte of the remaining mature graafian follicle to resume meiosis. This response can be observed visually about 15 hours after the beginning of the ovulatory surge in FSH and LH, when the membrane of the swollen germinal vesicle (nucleus) of the oocyte breaks down (Fig 1–8A). By

Figure 1-6. *A,* Schematic depiction of folliculogenesis and ovulation in the ovary. Five to 12 primordial follicles initially respond to the rising levels of follicle-stimulating hormone (FSH) and luteinizing hormone (LH), but only one matures. In response to the ovulatory surge in LH and FSH, the oocyte of this mature graafian follicle resumes meiosis, and the follicle ovulates. The final steps of meiosis take place only if the released oocyte is penetrated by a sperm. *B,* Scanning electron micrograph of a responding preovulatory follicle. The cumulus oophorus cells surrounding the oocyte have disaggregated in preparation for ovulation.

Figure 1–7. *A,* Scanning electron micrograph of the zona pellucida after removal of the cumulus cells. The zona consists of protein and mucopolysaccharide and forms a barrier that the sperm can penetrate only by means of its acrosomal enzymes. *B,* Scanning electron micrograph of the oocyte surface and cumulus oophorus, with the zona pellucida digested away. The cumulus cells maintain contact with the oocyte via thin cell processes that penetrate the zona pellucida and form gap junctions and intermediate junctions with the oocyte cell membrane. (*A,* From Phillips DM, Shalgi R. 1980. Surface architecture of the mouse and hamster zona pellucida and oocyte. J Ultrastruct Res 72:1. *B,* Photo courtesy of Dr. David Phillips.)

Cumulus cells

Cumulus cell process

Oocyte surface

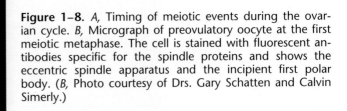

Figure 1–8. *A,* Timing of meiotic events during the ovarian cycle. *B,* Micrograph of preovulatory oocyte at the first meiotic metaphase. The cell is stained with fluorescent antibodies specific for the spindle proteins and shows the eccentric spindle apparatus and the incipient first polar body. (*B,* Photo courtesy of Drs. Gary Schatten and Calvin Simerly.)

20 hours, the chromosomes are lined up in metaphase. Cell division to form the secondary oocyte and first polar body rapidly ensues (see Fig. 1–8*B*). The secondary oocyte promptly begins the second meiotic division but, about 3 hours before ovulation, is arrested at the second meiotic metaphase.

The Cumulus Oophorus Expands in Response to the Ovulatory Surge in LH and FSH. Just at the same time that the germinal vesicle breaks down, the cumulus cells surrounding the oocyte lose their cell-to-cell connections and disaggregate (see Fig. 1–6). As a result, the oocyte and a mass of loose cumulus cells detach into the antral cavity. Over the next few hours, the cumulus cells secrete an abundant extracellular matrix, consisting mainly of hyaluronic acid, which causes the cumulus cell mass to expand severalfold. This process of **cumulus expansion** may play a role in several processes, including the regulation of meiotic progress and

ovulation. In addition, the mass of matrix and entrapped cumulus cells that accompanies the ovulated oocyte may play a role in the transport of the oocyte in the oviduct, in fertilization, and in the early development of the zygote.

Ovulation Depends on the Breakdown of the Follicle Wall. The process of **ovulation** (the expulsion of the secondary oocyte from the follicle) appears to be similar to an inflammatory response. The cascade of events that culminates in ovulation is believed to be initiated by the secretion of histamine and prostaglandins, well-known inflammatory mediators. Within a few hours after the ovulatory surge of FSH and LH, the follicle becomes more vascularized and is visibly pink and edematous in comparison with nonresponding follicles. The follicle is displaced to the surface of the ovary, where it forms a bulge (see Fig. 1–6*A*). As ovulation approaches, the projecting wall of the follicle begins to thin, resulting in the formation of a small, nipple-shaped protrusion called the **stigma.** Finally, a combination of tension produced by smooth muscle cells in the follicle wall plus the release of collagen-degrading enzymes and other factors by fibroblasts in the region causes the follicle to rupture. The rupture of the follicle is not explosive: The oocyte, accompanied by a large number of investing cumulus cells bound in the hyaluronic acid matrix and by some follicular fluid, is slowly extruded onto the surface of the ovary. Ovulation occurs about 38 hours after the beginning of the ovulatory surge of FSH and LH.

The sticky mass formed by the oocyte and cumulus is actively scraped off the surface of the ovary by the fimbriated mouth of the oviduct (Fig. 1–9). The cumulus-oocyte complex is then moved into the ampulla of the oviduct by the synchronized beating of the cilia on the oviduct wall. Within the ampulla, the oocyte may remain viable for as long as 24 hours before it loses its capacity to be fertilized.

The Ruptured Follicle Forms the Endocrine Corpus Luteum. After ovulation, the membrane granulosa cells of the ruptured follicular wall begin to proliferate and give rise to the **luteal cells** of the **corpus luteum** (see Figs. 1–6 and 1–9). As described later, the corpus luteum is an endocrine structure that secretes steroid hormones that maintain the uterine endometrium in a condition ready to receive an embryo. If no embryo implants in the uterus, the corpus luteum degenerates after

about 14 days and is converted to a scarlike structure called a **corpus albicans.**

ESTROGENS AND PROGESTERONE SECRETED BY THE FOLLICLE CONTROL THE UTERINE EVENTS OF THE MENSTRUAL CYCLE

Beginning on day 5 of the menstrual cycle, the thecal and follicle cells of responding follicles secrete steroid **estrogens.** These hormones in turn cause the endometrial lining of the uterus to proliferate and undergo remodeling. This **proliferative phase** begins at about day 5 of the cycle and is complete by day 14 (see Fig. 1–5).

After ovulation occurs, thecal cells in the wall of the corpus luteum continue to secrete estrogens, and the **luteal cells** that differentiate from the remaining follicle cells also begin to secrete high levels of a related steroid hormone, **progesterone.** Luteal progesterone stimulates the uterine endometrial layer to thicken further and to form glandular structures and increased vasculature. Unless an embryo implants in the uterine lining, this **secretory phase** of endometrial differentiation lasts about 13 days (see Fig. 1–5). At that point (near the end of the menstrual cycle), the corpus luteum shrinks and the levels of progesterone fall. The developed endometrium, which is dependent on progesterone, degenerates and begins to slough. The 4- to 5-day **menstrual phase,** during which

Figure 1–9. The ovulated oocyte clings to the surface of the ovary by the gelatinous cumulus oophorus and is actively scraped off by the fimbriated oviduct mouth. After ovulation, the membrana granulosa layer of the ruptured follicle proliferates to form the endocrine corpus luteum.

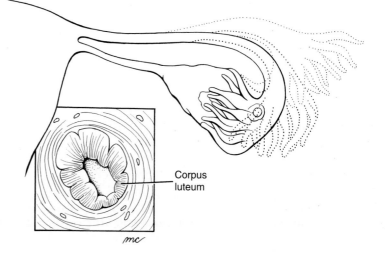

Corpus luteum

mc

the endometrium is sloughed (along with about 35 mL of blood and the unfertilized oocyte), is conventionally taken as the start of the next cycle.

AT FERTILIZATION, THE SPERM NUCLEUS ENTERS THE OOCYTE, THE OOCYTE COMPLETES MEIOSIS, AND THE CHROMOSOMES OF THE TWO MATURE GAMETES COMBINE

Fertilization Is a Complex Interaction Between Sperm and Oocyte

If viable spermatozoa encounter an ovulated oocyte in the ampulla of the oviduct, they surround it and begin forcing their way through the cumulus mass (Fig. 1–10*A*). When a spermatozoon reaches the tough zona pellucida surrounding the oocyte, it binds in a human-specific interaction with a glycoprotein sperm receptor molecule in the zona (ZP3), and then the acrosome is induced to release degradative enzymes that allow the sperm to penetrate the zona pellucida. When a spermatozoon successfully penetrates the zona pellucida and reaches the oocyte, the cell membranes of the two cells fuse (see Fig. 1–10*A, B*). This event immediately causes thousands of small **cortical granules** located just beneath the oocyte cell membrane to release their contents into the **perivitelline space** between the oocyte and the zona pellucida. The substances released from the cortical granules in-

teract with the zona pellucida in such a way as to alter the sperm receptor molecules, causing the zona to become impenetrable by additional spermatozoa. This mechanism prevents **polyspermy,** or the fertilization of the oocyte by more than one spermatozoon.

The fusion of the spermatozoon cell membrane with the oocyte membrane also causes the oocyte to resume meiosis. The oocyte completes the second meiotic metaphase and rapidly proceeds through anaphase, producing another polar body. Disregarding the presence of the sperm, the oocyte is now considered to be a **definitive oocyte.** Because the embryo now contains a diploid complement of chromosomes and a 2N quantity of DNA, this fertilized oocyte is called a **zygote** (Fig. 1–10*C*).

The chromosomes of the oocyte and sperm are then respectively enclosed within **female** and **male pronuclei,** but these membranes soon disappear as both maternal and paternal chromosomes are replicated in preparation for the first cleavage (see the next section).

DURING THE FIRST DAYS OF DEVELOPMENT, THE ZYGOTE TRAVELS DOWN THE OVIDUCT AND UNDERGOES CLEAVAGE

Cleavage Subdivides the Zygote Without Increasing Its Size

Within 24 hours after fertilization, the zygote embarks on a regulated series of mitotic cell divisions

Figure 1–10. Fertilization. *A,* Spermatozoa wriggle through the cumulus mass and release their acrosomal enzymes on contact with the zona pellucida. The acrosomal enzymes dissolve the zona pellucida and allow the sperm to reach the oocyte. As soon as the membranes of the sperm and oocyte fuse, the cortical granules of the oocyte release their contents, which cause the zona pellucida to become impenetrable to further sperm. The entry of the sperm nucleus into the cytoplasm induces the oocyte to complete the second meiotic diffusion. *B,* Scanning electron micrograph showing a human sperm fusing with a hamster oocyte that has been enzymatically denuded of the zona pellucida. The ability of a man's sperm to penetrate a denuded hamster oocyte is often used as a clinical test of sperm activity. *C,* The events of zygote formation. After the oocyte completes meiosis, the female pronucleus and the larger male pronucleus approach each other as DNA is doubled in maternal and paternal chromosomes to initiate the first mitotic division. The pronuclear membranes then break down and maternal and paternal chromosomes assemble on the metaphase plate. The centromeres then replicate, and homologous chromosomes are distributed to the first two cells of the embryo. (*B,* Photo courtesy of Dr. David Philips.)

Sperm penetration triggers second meiotic division

Release of acrosomal enzymes allows sperm to penetrate zona pellucida

Follicle cells

Zona pellucida

Cortical granule

Plasma membrane

Sperm penetration causes cortical granules to release their contents, which render the zona pellucida impenetrable to further sperm

Sperm penetrates oocyte

A

B

Polar bodies

Female pronucleus

Male pronucleus

Degenerating tail of sperm

Zona pellucida

C

Pronuclear stage

Pronuclear migration, chromosome doubling, and initiation of first cleavage

Metaphase of first cleavage

Anaphase of first cleavage

Figure 1–10 *See legend on opposite page*

called **cleavage** (Fig. 1–11). These divisions are not accompanied by cell growth, so they subdivide the large zygote into many smaller daughter cells called **blastomeres,** whereas the embryo as a whole does not change in size but remains enclosed in the zona pellucida. The first cleavage division divides the zygote along a plane at right angles to its equator and in line with the polar bodies. Subsequent cleavage divisions become somewhat asynchronous. The second division, which is complete at about 40 hours after fertilization, produces four equal blastomeres. By 3 days, the embryo consists of 6 to 12 cells, and by 4 days, it consists of 16 to 32 cells. By the 32 cell stage, the embryo has the appearance of a small mulberry and is therefore, called a **morula** (from Latin *morum*, mulberry).

The Segregation of Blastomeres Into Embryoblast and Trophoblast Precursors Occurs in the Morula

The cells of the morula will give rise not only to the embryo proper and its attached membranes but also to the placenta and related structures. The cells that will follow these different developmental paths become segregated during cleavage. Starting at the eight-cell stage of development, the originally round and loosely adherent blastomeres begin to flatten, developing an inside-outside polarity that maximizes cell-to-cell contact among the blastomeres at the center of the mass (Fig. 1–12). As differential adhesion develops, the outer surfaces of the cells become convex and their inner surfaces become concave. This reorganization, called **compaction,** involves the activity of cytoskeletal elements and adhesion of the blastomeres.

The development of differential adhesion between different groups of blastomeres also results in the segregation of some cells to the center of the morula and others to the outside. It is believed that the third- or fourth-generation blastomeres that divide earliest may be the ones displaced to the center of the morula. These centrally placed blastomeres are now called the **inner cell mass,** whereas the blastomeres at the periphery constitute the **outer cell mass.** Some exchange occurs between these groups. However, in general, the inner cell mass gives rise to most of the embryo proper

and is therefore called the **embryoblast.** The outer cell mass is the primary source for the membranes of the placenta and is therefore called the **trophoblast** (see Ch. 2).

The Morula Develops a Fluid-Filled Cavity and Is Transformed Into a Blastocyst

By 4 days of development, the morula, consisting now of about 30 cells, begins to absorb fluid. This fluid is thought to be taken up at first into intracellular vacuoles within the blastomeres, but it then begins to collect between the cells. Meanwhile, specialized cell-to-cell junctions called **tight junctions** and **gap junctions** begin to develop between many blastomeres, especially those of the outer cell mass. As a result of tight junction formation between cells of the outer cell mass, the fluid that continues to enter the morula collects mainly between the cells of the inner cell mass. As the hydrostatic pressure of this fluid increases, a large cavity called the **blastocyst cavity** forms within the morula (see Fig. 1–11). The embryoblast cells (inner cell mass) then form a compact mass at one side of this cavity, and the outer cell mass, or trophoblast, is organized into a thin, single-layered epithelium. The embryo is now called a **blastocyst.** The side of the blastocyst containing the inner cell mass is called the **embryonic pole** of the blastocyst, and the opposite side is called the **abembryonic pole.**

THE BLASTOCYST IMPLANTS IN THE UTERINE WALL ON ABOUT DAY 6

The Blastocyst Hatches From the Zona Pellucida Before Implanting

The morula reaches the uterus between 3 and 4 days of development. By day 5, the blastocyst hatches from the clear zona pellucida by enzymatically boring a hole in it and squeezing out (see Fig. 1–11). The blastocyst is now naked of all its original investments and can interact directly with the endometrium.

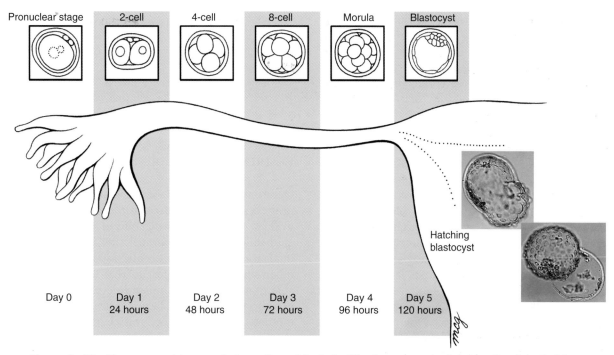

Figure 1–11. Cleavage and transport down the oviduct. Fertilization occurs in the ampulla of the oviduct. During the first 5 days, the zygote undergoes cleavage as it travels down the oviduct and enters the uterus. On day 5, the blastocyst hatches from the zona pellucida and is then able to implant in the uterine endometrium. (From Boatman DE. 1987. In vitro growth of nonhuman primate pre- and peri-implantation embryos. p. 273. In Bavister BD (ed): The Mammalian Preimplantation Embryo. Plenum, New York. Photo courtesy of Drs. Barry Bavister and D.E. Boatman.)

Figure 1–12. Compaction. *A,* Scanning electron micrograph of 10-cell human embryo before compaction. Note intercellular clefts. *B,* Scanning electron micrograph of 10-cell human embryo during process of compaction. Note the absence of intercellular clefts between some of the blastomeres (arrows). The zona pellucida was mechanically removed from both embryos. (From Nikas G, Asangla A, Winston RML, Handyside AH. 1996. Compaction and surface polarity in the human embryo in vitro. Biol Reprod 55:32. Photos courtesy of Dr. G. Nikas.)

Very soon after arriving in the uterus, the blastocyst becomes tightly adherent to the uterine lining (Fig. 1–13). The adjacent cells of the endometrial stroma respond to its presence and to the progesterone secreted by the corpus luteum by differentiating into metabolically active, secretory cells called **decidual cells.** This response is called the **decidual reaction** (see Fig. 15–1). The endometrial glands in the vicinity also enlarge, and the local uterine wall becomes more highly vascularized and edematous. It is thought that the secretions of the decidual cells and endometrial glands include growth factors and metabolites that support the growth of the implanting embryo.

The uterine lining is maintained in a favorable state and kept from sloughing partly by the progesterone secreted by the corpus luteum. In the absence of an implanted embryo, the corpus luteum normally degenerates after about 13 days. If an embryo implants, however, the cells of the trophoblast produce the hormone **human chorionic gonadotropin (hCG),** which supports the corpus luteum and thus maintains the supply of progesterone **(maternal recognition of pregnancy).** The corpus luteum continues to secrete sex steroids for 11 to 12 weeks of embryonic development, after which the placenta itself begins to secrete large amounts of progesterone and the corpus luteum slowly involutes, becoming a corpus albicans.

Implantation in an Abnormal Site Results in an Ectopic Pregnancy

Occasionally, a blastocyst implants in the peritoneal cavity, on the surface of the ovary, within the oviduct, or at an abnormal site in the uterus. The epithelium at these abnormal sites responds to the implanting blastocyst with increased vascularity and other supportive changes, so that the blastocyst is able to survive and commence development. These **ectopic pregnancies** often threaten the life of the mother because the blood vessels that form at the abnormal site are apt to rupture as a result of the growth of the embryo and placenta. The ectopic nature of a pregnancy is often revealed by symptoms of abdominal pain and/or vaginal bleeding. Surgical intervention may be required to remove the developing embryo.

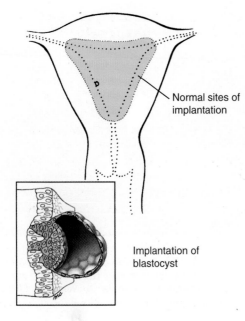

Normal sites of implantation

Implantation of blastocyst

Figure 1–13. Implantation. On about day 6.5 after fertilization, the trophoblast cells at the embryonic pole of the blastocyst proliferate to produce the syncytiotrophoblast, which is able to invade the uterine lining. The colored area indicates the normal sites of implantation in the uterine wall.

Clinical Applications

Chromosomal Anomalies, Contraceptive Techniques, and Strategies of Assisted Reproduction

Studies of the mechanisms that underlie human gametogenesis provide a basis for understanding (1) human chromosome anomalies, (2) contraceptive techniques, and (3) the strategies designed to assist reproduction in otherwise sterile couples.

Chromosomal Abnormalities Result in Spontaneous Abortion or Abnormal Development

It is estimated that one third of all conceptions in normal, healthy women abort spontaneously; approximately one fourth of these occur before pregnancy is detected. Chromosomal anomalies appear to cause about 40 to 50 percent of spontaneous abortions in cases in which the conceptus has been recovered and examined. Many chromosomal anomalies, however, allow the fetus to survive to term. The resulting infants display a variety of developmental abnormalities and syndromes, including Down, Turner, Klinefelter, Angelman, and Prader-Willi syndromes; Wilms' tumors of the kidney; and retinoblastoma.

Many Chromosomal Anomalies Arise During Gametogenesis and Cleavage

Abnormal chromosomes can be produced in the germ line of either parent through an error in meiosis or fertilization or can arise in the early embryo through an error in mitosis. The gametes or blastomeres that result from these events contain missing or extra chromosomes or chromosomes with duplicated, deleted, or rearranged segments. The absence of a specific chromosome in a gamete that combines with a normal gamete to form a zygote results in a condition known as **monosomy** (because the zygote contains only one copy of the chromosome rather than the normal two). Conversely, the presence of two of the same kind of chromosome in one of the gametes that forms a zygote results in **trisomy.**

Down Syndrome Is an Example of a Disorder Caused by an Error During Meiosis or Mitosis.

If the two copies of chromosome 21 fail to separate during the first or second meiotic anaphase of gametogenesis in either parent (a phenomenon called **nondisjunction**), half the resulting gametes will lack chromosome 21 altogether and the other half will have two copies (Fig. 1–14A). Embryos formed by fusion of a gamete lacking chromosome 21 with a normal gamete are called **monosomy 21** embryos. These embryos die rapidly; monosomies of autosomal chromosomes are invariably fatal during early embryonic development. If, on the other hand, a gamete with two copies of chromosome 21 fuses with a normal gamete, the resulting **trisomy 21** embryo may survive (Fig. 1–14B). Trisomy 21 infants display the range of abnormalities described as **Down syndrome.** In addition to recognizable facial characteristics and short stature, individuals with Down syndrome may exhibit congenital heart defects (atrioventricular septal defect is most common), mental retardation, propensity to development of leukemia, immune system defects, hearing loss, and duodenal obstruction. The defect in most Down syndrome individuals is the result of nondisjunction in the mother. Identification of the extra chromosome as maternal or paternal in origin was originally based on karyotyping analysis that compared banding patterns of the extra chromosome 21 with chromosome 21 of the mother and father. These early studies concluded that about 70 to 75 percent of Down syndrome occurred as a consequence of nondisjunction in the mother. By the late 1980s, more sensitive karyotype analysis, however, increased this frequency to 80 percent, and by the early 1990s, an even more sensitive molecular technique (Southern blot analysis of DNA polymorphisms) provided evidence that as much as 90 to 95 percent of Down syndrome arises through nondisjunction in the maternal germ line.

Occasionally, chromosome 21 nondisjunction

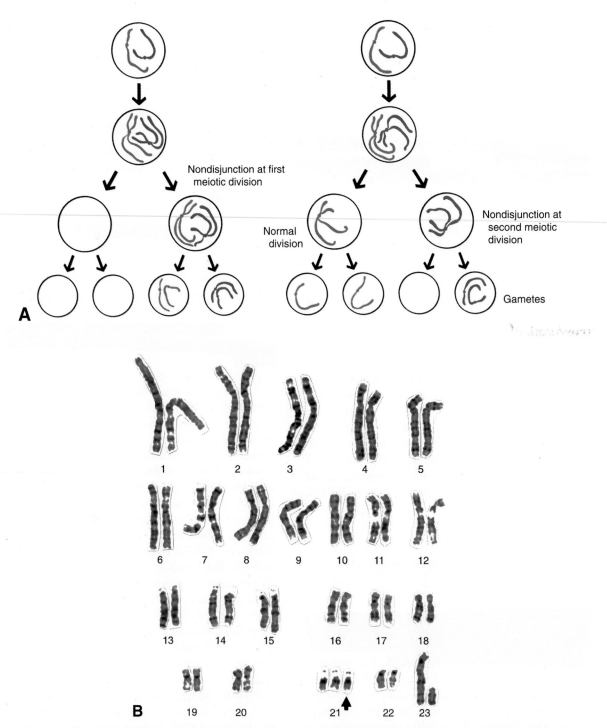

Figure 1–14. *A,* Mechanism of chromosomal nondisjunction in meiosis. Failure of like double-stranded chromosomes to separate before cytokinesis during the first meiotic division (left-hand panel) results in their distribution to only one of the secondary gonocytes (or first polar body). Failure of the two strands of a double-stranded chromosome to separate before cytokinesis during the second meiotic division (right-hand panel) results in their distribution to only one of the definitive gonocytes (or second polar body). *B,* Karyotype of a male with trisomy 21, causing Down syndrome. (*B,* Courtesy of Dr. Shirly Soukup.)

occurs in a single embryonic cell during cleavage. The resulting embryo develops as a **mosaic** of normal and trisomy 21 cells. About 2 to 5 percent of all individuals with Down syndrome are mosaics. Depending on the abundance and location of abnormal cells, these individuals may show very few features of Down syndrome. If the germ line is trisomic, however, such an apparently normal individual could produce several Down syndrome offspring. Meiosis of a trisomic germ cell yields gametes with a normal single copy of the chromosome as well as abnormal gametes with two copies, so normal offspring can also be produced.

Down syndrome does not always result from simple nondisjunction. Sometimes, a copy of chromosome 21 in a developing gamete becomes attached to the end of another chromosome, such as chromosome 14, during the first or second division of meiosis (Fig. 1–15). This event is called a **translocation.** The zygote produced by fusion of such a gamete with a normal partner will have two normal copies of chromosome 21 plus an abnormal chromosome 14 carrying a third copy of chromosome 21 (see Fig. 1–15). About 5 percent of all individuals with Down syndrome harbor such translocations.

Cases in which only a part of chromosome 21 is translocated have made it possible to determine which regions of the chromosome must be triplicated to produce Down syndrome. Indeed, the locations of genes responsible for the expression of specific features of Down syndrome have been defined by constructing "phenotypic maps" of chromosome 21 using molecular techniques. These studies implicate a **Down syndrome candidate region** on the long arm of chromosome 21 (21q 22.3) in the etiology of Down syndrome.

The incidence of Down syndrome increases significantly with the age of the mother but not with the age of the father. The risk of giving birth to a liveborn with Down syndrome at maternal age 30 is 1 in 1000. The risk increases to 9 in 1000 by maternal age 40. It is not clear, however, whether older women actually produce more oocytes with nondisjunction of chromosome 21 or whether the efficiency of aborting trisomy 21 embryos decreases with age.

Trisomies 18, 13, 8, and 9 also produce recognizable syndromes of abnormal development, as do abnormal numbers of sex chromosomes (Kline-

Figure 1–15. Karyotype of a male with Down syndrome caused by translocation of chromosome 21 onto chromosome 14. (Photo courtesy of Dr. Shirley Soukup.)

felter and Turner syndromes are discussed in the Clinical Applications and Experimental Principles sections of Ch. 10). **Triploid** or **tetraploid** embryos, in which multiple copies of the entire genome are present, can arise by errors in fertilization (see the Clinical Applications and Experimental Principles sections of Ch. 2).

Several Other Types of Chromosome Anomalies Are Produced at Meiosis. In some cases, errors in meiosis result in the deletion of just part of a chromosome or the duplication of small chromosome segments. **Partial monosomies** resulting from the deletion of parts of chromosomes 4, 5, and 9 produce recognizable syndromes; Wilms' tumors of the kidney are associated with the deletion of a specific region of chromosome 11. On the other hand, the **partial trisomy** produced by duplication of a small portion of chromosome 9 is associated with a syndrome involving facial abnormalities, muscular hypertonia, and stenosis of the pylorus. Other errors that can occur during meiosis are **inversions** of chromosome segments and the formation of **ring chromosomes.**

Chromosome Analysis Can Determine the Parental Source of the Defective Chromosome and Provides a Basis for Diagnosis and Possible Treatment

Genetic analysis of congenital defects is a very recent development. The normal human karyotype was not fully characterized until the late 1950s. Even more recently, special stains such as quinacrine have been used to visualize heritable patterns of chromosome banding in standard **karyotype analysis.** In the last few years, a technique called **Southern blotting,** which uses DNA probes with known sequences, has led to much finer analysis of DNA structure, making it possible to determine which parent is the source of a defective chromosome. These techniques are used in genetic counseling. Blood cells of a prospective parent can be checked for heritable chromosome anomalies, and embryonic cells obtained either from the amniotic fluid (**amniocentesis**) or from the chorionic villi (**chorionic villous sampling**) can be used to detect many disorders early in pregnancy. In a variation of the Southern blotting technique, DNA probes are linked to a fluorescent dye to directly label and identify specific loci on chromosomes in a method called **fluorescence in situ hybridization (FISH).** This technique is especially useful in detecting **aneuploidy** (an abnormal number of chromosomes) and translocations. In addition, these procedures, along with the use of animal mutants, transgenic animal models, and information derived from an ongoing project to sequence the entire human genome, will vastly increase our understanding of the role of genetic causes in human dysmorphology.

In a technique called **spectral karyotyping** or **chromosome painting,** human chromosomes can be stained with a combination of stains or **fluorochromes** so that each type of chromosome emits a unique spectrum of light. A computer is then used to display all of the chromosomes, each with its own assigned color (Fig. 1–16*A*). This technique is especially useful in revealing translocations (Fig. 1–16*B*, *C*).

Contraceptive Techniques Interfere With a Wide Variety of Reproductive Mechanisms

Despite the High Rate of Spontaneous Abortion, Human Reproductive Efficiency Is Very High. An average couple who do not practice contraception and have intercourse twice a week (timed randomly with respect to ovulation) have a better than 50 percent chance of fertilizing any given oocyte. Because about half of all embryos undergo spontaneous abortion, the chance that 1 month's intercourse will produce a term pregnancy is thus better than 25 percent. Healthy humans have astounding reproductive efficiency; it is not rare for couples who do not practice contraception to produce 10 to 20 offspring in a reproductive lifetime. The greatest officially recorded number of children is 69, born to a Russian woman in the 18th century. The *Guinness Book of World Records* cites a living Argentine woman who has given birth to 32 living children. Given present and projected birth and infant mortality rates, it is expected that the present world's population of 5.7 billion (1996) will double to more than 10 billion by 2050.

Contraception has played an important role in family planning for much of human history. Some of the oldest forms are simple **barrier contraceptives,** and these methods remain among the most frequently used today. Although progress in the development of new approaches to contraception has slowed in recent years, modern contraceptive research has been directed to developing strategies that interfere with many of the physiologic mechanisms discussed earlier that are required for successful conception.

Barrier Contraceptives Prevent the Sperm From Reaching the Egg. One of the oldest types of contraceptive device is the **male condom,** originally made of animal bladders or sheep cecum and now made of latex rubber and often combined with a chemical spermicide. The male condom is fitted over the erect penis just before intercourse. The **female condom** is a polyurethane sheath that is inserted to completely line the vagina as well as the perineal area. Use of the female condom has also been advocated to prevent the spread of sexually transmitted diseases (STDs). Other barrier devices, such as the **diaphragm** and **cervical cap,** are inserted into the vagina to cover the cervix and are usually used in conjunction with a spermicide. The **contraceptive sponge** is a spermicide-impregnated disc of polyurethane sponge that absorbs spermatozoa in the vagina.

The Birth Control Pill Prevents Ovulation. Knowledge of the endocrine control of ovulation led to the introduction of the birth control pill ("the Pill") in the early 1960s. These early pills released a daily dose of estrogen, which inhibited ovulation by preventing secretion of the gonadotropic hormones FSH and LH from the pituitary. In modern pills, the estrogen dosage has been reduced, the progesterone analog **progestin** has been added, and the doses of estrogen and progestin are usually varied over a 21-day cycle. Although the normal function of progesterone is to support pregnancy through its effect on the endometrium, it also interferes with the release of FSH and LH, thus preventing ovulation. In addition, it may interfere with oocyte transport down the oviduct or with sperm capacitation.

Injected or Implanted Sources of Progestin Deliver a Chronic Antiovulatory Dose. A **depot preparation** of medroxyprogesterone acetate (Depo-Provera) can be injected intramuscularly and will deliver antiovulatory levels of the hormone for 2 to 3 months. Alternatively, rods or capsules have been developed that are implanted subdermally and release a synthetic progestagen for a period of 1 to 5 years. Other devices act by releasing the hormone into the female reproductive tract rather than the bloodstream. Progesterone-containing **intrauterine devices** (IUDs) emit low levels of progesterone for a period of 1 to 4 years. **Vaginal rings** are inserted and removed by the user and, when in place around the cervix, release progestins continuously for 3 months.

Nonmedicated IUDs May Interfere With Conception Through Effects on Both Sperm and Egg. The mechanism by which nonmedicated loop-shaped or T-shaped IUDs prevent conception when inserted in the uterus is still unclear. Originally, they were thought to act by irritating the endometrium. However, when women who used IUDs and had intercourse during their fertile pe-

Figure 1–16. *A,* Spectral karyotyping of human chromosomes after the simultaneous hybridization of 24 combinatorially labeled chromosome painting probes. *B,* Karyotyping of chromosomes from the peripheral blood lymphocytes of a father of a child with mental retardation. Conventional banding analysis is insufficient to reveal a reciprocal translocation between chromosomes 1 and 11 (left panel) but is clearly shown with spectral karyotyping (right panel). *C,* High resolution Giemsa-banding of a patient with ataxia suggests that chromosome 4 material is translocated to chromosome 12 (left panel). This is confirmed by spectral karyotyping (right panel). (From Schrock E, du Manoir S, Veldman T, et al. 1996. Multicolor spectral karyotyping of human chromosomes. Science 272:494.)

riod were examined, no fertilized oocytes could be found in the uterus or fallopian tubes, in contrast to women who did not use an IUD. IUDs may, therefore, prevent fertilization through effects on the sperm or oocyte. Alternatively, they may interfere with preimplantation development of the zygote.

The Antiprogesterone Compound RU-486 Is an Abortifacient.

The mechanism of action of RU-486 (mifepristone) is not known, but this compound has potent antiprogesterone activity and may also stimulate prostaglandin synthesis. When taken within 8 weeks of the last menses, an adequate dose of RU-486 will initiate menstruation. If a conceptus is present, it will be sloughed along with the endometrial decidua. A large-scale French study in which RU-486 was administered along with a prostaglandin analog yielded an efficacy rate of 96 percent.

Sterilization Is Used by About One Third of American Couples.

Sterilization of the male partner (**vasectomy**) or female partner (**ligation of the fallopian tubes**) is an effective method of contraception and is often chosen by people who want no additional children. However, both methods involve surgery, and neither is reliably reversible.

New Methods of Contraception Are Needed.

Every method of birth control so far devised has drawbacks—some produce side effects; some may be considered objectionable or immoral; some are illegal in certain societies. For example, only 50 to 70 percent of women who begin to take the Pill are still taking it a year later. A greater variety of better contraceptives is urgently needed. Nevertheless, as a result of litigation, changing mores, and political inaction, contraceptive development overall has slowed in recent years. One consequence is that the rates of pregnancy and abortion among American teenagers are the highest in the industrial world. The abortion rates in several other countries with low contraceptive use (such as the Soviet Union) have also risen dramatically. Conversely, it has been suggested that low abortion rates in the Netherlands can be explained by widespread use of contraceptives.

Many other signs point to the need for better contraception: the explosive growth of the human population, the acquired immunodeficiency syndrome (AIDS) epidemic, rising rates of several other STDs, concern about chronic exposure to the steroids used in birth control pills, and the low efficacy of some existing contraception methods. Studies are under way on a number of new techniques. These include spermicides with antiviral activity (to help slow AIDS transmission), a once-a-month menses inducer, a reliable ovulation predictor for couples who want to practice "natural" family planning, reversible male sterilization, male contraceptive pills, and antifertility vaccines such as a vaccine against the hormone hCG.

The Maturation of Human Gametes and Early Embryos Can Now be Supported Outside the Body to Assist Infertile Couples

It is estimated that about 15 to 30 percent of American couples are infertile. A number of in vitro techniques are now used to assist reproduction when natural conception is not possible. The development of defined culture media and the use of modern tissue culture techniques have made it possible to maintain human gametes and cleavage-stage embryos outside the body. Gametes and embryos can also be successfully frozen and stored, adding to the options for assisted reproduction.

An Oocyte Can Be Fertilized In Vitro and Then Implanted in the Uterus.

The procedure of **in vitro fertilization (IVF) and embryo transfer** is widely used in cases in which scarring of the oviducts (a common consequence of pelvic infections) either prevents the sperm from reaching the ampulla or prevents the fertilized oocyte from passing to the uterus. In this technique, the woman's ovaries are first induced to **superovulate** (develop multiple mature follicles) by administration of an appropriate combination of hormones (usually human menopausal gonadotropin and pure FSH, sometimes combined with clomiphene citrate). Maturing oocytes are then harvested from the follicles. Harvesting is usually performed through a laparoscope, which can be inserted through a small puncture in the umbilical region, but an ultrasonography-guided needle inserted via the vagina can also be used. Once retrieved, the oocytes are allowed to mature in a culture medium to the second meiotic metaphase and are then fertilized with previously obtained and capacitated sperm. The resulting zygotes are allowed to develop in the culture medium to the two- to four-cell stage (or later) and are then inserted into the uterus.

Given the access provided to the oocyte and zygote in the IVF and embryo transfer technique, the use of polar bodies for genetic screening of patients who may fear the transmission of a heritable disease is under study. Either polar body may be removed without apparent harm to oocyte or zygote development and screened for aneuploidy or translocations with standard karyotypic analysis or FISH and for mutations with techniques like the **polymerase chain reaction (PCR)**. PCR amplifies DNA from a single polar body, producing many copies for sequence analysis. The drawbacks of polar body analysis include contamination from maternal cells, difficulties in analysis of both first and second polar bodies (which is more informative) and the lack of information regarding paternal contributions to the zygote. Similar genetic analyses, however, can be carried out on single blastomeres removed from the embryo during early cleavage stages, thus revealing possible defects of the paternal genome, but this technique carries risks for the embryo and is more costly. A significant advantage of polar body or blastomere biopsy, however, may be avoidance of abortion, which poses both ethical and medical dilemmas for parents.

Gametes or Zygotes Can Be Introduced Directly Into the Ampulla of the Oviduct. If the woman's oviduct is normal and the couple is infertile because of an innate deficiency in spermatozoon motility or for some other reason, a technique called **gamete intrafallopian transfer (GIFT)** is often used. Oocytes are harvested as described above and are then placed into a laparoscope catheter along with precapacitated spermatozoa. The oocytes and spermatozoa are introduced together directly into the ampulla of the oviduct, where fertilization takes place. Further development occurs by normal processes. In an alternative technique, **zygote intrafallopian transfer (ZIFT),** the oocytes are fertilized in vitro, and only fertilized pronuclear zygotes are introduced into the ampulla. In cases in which the male spermatozoa are unable to penetrate the zoma pellneida, a technique called **intracytoplasmic sperm injection (ICSI)** may be used. In this procedure, a single spermatozoan is selected under a microscope, aspirated into a needle, and injected into the oocyte cytoplasm. A possible risk to embryo development in this technique may exist because of an increased incidence of the chromosone anomalies or gene disruptions in the spermatozoa of some infertile men.

Experimental Principles

Genetic Regulation of Germ Cell Formation, Proliferation, Migration, and Development

A COMPLEX REGULATORY CASCADE CONTROLS DEVELOPMENT OF THE GERM LINE IN HUMANS

As discussed at the beginning of this chapter, the primordial germ cells (PGCs) in male and female humans arise within the primary ectoderm (epiblast), are translocated to the secondary yolk sac (see Ch. 2), and then, by ameboid movement, migrate through the gut wall and the dorsal mesentery and into the posterior body wall, where they participate in induction of the gonad. As in many other complex developmental processes, it is now clear that stages of germ line formation are controlled by a **regulatory gene cascade** (Fig. 1–17). This cascade comprises a sequential activation of genes that direct the initial induction and development, proliferation, survival, migration, and differentiation of the primordial germ cells.

Genes required for initiation of germ cell formation in lower animals are called **maternal effect genes** (see Experimental Principles Section of Ch. 3). The activation of these maternal genes regulates the segregation of the **germ plasm** (cyto-

Figure 1–17. Regulation gene cascade controlling the development of primordial germ cells.

plasm containing determinants of the germ line) to a specific region of the zygote so that it becomes incorporated during cleavage into a unique group of cells that will form the germ cell precursors. In contrast, it is likely that all early cells of the mammalian embryo, including the morula, are capable of forming pluripotent (ability to form many cell types) germ cells but that this capacity becomes restricted first to the inner cell mass and then to the epiblast. In mammals, therefore, **initiation of germ line development** requires the activation of genes that maintain pluripotency within the precursors that will form the germ line. One such gene appears to encode a POU domain transcriptional regulator (Oct-4). Its activity is present in all cells of the morula, but then only in the inner cell mass. It is then restricted to the epiblast and finally is expressed only in the presumptive germ cells themselves.

Further development of the germ line requires the activation of genes that initiate differentiation of primordial germ cells in the epiblast. This process appears to require an inductive signal

from the trophoblast (see discussion of induction in Experimental Principles section of Ch. 3). One such candidate signal is bone morphogenetic protein-4 (Bmp-4). Bmp-4 apparently activates genes such as germ cell-less (Gcl) within the presumptive germ cells of the epiblast.

As presumptive germ cells are translocated to the yolk sac (see Fig. 1–1A), their **proliferation and survival** is ensured by the expression of **trophic factors** within the PGCs or within associated cells. A trophic factor expressed by PGCs and required for their early survival and proliferation is the RNA-binding protein TIAR. Many other trophic factors appear to be required for the survival and proliferation of PGCs along their migratory pathway from the yolk sac to the gut and dorsal mesentery and then to the posterior body wall. These include several factors expressed by tissues along the pathway including c-kit ligand (stem cell factor), and members of the interleukin/Lif cytokine family.

Other factors, including extracellular matrix proteins, must also be expressed by cells along the pathway to **direct the migration of the PGCs** from the yolk sac to the gut and dorsal mesentery and then to the gonadal ridge (presumptive gonad) in the posterior body wall. One such factor may be tenascin c, but few other candidates have been identified in mammals.

Finally, once the PGCs have arrived within the presumptive gonad, numerous genes must be expressed to **regulate the final differentiation of cells of the germ line.** These include genes that encode the signalling factor Gas-6 and its receptor tyrosine kinase (Sky), the transcription factor Gata-4, and the zinc finger proteins Zfx (in females) and Zfy (in males). Several of these factors and others such as Sf-1 and Wt-1 are discussed in the Experimental Principles Section of Chapter 10.

Studies of PGC Regulatory Genes May Reveal Mechanisms of Teratoma Formation. Human extragonadal pluripotent teratomas are a rare class of tumors of variable phenotype and controversial origin. They may form in the sacrococcygeal region (most often in infants), in the mediastinum (most often in adult males), or at retroperitoneal, cervical, or cranial sites. Their pluripotency is exhibited by their ability to form a variety of definitive anatomic structures, including hair, teeth, pituitary gland, and even a fully formed eye. It has been argued that some teratomas may arise from primordial germ cells that atypically migrate to their definitive ectopic location from various sites along their normal pathway of migration. In other cases, it is thought that the teratoma may arise from transformed stem cells of the germ line within the gonad itself. Perhaps, as additional genes that regulate normal PGC development in humans are identified, it will be possible to utilize more specific genetic strategies to identify sites of origin and genetic disruptions that lead to the development of some of these tumors.

MANIPULATION OF THE MAMMALIAN GENOME

Recently, several lines of research have coalesced to yield techniques that make it possible to insert specific DNA sequences into their correct locations in the mammalian genome. These techniques give researchers the power to alter and manipulate the genome and to investigate its detailed functioning. Animal models of human genetic diseases can be created by disabling specific normal genes. Moreover, the ability to correct defective genes lays the groundwork for developing techniques to cure genetic disorders.

Figure 1–18. Technique of creating an injection chimera by introducing genetically modified ("targeted") embryonic stem cells (ES cells) into a blastocyst. The blastocyst is held at the end of a suction pipette, and the ES cells are injected into the blastocyst cavity through a very fine glass needle. The injected cells are incorporated into the inner cell mass of the host blastocyst. (Photos courtesy of Drs. Achim Gossler, Thomas Doetschman, and Rolf Kemler.)

Transgenic Animals Can Be Created by Injecting DNA Into the Male Pronucleus of the Fertilized Egg.

A **transgenic animal** is one whose genome has been altered by the integration of donor DNA sequences. The most direct way to create a transgenic animal is to inject many copies of the donor DNA sequence into the male pronucleus of a fertilized egg. (The male pronucleus is used because it is larger than the female pronucleus). The injected DNA sometimes integrates stably into the host chromosomes, and in many cases, the donor gene is expressed. In a pioneering experiment, for example, a zinc-dependent rat growth hormone gene was introduced into the genome of a series of mice. When zinc was added to the drinking water to induce the expression of the rat growth hormone gene, these transgenic mice grew at twice the rate of control animals.

DNA Can Be Targeted to a Specific Genomic Location.

Injection of DNA into the fertilized egg does not allow one to target the donor gene to a specific location in the host genome. That can be accomplished, however, by a technique in which the donor DNA is inserted into cells obtained from the inner cell mass of the blastocyst, and the rare cells in which the donor DNA has integrated correctly are identified and used to create a special type of transgenic animal called an **injection chimera.** In this approach, blastocysts are obtained from the oviducts of fertilized mice and are grown on a layer of fibroblasts in a culture dish. Culturing causes a cluster of cells from the inner cell mass to erupt from the blastocyst. These inner cell mass clusters are harvested and subcultured to produce stable lines of **embryonic stem (ES) cells,** which are **totipotent** (able to give rise to any tissue in the body).

Donor DNA sequences can be introduced into cultured ES cells by a technique called **electroporation,** in which a suspension of ES cells is mixed with many copies of the donor DNA and subjected to an electric current. The current apparently facilitates the movement of the donor DNA through the cell membrane, allowing the DNA to enter the nucleus. In a tiny fraction of these cells, the introduced DNA is incorporated into the desired target site on the genome by **homologous recombination.** Appropriate marker genes and screening techniques are used to isolate and subculture these rare "targeted" cells.

Injection Chimeras Can Be Produced by Injecting the Transgene-Containing ES Cells Into a Normal Blastocyst.

To create transgenic mice containing the new DNA, groups of 8 to 12 targeted ES cells are injected into the cavity of normal mouse blastocysts, where they combine with the inner cell mass and participate in the formation of the embryo (Fig. 1–18). The resulting blasto-

Figure 1–19. A litter of transgenic mice bred from a chimeric parent. The parent mouse on the left is an injection chimera produced by inserting cells from a black mouse into a blastocyst from an agouti (brown-and-white) strain. This chimeric animal displays the typical agouti coat pattern except for a telltale spot of black on the forehead (arrow). When the animal was bred with a black mouse (parent on the right), two of the offspring (bottom row) were black, showing that the germ line of the chimeric parent contains both black and agouti cells. (The agouti coat pattern is genetically dominant over the black coat pattern.) (Photo courtesy of Drs. Achim Gossler, Thomas Doetschman, and Rolf Kemler.)

cysts (called **chimeras** because they are composed of cells from two different sources) are then implanted in the uterus of a pseudopregnant mouse, where they develop normally. Depending on their location in the embryonic disc, the ES cells may contribute to almost any tissue of the chimeric mouse. When they contribute to the germ line, the donor genes can be passed on to the offspring (Fig. 1–19). Dominant donor genes may be expressed in the immediate offspring; if the donor genes are recessive (as they usually are), an inbreeding program is used to produce a homozygous strain that can express the gene.

Gene-Targeting Technology Will Have a Strong Impact on the Understanding and Treatment of Heritable Disorders. Gene-targeting techniques are being used to develop animal models of several human diseases, including neurofibromatosis, insulin-dependent diabetes mellitus, cystic fibrosis, Lesch-Nyhan syndrome, and retinoblastoma. Less advanced is the application of gene-targeting techniques to the actual correction of genetic disorders by the insertion of a normal gene. However, these techniques have been used to "cure" the germ lines of mice with various heritable disorders so that the offspring are healthy (see Ch. 15).

SUGGESTED READINGS

Descriptive Embryology

Aitken RJ. 1995. The complexities of conception. Science 269:39

Archer DF, Zeleznik AJ, Rockette HE. 1988. Ovarian follicular maturation in women. II. Reversal of estrogen inhibited ovarian folliculogenesis by human gonadotropin. Fertil Steril 50:555

Byskov AG. 1986. Differentiation of the mammalian embryonic gonad. Physiol Rev 66:71

Clermont Y. 1972. Kinetics of spermatogenesis in mammals: seminiferous epithelium cycle and spermatogonial renewal. Physiol Rev 52:198

DeSousa PA, Valdimarsson G, Nicholson BJ, Kidden GM. 1993. Connexin trafficking and the control of gap junction assembly in mouse preimplantation embryos. Development 117:1355

Eddy EM, Clark JM, Gong D, Fenderson BA. 1981. Origin and migration of primordial germ cells in mammals. Gamete Res 4:333

Enders AC, Hendrickx AG, Schlake S. 1983. Implantation in the rhesus monkey: initial penetration of the endometrium. Am J Anat 167:275

Gilman J. 1948. The development of the gonads in man, with consideration of the role of fetal endocrines and the histogenesis of ovarian tumors. Contrib Carnegie Inst 32:81

Hammen R. 1944. Studies on Impaired Fertility in Man with Special Reference to the Male. p. 206. Munksgaard and Milford, Copenhagen

Hertig AT, Rock J, Adams EC. 1956. A description of 34 human ova within the first 17 days of development. Am J Anat 98:435

Hillman N, Sherman MI, Graham C. 1972. The effect of spatial arrangement on cell determination during mouse development. J Embryol Exp Morphol 18:263

Lawson KA, Hage J. 1994. Clonal analysis of the origin of primordial germ cells in the mouse. CIBA Symp. 182. Germline Development. John Wiley and Sons, New York

Luckett WP. 1978. Origin and differentiation of the yolk sac and extraembryonic mesoderm in presomite human and rhesus monkey embryos. Am J Anat 152:59

O'Rahilly R. 1973. Developmental stages in human embryos. A. Embryos of the first three weeks (stages 1–9). Carnegie Inst Wash Publ, p. 531

Pedersen RA, Wu K, Balakier H. 1986. Origin of the inner cell mass in mouse embryos: cell lineage analysis by microinjection. Dev Biol 117:581

Pelletier RM, Friend DS. 1983. Development of membrane differentiations in the guinea pig spermatid during spermiogenesis. Am J Anat 167:119

Pincus G, Enzmann EV. 1935. The comparative behavior of mammalian eggs in vivo and in vitro. I. The activation of ovarian eggs. J Exp Med 62:665

Russell LD. 1980. Sertoli-germ cell interactions: a review. Gamete Res 3:179

Schultz RM, Endo Y, Mattei P, et al. 1988. Egg induced modifications of the mouse zona pellucida. Prog Clin Biol Res 284:77

Smith C, Moore HDM, Hearn JP. 1987. The ultrastructure of early implantation in the marmoset monkey (*Callitrix jacchus*). Anat Embryol 175:399

Tarkowski AK, Wroblewska J. 1967. Development of blastomeres of mouse eggs isolated at the 4- and 8-cell stage. J Embryol Exp Morphol 18:155

Wasserman PM. 1991. Elements of Mammalian Fertilization. Vol. I. Basic Concepts. CRC Press, Boca Raton, FL

Witschi E. 1948. Migration of the germ cells of human embryos from the yolk sac to the primitive gonadal folds. Contrib Embryol Carnegie Inst 32:67

Clinical Applications

Alvarez F, Brache V, Fernandez E, et al. 1988. New insights on the mode of action of intrauterine contraceptive devices in women. Fertil Steril 49:768

Bolton VN, Braude PR. 1987. Development of the human preimplantation embryo in vitro. Curt Top Dev Biol 23:93

Comhaire FH. 1994. Male contraception: hormonal, mechanical and other. Hum Reprod 9:22

Connell EB. 1989. Barrier contraceptives. Clin Obstet Gynecol 32:377

de Grouchy J, Turleau C. 1984. Clinical Atlas of Human Chromosomes. John Wiley & Sons, New York

Devroey P, Staessen C, Camus M, et al. 1989. Zygote intrafallopian transfer as a successful treatment for unexplained fertility. Fertil Steril 52:246

Diczfalusy E, Bygdeman M (eds). 1987. Fertility Regulation Today and Tomorrow. Raven Press, New York

Djerassi C. 1989. The bitter pill. Science 245:356

Edward RG. 1994. Implantation interception and contraception. Hum Reprod 9:73

Groner Y, Elroy-Stein O, Bernstein Y, et al. 1986. Molecular genetics of Down's syndrome: overexpression of transfected human Cu/Zn-superoxide dismutase gene and the consequent physiological changes. Cold Spring Harbor Symp Quant Biol L1:381

Hook EB. 1989. Issues pertaining to the impact and etiology of trisomy 21 and other aneuploidy in humans: a consideration of evolutionary implications, maternal age mechanisms, and other matters. Prog Clin Biol Res 311:1

Jones KL. 1988. Smith's Recognizable Patterns of Human Malformations. WB Saunders, Philadelphia

Ketting E, Visser AP. 1994. Contraception in the Netherlands: the low abortion rate explained. Patient Counseling Education 23:161

McFarlan D (ed). 1991. Guinness Book of World Records. p. 14. Bantam, New York

McKusick VA. 1989. Mapping and sequencing the human genome. N Engl J Med 320:910

McLaren A. 1988. The IVF conceptus: research today and tomorrow. Ann N Y Acad Sci 541:639

Morton NE, Chiu D, Holland C, et al. 1987. Chromosome anomalies as predictors of recurrence risk for spontaneous abortion. Am J Med Genet 28:353

Korenberg JR, Chen XN, Schipper R, et al. 1994. Down syndrome phenotypes: the consequence of chromosomal imbalance. Proc Natl Acad Sci U S A 91:4997

Silvestre L, Dubois C, Renault M, et al. 1989. Voluntary interruption of pregnancy with mifepristone (RU 486) and a prostaglandin analogue: a large scale French experience. N Engl J Med 322:645

Steptoe PC, Edwards RG. 1978. Birth after the implantation of a human embryo. Lancet ii:366

Stewart GD, Hassold TJ, Kurnit DM. Trisomy 21: molecular and cytogenetic studies of nondisjunction. Adv Hum Genet 17:99

Temmerman M. 1994. Sexually transmitted diseases and reproductive health. Sexually Transmitted Diseases 21:555

Tesarik J, Mendoza L. 1999. In vitro fertilization by intracytoplasmic sperm injection. Bioessays 21:791

Verlinsky Y, Kuliev A. 1994. Human preimplantation diagnosis: needs, efficiency and efficacy of genetic and chromosome analysis. [Review]. Baillieres Clin Obstet Gynaecol 8:177

Wapner RJ, Jackson L. 1988. Chorionic villous sampling. Clin Obstet Gynecol 31:328

Wilcox AJ, Weinberg CR, O'Connor JF, et al. 1988. Incidence of early loss of pregnancy. N Engl J Med 319:189

Wood EC. 1988. The future of in vitro fertilization. Ann N Y Acad Sci 541:715

Wu FCW. 1988. Male contraception: current status and future prospects. Clin Endocrinol 29:443

Zipursky A, Poon A, Doyle J. 1992. Leukemia in Down Syndrome: a review. Pediatr Hematol Oncol 9:139

Experimental Principles

Capecchi MR. 1989. The new mouse genetics: altering the genome by gene targeting. Trends Genet 5:70

Chagant RS, Houldsworth J. 1998. The cytogenetic theory of the pathogenesis of human adult male germ cell tumors. APMIS 106:80

Doetschman TC. 1989. Gene targeting in embryonic stem cells. p. 89. In First N, Haseltine FP (eds): Transgenic Animals in Medicine and Agriculture (The Biotechnology Series). Butterworth, Stoneham, MA

Doetschman T, Gregg RG, Maeda N, et al. 1987. Targeted correction of a mutant HPRT gene in mouse embryonic stem cells. Nature (London) 330:576

Frohman MA, Martin GR. 1989. Cut, paste, and save: new approaches to altering specific genes in mice. Cell 56:145

Gordon JW. 1989. Transgenic animals. Int Rev Cytol 115:171

Jaenisch R. 1988. Transgenic animals. Science 240:1468

Kim HS, Smithies O. 1988. Recombinant fragment assay for gene targeting based on the polymerase chain reaction. Nucleic Acids Res 16:8887

Piccolo S, Sasai Y, Lu B, De Robertis EM. 1996. Dorsoventral patterning in Xenopus: Inhibition of ventral signals by direct binding of chordin to BMP-4. Cell 86:589

Prather RS, Hageman LJ, First NL. 1989. Preimplantation mammalian aggregation and injection chimeras. Gamete Res 22:233

Robertson E, Bradley A, Kuehn M, Evans MJ. 1986. Germ-line transmission of genes introduced into cultured pluripotential cells by a retroviral vector. Nature (London) 323:445

Tarkowski AK. 1961. Mouse chimeras developed from fused eggs. Nature (London) 190:857

Tian Q, Frierson HF, Krystal GW, Moskaluk CA. 1999. Activating c-kit gene mutations in human germ cell tumors. Am J Pathol 154:1643

Wylie C. 1999. Germ cells. Cell 96:165

2

The Second Week

Summary

As discussed in the preceding chapter, the zygote undergoes cleavage during the first week to produce a blastocyst consisting of an inner cell mass or embryoblast and an outer cell mass or trophoblast. At the beginning of the second week, the embryoblast splits into two layers, the **epiblast** or **primary ectoderm** and the **hypoblast** or **primary endoderm.** This event reflects establishment of the dorsoventral axis of the embryo. A cavity, called the **amniotic cavity,** then develops within the epiblast as a layer of cells derived from the epiblast thins to become the **amniotic membrane.** The remainder of the epiblast and the hypoblast now constitute a **bilaminar germ disc** lying between the amniotic cavity and the blastocyst cavity. The cells of this germ disc develop into the **embryo proper** and also contribute to some of the **extraembryonic membranes.** During the second week, the hypoblast sends out two waves of endodermal cells that successively line the blastocyst cavity. The first of these waves transforms the blastocoel into the primary yolk sac, and the second transforms the primary yolk sac into the secondary or definitive yolk sac.

In the middle of the second week, the inner surface of the cytotrophoblast and the outer surface of the yolk sac and amnion become lined by a new tissue, the **extraembryonic mesoderm.** The source of this tissue is debated. A new cavity, the **chorionic cavity** or **extraembryonic coelom,** develops between the two layers of the extraembryonic mesoderm.

Meanwhile, implantation continues, mediated primarily by the trophoblast. The cellular trophoblast, now called the **cytotrophoblast,** actively invades the endometrium and pulls the blastocyst into the uterine wall. It also gives rise to an expanding peripheral syncytial layer, the syncytiotrophoblast. These trophoblast layers contribute exclusively to the extraembryonic membranes, not to the embryo proper. During the second week, the extraembryonic mesoderm, cytotrophoblast, and syncytiotrophoblast begin to collaborate with the uterus to form the **placenta.** The fetal tissues form outgrowths, the **chorionic villi,** which grow into maternal blood sinuses.

Many events occur in twos during the second week. Although it has exceptions, this "Rule of Twos" constitutes a handy mnemonic for remembering the events of the second week. During the second week, the embryoblast splits into two germ layers, the epiblast and hypoblast. The trophoblast also gives rise to two tissues, the cytotrophoblast and the syncytiotrophoblast. The blastocyst cavity is remodeled twice, changing first into the primary yolk sac and then into the definitive yolk sac. Two novel cavities appear, the amniotic cavity and the chorionic cavity, and the extraembryonic mesoderm splits into the two layers that line the chorionic cavity.

Development of the Bilaminar Germ Disc and Establishment of the Uteroplacental Circulation

The trophoblast differentiates to produce the syncytiotrophoblast, and begins to implant the blastocyst into the uterine endometrium. The germ disc is bilaminar

The amniotic cavity appears within the epiblast; the syncytiotrophoblast expands

The hypoblast proliferates to produce Heuser's membrane, which migrates out to line the blastocyst cavity (now the primary yolk sac cavity). Lacunae appear within the syncytiotrophoblast. Implantation is complete; syncytiotrophoblast surrounds the embryo

The acellular extraembryonic reticulum is secreted between the cytotrophoblast and Heuser's membrane. Extraembryonic mesoderm then appears and forms the outer covering of the primary yolk sac and the inner lining of the cytotrophoblast; between these layers the extraembryonic reticulum breaks down to form the chorionic cavity. The trophoblastic lacunae anastomose with maternal blood sinusoids

Proliferation of the hypoblast produces the secondary yolk sac endoderm, which migrates out to line the inside of the extraembryonic mesoderm, forming the definitive yolk sac. The primary yolk sac is pushed aside and begins to collapse

The primary yolk sac is reduced to a transient collection of vesicles at the abembryonic pole of the chorionic cavity

The embryo proper is attached to the wall of the chorionic cavity by the connecting stalk

Timeline. The second week of development.

THE SYNCYTIOTROPHOBLAST HELPS TO IMPLANT THE EMBRYO IN THE ENDOMETRIUM

As described in Chapter 1, the blastocyst adheres to the uterine wall at the end of the first week. Contact with the uterine endometrium induces the trophoblast at the embryonic pole to proliferate. Some of these proliferating cells lose their cell membranes and coalesce to form a syncytium (a mass of cytoplasm containing numerous dispersed nuclei) called the **syncytiotrophoblast** (Fig. 2–1).

By contrast, the cells of the trophoblast, forming the wall of the blastocyst, retain their cell membranes and constitute the **cytotrophoblast.** The syncytiotrophoblast increases in volume throughout the second week as cells detach from the proliferating cytotrophoblast at the embryonic pole and fuse with the syncytium (Figs. 2–2 and 2–3).

Between days 6 and 9, the embryo becomes completely implanted in the endometrium, largely as a result of the activities of the highly invasive subpopulation of the cytotrophoblast. Proteolytic enzymes, including several metalloproteinases, are secreted by the cytotrophoblast to break down the extracellular matrix between the endometrial cells. Active processes extending from the syncytiotrophoblast then penetrate between the separating endometrial cells and pull the embryo into the endometrium of the uterine wall (see Figs. 2–1 and 2–2). As implantation progresses, the expanding syncytiotrophoblast gradually envelops the blastocyst. By day 9, the entire blastocyst, except for a small region at the abembryonic pole, is blanketed by a thick layer of syncytiotrophoblast (see Fig. 2–3). The small hole marking the point in the endometrial epithelium where the blastocyst implanted is sealed by a plug of acellular material is called the **coagulation plug.**

THE EMBRYOBLAST SPLITS INTO EPIBLAST AND HYPOBLAST

Even before implantation occurs, cells of the embryoblast begin to differentiate into two layers. By day 8, the embryoblast consists of a distinct external layer of columnar cells, called the **epiblast,** or **primary ectoderm,** and an internal layer of cuboidal cells, called the **hypoblast** or **primary endoderm** (see Fig. 2–2). It is thought that the relative position of a cell in the inner cell mass of the morula determines whether it differentiates into epiblast or hypoblast; the evidence supports the idea that the epiblast arises from the innermost, apolar cells of the inner cell mass. An extracellular basement membrane is laid down between the two

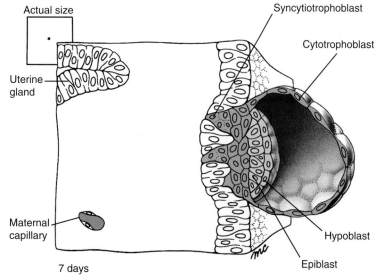

Figure 2–1. At 7 days, the newly hatched blastocyst contacts the uterine endometrium and begins to implant. The trophoblast at the embryonic pole of the blastocyst proliferates to form the invasive syncytiotrophoblast, which insinuates itself among the cells of the endometrium and begins to draw the blastocyst into the uterine wall. The germ disc is bilaminar, consisting of hypoblast and epiblast layers.

Actual size

Uterine gland

Maternal capillary

7 days

Syncytiotrophoblast

Cytotrophoblast

Hypoblast

Epiblast

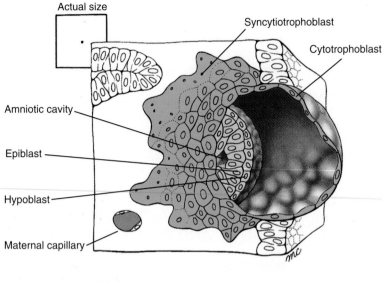

Actual size

Syncytiotrophoblast

Cytotrophoblast

Amniotic cavity

Epiblast

Hypoblast

Maternal capillary

8 days

Figure 2–2. By 8 days, the amniotic cavity has appeared within the epiblast, and some epiblast cells begin to differentiate into the amnioblasts that will form the amniotic membrane. Implantation continues, and the growing syncytiotrophoblast expands to cover more of the blastocyst.

layers immediately after they become distinct. The resulting two-layered embryoblast is called the **bilaminar germ disc.**

THE AMNIOTIC CAVITY DEVELOPS WITHIN THE EPIBLAST

The first new cavity to form during the second week—the **amniotic cavity**—appears on day 8 as fluid begins to collect between cells of the epiblast (see Fig. 2–2). A layer of epiblast cells is gradually displaced toward the embryonic pole by the accumulating fluid and differentiates into a thin membrane separating the new cavity from the cytotrophoblast. This membrane is the **amniotic membrane,** and the new cavity is the **amnion** (see Fig. 2–3). The cells that form the amniotic membrane are called **amnioblasts.** Although the amniotic cavity is at first smaller than the blastocyst

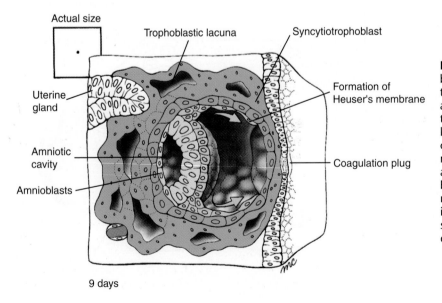

Actual size

Trophoblastic lacuna

Syncytiotrophoblast

Uterine gland

Formation of Heuser's membrane

Amniotic cavity

Amnioblasts

Coagulation plug

9 days

Figure 2–3. By 9 days, the embryo is completely implanted in the uterine endometrium. The amniotic cavity is expanding, and the hypoblast has begun to proliferate and migrate out over the cytotrophoblast to form Heuser's membrane. Trophoblastic lacunae appear in the syncytiotrophoblast, which now completely surrounds the embryo. The point of implantation is marked by a transient coagulation plug in the endometrial surface.

cavity, it expands steadily; by the eighth week, the amnion encloses the entire embryo (see Fig. 6–12).

THE FORMATION OF THE YOLK SAC AND CHORIONIC CAVITY IS NOT FULLY UNDERSTOOD

Two successive membranes migrate out from the hypoblast to line the blastocyst cavity, transforming it first into a primary yolk sac and then into the definitive yolk sac; a novel space, the chorionic cavity, separates the embryo with its attached amnion and yolk sac from the outer wall of the blastocyst, now called the **chorion.**

The Hypoblast Gives Rise to the Extraembryonic Endoderm That Lines the Primary Yolk Sac

On day 8, cells at the periphery of the newly formed hypoblast begin to migrate out over the inner surface of the cytotrophoblast, becoming flattened and squamous. By day 12, these cells form a thin membrane of **extraembryonic endoderm** completely lining the former blastocyst cavity (Fig. 2–4A). This membrane is called the **exocoelomic membrane** or **Heuser's membrane,** and the former blastocyst cavity is now called the **primary yolk sac** or **exocoelomic cavity.** As soon as the primary yolk sac forms, a thick, loosely reticular layer of acellular material called the **extraembryonic reticulum** is secreted between Heuser's membrane and the cytotrophoblast (see Fig. 2–4A).

The Chorionic Cavity Is Produced in Conjunction With the Development of the Extraembryonic Mesoderm

Although the extraembryonic reticulum contains some cells of hypoblast origin, there is evidence that a distinctive population of **extraembryonic mesoderm** cells appears within it on about day 12 or 13. Debate surrounds both the origin of this tissue and the mechanism by which it comes to be distributed into two layers lining the new **chori-**onic cavity (extraembryonic coelom) that forms between the yolk sac and the cytotrophoblast. According to one theory, the extraembryonic mesoderm cells arise from the epiblast at the caudal end of the bilaminar germ disc and migrate out to form two layers, one coating the outer surface of Heuser's membrane and the other lining the inner surface of the cytotrophoblast (Fig. 2–4B). The extraembryonic reticulum trapped between the two layers of extraembryonic mesoderm then breaks down and is replaced by fluid, forming the chorionic cavity (Figs. 2–4C and 2–5A).

As the chroionic cavity expands during the second week, the growth and migration of the extraembryonic mesoderm gradually separate the amnion from the cytotrophoblast. By day 13, the embryonic disc with its dorsal amnion and ventral yolk sac is suspended in the chorionic cavity solely by a thick stalk of mesoderm called the **connecting stalk** (Fig. 2–6).

THE DEFINITIVE YOLK SAC IS FORMED BY A NEW WAVE OF CELLS THAT MIGRATE FROM THE HYPOBLAST AND DISPLACE HEUSER'S MEMBRANE

By day 12, cells of the hypoblast again begin to proliferate and migrate outward (Fig. 2–5A). As this new wave of cuboidal cells spreads out over the inner surface of the extraembryonic mesoderm, the old primary yolk sac is pushed away toward the abembryonic pole. It then detaches from the embryo as it disintegrates into a collection of **exocoelomic vesicles** (see Fig. 2–5B). By day 13, these exocoelomic vesicles can be seen lying at the abembryonic pole, where they ultimately degenerate (Figs. 2–5C and 2–6). The space that constituted the blastocyst cavity and then the primary yolk sac thus becomes the **secondary** or **definitive yolk sac.**

The definitive yolk sac remains a major structure of the embryo through the fourth week and performs a number of important early functions. The extraembryonic mesoderm forming the outer layer of the yolk sac wall is a major site of **hematopoiesis** (blood formation). Cells giving rise to these first endothelial cells and hematopoietic stem cells migrate into the yolk sac from the pri-

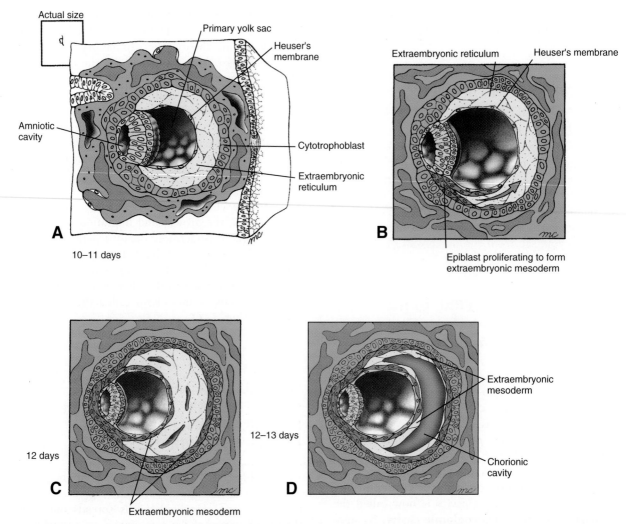

Figure 2–4. The extraembryonic mesoderm is formed in the middle of the second week. *A,* On days 10 to 11, an acellular extraembryonic reticulum forms between Heuser's membrane and the cytotrophoblast. At the same time, the trophoblastic lacunae begin to anastomose with maternal capillaries and become filled with blood. *B,* On days 11 and 12, the extraembryonic reticulum is rapidly invaded by the extraembryonic mesoderm. According to the theory illustrated here, the extraembryonic mesoderm originates from the epiblast. Other theories hold that it arises from the cytotrophoblast or the hypoblast. *C,* By day 12, the extraembryonic mesoderm becomes organized to form a layer coating the outside of Heuser's membrane and a layer lining the inside of the cytotrophoblast. Lacunae appear in the extraembryonic reticulum between these layers and (*D*) coalesce to form the chorionic cavity. Heuser's membrane and its overlying layer of extraembryonic mesoderm constitute the primary yolk sac.

mary ectoderm. The coordinated development of these cells into the **vitelline vasculature** is called **blood island** formation (see Fig. 2–6 and Ch. 8). The endoderm lining the yolk sac wall may produce serum proteins, and the definitive yolk sac may also play a limited role in the metabolism of embryonic nutrients. As described in Chapter 1,

the yolk sac also gives rise to the germ cells that populate the developing gonads. After the fourth week, the yolk sac is rapidly overgrown by the developing embryonic disc. The yolk sac normally disappears before birth, but rarely it persists in the form of a digestive tract anomaly called **Meckel's diverticulum** (see Ch. 9).

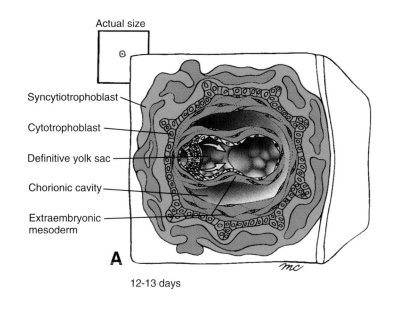

Actual size

Syncytiotrophoblast

Cytotrophoblast

Definitive yolk sac

Chorionic cavity

Extraembryonic
mesoderm

A

12-13 days

Cytotrophoblast

Chorionic
cavity

Definitive
yolk sac

Extraembryonic
mesoderm

B

13 days

Definitive yolk sac

C

Remnants of
primary yolk
sac

Figure 2–5. *A,* On day 12, a second wave of proliferation in the hypoblast produces a new membrane that migrates out over the inside of the extraembryonic mesoderm, pushing the primary yolk sac in front of it. This new layer becomes the endodermal lining of the definitive (secondary) yolk sac. *B, C,* As the definitive yolk sac develops on day 13, the primary yolk sac breaks up and is reduced to a collection of vesicles at the abembryonic end of the chorionic cavity.

THE UTEROPLACENTAL CIRCULATORY SYSTEM BEGINS TO DEVELOP DURING THE SECOND WEEK

During the first week of development, the embryo obtains nutrients and eliminates wastes by simple diffusion. The growth of the embryo rapidly makes a more efficient method of exchange imperative. This need is filled by the **uteroplacental circulation**—the system by which maternal and fetal blood flowing through the **placenta** come into close contact and exchange gases and metabolites by diffusion. This system begins to form on day 9 as vacuoles called **trophoblastic lacunae** open within the syncytiotrophoblast (see Fig. 2–3). Ma-

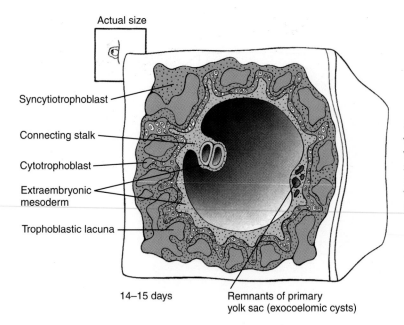

Actual size

Syncytiotrophoblast

Connecting stalk

Cytotrophoblast

Extraembryonic
mesoderm

Trophoblastic lacuna

14–15 days

Remnants of primary
yolk sac (exocoelomic cysts)

Figure 2–6. By the end of the second week, the definitive yolk sac loses contact with the remnants of the primary yolk sac (exocoelomic cysts), and the bilaminar germ disc with its dorsal amnion and ventral yolk sac is suspended in the chorionic cavity by a thick connecting stalk.

ternal capillaries near the syncytiotrophoblast then expand to form **maternal sinusoids** that rapidly anastomose with the trophoblastic lacunae (Figs. 2–4*A* and 2–7*A*). Between days 11 and 13, as these anastomoses continue to develop, the cytotrophoblast proliferates locally to form extensions that grow into the overlying syncytiotrophoblast (see Figs. 2–5*A* and 2–7*A*). The growth of these protrusions is thought to be induced by the underlying newly formed extraembryonic mesoderm. These extensions of cytotrophoblast grow out into the blood-filled lacunae, carrying with them a covering of syncytiotrophoblast. The resulting outgrowths are called **primary stem villi** (see Fig. 2–7*A*).

It is not until day 16 that the extraembryonic mesoderm associated with the cytotrophoblast penetrates the core of the primary stem villi, thus

transforming them into **secondary stem villi** (see Fig. 2–7*B*). By the end of the third week, this villous mesoderm has given rise to blood vessels that connect with the vessels forming in the embryo proper, thus establishing a working uteroplacental circulation. Villi containing differentiated blood vessels are called **tertiary stem villi** (see Fig. 2–7*C*). As can be seen from Figure 2–7*C*, the gases, nutrients, and wastes that diffuse between the maternal and fetal blood must cross four tissue layers: the endothelium of the villus capillaries, the loose connective tissue in the core of the villus, a layer of cytotrophoblast, and a layer of syncytiotrophoblast. The endothelial lining of the maternal blood vessels does not invade the trophoblastic lacunae. Further differentiation of the placenta and stem villi during fetal development is discussed in Chapter 15.

Clinical Applications

HYDATIDIFORM MOLE

A Complete Hydatidiform Mole Is a Pregnancy Without an Embryo

In a normal pregnancy, the embryoblast gives rise to the embryo, and the trophoblast gives rise to

the placenta. In approximately 0.1 to 0.5 percent of pregnancies, however, the fetus is entirely missing, and the conceptus consists only of placental membranes. A conceptus of this type is called a **complete hydatidiform mole** (Fig. 2–8). Because the fetal vasculature that would normally drain off the fluid taken up from the maternal circulation is

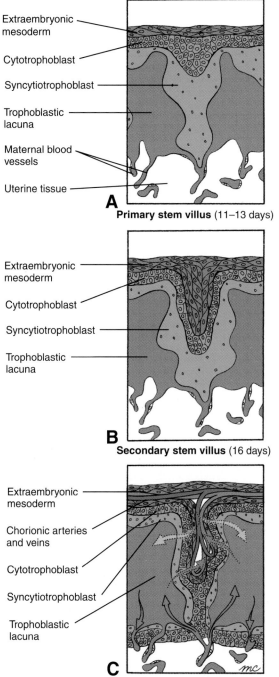

A
Primary stem villus (11–13 days)

Extraembryonic mesoderm

Cytotrophoblast

Syncytiotrophoblast

Trophoblastic lacuna

Maternal blood vessels

Uterine tissue

B
Secondary stem villus (16 days)

Extraembryonic mesoderm

Cytotrophoblast

Syncytiotrophoblast

Trophoblastic lacuna

C
Tertiary stem villus (21 days)

Extraembryonic mesoderm

Chorionic arteries and veins

Cytotrophoblast

Syncytiotrophoblast

Trophoblastic lacuna

Figure 2–7. Formation of the chorionic villi. *A,* The primary stem villi appear on days 11 to 13 as cytotrophoblastic proliferations that bud into the overlying syncytiotrophoblast. *B,* By day 16, the extraembryonic mesoderm begins to proliferate and invade the center of each primary stem villus, transforming each into a secondary stem villus. *C,* By day 21, the mesodermal core differentiates into connective tissue and blood vessels, forming the tertiary stem villi.

Figure 2–8. This complete, hydatidiform mole has been "dissected" to show the clear, swollen villi characteristic of these structures. (Photo courtesy of Dr. Tariq Siddiqi.)

absent, the placental villi of a complete mole are swollen and vesicular, resembling bunches of grapes ("hydatid" is from the Greek *hydatidos*, drop of water). No evidence of an embryo can be found; if an embryoblast forms at all, it must degenerate almost immediately. Complete moles often abort early in pregnancy. If they do not abort, they may be discovered by the physician because they cause characteristic symptoms of hypertension, edema, and vaginal bleeding in the mother.

Like normal trophoblastic tissue, moles secrete the hormone human chorionic gonadotropin (hCG). Moles and mole remnants are readily diagnosed on the basis of an abnormally high level of plasma hCG. Definitive identification of hydatidiform moles requires cytogenetic analysis. Molar pregnancies are somewhat more common in younger than in older women.

Complete Hydatidiform Moles Are Diploid but Contain Only Paternal Chromosomes

Chromosome analysis has shown that even though the cells of a complete mole have a normal, diploid karyotype, all the chromosomes are derived from the father. Further studies demonstrated that this situation usually arises in one of two ways. Two spermatozoa may fertilize an oocyte that lacks its own nucleus **(dispermic fertilization),** and the two male pronuclei may then fuse to form a diploid nucleus. Alternatively, if a single spermatozoon inseminates an oocyte that lacks its own nucleus **(monospermic fertilization),** the resulting male pronucleus may undergo an initial mitosis without cleavage to produce a diploid nucleus (Fig. 2–9). Complete moles produced by *dispermic* fertilization may have either an XX or an XY karyotype. All complete moles produced by *monospermic* fertilization, in contrast, are XX, because YY zygotes lack essential genes located on the X chromosome and cannot develop. Karyotyping surveys show that most complete hydatidiform moles are XX, indicating that monospermic fertilization is the dominant mode of production.

Partial Hydatidiform Moles Are Triploid, With a Double Dose of Paternal Chromosomes, and Show Partial Development of an Embryo

In contrast to the complete hydatidiform mole, some evidence of embryonic development is usually found in **partial hydatidiform moles.** Even if no embryo remnant can be found at the time the mole aborts or is delivered, the presence of typical nucleated embryonic erythroblasts in the molar villi indicates that an embryo was present. On rare occasions, an abnormal fetus is delivered. The swollen villi that are the hallmark of a complete mole are present only in patches, and the clinical symptoms that indicate a molar pregnancy—hypertension, edema, and vaginal bleeding—are usually milder and slower to develop than in the case of complete moles. Spontaneous abortion usually does not occur until the second trimester (4 to 6 months).

Karyotype analysis indicates that conceptuses of this type are usually triploid, with two sets of chromosomes from the father. The sex chromosome karyotype is XXX, XXY or XYY. Studies have shown that these moles result from the insemination of an oocyte containing a female pronucleus by two spermatozoa or possibly by a single abnormal diploid sperm (Fig. 2–10).

Hydatidiform Moles Can Give Rise to Persistent Trophoblastic Disease or to Choriocarcinoma

Residual trophoblastic tissue remaining in the uterus after the spontaneous abortion or surgical removal of a hydatidiform mole may give rise to a condition known as **persistent trophoblastic dis-**

An oocyte is inseminated by a single sperm and the female pronucleus is lost

The single male pronucleus divides to form two haploid nuclei, which combine to form a diploid nucleus

An oocyte is inseminated by two sperm and the female pronucleus is lost

The two male pronuclei combine to form a diploid nucleus

Figure 2–9. Formation of complete hydatidiform mole. A complete mole is produced when an oocyte that has lost its female pronucleus acquires two male pronuclei. Two mechanisms are shown.

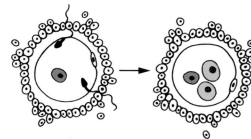

Figure 2–10. A partial hydatidiform mole is produced when a normal oocyte acquires two male pronuclei (or a diploid male pronucleus).

An oocyte is inseminated by two sperm (or by an abnormal diploid sperm)

The female pronucleus and two male pronuclei combine to form a triploid nucleus

ease, in which the mole remnant grows to form a tumor. Tumors arising from partial moles are usually benign. When tumors arising from complete moles become malignant, they may grow either as an **invasive mole** or as metastatic **choriocarcinoma.** All forms of persistent mole, benign and malignant, secrete high levels of hCG.

Only a few years ago, the mortality rate for patients with invasive moles was about 60 percent, and the mortality for choriocarcinoma was approximately 100 percent. Today, effective chemotherapy has resulted in a cure rate for nonmetastatic and low-risk metastatic disease that approaches 100 percent, whereas the cure rate for high-risk metastatic disease is about 80 percent. The dramatic success of these chemotherapeutic cures came about because of the concerted development of sensitive radioimmunoassays for plasma hCG and cytogenetic and molecular techniques that provided a means to identify the parental source of chromosomes within the trophoblastic tissues.

The cytogenetic analysis of hydatidiform moles suggests that the paternal genetic complement is responsible for the early development of the placenta and that the maternal genetic complement is responsible for the early development of the embryo. The following Experimental Principles section discusses experiments that confirm this hypothesis and that have begun to reveal molecular differences between the paternal and maternal chromosomes.

Experimental Principles

GENOMIC IMPRINTING

The Maternal Chromosomes Regulate Embryoblast Development, and the Paternal Chromosomes Regulate Trophoblast Development

As discussed in the preceding Clinical Applications section, the cytogenetic analyses of human hydatidiform moles suggest that the maternal and paternal genome complements play different roles in early development. These roles have been studied with mouse oocytes experimentally manipulated to contain either two male or two female pronuclei. Oocytes of this type can be produced in several ways. Fertilized mouse oocytes can be removed from the ampulla of the oviduct at the pronuclear stage of development and held by light suction at the end of a glass pipette. Either the female pronucleus or the somewhat larger male pronucleus can then be removed with a very fine pipette and replaced with a pronucleus of the opposite type. Another technique involves removing the male or female pronucleus from a fertilized oocyte and then blocking cleavage with an appropriate blocking agent while a single mitosis takes place, thus producing a diploid zygote. Oocytes with two male pronuclei may also be produced by removing the female pronucleus from an unfertilized oocyte and fertilizing the enucleated oocyte with an abnormal diploid sperm.

When an experimental zygote containing two male pronuclei (possessing between them at least one X chromosome) is implanted into a pseudopregnant female mouse, it develops as a trophoblast and gives rise to a mass of placental membranes resembling a human hydatidiform mole. Very rarely, an embryo appears and develops to a stage comparable to approximately the 3-week stage of human development. In contrast, zygotes containing two female pronuclei develop as small but recognizable embryos with reduced placental membranes. These parthenogenic embryos never survive to term. It is important to emphasize that these developmental patterns do not depend on the sex chromosomes present in the zygote (XX or XY), but only on the sex of the parent from whom the genome is inherited.

Early Gene Expression May Depend on Genomic Imprinting

What mechanism underlies the independent expression of maternal and paternal genomes during early development? This question has been approached by studying the expression of a marker viral oncogene, the *myc* oncogene, which was introduced into a line of *transgenic* mice (mice whose genome contains a foreign DNA sequence). In theory, mice carrying this integrated transgene should express its gene product when appropriately stimulated. It was found, however, that the gene product was produced only when the gene had been inherited from the father, not when it had been inherited from the mother. Further investigation revealed a subtle but significant difference between the DNA of the male and female germ line cells: the DNA of the female germ line is more highly **methylated** (carries more methyl groups) than the DNA of the male germ line.

Further investigations were done with several different lines of transgenic mice carrying foreign transgenes at various locations in the genome. In most (although not all) cases, these transgenes showed a characteristic "male" or "female" degree of methylation, and the pattern of methylation displayed in the somatic cells depended on the parent from which the gene had been inherited. Thus, a transgene showed the female pattern of methylation in the somatic cells of both sons and daughters if it was inherited from the mother. However, when one of these sons passed the gene to his offspring, their somatic cells showed the male pattern of methylation. The analogous reversal of methylation patterns also occurs when a grandfather's transgene is transmitted to grandchildren through a daughter.

Methylation of DNA also appears to play a role in the imprinting and expression of endogenous genes, particularly in several genes implicated in regulation of intrauterine growth (e.g., *H19, IGF2, IGF2r, MASH2*). This is an intriguing correlation, because imprinting of autosomal chromosomes does not occur in oviparous (egg laying) vertebrates. Although about 30 to 40 imprinted genes have been described, it has been suggested that as many as 100 to 200 may exist within the human genome and that they will be clustered, possibly reflecting mechanisms regulating the imprinting process in the haploid gamete and the relaxation of imprinting that occurs during earlier stages of gametogenesis.

The sites of DNA methylation are cytosine bases that immediately precede guanosine bases. The mechanisms controlling this modification of the chromatin are not understood and are the focus of considerable research. Moreover, it appears that the methylation of some genes may lead to their silencing, whereas others may be activated by methylation. There is evidence that differential methylation takes place during the early development of the gametes, but the molecular basis of this difference in the preprogramming or **genomic imprinting** of autosomes of the male and female germ lines is not understood.

DNA Methylation Leads to Inactivation of Genes on One X Chromosome in Every Female Cell

To compensate for the presence of only one X chromosome in the cells of males (46,XY), one of the two active X chromosomes in each cell of the female blastocyst (46,XX) is stably inactivated. The inactivation is random with respect to the parental source of the X chromosome in the embryoblast, but only paternally derived X chromosomes are inactivated in the trophoblast. Inactivation of X chromosomes in female embryos requires expression of a specific X chromosome locus, the **XIST** locus, which produces an RNA that remains associated with the chromosome. Moreover, the expression of XIST leads to the methylation of CpG islands at the 5′ ends of the inactivated genes on this chromosome. The inactivated X chromosome also lacks histone H4 acetylation, and, ultimately, the chromosome condenses into a recognizable structure called a **Barr body.** Although this X chromosome remains inactive in all somatic cells of the female, inactivated X chromosomes in the oogonia of the female germ line are reactivated during early fetal life. Thus, the male zygote obtains a single active X chromosome from the mother, and the female zygote obtains two active X chromosomes, one from the mother and one from the father. Both of the X chromosomes in each cell of the early female embryo then remain active until one of them is again inactivated at the blastocyst stage (see earlier).

GENOMIC IMPRINTING AFFECTS THE INHERITANCE OF CONGENITAL DISEASE

One consequence of random X inactivation in female cells is that all females are **genetic mosaics.** Some cells only express the X-linked genes inherited from the mother and some cells only express X-linked genes inherited from the father. Thus, in cases in which the female offspring inherits a recessive X-linked mutation from one parent and a wild-type allele from the other, she does not exhibit symptoms of the disease because of compensation by cells in her body that express the wild-type allele. This individual is called a **silent carrier.** Examples of such X-linked recessive disease include **Duchenne muscular dystrophy** (progressive dystrophy and degeneration of myofibers of proximal skeletal muscles, cardiomyopathy, mild mental retardation) and **Simpson-Golabi-Behmel syndrome** (protruding jaw, broad nasal bridge, short hands and fingers, heart defects, renal de-

fects, hypogonadism). In contrast, offspring who inherit a dominant X-linked mutation from one parent exhibit some symptoms of the disease, because the expression of the wild-type allele in other cells cannot fully compensate. These include diseases such as **Goltz syndrome** (skin atrophy and skeletal malformations) and **incontinentia pigmenti** (spotty pigmentation).

The pattern of inheritance of some human genetic disease may also be dependent on **imprinting differences in male and female autosomes.** For example, deletions in a region of human chromosome 15 (15q11-q13) results in **Prader-Willi syndrome** when inherited from the father and **Angelman syndrome** when inherited from the mother. These two syndromes are characterized by vastly different symptoms. Symptoms of Prader-Willi syndrome include feeding problems in infancy and rapid weight gain in childhood, hypogonadism, and mild mental retardation. Symptoms of Angelman syndrome include developmental delay, speech and balance disorders, and a unique happy demeanor. Many imprinted genes are located in the 15q11-q13 region of chromosome 15, including SNRPN (small nuclear protein N), ZNF 127 (a zinc finger protein), IPW, PAR1, PAR5, PW71, P, GABRB3, GABRA5, GABRG3, EGAP, and IC (the imprinting center that controls the imprinting of imprinted genes in the 15q11-q13 region). Most cases of Prader-Willi syndrome and Angelman syndrome result from large deletions in the 15q11-q13 region of chromosome 15. However, specific mutations of IC in the paternally inherited chromosome may cause Prader-Willi syndrome, whereas mutations of the maternal IC gene may cause Angelman syndrome. A small percentage of Prader-Willi syndrome results from maternal uniparental disomy of chromosome 15, whereas a small percentage of Angelman syndrome results from paternal uniparental disomy of chromosome 15. **Uniparental disomy** is a condition in which both chromosomes of a given pair are inherited from the same parent. Angelman syndrome may also result from specific mutation of EGAP on the maternal chromosome in the 15q11-q13 region.

The development of several congenital **overgrowth syndromes** may also result from abnormal imprinting of human autosomes. For example, translocations, duplications, or mutations of human chromosome 11p15 may lead to overexpression of insulin-like growth factor 2 (IGF2) and renal hyperplasia and nephroblastoma in **Beckwith-Wiedemann syndrome** (see Ch. 10). Disruption of normal imprinting may also lead to development of cancers, including **renal** and **cervical carcinoma.**

SUGGESTED READING

Descriptive Embryology

Cross JC, Werb Z, Fisher SJ. 1994. Implantation and the placenta: key pieces of the developmental puzzle. Science 266:1508

Enders AC, King B. 1988. Formation and differentiation of extraembryonic mesoderm in rhesus monkey. Am J Anat 181:327

Fleming TP. 1987. A quantitative analysis of cell allocation to trophectoderm and inner cell mass of the mouse. Dev Biol 119:520

Gardner RL. 1983. Origin and differentiation of extraembryonic tissues in the mouse. Int Rev Exp Pathol 24:63

Hertig AT. 1935. Angiogenesis in the early human chorion and in the primary placenta of the macaque monkey. Contrib Embryol Carnegie Inst 25:37

Hertig AT, Rock J. 1941. Two human ova of the previllous stage, having a developmental age of about eleven and twelve days respectively. Contrib Embryol Carnegie Inst 29:127

Hertig AT, Rock J. 1945. Two human ova of the previllous stage, having a developmental age of about seven and nine days respectively. Contrib Embryol Carnegie Inst 31:65

Hertig AT, Rock J. 1949. Two human ova of the previllous stage, having a developmental age of about eight and nine days respectively. Contrib Embryol Carnegie Inst 33:169

Hertig AT, Rock J, Adams EC. 1956. A description of 34 human ova within the first seventeen days of development. Am J Anat 98:435

Hertig AT, Rock J, Adams EC, Menkin MC. 1959. Thirty-four fertilized human ova, good, bad, and indifferent, recovered from 210 women of known fertility. Pediatrics 23:202

Lawson KA, Meneses JJ, Pedersen RA. 1986. Cell fate and cell lineage in the presomite mouse embryo, studied with an intracellular tracer. Dev Biol 115:325

Lawson KA, Pedersen R. 1992. Clonal analysis of cell fate during gastrulation and early neurulation in the mouse. CIBA Symp. 165. Postimplantation Development in the Mouse. John Wiley & Sons, New York

Luckett WP. 1971. The origin of the extraembryonic mesoderm in the early human and rhesus monkey embryos. Anat Rec 169:369

Luckett WP. 1973. Amniogenesis in the early human and rhesus monkey embryos. Anat Rec 175:375

Luckett WP. 1975. The development of primordial and definitive amniotic cavities in early rhesus monkey and human embryos. Am J Anat 144:149

Luckett WP. 1978. Origin and differentiation of the yolk sac and extraembryonic mesoderm in presomite human and rhesus monkey embryos. Am J Anat 152:59

Streeter GL. 1942. Developmental horizons in human embryos. Description of age group XI, 13 to 20 somites, and age group XII, 21 to 29 somites. Contrib Embryol Carnegie Inst 30:211

Vogler H. 1987. Human blastogenesis. Formation of the extraembryonic cavities. Bibl Anat 30:1

Clinical Applications

Bracken MB. 1987. Incidence and aetiology of hydatidiform mole: an epidemiological review. Br J Obstet Gynaecol 94:1123

Chatkupt S, Antonowicz M, Johnson WG. 1995. Parents do matter: genomic imprinting and parental sex effects in neurological disorders. J Neurol Sci 130:1

Kajii T, Ohama K. 1977. Androgenetic origin of hydatidiform mole. Nature 264:633

Lawler SD, Fisher RA. 1987. Genetic studies in hydatidiform mole with clinical correlations. Placenta 8:77

Leighton PA, Saam JS, Ingram RD, Tilghman SM. 1996. Genomic imprinting in mice: its function and mechanism. Biol Reprod 54:273

Lewis JL Jr. 1993. Diagnosis and management of gestational trophoblastic disease. Cancer 71:1639

Rose PG. 1995. Hydatidiform mole: diagnosis and management. Semin Oncol 22:149

Szulman AE. 1987. Clinicopathologic features of partial hydatidiform mole. J Reprod Meal 32:640

Experimental Principles

Barlow DP. 1995. Gametic imprinting in mammals. Science 270:1610

Cassidy SB. 1995. Uniparental disomy and genomic imprinting as causes of human genetic disease. Environ Mol Mutagen 25:13

Hadchoucl M, Farza H, Simon D, Tillais P, Pourecl C. 1987. Maternal inhibition of hepatitis B surface antigen gene expression in transgenic mice correlates with de novo methylation. Nature 329:454

Kent-First M. 1997. A lesson from mosaics: don't leave the genetics out of molecular genetics. J NIH Res 9:29

Li E, Beard C, Jaenisch R. 1993. Role for DNA methylation in genomic imprinting. Nature 366:362

Li M, Squire JA, Weksberg R. 1998. Overgrowth syndrome and genomic imprinting: from mouse to man. Clin Genet 53:165

Lyon MF. 1993. Epigenetic inheritance in mammals. TIG 9:123

McGrath J, Solter D. 1984. Completion of mouse embryogenesis requires both the maternal and paternal genomes. Cell 37:179

Morison IM, Reeve AE. 1998. A catalogue of imprinted genes and parent of origin effects in humans and animals. Hum Mol Genet 7:1599

Reik W. 1989. Genomic imprinting and genetic disorders in man. Trends Genet Sci 5:331

Sapienza C. 1990. Parental imprinting of genes. Sci Am 263:52

Strain L, Warner JP, Johnston T, Bonthron DT, 1995. A human parthenogenetic chimera. Nature Genet 11:164

Surani MAH, Barton SC, Norris ML. 1984. Development of reconstituted mouse eggs suggests imprinting of the genome during gametogenesis. Nature 308:548

Swain II, Stewart TA, Leder P. 1987. Parental legacy determines methylation and expression of an autosomal transgene: a molecular mechanism for parental imprinting. Cell 50:719

Tartoff KD, Bremer M. 1990. Mechanisms for the construction and developmental control of heterochromatin formation and imprinted chromosome domains. Development (Suppl):35

3

The Third Week

Summary

The first major event of the third week, **gastrulation,** commences with the appearance of a faint midline structure, the **primitive streak,** in the epiblast near the caudal end of the bilaminar germ disc. The superior end of the primitive streak contains a depression called the **primitive pit** that is surrounded by a small elevation of epiblast called the **primitive node.** Epiblast cells begin to detach along the primitive streak and migrate down into the potential space between the epiblast and hypoblast. Some invade the hypoblast, displacing the original hypoblast cells and replacing them with a layer of **definitive** or **secondary endoderm.** Others migrate laterally or cranially between the endoderm and the epiblast and coalesce to form a third germ layer, the **intraembryonic mesoderm.** After gastrulation is complete, the epiblast is called the **ectoderm.**

As gastrulation converts the bilaminar germ disc into a **trilaminar germ disc,** it brings subpopulations of cells into proximity so they can interact via induction to produce the tissue precursors or embryonic anlagen that give rise to the organ systems of the body. A block of mesoderm that is formed in the cranial midline of the embryo, called the **prechordal plate,** and another midline structure, the **notochordal process,** induce the development of the **neural plate.** Induction of mesoderm by underlying endoderm results in formation of blood vessels and other mesodermal organs, including the urogenital system and the lining of the viscera and the body wall.

The events of the third week set the stage for the period of **organogenesis** from week 4 to week 8, during which the major organ systems differentiate. The two most prominent precursor structures that arise during the third week are the **somites** and the **neural plate.** The somites are a series of blocklike mesodermal condensations that develop in the paraxial mesoderm on either side of the notochord. They form in craniocaudal succession from whorls of paraxial mesoderm called **somitomeres.** The somites later subdivide into **sclerotomes, myotomes,** and **dermatomes,** which give rise to the vertebral column, skeletal musculature, and dermis, respectively. The neural plate appears as a thickening in the ectoderm on either side of the midline, cranial to the primitive node. During the fourth week, this plate will indent along the midline and then fold into a tube, the **neural tube,** which is the precursor of the central nervous system.

Gastrulation, Formation of the Trilaminar Germ Disc, and Initial Development of the Somites and Neural Tube

Week Day

15   The primitive streak and primitive node form along the caudal midline of the bilaminar germ disc

16   During gastrulation, epiblast cells ingress along the primitive streak. The first cells to ingress replace the hypoblast and form the definitive endoderm. Subsequent ingressing cells migrate between epiblast and endoderm to form the mesoderm

17   A tube of mesoderm extends cranially from the primitive node to form the notochordal process, while the mesoderm lateral to the midline becomes the paraxial, intermediate, and lateral plate mesoderm. Cavities appear within the lateral plate mesoderm

3   18   The paraxial mesoderm begins to organize into somitomeres. The cavities in the lateral plate mesoderm coalesce to form the presumptive intraembryonic coelomic cavity. This cavity splits the lateral plate mesoderm into two layers: somatopleuric and splanchnopleuric

19

The buccopharyngeal and cloacal membranes are clearly visible, and the neural plate appears. The expanded cranial part of the neural plate represents the future brain, and the narrow caudal part represents the future spinal cord

20

The notochordal process fuses transiently with the endoderm to form the notochordal plate

4   21

The 8th somitomere differentiates to become the first occipital somite; the subsequent somites (42 to 44 total) begin to form in craniocaudal succession

22   The notochordal plate separates from the endoderm to form the solid notochord

Timeline. The third week of development.

Syncytiotrophoblast

Cytotrophoblast

Extraembryonic mesoderm

Amniotic cavity

Definitive yolk sac

Bilaminar germ disc

Epiblast

Hypoblast

Primitive groove

Amniotic cavity

Buccopharyngeal membrane

Primitive pit

Primitive node

Primitive streak

Primitive groove

Cloacal membrane

Definitive yolk sac

Extraembryonic mesoderm

15 days

Figure 3–1. View of the dorsal surface of the bilaminar germ disc through the sectioned amnion and yolk sac. The inset at the upper left shows the relation of the embryo to the wall of the chorionic cavity. The primitive streak, now 1 day old, occupies 50 percent of the length of the germ disc. The buccopharyngeal and cloacal membranes are present.

THE PRIMITIVE STREAK APPEARS AT THE BEGINNING OF THE THIRD WEEK

On about day 15 of development, a faint groove appears along the longitudinal midline of the germ disc, which has now assumed an oval shape (Fig. 3–1). Over the course of the next day, this groove becomes deeper and elongates to occupy about half the length of the embryo. On day 16, a deeper depression surrounded by a slight mound of epiblast appears at the presumptive cranial end of the groove, near the center of the germ disc. This groove is called the **primitive groove,** the depression is called the **primitive pit,** and the mound surrounding it is called the **primitive node.** The entire structure is the **primitive streak.**

The future head will form at the end of the germ disc near the primitive pit, and the surface of the epiblast in the region adjacent to the midline will form the dorsal surface of the embryo. The appearance of the primitive streak establishes the longitudinal axis and thus the bilateral symmetry of the future adult: the tissues to the right of this structure give rise to the right side of the body, and the tissues to the left of it give rise, in general, to the left side of the body. Although the form of the primary germ layers will change with folding of the embryo in the fourth week (see Ch. 6), the fundamental cranial/caudal, left/right, and ventral/dorsal axes of the body are thus definitively established early in the third week of development.

THE DEFINITIVE ENDODERM AND INTRAEMBRYONIC MESODERM FORM BY GASTRULATION THROUGH THE PRIMITIVE STREAK

On day 16, the epiblast cells near the primitive streak begin to proliferate, flatten, and lose their connections with each other (Fig. 3–2). These flattened cells develop long, footlike processes called **pseudopodia,** which allow them to migrate through the primitive streak into the space between the epiblast and the hypoblast. This process of involution and ingress is called **gastrulation.** Some of the ingressing epiblast cells invade the

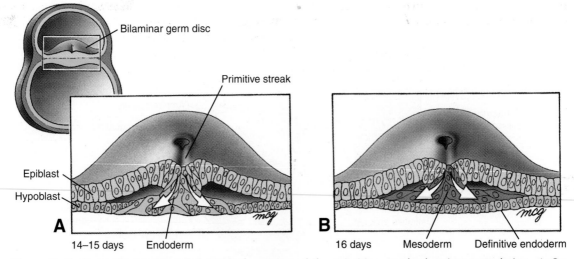

Figure 3–2. Germ discs sectioned through the region of the primitive streak, showing gastrulation. *A,* On days 14 and 15, the ingressing epiblast cells replace the hypoblast to form the definitive endoderm. *B,* The epiblast that ingresses on day 16 migrates between the endoderm and epiblast layers to form the intraembryonic mesoderm.

hypoblast and displace its cells, so that the hypoblast eventually is completely replaced by a new layer of cells, the **definitive endoderm** or **entoderm** (see Fig. 3–2). The definitive endoderm gives rise to the lining of the future gut and gut derivatives.

Starting on day 16, some of the epiblast cells migrating through the primitive streak diverge into the space between the epiblast and the nascent definitive endoderm to form a third germ layer, the **intraembryonic mesoderm** (see Fig. 3–2). Some of these mesoderm cells migrate laterally or cranially, whereas others are deposited on the midline near their site of entry (Figs. 3–2 and 3–3). The cells that migrate through the primitive pit and come to rest on the midline form two structures: first, the **prechordal plate,** a compact mass of mesoderm cranial to the primitive pit, and then a dense midline tube called the **notochordal process** (see Fig. 3–6). On either side of the midline, the mesoderm cells spread out to form a loose network or sheet that remains distinct from the epiblast and the endoderm (see Figs. 3–6 and 3–7).

When the intraembryonic mesoderm and definitive endoderm have formed, the epiblast takes on a new name, the **ectoderm.** The three definitive layers of the **trilaminar germ disc**—the ecto-

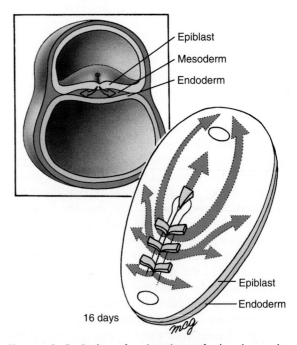

Figure 3–3. Paths of migration of the ingressing mesoderm. The epiblast cells that ingress through the primitive node migrate directly cranially to form the prechordal plate and notochordal process. The cells that ingress through the primitive groove migrate to form the mesoderm lying on either side of the midline.

derm, mesoderm, and definitive endoderm—thus are all derived from the epiblast.

The Primitive Streak Retreats and Disappears, and the Caudal Eminence Gives Rise to Caudal Structures of the Body

On day 16, the primitive streak spans about half the length of the embryo. As gastrulation proceeds, however, it regresses caudally, becoming gradually shorter (Fig. 3–4). By day 22, the primitive streak represents about 10 to 20 percent of the embryo's length; by day 26, it disappears. On about day 20, however, the streak produces a caudal midline mass of mesoderm called the **caudal eminence,** which will give rise to the caudal mesodermal structures of the body, as well as the caudalmost portion of the neural tube (see Ch. 4).

The Mechanics of Gastrulation Are Not Well Understood

The fact that gastrulation can be arrested by drugs that interfere with the function of actin microfila-ments suggests that an actin-mediated contractile system aids the migration of epiblast cells, but other forces may also participate. Moreover, the source of all the cells ingressing at the streak is not clear. The streak may act strictly as a conveyor belt for epiblast cells arising in more lateral regions of the epiblast, but it is possible that cells produced by proliferation within the streak itself also contribute.

The Fate of Gastrulating Epiblast Cells Can Be Predicted From Their Site of Origin

It is thought that somewhat different regions of the primitive streak are responsible for producing the extraembryonic mesoderm, the various sub-populations of the intraembryonic mesoderm, and the definitive endoderm. For example, as men-tioned above, cells migrating through the caudal end of the primitive streak give rise to the caudal eminence. The fate of various populations of mi-grating epiblast cells can be studied in experimen-tal animals by the technique of **cell tracing** or in **cell lineage studies.**

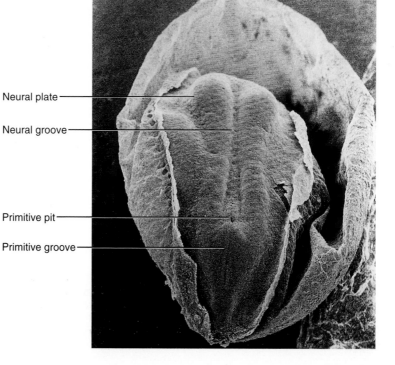

Figure 3–4. Scanning electron micro-graph showing the ectodermal surface of a trilaminar germ disc comparable to a 19-day human embryo (cranial end at the top). The neural plate and neural groove are discussed at the end of this chapter and in Chapter 4. (From Tamarin A. 1983. Stage 9 ma-caque embryos studied by electron microscopy. J Anat 137:765.)

Neural plate

Neural groove

Primitive pit

Primitive groove

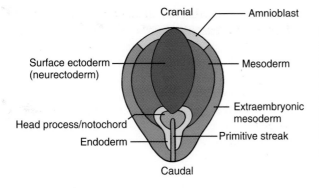

Figure 3–5. Fate map of the epiblast of a mouse embryo, showing the zones of epiblast that ingress through the primitive streak and form the major structures of the trilaminar germ disc. This map was deduced on the basis of cell lineage studies, in which epiblast cells were injected with tracer molecules and their labeled descendants later located. (Modified from Lawson KA, Peterson R. 1992. Clonal analysis of cell fate during gastrulation and early neurulation in the mouse. Symp. 165. John Wiley and Sons, New York.)

Cell tracing and cell lineage studies (discussed in detail in the Experimental Principles section of Chapter 5) make it possible to construct a **fate map** showing the developmental destinies of specific regions of the epiblast (Fig. 3–5). It appears that the most caudal region of the streak produces the extraembryonic mesoderm; the mid-region of the streak produces the mesoderm that migrates to the lateral parts of the germ disc; and the cranial regions of the streak produce the meso-derm that comes to rest on and adjacent to the midsagittal axis, as well as the definitive endoderm. Cell lineage studies indicate that most epiblast cells, including those that migrate in through the primitive streak, are **pluripotent**—that is, innately capable of developing into almost any cell type of the organism—and that their developmental fate is determined by the location to which they migrate in the embryo.

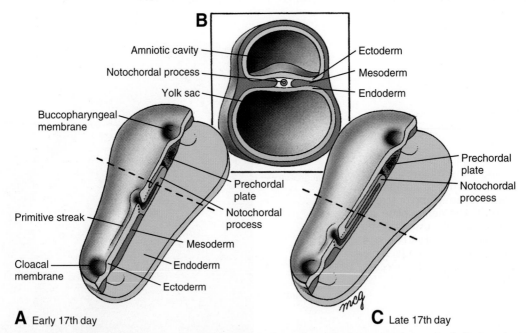

Figure 3–6. Formation of the notochordal process and prechordal plate mesoderm. *A, C,* Stages showing the hollow notochordal process growing cranially from the walls of the primitive pit. Note the changes in the relative length of the notochordal process and primitive streak as the embryo grows. Also note the fusion of ectoderm and endoderm in the buccopharyngeal and cloacal membranes. *B,* Cross-section of the germ disc at the level indicated by the dotted line.

The Notochord Is Produced by Cells That Ingress Through the Primitive Node

Just caudal to the newly formed prechordal plate, the primitive node sprouts a hollow mesodermal tube, the **notochordal process.** This tube grows in length as cells proliferating in the region of the primitive node add on to its proximal end and as the primitive streak regresses (Fig. 3–6). When the notochordal process is completely formed on about day 20, several dramatic structural transformations take place that convert it from a hollow tube to a solid rod (Fig. 3–7). First, the ventral floor of the tube fuses with the underlying endoderm. The tube then unzippers ventrally, starting in the region of the primitive pit. The yolk sac cavity thus transiently communicates with the amniotic cavity through an opening at the primitive pit called the **neurenteric canal** (see Fig. 3–7B). The unzippering of the tube floor converts the **notochordal**

process to a flattened, midventral bar of mesoderm called the **notochordal plate** (see Fig. 3–7A, B). It is not until days 22 to 24 that the notochordal plate completely detaches from the endoderm and retreats into the mesoderm-containing space between ectoderm and endoderm, changing as it does so into a solid cylinder called the **notochord** (see Fig. 3–7C). During this process, some cells of endodermal origin may become incorporated into the notochord.

The Ultimate Fate of the Notochord Is Debated

The rudiments of the vertebral bodies initially coalesce around the notochord, and it is commonly stated that the notochord gives rise to the nucleus pulposus at the center of the vertebral discs. Certainly, this is true in the embryo, the fetus, and young children. There is evidence, however, that

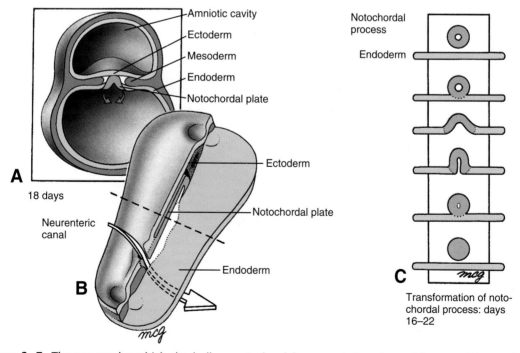

Figure 3–7. The process by which the hollow notochordal process is transformed into a solid notochord between days 16 and 22. A, B, First, the ventral wall of the notochordal process has begun to fuse with the endoderm to form the notochordal plate. As shown in B, this process commences at the caudal end of the notochordal process and proceeds cranially (the dotted line marks the level of A). An open neurenteric canal is briefly created between the amniotic cavity and the yolk sac cavity. C, The stages by which the notochordal process becomes the notochordal plate and then the notochord.

in early childhood the nucleus pulposus cells of notochordal origin degenerate and are replaced by adjacent mesodermal cells. The notochord does not contribute to the bony elements of the spinal column: Notochordal cells trapped in the centers of the developing vertebral bodies die and disappear. The notochord plays an important role in the induction of the vertebral bodies, however, and failure of this inductive interaction results in various vertebral column abnormalities including spina bifida and scoliosis (see the Clinical Applications section of Ch. 4).

Mesoderm Is Excluded From the Buccopharyngeal and Cloacal Membranes

During the third week of development, two faint depressions appear in the ectoderm, one at the cranial end of the embryo adjacent to the prechordal plate and the other at the caudal end behind the primitive streak. Late in the third week, the ectoderm in these areas fuses tightly with the underlying endoderm, excluding the mesoderm and forming a bilaminar membrane. The cranial membrane is called the **buccopharyngeal membrane,** and the caudal membrane is the **cloacal membrane.** The buccopharyngeal and cloacal membranes later become the blind ends of the gut tube. The buccopharyngeal membrane breaks down in the fourth week to form the opening to the oral cavity, whereas the cloacal membrane disintegrates later, in the seventh week, to form the openings of the anus and the urinary and genital tracts (see Chs. 9 and 10).

PARAXIAL, INTERMEDIATE, AND LATERAL PLATE MESODERM ARE FORMED BY CELLS MIGRATING LATERALLY FROM THE PRIMITIVE STREAK

As the primitive streak regresses during the third week, the mesoderm cells that migrated laterally

Figure 3–8. Sections through a 17-day embryo showing the differentiation of the mesoderm on either side of the midline. *A,* Early on day 17, the mesoderm has begun to differentiate into paraxial, intermediate, and lateral plate mesoderm. *B,* Sagittal cutaway showing the rodlike condensations of paraxial and intermediate mesoderm. The dotted line marks the plane of the two transverse sections. *C,* Later on day 17, the lateral plate begins to vacuolate to form the rudiment of the intraembryonic coelom.

from it begin to condense into rod- and sheetlike structures on either side of the notochord (Fig. 3–8). This process commences at the cranial end of the embryo and proceeds posteriorly, continuing throughout the third and fourth weeks. The mesoderm lying immediately on either side of the notochord forms a pair of cylindric condensations called the **paraxial mesoderm.** A less pronounced pair of cylindric condensations, the **intermediate mesoderm,** forms just lateral to the paraxial mesoderm. The remainder of the lateral mesoderm forms a flattened sheet and is called the **lateral plate mesoderm.**

These three divisions of mesoderm give rise to specific structures in the adult. The **paraxial mesoderm** differentiates into the axial skeleton, voluntary musculature, and part of the dermis of the skin, as described below. The **intermediate mesoderm** produces the urinary system and parts of the genital system (see Ch. 10). Starting on day 17, the **lateral plate mesoderm** splits into two layers: a ventral layer associated with the endoderm and a dorsal layer associated with the ectoderm (see Fig. 3–8C). The layer adjacent to the endoderm gives rise to the mesothelial covering of the visceral organs (viscera) and hence is called the **splanchnopleuric mesoderm** (from the Greek *splanchnon*, viscera). The layer adjacent to the ectoderm gives rise to the inner lining of the body

wall, to parts of the limbs, and to most of the dermis and hence is called the **somatopleuric mesoderm** (from the Greek *soma*, body). The further development of the lateral plate mesoderm is covered in Chapters 6 and 14.

The Paraxial Mesoderm Develops Into Somitomeres and Then Into Somites

As soon as it forms, the cells of the paraxial mesoderm begin to form a series of rounded, whorl-like structures called **somitomeres.** The early development of these structures in humans has been inferred largely from studies on other animals. Scanning electron microscopic analyses on embryos of animals ranging from fish to mice show that somitomeres first appear as a faint segmentation in the most cranial paraxial mesoderm, just on either side of the notochordal plate, at a stage corresponding to the 18th or 19th day of human development. Close inspection reveals that the somitomeres consist of disclike whorls of paraxial mesoderm cells (Fig. 3–9). Formation of somitomeres continues throughout the third and fourth weeks, starting with several pairs in the presumptive cranial region and proceeding craniocaudally through the cervi-

Figure 3–9. *A,* Scanning electron micrograph. *B,* Matching sketch of a somitomere. The concentric architecture of these structures is easiest to discern in stereophotographs. (Photo courtesy of Dr. Antone Jacobson.)

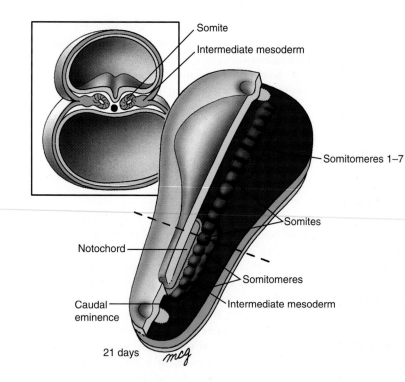

Somite

Intermediate mesoderm

Somitomeres 1–7

Somites

Notochord

Somitomeres

Caudal eminence

Intermediate mesoderm

21 days

Figure 3–10. Sections through a 21-day embryo. The cranial and caudal portions of the paraxial mesoderm have become organized into somitomeres, and the four occipital and first two cervical somitomeres have differentiated into somites. The seven most cranial somitomeres never become somites. The dotted line indicates the level of the transverse section. At this level, the lateral plate mesoderm contains the rudiment of the intraembryonic coelom.

cal, thoracic, lumbar, sacral, and coccygeal regions (Fig. 3–10).

Most of the somitomeres develop further to form discrete blocks of segmental mesoderm called **somites** (Figs 3–11 and 3–12). In all species studied, however, the first seven pairs of somitomeres do not go on to form somites. These seven pairs of somitomeres eventually give rise to the striated muscles of the face, jaw, and throat. As described in Chapter 12, these muscles differentiate within the segmental pharyngeal arches, which

develop on either side of the pharynx. The pharyngeal arches are central elements in the development of the neck and face (see Ch. 12).

The First Somites Appear on Day 20 in the Region of the Future Base of the Skull

Assuming that the human embryo develops in the same way as a wide evolutionary spectrum of ani-

Figure 3–11. Scanning electron micrograph of an embryo with the ectoderm removed to show somites and, more caudally, the paraxial mesoderm that has not yet segmented. Arrows indicate the region of somitomere formation. (From Bellairs R. 1986. The primitive streak. Anat Embryol 174:1.)

Figure 3–12. Scanning electron micrograph of a transversely sectioned embryo showing a somite and the intermediate mesoderm. Note also the notochord and the developing neural tube. (Photo courtesy of Dr. Kathryn Tosney.)

mals, the eighth, ninth, and tenth pairs of somitomeres differentiate into the first, second, and third pairs of somites on day 20 (see Fig. 3–10). The rest of the somites form in craniocaudal progression at a rate of about three or four a day, finishing on about day 30. In the human, approximately 42 to 44 pairs of somites form, flanking the notochord from the occipital (skull base) region to the embryonic tail. The caudalmost several somites eventually disappear, however, giving a final count of approximately 37 pairs.

The Somites Establish the Segmental Organization of the Body

The somites give rise to most of the axial skeleton, including the vertebral column and part of the oc-

cipital bone of the skull; to the voluntary musculature of the neck, body wall, and limbs; and to part of the dermis of the neck and trunk. It should be apparent, therefore, that the organization and migrations of the somites are of major importance in the development of the overall body plan.

The first four pairs of somites form in the occipital region. These somites contribute to the development of the occipital part of the skull; to the bones that form around the nose, eyes, and inner ears; to the extrinsic ocular muscles; and to muscles of the tongue (see Ch. 12). The next eight pairs of somites form in the presumptive **cervical** region. The most cranial cervical somite also contributes to the occipital bone, and others form the cervical vertebrae and associated muscles, as well as part of the neck dermis (see Ch. 4). The next 12 pairs, the **thoracic somites,** form thoracic vertebrae; the musculature and bones of the thoracic

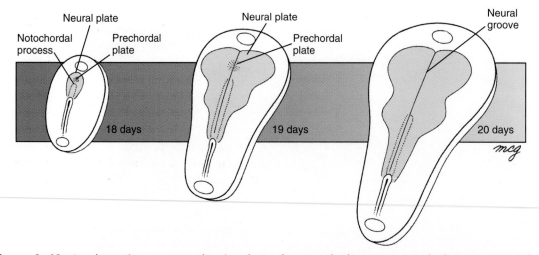

Neural plate · Notochordal process · Prechordal plate · 18 days

Neural plate · Prechordal plate · 19 days

Neural groove · 20 days

Figure 3–13. A schematic sequence showing how the neural plate grows and changes proportions between day 18 and day 20. The primitive streak shortens only slightly, but it occupies a progressively smaller proportion of the length of the embryonic disc as the neural plate and embryo grow.

wall; part of the thoracic dermis; and part of the abdominal wall. Cells from cervical and thoracic somites also invade the upper limb buds to form the limb musculature (see Ch. 11).

Caudal to the thoracic somites, the five **lumbar somites** form the abdominal dermis, abdominal muscles, and lumbar vertebrae, and the five **sacral somites** form the sacrum with its associated dermis and musculature. Cells from lumbar somites invade the lower limb buds to form the leg musculature. Finally, the three **coccygeal somites** that remain after degeneration of the caudalmost somites form the coccyx.

THE AXIAL MESODERM INDUCES THE OVERLYING ECTODERM TO FORM THE NEURAL PLATE

The first event in the formation of the future central nervous system is the appearance on day 18 of a thickened **neural plate** in the epiblast along the midsagittal axis cranial to the primitive pit (Figs. 3–13 and 3–14). It is likely that the neural plate develops in response to **inducing substances** secreted by the underlying axial mesodermal structures; that is, by the prechordal plate and the cranial portion of the notochordal plate. These substances diffuse to the overlying epiblast cells, in which they activate specific genes that cause the cells to differentiate into a thick plate of columnar, pseudostratified **neuroepithelial cells (neurectoderm).** The neural plate appears first at the cranial

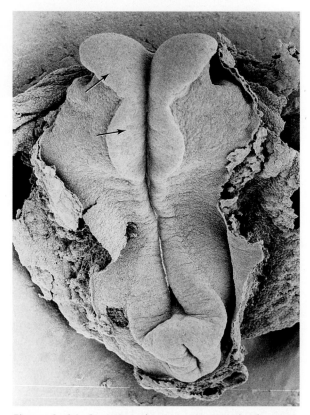

Figure 3–14. Scanning electron micrograph of an embryo comparable with a 20-day human embryo. The neural plate is clearly visible, and the expansions that will become the major subdivisions of the brain are apparent (arrows). Only a small region of the primitive streak remains. The primitive streak will disappear on day 25. (From Tamarin A. 1983. Stage 9 macaque embryos studied by electron microscopy. J Anat 137: 765.)

end of the embryo and differentiates craniocaudally. As described in Chapter 4, the neural plate folds during the fourth week to form a neural tube that is the precursor of the central nervous system. The lateral lips of the neural plate also give rise to an extremely important population of cells, the **neural crest,** which detaches during formation of the neural tube and migrates into the embryo to form a variety of structures.

The Neural Plate Forms the Brain and Spinal Cord

The neural plate is broad cranially and tapered caudally. The expanded cranial portion gives rise to the brain. Even at this very early stage of differentiation, the presumptive brain is visibly divided into three regions: the future forebrain, midbrain, and hindbrain (see Fig. 3–14). The narrow caudal portion of the neural plate, which overlies the notochord and is flanked by the developing somites, gives rise to the spinal cord (Figs. 3–12 through 3–14).

The role of gastrulation in the induction of the central nervous system was first demonstrated by Mangold and Spemann in amphibian embryos. Their experiments and others that led to our present understanding of inductive interactions are described in the Experimental Principles section of this chapter and of Chapter 4.

Clinical Applications

ABNORMAL GASTRULATION

A Spectrum of Human Caudal Malformations Poses a Developmental Puzzle

In 1961, Duhamel described a syndrome he called **caudal regression,** characterized by varying degrees of (1) flexion, inversion, and lateral rotation of the lower extremities; (2) anomalies of lumbar and sacral vertebrae; (3) imperforate anus; (4) agenesis of the kidneys and urinary tract; and (5) agenesis of the internal genital organs except for the gonads. In some extreme cases, the deficiency in caudal development led to fusion of the lower limb buds during early development, resulting in a "mermaid-like" habitus called **sirenomelia** (Fig. 3–15). Several similar syndromes were later reported. This entire constellation of syndromes, ranging in severity from relatively minor lesions of the coccygeal vertebrae to sirenomelia, has been referred to as **caudal agenesis, sacral agenesis,** and **caudal dysplasia.** Individuals with skeletal and visceral malformations of this type also tend to exhibit varying degrees of neurologic deficit, particularly in the caudal regions. Because the etiology of this constellation of defects has not been established, the mechanistically neutral terms "caudal dysplasia" and "caudal dysgenesis" are the most prudent designations.

In some individuals, caudal malformations are associated with more cranial abnormalities. One of these associations is called the VATER association because it includes some or all of the following anomalies: *v*ertebral defects, *a*nal atresia, *t*racheal-*e*sophageal fistula, and *r*enal defects and *r*adial forearm anomalies. An extension of this association, the VACTERL association, also includes *c*ardiovascular anomalies and *l*imb defects. A number of other syndromes may be related to these associations.

Are These Diverse Anomalies Developmentally Related?

The diversity of the anomalies in these associations does not, at first sight, support the idea that they might arise by a single mechanism. It has been argued, however, that these malformations are found in association much more often than would be expected if they were unrelated and occurred together merely by chance. It also seems unlikely that the relatively large number of individuals afflicted with these similar spectra of multiple malformations can be accounted for by the independent actions of chemical teratogens, because two or three different teratogens would have to act on

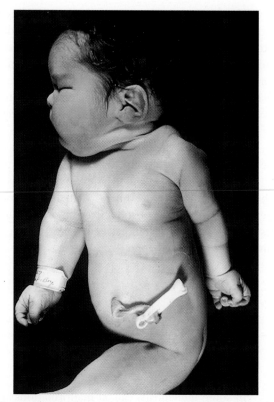

Figure 3–15. Sirenomelia. Severe reduction of the caudal structures has resulted in fusion of the lower extremity limb buds. (Photo courtesy of Children's Hospital Medical Center, Cincinnati, OH.)

different organ anlagen during their specific periods of sensitivity. Closer scrutiny, taking into account both the timing of genesis of the anomalous structures and the mechanisms by which they form, suggests that many of these malformations are related to defects in the growth and migration of mesoderm during the third week.

Defective Gastrulation May Cause Caudal Dysplasia and Associated Mesodermal Anomalies

Mesodermal structures formed during the third and fourth weeks participate in the development of most of the structures involved in caudal dysplasia and associated malformations. For example, the sa-

cral and coccygeal vertebrae form from structures called **sclerotomes** that develop from the sacral and caudal somites (see Ch. 4). The intermediate mesoderm differentiates into kidneys in response to induction by the ingrowing mesodermal ureteric buds. Imperforate anus may result from the incomplete migration of mesodermal septa, whereas tracheoesophageal fistulas may be caused by defective interaction between the endodermal foregut anlage and mesoderm (see the Clinical Applications section of Ch. 6). Radial forearm malformations apparently result from anomalous migration and differentiation of lateral plate mesoderm. It thus makes sense that a derangement of gastrulation that disturbs the migration and differentiation of mesoderm could cause an array of defects like those under discussion.

Both Environmental and Genetic Causes Have Been Implicated in the Etiology of Caudal Dysplasia

A spectrum of caudal mesodermal defects similar to those described in humans can be induced in chick embryos by injecting insulin into the egg during gastrulation. Another clue that abnormal gastrulation is involved in the genesis of these defects is the fact that direct irradiation of the primitive streak in chick embryos produces sirenomelia. On the other hand, a genetic basis for caudal dysplasia in humans is implied by the results of genetic and molecular characterization of a series of short-tail brachyuric and tailless anuric mouse mutants that were discovered in the 1920s and 1930s. In addition to malformations of the tail, these mice display a range of mesodermal defects and disruptions of gastrulation that are very similar to the abnormalities observed in human caudal dysplasia.

Brachyury and Anury in Mice Are Caused by Mutations in Genetic Loci Involved in Gastrulation and Notochord Development

The defects in brachyuric and anuric mice have been mapped to two areas, called *T* and *t*, on chromosome 17. The *T* locus is a well-defined genetic unit near the centromere. The *t* alleles, in contrast, seem to represent mutations in several loci within a small region of chromosome 17. These *t* loci appear always to be transmitted together.

Genetic analysis shows that the *T* and *t* loci influence very early embryonic development as well as the induction of the vertebrae and neural tube. Some embryos homozygous for the dominant *T* mutant allele (*T/T*) fail to form viable blastocysts or to implant; those that do implant show disruptions in mesoderm migration and notochord formation and die in early development. Histologic studies indicate that the *T* mutation interferes with gastrulation by preventing the normal ingression of epiblast cells through the primitive streak. In contrast to the *T* allele, the *t* alleles are recessive. All the *t/t* homozygotes so far described display aberrations similar to those of *T/T* mutants and die early in development. *T/+* heterozygotes (+ indicating the normal or wild-type allele) and animals with a *t/+* genotype are viable but display defects of notochord development that typically involve ei-ther failure of the notochord to separate from the endoderm or secondary fusion of the notochord with the neural tube. It has been suggested that the disturbances in gastrulation and in the behavior of notochord mesodermal cells displayed by mice with *T* and *t* mutations are caused by excessively strong cell-cell adhesion in epiblast and mesoderm during early development.

It is not known just what role the *T* gene protein plays in the formation of mesoderm, but the expression of this gene in the primitive streak and gastrulating mesoderm makes it clear how a mutation in the gene could cause the widespread axial mesoderm abnormalities observed in mice with a mutant *T* allele. The similarity between the defects in *T* and *t* mutant mice and the defects in humans with caudal dysplasia suggests, at the very least, that continued study of this model will provide useful information related to the mechanisms of mesoderm production in humans. Additional insights will undoubtedly result from studies of the newly discovered members of the growing family of T-box transcription factors (see Experimental Principles section of this chapter).

Experimental Principles

REGULATION OF DEVELOPMENT BY CASCADES OF GENE EXPRESSION

Development of the Human Embryo Is Regulated by Gene Cascades Modified From Those Used by Lower Organisms

Human embryos, like those of lower organisms, develop their intricate definitive characters through the gradual alteration of simpler precursors. This developmental process is called **epigenesis.**

It is now becoming clear that **epigenetic development** of the human body is regulated by **cascades** of **gene expression;** that is, early-acting regulatory genes initiate the developmental process and directly or indirectly induce expression of other "downstream" genes. The activities of these genes then induce the expression of yet additional genes and so on until the genes that encode the actual structural and functional characteristics of specific cells and tissues of the embryo are activated. Although these cascades have been described in some detail in organisms such as the fruitfly ***Drosophila,*** we know far less about their details in vertebrate embryos. There is dramatic evidence, however, that many aspects of the genetic hierarchy of development have been remarkably well conserved during evolution.

In *Drosophila*, the epigenetic cascade is initiated by genes expressed before fertilization, or **maternal effect genes.** These genes encode signals, establishing the axes of the embryo, including the anteroposterior axis (cranial/caudal axis in humans), the dorsoventral axis, and the left/right axis. In fruitflies, maternal effect genes encode **growth factors** or **transcription factors** that impart differences to subregions of the oocyte, zygote, and early embryo along the respective axes. Although such localized **cytoplasmic determinants** are important in development of *Drosophila* and some vertebrates, such as the frog *Xenopus*, there is evidence indicating that the mammalian oocyte cytoplasm is relatively homogeneous in composition.

During early embryonic development, the expression of maternal effect genes is superseded by a class of genes called **zygotic genes.** In *Drosophila*, one class of zygotic genes is called **segmentation genes** because their expression results in subdivision of fly embryos into several virtually identical segments. Many of these genes encode **transcription factors,** which can switch other genes on or off by binding to regulatory regions of their DNA. Likewise, several genes containing nucleotide sequences related to the segmentation genes of *Drosophila* have been identified in mammals, and the conversion from "maternal effect" to "zygotic" gene expression also occurs during early cleavage stages in these higher organisms. As is the case in *Drosophila*, some of these mammalian genes may also play a role in segmentation. For example, segmentation of the mammalian hindbrain (see Chs. 5, 12, and 13), the pharyngeal arches of the head and neck region (see Ch. 12), and the somites of the trunk (see Ch. 4) is genetically regulated.

Next, the fruitfly segmentation genes and the

Figure 3–16. Alignment of the four vertebrate *Hox* complexes with the *Drosophila* homeotic complex. (Adapted from Krumlauf R. 1993. *Hox* genes and pattern formation in the branchial region of the vertebrate head. Trends Genet 9:106.)

developmental changes they bring about induce expression of the **homeotic** genes. These genes contain a highly conserved 183 base pair region of DNA called the **homeobox,** which encodes the 61 amino acid **homeodomain,** which in turn recognizes and binds to specific DNA sequences of other genes. These encoded proteins thus function as transcription factors that regulate the activity of many "downstream" genes and as a consequence are often referred to as **master control genes.** A special subset of *Drosophila* homeobox genes are organized in two clusters on chromosome 3 and are collectively called the **homeotic complex, or HOM-C** (Fig. 3–16). Apparently, a common ancestor of this complex was duplicated once, and then each resulting complex was duplicated again during the evolution of mammals. The four complexes of homeobox genes in mammals are called *Hox* genes.

In *Drosophila,* mutations of homeotic genes often result in remarkable transformations of body parts. A mutation resulting in misexpression of the *Antennapedia* gene during development, for example, can cause cells that would normally form antennae to instead develop into legs, which now protrude from the head. Similarly, a mutation in the *Ultrabithorax* gene can result in homeotic transformation of the third thoracic segment into an additional second thoracic segment, giving a fruitfly with four wings instead of the normal two.

The *Drosophila* HOM-C and mammalian *Hox* genes have been extremely well conserved during evolution at the levels of clustered organization, sequence, expression, and function. Although the mammalian *Hox* genes have been individually altered through evolution, they retain significant sequence homology to the insect HOM-C genes. The order of the *Hox* genes in the mammalian clusters parallels that observed in the *Drosophila* HOM-C. The amino acid sequences of the encoded homeodomains of the *Drosophila* genes and their mammalian **orthologues,** or corresponding genes, are often greater than 90 percent identical. In addition, in both mammals and fruitflies, these genes exhibit the property of co-linearity, with the position of a gene within the cluster reflecting its expression domain in the developing embryo. As shown in Figure 3–16, genes located in more 5′ positions within clusters are expressed in more caudal regions of the embryo.

Transgenic fruitflies, carrying experimentally added genes, have been used to demonstrate an unexpected level of functional conservation between the *Drosophila* HOM-C and mammalian *Hox* genes. For example, misexpression of the mammalian orthologue of the *Antennapedia* gene in the developing fruitfly also causes homeotic transformation of antennae into legs. This suggests that both the *Drosophila* and mammalian genes are capable of recognizing the same downstream gene targets and initiating the same genetic cascade. It is interesting to note that misexpression of either the *Drosophila Antennapedia* gene or the corresponding mammalian gene results in the formation of ectopic *Drosophila* legs and not mammalian legs. This is because within the genetic context of the fruitfly, the downstream target genes are only capable of programming the development of a fly leg.

GASTRULATION IN MAMMALS IS A REGULATED MULTISTEP PROCESS CARRIED OUT BY ACTIVITIES OF THE PRIMITIVE STREAK

The Mammalian Primitive Streak Forms Early in Development

The three main axes of the human embryo are well established by the end of the second week of development. The cranial end is distinguished by a buccopharyngeal membrane and the caudal end by a distinct cloacal membrane. The epiblast covers the dorsal surface, and the hypoblast covers the ventral surface of the embryo. In addition, a structure called the **primitive streak,** with its **primitive node** and **primitive groove,** divides the left from the right side of the mammalian embryo (see Fig. 3–1). Other vertebrate embryos form structures that are homologous to the mammalian primitive streak, such as the **ectopic shield** of fish, the **dorsal blastopore lip** of amphibians, and **Henson's node** of birds.

The Primitive Node Is an Embryonic Organizer

The function of the **primitive node** and homologous structures in other animals is truly remarkable. As discussed in the descriptive section of this chapter, the primitive node and other regions of the primitive streak, through a process called **gastrulation,** constitute the mechanism that generates all three definitive germ cell layers from the epiblast: the definitive endoderm, the mesoderm, and the definitive ectoderm. But an even more amazing fact is that the primitive node has the capacity to induce an entire secondary embryonic axis if grafted onto an ectopic site of another embryo (Fig. 3–17A). This phenomenon was first discovered by Hilda Mangold and Hans Spemann, who were working on frog embryos in 1924. Because the grafted blastopore lip could induce development of an entire frog embryo, it was called the **embryonic organizer** and now is often called the **Spemann organizer.**

Genetic/Molecular Analysis Reveals Critical Steps in the Process of Gastrulation

The initial discovery of the embryonic organizer stimulated a search for the organizing substance(s) within the blastopore and primitive streak. In the last few years especially, the genetic/molecular analysis of the organizer in a variety of organisms has begun to reveal the identity and functions of controlling elements of the regulatory cascade that direct different steps in the process of gastrulation as shown in Figure 3–18. These studies have revealed new and unsuspected functions of the organizer, such as the initiation of development of handed asymmetry of the embryo (see Ch. 9). They have also more clearly elucidated other functions, such as the induction of the head, the trunk, and the tail by different subregions of the organizer, and the synergistic interactions of dorsalizing and ventralizing factors that lead to **establishment of the basic body plan.** Finally, these studies have shown how disruption of some of these regulatory genes may lead to the pathogenesis of specific human congenital diseases.

The Primitive Streak Is Initially Induced in the Epiblast by the Activities of Maternal Effect Genes

Studies of amphibian gastrulation show that one of the primary requirements for the initiation of gastrulation is the expression and release of factors from a specific region of the oocyte called the **Nieukoop center.** This region of the cytoplasm contains messenger RNAs previously transcribed by maternal effect genes. In mammals, it is likely that equivalent factors such as **β-catenin**

Figure 3–17. *A,* A donor blastopore grafted onto a host frog embryo induces formation of a complete secondary body axis resulting in formation of "conjoined" twins. *B,* A frog embryo was irradiated with ultraviolet light to abolish "organizer" activity, and then two blastomeres were injected with goosecoid mRNA resulting in induction of two embryonic axes. (*A,* Photo courtesy of Dr. Douglas Melton. *B,* From Steinbeisser H, De Robertis EM, Ku M, et al. 1993. *Xenopus* axis formation: induction of goosecoid by injected X-wnt-8 and activin mRNAs. Development 118:499.)

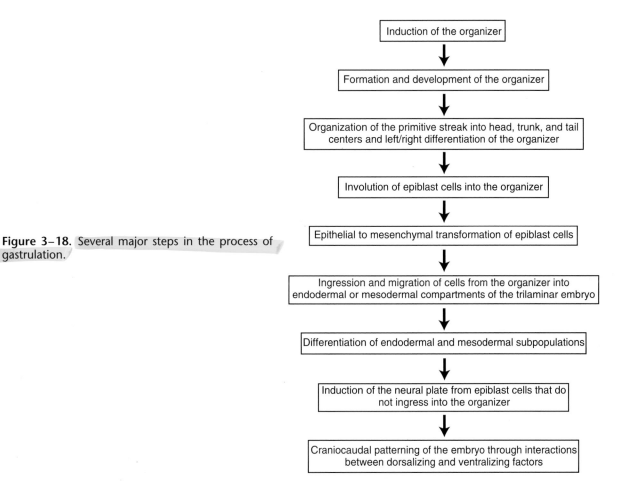

Figure 3–18. Several major steps in the process of gastrulation.

and members of the **transforming growth factor-β** (TGF-β) family, such as **bone morphogenetic protein-4 (BMP-4)** and **activin,** are first expressed in the hypoblast in a cranial region of the embryo where they induce the epiblast to form the primitive streak (see Fig. 3–18). Other factors thought to play a role in initial induction of the organizer in mammals include secreted signaling molecules of the **Wnt family,** such as **Wnt-3,** the paired-type homeobox transcription factor **MIX,** and members of the **fibroblast growth factor family** (FGF). From work in amphibians, it is thought that TGF-β and Wnt signals work together, as TGF-β signals impart competence to the epiblast to form the ectoderm, the endoderm, and the mesoderm, whereas Wnt signals provide instructions to the epiblast for organizer formation.

Development of the Primitive Streak Requires the Expression of Zygotic Genes

One of the first zygotic genes expressed by the epiblast is a homeobox gene **goosecoid.** Goosecoid genes have been characterized in frogs, chicks, mice, and humans. In all cases, they contain sequences homologous to regions within the fruitfly genes gooseberry and bicoid. **In situ hybridization studies** have shown that goosecoid mRNA is first expressed in epiblast cells of the mouse just before the appearance of the primitive streak. After formation of the primitive streak, however, it is specifically localized to the primitive node, suggesting an active role in the process of gastrulation. Findings from other experimental studies support this hypothesis. For example, when **antisense**

mRNA was injected into blastomeres of frog embryos that normally express goosecoid, the development of the organizer and the body axis were disrupted. More direct evidence for a role of goosecoid gene products in gastrulation was obtained by injection of goosecoid mRNA into two blastomeres of a frog embryo previously treated with ultraviolet light to abolish innate organizer activity. In these experiments, each of the blastomeres gave rise to a complete embryonic axis, supporting the view that goosecoid plays a significant role in the initiation of organizer activity (see Fig. 3–17B). On the other hand, results of experiments with transgenic mice with mutations of goosecoid are somewhat puzzling with respect to goosecoid's role in gastrulation. In these studies, goosecoid was targeted by **homologous recombination,** producing a **null allele** or **transgenic knockout** for this locus (see Experimental Principles section of Ch. 1). Unexpectedly, however, the knockout mice did not exhibit any apparent disruptions of gastrulation. For example, in one study, the goosecoid-null mice gastrulated normally but exhibited craniofacial abnormalities and anomalies of the sternum and ribs. In other studies, the goosecoid knockouts exhibited midline anomalies of the base of the skull and malformations of shoulder and hip articulations. In other studies, the mice were completely normal. These results may be explained by the fact that other genes of a **goosecoid family** of genes may be able to partially compensate for the knockout of a single member of the family. Indeed, at least three goosecoid genes have now been identified in mice. Such compensation for the knockout of one gene by related genes is not an unusual result. Thus, although definitive and expected phenotypic effects of gene knockouts provide strong inferences for the function of a particular gene, negative results must be treated with caution.

Another pathway that appears to play a role in development of the primitive streak is the **activin signaling pathway.** Knockout studies in mice have shown that both activin type 1 and activin type 2 receptors are required for appropriate development and elongation of the primitive streak.

The Primitive Streak Is Organized Into Three Regions: Head, Trunk, and Tail Organizing Centers

Once the primitive streak has formed, it will give rise to the endoderm and mesoderm of three dis-

Figure 3–19. Headless mice. The development and maintenance of the "head organizing center" requires the expression of the homeobox gene *Lim-1*. Knockout of *Lim-1* results in headless mice.

tinct regions of the body: head, trunk, and tail. Moreover, the endoderm and mesoderm subpopulations that migrate into each of these regions are formed at different times and by different subregions of the primitive streak. The mesoderm of the heart, brain, and eye is formed early in gastrulation by a "head center" at the cranial end of the primitive streak, whereas the endoderm of most of the gut and the paraxial mesoderm of the trunk somites and the lateral plate mesoderm are formed later by a middle "trunk center" of the streak. Finally, the endoderm of the cloaca, the mesoderm of the pelvic organs, and the caudal end of the neural tube are formed by a caudal "tail center" of the primitive streak.

The arrangement of the head, trunk, and tail organizing centers along the craniocaudal axis of the primitive streak apparently depends upon the expression of *Cripto*, a gene belonging to the *EGF-CFC* family of growth factors. Knockouts of *Cripto* in mice lead to disorganization of the craniocaudal sequence of embryo development. In addition, development and maintenance of the "head organizing center" (see Fig. 3–18) requires the expression of the homeobox gene *Lim-1*. Indeed, the knockout of *Lim-1* produces a dramatic result: a mouse without a head (Fig. 3–19). Apparently the head-forming actions of *Lim-1* are partly assisted by its interaction with the gene hepatic nuclear factor-3 *(HNF-3)* and the induction of genes *Otx-1* and *Otx-2,* which are homologous to the *Drosophila orthodenticle* gene (see discussion of neurulation later). The expression of *nodal* (a member of the *TGF-β* family) is also important for the development of cranial elements. In addition, in conjunction with the expression of many other genes, *nodal* plays a role in the establishment of left-/right-handed asymmetry of the embryo (see later and in Ch. 9). As noted above, the "trunk organizing center" directs the production of the paraxial and lateral plate mesoderm of the neck, thorax, and abdomen. A few genes responsible for the formation of trunk paraxial mesoderm have been identified in mice, including *Tbx-6* and *brachyury* (both T-box genes). However, many other trunk center genes have also been identified in zebrafish, suggesting the existence of a more complex system in higher organisms. Finally, a "tail organizing center" has been identified, which is responsible for formation of the mesoderm of the sacral region and the most caudal segment of the neural tube

(see Ch. 4). Genes of the tail organizing center in mice include *brachyury, Wnt-5a* and *Wnt-5b, Evx-1,* and HNF-3α, to name a few. It is thought that disturbances of caudal trunk and tail organizing centers are responsible for the spectrum of anomalies in humans called **caudal dysplasia** or **caudal dysgenesis.** Specifically, the mutation of T-box genes such as *brachyury* is thought to be central to the pathogenesis of these caudal malformations (see Clinical Applications section earlier).

The Primitive Streak Defines Left and Right Sides of the Embryo

As noted above, several genes expressed in the primitive streak of mice, including *nodal,* play a central role in the development of handed asymmetry of the mammalian body plan (see Fig. 3–18). **Handed asymmetry** is the term that denotes anatomic differences on the left and right sides of the body. For example, in humans, the gastrointestinal tract folds during development so that the stomach is on the left and the liver is on the right. The heart loops so that its apex points to the left, whereas its base is directed to the right. The right lung has three lobes and the left lung has two lobes. The establishment and significance of handed asymmetry are described in detail in the Experimental Principles section of Chapter 9.

Zygotic Genes Regulate the Involution of Epiblast Cells Into the Primitive Streak and Their Ingression Into the Space Between the Epiblast and the Hypoblast

Cells of the epiblast become incorporated into the primitive streak by a process of **involution** (see Figs. 3–18 and 3–5). Cell-tracing experiments show that cells on the left side of the epiblast tend to involute into the left side of the primitive streak, whereas cells of the right side of the epiblast involute into the right side of the primitive streak. Very little crossing over between left and right side cells occurs within the primitive streak itself. It is thought that **goosecoid family members** may play a role in involution as well as **friz-**

Figure 3–20. Autoradiograph showing localization of *slug*, a vertebrate gene encoding a zinc-finger protein of the snail family. *Slug* is expressed in flask-shaped cells lining the primitive streak. *Slug* mRNA transcripts are localized by the in situ hybridization technique. (From Nieto MA, Sargent MG, Wilkinson DG, Cooke J. 1994. Control of cell behavior during vertebrate development by slug, a zinc finger gene. Science 264:835.)

streak is *slug,* a zinc-finger transcription factor (Fig. 3–20). Under its influence, expression of cell-to-cell adhesion molecules such as E-cadherin may temporarily cease, whereas the expression of cytoskeletal proteins such as vimentin is induced. The epithelial to mesenchymal transformation of epiblast cells is essential for their ability to **ingress** or migrate through the primitive streak and into the space between the epiblast and the hypoblast to produce the definitive endoderm and the mesoderm. In addition to *slug,* genes that regulate these **morphogenetic movements** are a variety of growth factors, transcription factors, and adhesion or counteradhesion factors. For example, in null mutations of the **fibroblast growth factor receptor 1 (FGFR1),** involuting cells lose their ability to migrate, and, as a consequence, simply accumulate within the primitive streak. A member of the *Rho* gene family and the *Ras* gene superfamily, **Rac1,** is required for the organization of actin and the development of lamellipodia of gastrulating cells within the primitive streak. When its expression is disrupted, cells accumulate and die within the space between the epiblast and the hypoblast. As might be predicted, knockouts of a variety of **cytoskeletal/adhesion molecules** disrupt the process of ingression. These include **afadin,** an actin filament-binding protein, **N-cadherin,** a cell-cell adhesion molecule, and *β***-catenin,** a cytoplasmic component of the cadherin/catenin adhesion complex.

zled proteins, which are receptors for the Wnt family of secreted signaling molecules. Involution apparently ceases with closure of the caudal neuropore.

Cells Involuting Into the Primitive Streak Undergo an Epithelial to Mesenchymal Transformation

Involuting epiblast cells quickly undergo an **epithelial to mesenchymal transformation** within the streak where their predominant adhesive activity shifts from cell to cell to cell to substratum. One gene responsible for repressing ectodermal characteristics in the mesenchymal cells of the

Cells Ingressing Through the Primitive Streak Produce the Definitive Endoderm and Mesoderm and Their Derivatives

The expression of *HNF/forkhead* genes has been shown to be necessary for **development of the definitive endoderm** and its derivatives, such as the intestinal epithelium and liver hepatocytes in mouse embryos. Unfortunately, however, very little other than this is known about the regulation of formation of definitive endoderm in mammals. However, it is possible that mechanisms of endoderm formation in mice are similar to those elucidated in amphibians. In *Xenopus,* for example, endoderm formation requires the expression of a maternal T-box gene. This transcription factor then induces expression of members of the *Bix* family (brachyury-inducible, homeobox-containing genes). In addition, TGF-β signaling pathways may trigger expression of *nodal*-related genes required for endoderm formation in frogs.

The **development of intraembryonic mesoderm** has been more comprehensively studied in mammals. Moreover, it has become apparent that one particular family of genes, the **T-box genes**, plays an especially significant role in formation of mesoderm and in the differentiation of mesodermal derivatives in mammals. For example, *Tbx-6*, a mouse T-box transcription factor gene that is closely related to the prototypical T-box gene *brachyury* (see next sentence and Clinical Applications section of this chapter), is required for the formation of **paraxial mesoderm.** The product encoded by the *brachyury* or **T gene** itself **(T protein)** is required for the formation of **caudal mesoderm** including the notochord. It is thought that *brachyury* may regulate downstream gene expression through its activation of the *eFGF* gene. Formation of more **cranial mesoderm** may be regulated by other T-box genes, *Wnt-13*, *Tlx-2* (a homeobox gene), and serum response factor (SRF) and by recently discovered novel factors encoded by the *Msg1* and *Mrg1* genes. *Mrg1* is thought to play a pivotal role in induction of the most cranial mesoderm formed in the mammalian embryo, the mesoderm of the septum transversum (see Ch. 6). Finally, **fibroblast growth factor-9 (FGF-9)** appears to play a central role in the formation of **intermediate mesoderm,** whereas expression of the basic helix-loop-helix (bHLH) transcription factor **scleraxis** is required for the development of somite-derived chondrogenic lineages of the paraxial mesoderm.

Cells Within the Epiblast Give Rise to Surface Ectoderm and the Neural Plate

Cells that remain within the epiblast at the conclusion of gastrulation give rise to **surface ectoderm** or to the **neurectoderm of the neural plate.** Indeed, the alternative development of one or the other of these tissue types from the epiblast appears to be highly regulated by both inductive and suppressive factors, originating at first from the underlying hypoblast and later from the underlying mesoderm. For example, studies in amphibians show that the protein encoded by the gene *chordin* induces expression of a zinc-finger transcription factor **zic-related-1 (zic-r1)** and an Sry-related HMG factor, **Sox-2,** which in turn are required for the activation of the proneural gene *neurogenin.* In contrast, the bone morphogenetic protein encoded by **BMP-4** suppresses the expression of *zic-r1* and *Sox-2,* leading to development of surface ectoderm. A further level of control of this process is demonstrated by the ability of **chordin, noggin, gremlin,** and **follistatin** to block BMP-2 and BMP-4 signaling, thus favoring neurulization of the epiblast. In addition, direct inducers of neural plate development include **geminin** and **FGF-2.** Geminin induces expression of neurogenin-related-1 factor, which induces neural development. Likewise, the growth factor FGF-2 induces expression of the orthodenticle-related genes *Otx-1* and *Otx-2,* which play pivotal roles in the actions of the head organizing center during gastrulation (see earlier) and in neural development.

Synergistic Interactions of Dorsalizing and Ventralizing Factors Regulate Differentiation of the Embryo in the Craniocaudal Axis

It should be apparent from the discussion above that the craniocaudal differentiation of the mammalian embryo is partly dependent on the expression of one group of specific factors in the cranial region of the primitive streak and the expression of other factors in the middle and caudal regions of the primitive streak. However, it is also likely that the full and graded range of development along the craniocaudal axis depends to a large degree upon synergistic interactions between the cranially expressed "dorsalizing factors" and more caudally expressed "ventralizing factors." As noted in the discussion of neurulation earlier, **dorsalizing factors** include the products of *chordin*, *nodal*, and *follistatin* genes, whereas BMP-2 and BMP-4 act as **ventralizing factors.** Other dorsalizing factors include Lim-1, goosecoid, noggin, Otx-1, Otx-2, and activin, and other ventralizing factors include glycogen synthase kinase-3, FGF-2, and Wnt-3a.

Evidence for the synergistic interactions of dorsalizing and ventralizing substances in early development has been obtained in a variety of experiments. For example, several studies have shown that a combination of dorsalizing and ventralizing factors is typically required to induce more complete development of neural or mesodermal tissues from undifferentiated precursors. Numerous studies have also shown that disruption of a dorsalizing factor often results in ventralization and vice versa. Moreover, graded disruptions or suppression of dorsalizing or ventralizing factors along the craniocaudal axis also result in their graded expression, resulting in the differentiation of cranial, trunk, and tail mesodermal phenotypes. For example, *Evx-1* (homologue of *Drosophila* zygotic pair-rule gene, *even-skipped*) is expressed within the primitive streak in a graded pattern that is correlated with the production of different mesodermal types in different regions of the streak. Consistent with this finding, it has been shown that direct injections of low to high concentrations of goosecoid mRNA into *Xenopus* blastomeres results in development of different kinds of mesodermal descendants. For example, blood and embryonic kidney form at lower concentrations, and muscle and notochord develop at higher concentrations. Likewise, when low levels of *brachyury* mRNA are injected into explanted *Xenopus* tissue, smooth muscle and mesenchyme are produced, whereas injections of high concentrations of *brachyury* result in the formation of somites.

Mutations of Genes in the Gastrulation Cascade Result in Human Congenital Disease

An important lesson from these recent experimental findings is that the disruption of any one of a large number of genes that regulate gastrulation could, theoretically, have devastating consequences for human development. Indeed, a number of human congenital malformations have now been shown, or are suspected, to have resulted from mutations of genes that regulate the gastrulation mechanism. Mutations of *brachyury*, for example, are thought to cause the spectrum of anomalies called **caudal dysplasia** (see Clinical Applications section of this chapter). Mutations of another, more recently discovered T-box gene, *TBX5*, have been shown to result in **Holt-Oram syndrome** (see Ch. 11), whereas mutations of *TBX3* result in **ulnar-mammary syndrome** (see Chs. 11 and 14). More recently, it has been suggested that mutations of the T-box gene *TBX15* could be responsible for the pathogenesis evident in **acromegaloid facial appearance syndrome.** Finally, goosecoid (perhaps in conjunction with another closely linked factor) is a candidate gene for **velocardiofacial** and **DiGeorge syndromes** (see Ch. 12).

SUGGESTED READING

Descriptive Embryology

Bellairs R. 1986. The primitive streak. Anat Embryol 174:1

Meier S, Tam PPL. 1982. Metameric pattern development in the embryonic axis of the mouse. I. Differentiation of cranial segments. Differentiation 21:95

Müller F, O'Rahilly R. 1983. The first appearance of the major divisions of the human brain at stage 9. Anat Embryol 168:419

O'Rahilly R. 1973. Developmental Stages in Human Embryos. Part A. Embryos of the First 3 Weeks (Stages 1–9). Carnegie Institute of Washington, Washington, DC

Rosenquist GC. 1966. A radioautographic study of labelled grafts in the chick blastoderm: development from primitive streak to stage 12. Contrib Embryol Carnegie Inst 38:71

Snow MHL. 1981. Growth and its control in early mammalian development. Br Med Bull 37:221

Tam PPL, Beddington RSP. 1987. The formation of mesodermal tissues in the mouse embryo during gastrulation and early organogenesis. Development 99:109

Tam PPL, Meier S, Jacobson A. 1982. Differentiation of the metameric pattern in the embryonic axis of the mouse. II. Somitomeric organization of the presomitic mesoderm. Differentiation 21:109

Clinical Applications

Duhamel B. 1961. From the mermaid to anal imperforation: the syndrome of caudal regression. Arch Dis Child 36:152

Kallen B, Winberg J. 1974. Caudal mesoderm pattern of anomalies: from renal agenesis to sirenomelia. Teratology 9:99

Kalter H. 1993. Case reports of malformations associated with maternal diabetes: a history and critique. Clin Genet 43:174

Khoury MJ, Cordero JF, Greenberg F, et al. 1983. A population study of the VACTERL association: evidence for its etiological heterogeneity. Pediatrics 71:815

Quan L, Smith DW. 1973. The VATER association. J Pediatr 82:104

Russell LJ, Weaver DD, Bull MJ. 1981. The axial mesoderm aplasia syndrome. Pediatrics 67:176

Stott D, Kispert A, Herrmann BG. 1993. Rescue of the tail defect in brachyury mice. Genes Dev 7:197

Experimental Principles

Barnes JD, Crosby JL, Jones CM, et al. 1994. Embryonic expression of *Lim-1*, the mouse homolog of *Xenopus Xlim-1*, suggests a role in lateral mesoderm differentiation and neurogenesis. Dev Biol 161:168

Bennett D. 1975. The *T*-locus of the mouse. Cell 6:441

Blum M, DeRobertis EM, Kojis T, et al. 1994. Molecular cloning of the human homeobox gene goosecoid (*GSC*) and mapping of the gene to human chromosome 14q32.1. Genomics 21:383

Dush M, Martin G. 1992. Analysis of mouse *Evx* genes: *Evx-1* displays graded expression in the primitive streak. Dev Biol 151:273

Faust C, Magnuson T. 1993. Genetic control of gastrulation in the mouse. Curr Opin Genet Dev 3:491

Graff JM, Bansal A, Melton DA. 1996. Xenopus Mad proteins transduce distinct subsets of signals for the TGF-β superfamily. Cell 85:479

Hahn SA, Schutte M, Hoque AT, et al. 1996. DPC4, a candidate tumor suppressor gene at human chromosome 18q21.1. Science 271:350

He X, Saint-Jeannet JP, Woodgett JR, et al. 1995. Glycogen synthase kinase-3 and dorsoventral patterning in *Xenopus* embryos. Nature 374:617

Hemmati-Brivanlou A, Thomsen GH. 1995. Ventral mesodermal patterning in *Xenopus* embryos: expression patterns and activities of BMP-2 and BMP-4. Dev Genet 17:78

Herrmann BG, Labeit S, Poustka A, et al. 1990. Cloning of the *T* gene required in mesoderm formation in the mouse. Nature 343:617

Hogan B, Blessing M, Winnier GE, et al. 1994. Growth factors in development: the role of TGF-B related polypeptide signalling molecules in embryogenesis. Development (suppl) 53–60

Holley SA, Jackson PD, Sasai Y, et al. 1995. A conserved system for dorsal-ventral patterning in insects and vertebrates involving sog and chordin. Nature 376:249

Ivens A, Moore G, Williamson R. 1988. Molecular approaches to dysmorphology. J Med Genet 25:473

Kessler DS, Melton DA. 1994. Vertebrate embryonic induction: mesoderm and neural patterning. Science 266:596

Knecht AK, Good PJ, Dawid IB, et al. 1995. Dorsal-ventral patterning and differentiation of noggin-induced neural tissue in the absence of mesoderm. Development 121:1927

Krumlauf R. 1993. *Hox* gene and pattern formation in the branchial region of the vertebrate head. TIG 9:106

Lamb TM, Harland RM. 1995. Fibroblast growth factor is a direct neural inducer, which combined with noggin generates anterior-posterior neural pattern. Development 121:3627

Liu F, Hata A, Baker JC, et al. 1996. A human Mad protein acting as a BMP-regulated transcriptional activator. Nature 381:620

Mayer R, Morgan R, Sargent MG. 1995. Induction of the prospective neural crest of *Xenopus*. Development 121:767

Mishina Y, Suzuki A, Ueno N, Behringer RR. 1995. *Bmpr* encodes a type I bone morphogenetic protein receptor that is essential for gastrulation during mouse embryogenesis. Genes Dev 9:3027

Moos M Jr, Wang S, Krinks M. 1995. Anti-dorsalizing morphogenetic protein is a novel TGF-β homolog expressed in the Spemann organizer. Development 121:4293

Niehrs C, Steinbeisser H, De Robertis EM. 1994. Mesodermal patterning by a gradient of the vertebrate homeobox gene goosecoid. Science 263:817

Nieto MA, Sargent MG, Wilkinson DG, Cooke J. 1994. Control of cell behavior during vertebrate development by slug, a zinc finger gene. Science 264:835

Nothias JY, Majumber S, Kaneko KJ, DePamphilism L. 1995. Regulation of gene expression at the beginning of mammalian development. J Biol Chem 270:22077

Nüsslein-Volhard C. 1994. Of flies and fishes. Science 266:572

O'Reilly MA, Smith JC, Cunliffe V. 1995. Patterning of the mesoderm in *Xenopus*: dose dependent and synergistic effects of brachyury and Pintallavis. Development 121:1351

Rashbass P, Wilson V, Rosen B, Beddington RS. 1994. Alterations of gene expression during mesoderm formation and axial patterning in brachyury (*T*) embryos. Int J Dev Biol 38:35

Riou JF, Clavilier L, Boucaut JC. 1996. Early regionalized expression of a novel *Xenopus* fibroblast growth factor receptor in neuroepithelium. Biochem Biophys Res Commun 218:198

Rivera-Perez JA, Mallo M, Gendron-Macquire M, et al. 1995. Goosecoid is not an essential component of the mouse gastrula organizer but is required for craniofacial and rib development. Development 121:3005

Sasai Y, Lu B, Steinbeisser H, et al. 1994. *Xenopus* chordin: a novel dorsalizing factor activated by organizer-specific homeobox genes. Cell 79:779

Sasai Y, Lu B, Steinbeisser H, De Robertis EM. 1995.

Regulation of neural induction by the Chd and BMP-4 antagonistic patterning signals in *Xenopus*. Nature 376:333

Schmidt J, Francois V, Bier E, Kimelman D. 1995. *Drosophila* short gastrulation induces an ectopic axis in *Xenopus:* evidence for conserved mechanisms of dorsal-ventral patterning. Development 121:4319

Shawlot W, Behringer RR. 1995. Requirement for *Lim1* in head-organizer function. Nature 374:425

Shawlot W, Wakamiya M, Kwan KM, et al. 1999. Lim1 is required in both primitive streak-derived tissues and visceral endoderm for head formation in the mouse. Development 126:4925

Shin HS. 1989. The *T/T* complex and the genetic control of mouse development. p. 443. In Litwin SD (ed): Human Immunogenetics: Basic Principles and Clinical Relevance. Marcel Dekker, New York

Smith WC, Knecht AK, Wu M, Harland RM. 1993. Secreted noggin protein mimics the Spemann organizer in dorsalizing *Xenopus* mesoderm. Nature 361:547

Smith WC, McKendry R, Ribisi S Jr, Harland RM. 1995. A nodal-related gene defines a physical and functional domain within the Spemann organizer. Cell 82:37

Steinbeisser H, Fainsod A, Niehrs C, et al. 1995. The role of gsc and BMP-4 in dorsoventral patterning of the marginal zone of *Xenopus:* a loss of function study using antisense RNA. EMBO J 14:5230

Taira M, Otani H, Saint-Jeannet JP, Dawid IB. 1994.

Role of the *LIM* class homeodomain protein Xlim-1 in neural and muscle induction by the Spemann organizer in *Xenopus*. Nature 372:677

Toyama R, O'Connell ML, Wright CV, et al. 1995. Nodal induces ectopic goosecoid and lim1 expression and axis duplication in zebrafish. Development 121:383

Watanabe T, Kim S, Candia A, et al. 1995. Molecular mechanisms of Spemann's organizer formation: conserved growth factor synergy between *Xenopus* and mouse. Genes Dev 9:3038

Wilkinson DG, Bhatt S, Herrmann BG. 1990. Expression pattern of the mouse *T* gene and its role in mesoderm formation. Nature 343:657

Wilson V, Manson L, Skarnes WC, Beddington RSP. 1995. The *T* gene is necessary for normal mesodermal morphogenetic movements during gastrulation. Development 121:877

Winnier G, Blessing M, Labosky PA, Hogan BL. 1995. Bone morphogenetic protein-4 is required for mesoderm formation and patterning in the mouse. Genes Dev 9:2105

Yamada G, Mansouri A, Torres M, et al. 1995. Targeted mutation of the murine goosecoid gene results in craniofacial defects and neonatal death. Development 121:2917

Yang JT, Rayburn H, Hynes RO. 1993. Embryonic mesoderm defects in 25 integrin-deficient mice. Development 119:1079

4

The Fourth Week

Summary

During the fourth week, the tissue layers laid down in the third week differentiate to form the primordia of most of the major organ systems of the body. Simultaneously, the embryonic disc undergoes a process of folding that creates the basic vertebrate body form. Embryonic folding is covered in Chapter 6. This chapter describes the differentiation of the structures that arise along the embryonic axis during the third week—the somites and the neural plate.

Somites continue to segregate from the paraxial mesoderm in craniocaudal progression until day 30. Meanwhile, beginning in the cervical region, the somites subdivide into three kinds of mesodermal primordium: **myotomes, dermatomes,** and **sclerotomes.** The myotomes develop into the segmental musculature of the back and the anterolateral body wall; the dermatomes form some of the dermis of the scalp, neck, and trunk; the sclerotomes give rise to the vertebral bodies and vertebral arches and also contribute to the base of the skull.

During the fourth week, a process of folding called **neurulation** converts the neural plate to a hollow **neural tube** that sinks into the body wall and begins to differentiate into the brain and spinal cord. The caudal-most portions of the neural tube are formed by a separate process of **secondary neurulation** involving the mesodermal caudal eminence. Even before the end of the fourth week, the major regions of the brain become apparent, and neurons and glia begin to differentiate from the neuroepithelium of the neural tube. As neurulation occurs, a special population of cells, the **neural crest,** detaches from the lateral lips of the neural folds and migrates to numerous locations in the body, where the cells differentiate to form a wide range of structures and cell types.

With the exception of some cranial nerve sensory ganglia (discussed in Ch. 13), ganglia of the peripheral nervous system are derived from neural crest. Sensory **dorsal root ganglia** condense next to the spinal cord in register with the somites. These ganglia house the sensory neurons that relay information from somatic and visceral sense receptors to the central nervous system. A linked series of **sympathetic chain ganglia** develops along the entire length of the spinal cord; in addition, a few **prevertebral sympathetic ganglia** develop in association with branches of the abdominal aorta. These ganglia house peripheral neurons of the two-neuron sympathetic pathways and are innervated by central sympathetic fibers originating in the thoracolumbar spinal cord. The peripheral neurons of the parasympathetic system are housed in **parasympathetic ganglia** that develop in association with the viscera and cranial nerves. These ganglia are innervated by central parasympathetic fibers originating in the midbrain, hindbrain, and sacral spinal cord.

Neural crest cells also give rise to numerous non-neuronal structures, including the melanocytes (pigment cells) of the epidermis, certain components of the heart, and the cartilages of the pharyngeal arches.

Differentiation of the Somites and the Nervous System

Segmental Development and Integration

Weeks	Days		
	22	Neural crest begins to migrate, commencing in the cervical region	Neurulation begins
	26		Cranial neuropore closes
4	28	Sclerotome cells surround the neural tube and notochord	Caudal neuropore closes and primitive streak disappears
	33	Costal processes appear on the vertebral bodies	
5	35	In the thoracic region, costal processes elongate to form ribs	
	40	Mesodermal sternal bars appear	The myotome splits into epimere and hypomere
6	42	Costovertebral joints begin to develop	The caudal end of the neural tube develops from the caudal eminence by the process of secondary neurulation
	45	Ribs connect with sternal bars; sternal bars begin to fuse	Sacral vertebrae fuse to form sacrum
7	50		
8	60	Sternal bars are completely fused	Epimere and hypomere give rise respectively to the spinal musculature and to the trunk wall muscle layers

Epimere

Hypomere

Intervertebral discs are distinct and consist of an annulus fibrosus and nucleus pulposus

Timeline. Development of the somites and the neural tube.

THE SOMITES DIFFERENTIATE INTO SCLEROTOME, MYOTOME, AND DERMATOME

The Sclerotome Cells Surround the Notochord and Neural Tube

Shortly after forming, each somite separates into subdivisions that give rise to specific mesodermal components. The first of these subdivisions to appear are the **sclerotomes,** which will develop into the vertebrae. The sclerotomes arise as follows. Each newly formed somite develops a central cavity that becomes occupied by a population of loose **core cells** (Fig. 4–1). The somite then ruptures on its medial side, and the core cells, plus some additional cells from the ventromedial wall of the somite, remain in the vicinity of the notochord and developing neural tube as the dermomyotome is displaced laterally by expansion of the dorsolateral body wall. This group of ventromedial and core cells is the **sclerotome.** The ventral portion of the sclerotome surrounds the notochord and forms the rudiment of the vertebral body. The dorsal portion of the sclerotome surrounds the neural tube and forms the rudiment of the vertebral arch.

Transplantation experiments have established that sclerotome cells differentiate to form either a vertebral body or a vertebral arch in response to specific inducing substances. Vertebral bodies are formed in response to substances produced by the notochord and floor plate of the neural tube, whereas induction of vertebral arches also requires interaction with the surface ectoderm (see the Experimental Principles section of this chapter).

A number of spinal defects are caused by abnormal induction of the sclerotomes and the neural tube. Defective induction of vertebral bodies on one side of the body may result in a severe lateral **scoliosis** (lateral bending of the spinal column), which must be surgically corrected. The Clinical Applications section of this chapter also describes a range of defects, called **spina bifida, anencephaly,** and **rachischisis,** which are caused by abnormal induction of the vertebral arch rudiments by the neural tube or by failure of the caudal neuropores to close.

Figure 4–1. Initial subdivision of the somitic mesoderm. The ventromedial and core cells of the somite, constituting the sclerotome, migrate toward the midline of the embryo to enclose the neural tube and notochord, where they subsequently form the vertebral arches and vertebral bodies, respectively. The remaining dorsolateral cells of the somite form the dermomyotome.

The Segmental Sclerotomes Split and Recombine to Form Intersegmental Vertebral Rudiments. The spinal nerves develop **segmentally;** that is, each spinal nerve emerges at the same level as the corresponding somite. Because the vertebral arches completely enclose the neural tube during the period when the spinal nerves sprout, one may wonder how the spinal nerves escape from the developing vertebral canal. A related question is why eight cervical sclerotomes produce seven cervical vertebrae, whereas in the rest of the vertebral column there is a one-to-one correspondence of sclerotomes to vertebrae.

The answer to these questions is that the sclerotomes split and recombine to produce vertebral rudiments that lie **intersegmentally.** Figure 4–2 illustrates this process. As the sclerotome surrounds the notochord and neural tube, it splits into a cranial half and a caudal half, and the caudal half of each sclerotome fuses with the cranial half of the succeeding sclerotome. The resulting composite structures thus produce vertebrae that lie intersegmentally.

Seven cervical vertebrae form from eight cervical somites because the cranial half of the first cervical sclerotome fuses with the caudal half of the fourth occipital sclerotome and contributes to the formation of the base of the skull (Fig. 4–3). The caudal half of the first cervical sclerotome then fuses with the cranial half of the second cervical sclerotome to form the first cervical vertebra (the atlas), and so on down the spine. The eighth cervical sclerotome thus contributes its cranial half to the seventh cervical vertebra and its caudal half to the first thoracic vertebra.

As a result of sclerotomal resegmentation, the segmental spinal nerves exit between the vertebrae. It is important to remember, however, that even though there are seven cervical vertebrae, there are eight cervical spinal nerves: The first spinal nerve exits between the base of the skull and the first cervical vertebra (in alignment with the first cervical somite), and thus the eighth spinal nerve exits above the first thoracic vertebra (in alignment with the eighth cervical somite). From this point onward, each spinal nerve exits just below the vertebra of the same number (see Fig. 4–3).

The fibrous intervertebral discs form between the vertebral bodies at segmental levels (Fig. 4–4). The original core of each disc, the **nucleus pulposus,** is composed of cells of notochordal origin, whereas the surrounding **annulus fibrosus** develops from sclerotomal cells that are left in the region of sclerotome splitting during resegmentation.

The Ribs Develop From Costal Processes of the Developing Thoracic Vertebrae. Small lateral mesenchymal condensations called **costal pro-**

Figure 4–2. Recombining of the sclerotomes to form vertebrae. Each sclerotome splits into cranial and caudal segments. As the segmental spinal nerves grow out to innervate the myotomes, the cranial segment of each sclerotome recombines with the caudal segment of the next superior sclerotome to form a vertebral rudiment.

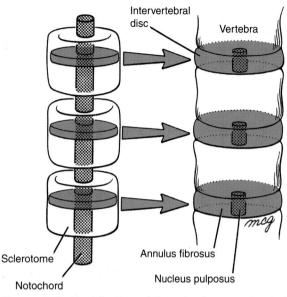

Figure 4–4. Contribution of the sclerotome and notochord to the intervertebral disc. When the sclerotome splits, cells remaining in the plane of splitting coalesce to form the annulus fibrosus of the disc, and the notochordal cells enclosed by this structure differentiate to form the nucleus pulposus of the disc. The regions of the notochord enclosed by the developing vertebral bodies degenerate and disappear.

cesses develop in association with the vertebral arches of all the developing neck and trunk vertebrae (Fig. 4–5A). Concomitantly, the slightly more dorsal transverse processes grow laterally along the dorsal side of each costal process. Only in the thoracic region, however, do the distal tips of the costal processes lengthen to form ribs. The ribs begin to form and lengthen on day 35. The first seven ribs connect ventrally to the sternum via **costal cartilages** by day 45 and are called the **true ribs.** The five lower ribs do not articulate directly with the sternum and are called the **false ribs.** The ribs develop as cartilaginous precursors that later ossify; this process of **endochondral ossifica-**

Figure 4–3. The mechanism by which the cervical region develops eight cervical nerves but only seven cervical vertebrae. Each somite induces a ventral root to grow out from the spinal cord. When the sclerotomes recombine, however, the cranial half of the first sclerotome fuses with the occipital bone of the skull. In the thoracic, lumbar, and sacral regions, the number of spinal nerves matches the number of vertebrae.

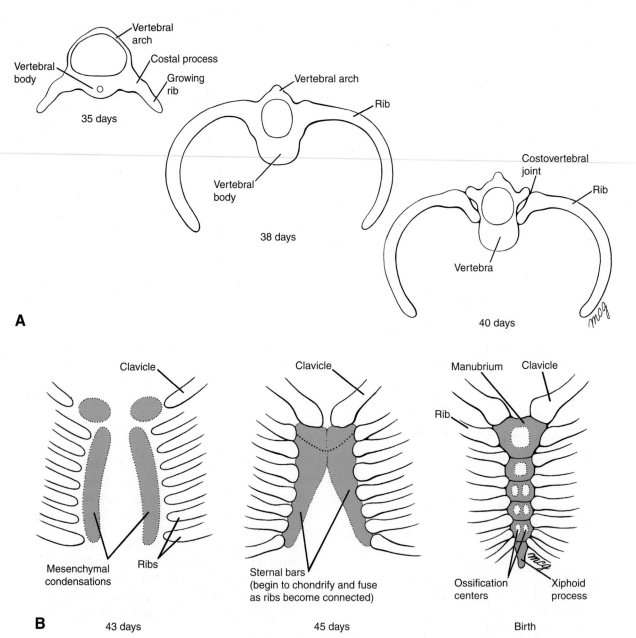

Figure 4–5. Development of the ribs and sternum. *A,* The costal processes of the vertebrae in the thoracic region begin to elongate in the fifth week to form ribs. Late in the sixth week, the costovertebral joints form and separate the ribs from the vertebrae. *B,* Paired mesenchymal condensations called sternal bars form within the ventral body wall at the end of the sixth week. These bars quickly fuse together at their cranial ends while their lateral edges connect with the distal ends of the growing ribs. The sternal bars then zipper together in a craniocaudal direction. Ossification centers appear within the sternum as early as 60 days, but the xiphoid process does not ossify until birth.

tion is discussed in more detail in Chapter 11. Primary ossification centers appear near the angle of each rib in the sixth week, and further ossification occurs in a distal direction. Secondary ossification centers develop in the tubercles and heads of the ribs during adolescence.

The costal processes of the cervical vertebrae give rise to the lateral boundary, and the transverse processes give rise to the medial boundary of the foramina transversaria that transmit the vertebral arteries. In the lumbar region, the costal processes become the transverse processes of the lumbar vertebrae. The costal processes of the first two or three sacral vertebrae contribute to the development of the lateral sacral mass or ala of the sacrum.

The sternum develops from a pair of longitudinal mesenchymal condensations, the **sternal bars,** that form in the ventrolateral body wall (Fig. 4–5B). As the most cranial ribs make contact with them in the seventh week, the sternal bars meet along the midline and begin to fuse. Fusion commences at the cranial end of the sternal bars and progresses caudally, finishing with the formation of the xiphoid process in the ninth week. Like the ribs, the sternal bones ossify from cartilaginous precursors. The sternal bars ossify in craniocaudal succession from the fifth month until shortly after birth, producing the definitive bones of the sternum: the manubrium, the body, and the xiphoid process.

The Myotomes and Dermatomes Develop at Segmental Levels

The portion of the somite that is translocated dorsolaterally while the sclerotome remains in its original medial location is called the **dermomyotome.** This structure quickly separates into two structures: a **dermatome** and a **myotome** (Fig. 4–6). The dermatomes contribute to the dermis (including fat and connective tissue) of the neck, the back, and the ventral and lateral trunk. As discussed in Chapter 14, however, most of the dermis is derived from somatopleuric lateral plate mesoderm.

The myotomes differentiate into myogenic (muscle-producing) cells. Each myotome splits into two structures: a dorsal **epimere** and a ventral **hypomere.** The epimeres give rise to the deep epax-

ial muscles of the back, including the erector spinae and transversospinalis groups. The hypomeres form the hypaxial muscles of the lateral and ventral body wall in the thorax and abdomen (see Fig. 4–6). These include three layers of intercostal muscles in the thorax, the homologous three layers of the abdominal musculature (the external oblique, internal oblique, and transversus abdominis), and the rectus abdominis muscles that flank the ventral midline. The rectus column is usually limited to the abdominal region, but occasionally it develops on either side of the sternum as a sternalis muscle. In the cervical region, hypaxial myoblasts form the strap muscles of the neck, including the geniohyoid, scalene, and infrahyoid muscles. In the lumbar region, the hypomeres form the quadratus lumborum muscles. Somitic myoblasts also invade the developing limb buds and give rise to the limb musculature. The remaining mesodermal structures of the limb, including the appendicular skeleton, are derived from the somatopleuric lateral plate mesoderm (see Ch. 11).

Surprisingly, it appears that myotomes do not contribute to the formation of the tendons and internal connective tissue of the body wall muscles. Cell marking experiments indicate that these structures arise from somatopleuric lateral plate mesoderm.

THE NEURAL PLATE DIFFERENTIATES INTO BRAIN AND SPINAL CORD REGIONS AND FOLDS TO FORM THE NEURAL TUBE

The Future Spinal cord and the Divisions of the Brain Are Apparent in the Neural Plate at the Beginning of the Fourth Week

By the beginning of the fourth week, the neural plate consists of a broad cranial portion that will give rise to the brain and a narrow caudal portion that will give rise to the spinal cord. On about day 22, the cephalic end of the embryo begins to flex sharply ventrally (Fig. 4–7). This flexure marks the site of the future mesencephalon or midbrain and therefore is called the **mesencephalic flexure.** The portion of the future brain cranial to the mes-

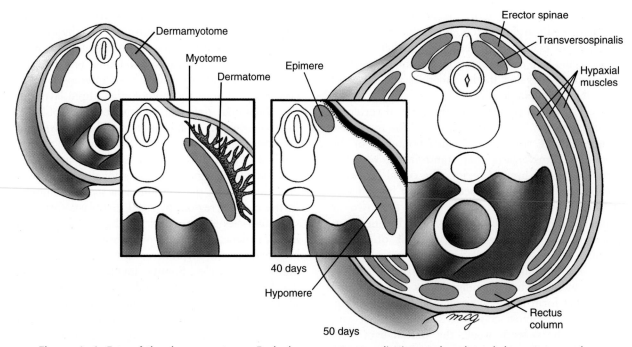

Figure 4–6. Fate of the dermomyotome. Each dermomyotome splits into a dorsolateral dermatome and a myotome. Dermatome cells migrate to the surface ectoderm of the corresponding segmental region, where they collaborate with lateral plate mesoderm to form the dermis. Each myotome splits first into a dorsal epimere and ventral hypomere. The epimere forms deep muscles of the back. In the thoracic region, the hypomere splits into three layers of anterolateral muscles; in the abdominal region, a fourth ventral segment also differentiates and forms the rectus abdominis muscle.

encephalic flexure becomes the **prosencephalon** or forebrain, and the portion caudal to the flexure becomes the **rhombencephalon,** or hindbrain. Even at this early stage of differentiation, the rhombencephalon is divided into segments by faint constrictions. These segments are called **neuromeres** or, more specifically, **rhombomeres.** On day 22, four rhombomeres are visible; by day 26, there are seven or eight rhombomeres. The development of the brain is covered in Chapter 13, and brain segmentation and its relationship to development of the pharyngeal arches is discussed in the Experimental Principles section of Chapter 12.

On day 22 (eight pairs of somites), the narrow caudal portion of the neural plate—the future spinal cord—represents only about 25 percent of the length of the neural plate. As somites continue to develop, however, the spinal cord region lengthens faster than the cephalic neural plate. By day 23 or 24 (12 and 20 pairs of somites, respectively), the future spinal cord occupies about 50 percent of the length of the neural plate, and by day 26 (25 pairs

of somites), it occupies about 60 percent. The rapid lengthening of the neural plate during this period is thought to depend on the elongation of the underlying notochord.

Formation of the Neural Tube Begins on Day 22 at the Level of the First Five Somites

One of the most important events of the fourth week is the conversion of the neural plate into a **neural tube** by a process of folding called **neurulation.** Neurulation commences as the neural plate begins to crease ventrally along its midline. This crease develops along the midline neural groove (see Ch. 3). The neural groove, which is thought to develop in response to induction by the closely apposed notochord, acts as a hinge region, and the two thick neural folds rotate around it like the leaves of a closing book (Fig. 4–8). The neural folds become concave as they rotate, so that the

Mesencephalon   Rhombencephalon

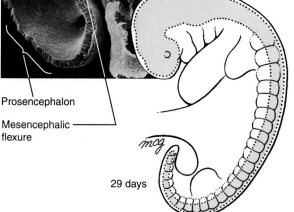

Rhombomere

Prosencephalon

Mesencephalic
flexure

29 days

Figure 4–7. The anlage of the central nervous system, the neural tube, is present by the end of the fourth week. It is formed by the process of neurulation described at the end of Chapter 3. Even at this early stage, the primary vesicles of the brain, two of its three flexures, and the rhombomeric subdivisions of the hindbrain can be identified. (Photo courtesy of Drs. Antone Jacobson and Patrick Tam.)

lateral lips of the folds meet dorsally to form a tube enclosing a space called the **neural canal.** As the lips of the neural tube fuse, the junction between the neuroepithelium and the adjacent surface ectoderm is pulled dorsally, and the opposing margins of surface ectoderm also meet and fuse. As soon as the surface ectoderm fuses, the neural tube separates from it and sinks into the mesenchyme of the posterior body wall.

A number of forces apparently cooperate in causing the neural plate to fold. It has been suggested that the rapid growth of the embryonic axis physically stretches the neural plate and that this action contributes to formation of the crease in the neural plate in the same way that stretching an elastic sheet causes it to warp down the middle. Other forces that probably contribute to folding include differential growth of specific regions of neurectoderm, changes in the conformation of

neuroepithelial cells, and the activity of cytoskeletal and cytomuscular elements such as microtubules and microfilaments.

Closure of the Neural Tube Proceeds Bidirectionally, Ending With Closure of the Cranial and Caudal Neuropores

The lips of the neural folds first make contact on day 22 in the area of the four occipital somites and first cervical somite (Figs. 4–9 and 4–10). The newly formed neural canal communicates with the amniotic cavity at either end through large openings called the **cranial** and **caudal neuropores.** The neural folds may initially fuse at several separate points in the occipital region, but the small intervening openings rapidly fill in to produce a continuous canal. As neurulation continues, the cranial and caudal neuropores gradually diminish in size. The cranial neuropore finally closes on day 24, and the caudal neuropore closes on day 26. Closure of the cranial neuropore is actually bidirectional, and final closure occurs in the area of the future forebrain. Closure of the caudal neuropore is strictly craniocaudal and finishes at the level of the second sacral segment (the level of somite 31).

Abnormalities of neural tube closure not only affect the development of the central nervous system but also interfere with vertebral arch and cranial vault morphogenesis. Disturbances of neural tube closure underlie the spina bifida, anencephaly and rachischisis defects discussed in the Clinical Applications section of this chapter.

The Caudalmost Portion of the Neural Tube Is Formed by Secondary Neurulation of the Caudal Eminence

The neural tube formed by closure of the caudal neuropore terminates at somite 31. How do the more caudal portions of the neural tube—the inferior sacral and coccygeal levels—form? Recall from Chapter 3 that gastrulation through the regressing tail center of the primitive streak produces the mesodermal caudal eminence by day 20. Both experimental studies and the examination of human embryos support the hypothesis that it is the cau-

Figure 4–8. Neurulation. *A–C,* Neurulation begins in the occipitocervical region as the neural plate is thrown into neural folds. *D,* The lateral edges of the neural folds meet in the midline and fuse while simultaneously detaching from the surface ectoderm. *D, E,* These detaching edges of surface ectoderm then fuse with each other to enclose the neural tube completely. (A–D From Schoenwolf GC. 1982. On the morphogenesis of the early rudiments of the developing central nervous system. Scanning Microsc 1: 289. *E,* Photo courtesy of Dr. Kathryn Tosney.)

dal eminence rather than the neural plate that gives rise to the caudal neural tube and to the caudal extension of the spinal cord coverings (Fig. 4–11). This process is called **secondary neurulation.** Apparently, a central mass of pluripotent tissue within the caudal eminence first forms a solid **neural cord.** This cord then cavitates along its central axis, and the newly formed lumen joins with the neural canal. The formation of the caudal end of the neural tube is completed by about 8 weeks of development. The caudal extension of the dural and pial components of the spinal cord coverings, the filum terminale, is formed later by regression of the caudalmost part of the neural tube. The caudal eminence also produces the somites at the most inferior levels of the embryo.

NEURAL CREST CELLS ORIGINATE IN THE NEURAL FOLDS, MIGRATE TO SPECIFIC LOCATIONS IN THE BODY, AND GIVE RISE TO NUMEROUS STRUCTURES

Neural Crest Cells Detach From the Lips of the Neural Folds During Neurulation

The **neural crest** is a special population of cells that arises along the lateral margins of the neural folds. During neurulation, these cells detach from the neural plate and migrate to many specific locations in the body, where they differentiate into a

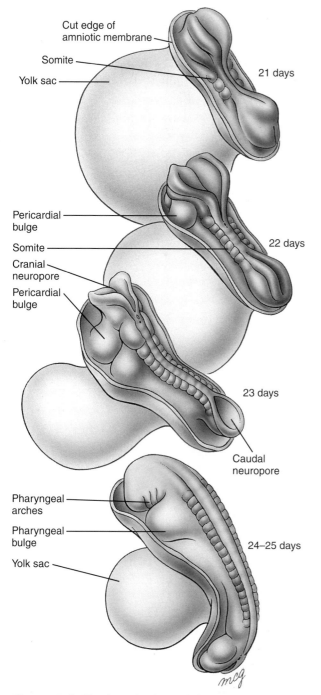

Cut edge of amniotic membrane

Somite

Yolk sac

21 days

Pericardial bulge

Somite

22 days

Cranial neuropore

Pericardial bulge

23 days

Caudal neuropore

Pharyngeal arches

Pharyngeal bulge

Yolk sac

24–25 days

Figure 4–9. The lateral edges of the neural folds first begin to fuse in the occipitocervical region on day 22, leaving the cranial and caudal neuropores open at each end. The neural tube increases in length as it zippers up both cranially and caudally, and the neuropores become progressively smaller. The cranial neuropore closes on day 24, and the caudal neuropore closes on day 26.

Figure 4–10. This embryo is comparable to a day 22 or day 23 human embryo. The cranial and caudal neuropores are both open. (Photo courtesy of Dr. T. H. Shepard.)

remarkable variety of structures (Fig. 4–12; see also Fig. 4–14 later). This unusual tissue type first arose during the early evolution of the vertebrates.

Neural crest cells differentiate first in the mesencephalic zone of the future brain. These cephalic neural crest cells associated with the developing brain begin to detach and migrate before closure of the cranial neuropore, even while the neural folds are still widely open. In the spinal cord portion of the neural tube, the neural crest cells detach as the lateral lips of the tube fuse. Some neural crest cells at the caudal end of the neural tube are produced even after the caudal neuropore closes on day 26. Thus, detachment and migration of the neural crest cells occur in a craniocaudal wave, from the mesencephalon to the caudal end of the spinal neural tube. (Fig. 4–13*A*).

Caudal eminence

Neural tube

Lumen develops

Lumen of caudal eminence becomes continuous with neural canal

Neural canal

20 days

40 days

Figure 4–11. Formation of the neural tube inferior to the second sacral level by secondary neurulation. Mesoderm invading this region during gastrulation condenses into a solid rod called the caudal eminence, which later develops a lumen. At the end of the sixth week, this structure fuses with the neural tube.

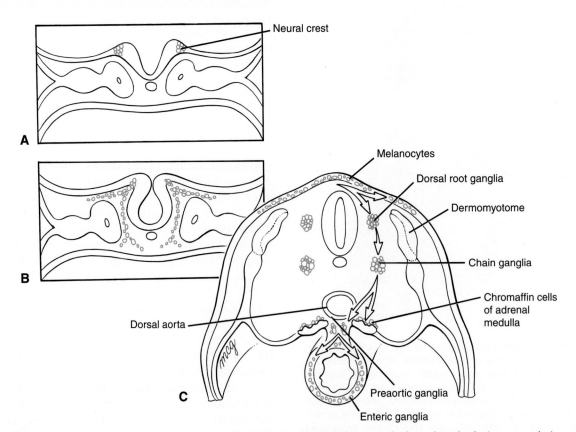

Neural crest

A

B

Melanocytes

Dorsal root ganglia

Dermomyotome

Chain ganglia

Chromaffin cells of adrenal medulla

Dorsal aorta

Preaortic ganglia

Enteric ganglia

C

Figure 4–12. Neural crest cells arising at the lateral edges of the neural plate detach during neurulation and migrate throughout the embryo to form many different tissues.

Figure 4–13. *A,* This scanning electron micrograph illustrates the craniocaudal sequence of release of neural crest cells from the neural tube. At this stage of development, neural crest cells have already begun to migrate from the neural tube in more cranial regions (solid arrow) but have not yet separated from the neural tube in more caudal regions (open arrow). *B,* High magnification scanning electron micrograph showing neural crest cells migrating onto the surface of the somite. Their migration paths become segmental (arrow) as they approach the boundary between the sclerotome and the dermomyotome. (*A,* From Tosney K. 1978. The early migration of neural crest cells in the trunk region of the avian embryo. Dev Biol 62:317. *B,* From Tosney K. 1988. Somites and axon guidance. Scanning Microsc 2:427.)

Cell Tracing Studies Are Used to Study Neural Crest Migration

The migration routes of the crest cells from various parts of the neural plate have been mapped by cell tracing studies in bird and mouse embryos. As described in the Experimental Principles section of Chapter 5, these studies use natural or artificial markers to follow the path of migrating cells and cell lineages. It has been argued that one component of neural crest migration is largely passive, because inert latex beads injected at sites of neural crest origin are carried along normal routes of crest cell migration. Nevertheless, it seems likely

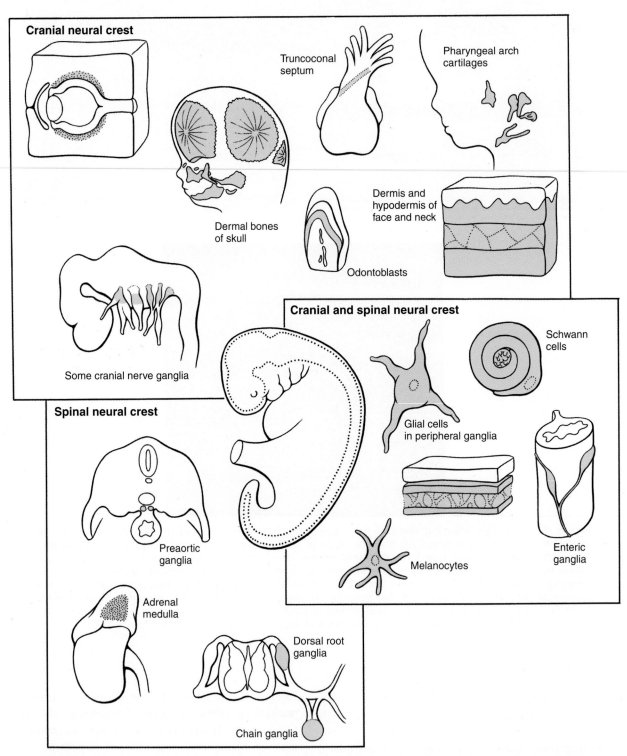

Figure 4–14. Neural crest cells migrating from both cranial and trunk regions of the neural tube give rise to a variety of tissues in the embryo.

that crest cells also migrate actively and that they are guided by molecules in the extracellular matrix such as fibronectin and glycosaminoglycans (see Figs. 4–12 and 4–13*B*). (See the Experimental Principles section of Ch. 5 for a discussion of the pathfinding capacities of neural crest cells.) Studies of staged human embryos have also provided information about the migration and developmental fate of human neural crest cells. Figure 4–14 summarizes the structures derived from neural crest cells originating at various levels of the neural plate.

The Cephalic Neural Crest Gives Rise to Diverse Structures of the Head and Neck

When the cephalic neural crest cells migrate away from the neural folds, they travel through the space just deep to the ectoderm and within the loose mesoderm or mesenchyme of the head and neck. Crest cells from different levels of the cephalic neural plate are trapped at specific sites, where they differentiate to form the appropriate structures. Whether and to what extent the fate of a crest cell either is predetermined before the crest cell leaves the neural fold or is determined by cues along the route of migration and at the site of differentiation is a major topic of neural crest research (see Chs. 12 and 13 and the Experimental Principles section of Ch. 5).

Neural crest cells from the mesencephalon and caudal prosencephalon regions give rise to the parasympathetic ganglion of cranial nerve III, to the connective tissue around the developing eyes and optic nerves, to the muscles of the pupil and ciliary body in the optic globe, and to the head mesenchyme cranial to the level of the mesencephalon (see Chs. 12 and 13). Neural crest gives rise to the pia mater and arachnoid of the occipital region; the dura mater is thought to arise largely from paraxial mesoderm.

Neural crest cells from the mesencephalon and rhombencephalon regions also give rise to structures in the developing **pharyngeal arches** of the head and neck (see Ch. 12 and the Experimental Principles section of this chapter). These structures include cartilaginous rudiments of several bones of the nose, face, middle ear, and neck. The mesencephalon and rhombencephalon crest cells

form the dermis, smooth muscle, and fat of the face and ventral neck and the odontoblasts of the developing teeth. Neural crest cells arising from the caudalmost rhombencephalon may give rise to C cells of the thyroid (see Ch. 12).

The rhombencephalic neural crest also contributes some of the cranial nerve ganglia (see Ch. 13). Rhombencephalic neural crest cells give rise to neurons and glial cells in parasympathetic ganglia of cranial nerves VII, IX, and X and to some neurons and all glial cells in the sensory ganglia of cranial nerves V, VII, VIII, IX, and X. Some of the distal sensory neurons of these cranial nerves, however, arise from placodes originating in the surface ectoderm, as do the more distal neurons of the olfactory system. (Ectodermal placodes and some of their other derivatives, including the lens and the inner ear, are described in Chs. 12 and 13.)

Occipital and Spinal Neural Crest Also Produce Major Components of the Peripheral Nervous System

The peripheral nervous system of the neck, trunk, and limbs includes the following three types of peripheral neurons: the peripheral sensory neurons, the cell bodies of which reside in the dorsal root ganglia, and the parasympathetic and sympathetic peripheral motor neurons, the cell bodies of which reside, respectively, in the sympathetic and parasympathetic ganglia. All three types of peripheral neurons, plus their associated glia, are derived from neural crest cells. This chapter describes the origin of these structures; their further development is covered in Chapter 5.

The Dorsal Root Ganglia Are Derived From Spinal Neural Crest. Some of the neural crest cells arising from the spinal neural tube come to rest in the space between the dorsal neural tube and the developing somites, where they aggregate to form small clumps in register with the somites (see Fig. 4–12). These clumps then differentiate into the segmental **dorsal root ganglia** of the spinal nerves, which house the sensory neurons that conduct impulses to the spinal cord from end organs in the viscera, body wall, and extremities. Experiments with the quail-chick chimera system demonstrate that most of the cells in each ganglion are derived from the neural tube at the corresponding level, although some may originate in neural crest adjacent to the caudal portion of the preceding somite.

It has been demonstrated that migrating neural crest cells prefer to migrate through the rostral half of sclerotomes. This preference is mediated by the repulsive effects of particular members of the **ephrin** family of proteins that are expressed by cells in the caudal portion of the sclerotome and recognized by receptors **(Eph tyrosine kinases)** expressed by neural crest cells. Experimental evidence also indicates that the survival and differentiation of the dorsal root ganglion anlagen may depend on a small protein called **brain-derived neurotrophic factor (BDNF),** which is secreted by the adjacent neural tube as well as other growth factors, including members of the **bone morphogenic protein (BMP)** family.

A pair of dorsal root ganglia develops at every segmental level except the first cervical and the second and third coccygeal levels (Fig. 4–15; also see Figs. 4–12 and 4–13B). Thus, there are 7 pairs of cervical, 12 pairs of thoracic, 5 pairs of lumbar, 5 pairs of sacral, and 1 pair of coccygeal dorsal root ganglia. The most cranial pair of cervical dorsal root ganglia (adjacent to the second cervical somite) appears on day 28, and the others form in craniocaudal succession over the next few days.

Postganglionic Parasympathetic Neurons of the Viscera Are Derived From the Occipitocervical and Sacral Neural Crests. Some peripheral motor neurons of the "two-neuron" parasympathetic autonomic nervous system arise from neural crest cells that migrate into the walls of the developing viscera, such as the heart, stomach, and bladder. The cell bodies of these neurons reside in

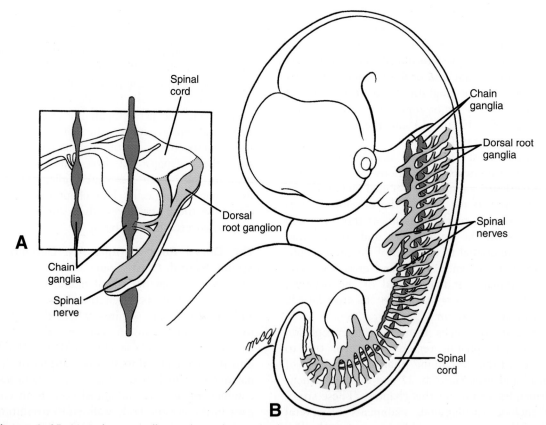

Figure 4–15. Neural crest cells produce chain ganglia and dorsal root ganglia at almost every spinal segment.

the peripheral **parasympathetic ganglia,** which provide parasympathetic motor innervation to the adjacent viscera. Crest cells originating from the occipitocervical region of the neural tube (the "vagal region") migrate in the gut wall mesenchyme to innervate all regions of the gut tube from the esophagus to the rectum. The parasympathetic ganglion cells in the most inferior regions of the gut, however, have a dual origin: Some arise from the occipitocervical neural crest, but others arise from the sacral neural crest.

The peripheral parasympathetic ganglia in the wall of the gut tube and its derivatives (collectively called **enteric ganglia**) may be connected to the central nervous system by axons that course either in the vagus nerve (cranial nerve X) or in pelvic splanchnic nerves from sacral levels 2, 3, and 4. The parasympathetic system is active during periods of "peace and relaxation" and stimulates the visceral organs to carry out their routine functions of housekeeping and digestion. Because the proximal neurons of the system are located in the cranial and sacral regions of the central nervous system, the parasympathetic system is called a **craniosacral system** (see Ch. 5).

The Sympathetic Chain Ganglia Are Innervated by Preganglionic Sympathetic Thoracolumbar Fibers. Some spinal cord neural crest cells migrate to a zone just ventral to the future dorsal root ganglia, where they form a series of condensations that develop into the **chain ganglia** of the sympathetic autonomic system (see Figs. 4–12C and 4–15). In the thoracic, lumbar, and sacral regions, one pair of chain ganglia forms in register with each pair of somites. In the cervical region, however, only three larger chain ganglia develop, and the coccygeal region has only a single chain ganglion, which forms at the first coccygeal level. Quail-chick cell marking experiments indicate that the neural crest cells that give rise to the cervical chain ganglia originate along the cervical neural tube, whereas the thoracic, lumbar, and sacral ganglia are formed by crest cells from these corresponding levels of the neural tube. Unlike the dorsal root ganglia, the chain ganglia do not depend on BDNF for survival, but they may depend on other growth factors such as **insulin-like growth factors (IGFs)** and **nerve growth factor (NGF).**

The neurons that develop in the chain ganglia become the peripheral neurons of the two-neuron sympathetic system. The sympathetic system provides autonomic motor innervation to most of the same structures as the parasympathetic system and exerts control over involuntary functions such as heartbeat, glandular secretions, and intestinal movements. By and large, however, the sympathetic system is activated during conditions of "fight or flight" and, therefore, has effects opposite to those of the parasympathetic system. Like the parasympathetic system, the sympathetic system consists of "two-neuron" pathways: the viscera are innervated by axons from the peripheral sympathetic neurons, which in turn receive axons from central sympathetic motor neurons in the spinal cord. These central sympathetic motor neurons are located at all 12 thoracic levels and at the first 3 lumbar levels. For that reason, the sympathetic system (central and peripheral) is called a **thoracolumbar system.**

Not all peripheral sympathetic neurons are located in the chain ganglia. The peripheral ganglia of some specialized sympathetic pathways develop from neural crest cells that congregate next to major branches of the dorsal aorta (see Fig. 4–12C and Ch. 5). One pair of these **prevertebral** or **preaortic ganglia** originates from the cervical neural crest and forms at the base of the celiac artery. Other, more diffuse ganglia develop in association with the superior mesenteric artery, the renal arteries, and the inferior mesenteric artery. These are formed by thoracic and lumbar neural crest cells.

The Spinal Cord Neural Crest Forms a Variety of Non-neuronal Structures in the Body

Spinal neural crest cells in humans are thought to form the inner and middle meningeal coverings of the spinal cord (the pia mater and arachnoid mater), as well as glial cells of the ganglia derived from the spinal neural crest (see Fig. 4–14). Some of the neural crest cells may differentiate into Schwann cells, which form the myelin sheaths (neurilemma) of peripheral nerves. Spinal neural crest cells also differentiate into the neurosecretory chromaffin cells of the adrenal medulla and into neurosecretory cells of the heart and lungs. The

Figure 4–16. Cytodifferentiation of the neural tube. *A, B,* Neuroepithelial cells within the primitive neural tube elongate just before mitosis. Initial waves of mitosis and differentiation form first the neuroblasts, which will become the neurons of the central nervous system. *A, C,* As neurons form, the neural tube becomes stratified into a ventricular layer (adjacent to the neural canal), a mantle layer (containing neuronal cell bodies), and a marginal layer (containing nerve fibers). Subsequent waves of mitosis and differentiation produce the glioblasts, which form several types of supporting cells of the central nervous system. The radial glia may provide pathways for neuroblast migration within the developing neural tube. (*A,* Modified from Rakic P. 1982. Early developmental events: cell lineages, acquisition of neuronal positions, and areal and laminar development. Neurosci Res Prog Bull 20:439. *B,* Photo courtesy of Dr. Kathryn Tosney.)

neural crest also gives rise to the melanocytes (pigment cells) of the skin and contributes to the outflow tracts of the heart (see Ch. 7).

THE NEURONS, GLIA, AND EPENDYMA OF THE CENTRAL NERVOUS SYSTEM DIFFERENTIATE FROM THE NERVE EPITHELIUM ADJACENT TO THE NEURAL CANAL

Neuroblasts Appear in the Rhombencephalic Region on Day 24

Cytodifferentiation of the neural tube commences in the rhombencephalic region just after the occipitocervical neural folds fuse and proceeds cranially and caudally as the tube zippers up. The precursors of most of the cell types of the future central nervous system—the neurons, some types of glial cells, and the ependymal cells that line the central canal of the spinal cord and the ventricles of the brain—are produced by proliferation in the layer of neuroepithelial cells that immediately surrounds the neural canal (Fig. 4–16). This layer of proliferating cells is called the **ventricular layer** of the differentiating neural tube. The first wave of cells produced in the ventricular layer consists of the **neuroblasts,** which will give rise to the neurons of the central nervous system. These neuroblasts migrate peripherally to establish a second layer, the **mantle layer,** external to the ventricular layer (see Fig. 4–16A, C). This neuron-containing layer develops into the **gray matter** of the central nervous system. The neuronal processes that sprout from the mantle layer neurons grow peripherally to establish a third layer, the **marginal layer,** which contains no neuronal cell bodies and becomes the **white matter** of the central nervous system.

The rearrangements of the mantle and marginal layers that take place during the maturation of the spinal cord are relatively simple and are described in the next section. The much more complex alterations that occur in the developing brain are discussed in Chapter 13.

Glioblasts and Ependymal Cells Are Produced After the Formation of Neuroblasts Ceases

As soon as the neuroepithelial layer lining the neural canal ceases to produce neuroblasts, it begins to produce a new cell type, the **glioblast** (see Fig. 4–16A). These cells differentiate into a variety of types of glial cells, including **astrocytes** and **oligodendrocytes.** The glia provides metabolic and structural support to the neurons of the central nervous system. Finally, the neuroepithelial layer differentiates in place to produce the specialized **ependymal cells** that line the cerebral ventricles and the central canal of the spinal cord (Fig. 4–16A, C). Elaborations of the ependyma are responsible for producing the cerebrospinal fluid (CSF), which fills the cerebral ventricles, the central canal of the spinal cord, and the subarachnoid space that surrounds the central nervous system. The CSF is under pressure and thus provides a fluid jacket that protects and supports the brain.

Dorsal and Ventral Columns Begin to Form in the Mantle Layer of the Spinal Cord at the End of the Fourth Week

Starting at the end of the fourth week, the neuroblasts in the mantle layer of the spinal cord become organized into four columns that run the length of the cord: a pair of **dorsal** or **alar columns** and a pair of **ventral** or **basal columns** (Fig. 4–17). Laterally, the alar and basal columns are separated by a groove called the **sulcus limitans;** dorsally and ventrally they are separated by acute thinnings of the neural tissue called, respectively, the **roof plate** and the **floor plate.** The cells of the ventral columns become the **somatic motor neurons** of the spinal cord and innervate somatic motor structures such as the voluntary (striated) muscles of the body wall and extremities. The cells of the dorsal columns develop into **association neurons,** which will interconnect the motor neurons of the ventral columns with neuronal processes that soon grow into the cord from the

Ventral (basal) columns

Dorsal (alar) columns

Intermediolateral cell columns (T1–L3 and S2–S4 only)

Figure 4–17. Neurons within the mantle layer of the neural tube become organized into two ventral motor (basal) columns and two dorsal sensory (alar) columns throughout most of the spinal cord and hindbrain. Intermediolateral cell columns also form at spinal levels T1–S4 and S2–S4.

sensory neurons of the dorsal root ganglia. In most regions of the cord—at all 12 thoracic levels, at lumbar levels L1 and L2, and at sacral levels S2 through S4—the neuroblasts in more dorsal regions of the basal columns segregate to form **intermediolateral cell columns** (see Fig. 4–17). The thoracic and lumbar intermediolateral cell columns contain the central autonomic motor neurons of the sympathetic system, whereas the intermediolateral cell columns in the sacral region contain central autonomic motor neurons of the parasympathetic system. The structure and function of these systems are discussed in the next chapter. In general, at any given level of the brain or spinal cord, the motor neurons form before the sensory elements appear.

Clinical Applications

MALFORMATIONS OF NEURAL TUBE CLOSURE

Neural Tube Defects Originate During the Third Week of Development

A failure of part of the neural tube to close **(spinal dysraphism)** disrupts both the differentiation of the central nervous system and the induction of the vertebral arches and can result in a number of developmental anomalies. These malformations generally involve the cranial or caudal neuropore, resulting in a defect of the cranial or lower lumbar and sacral regions of the central nervous system.

Failure of the neural tube to close disrupts the induction of the overlying vertebral arches so that the arches remain underdeveloped and fail to fuse along the dorsal midline to enclose the vertebral canal. The resulting open vertebral canal is a condition called **spina bifida.** In some cases of

spina bifida, the contents of the vertebral canal bulge into a membranous sac or **cele** that is continuous with the surrounding skin. The fact that spina bifida is quite common in the lower lumbar and upper sacral region suggests that neuropore closure or secondary neurulation may be involved in the etiology of these malformations.

Approximately 2500 infants with these defects are born each year in the United States. An additional 1500 fetuses afflicted with these malformations are aborted. Approximately 400,000 infants with spina bifida are born worldwide each year.

Spina Bifida and Related Defects of Cranial Neuropore Closure Result in a Range of Malformations

The clinical consequences of a defect in neural tube closure range from mild to fatal.

At the mildest extreme of spina bifida, the vertebral arches of a single vertebra fail to fuse, but the underlying neural tube differentiates normally and does not protrude from the vertebral canal. This condition, known as **spina bifida occulta,** may occur anywhere along the spinal cord but is most common at lower lumbar or sacral levels. The location of the defect is frequently indicated by a tuft of hair induced by the underlying abnormality, or by an angioma, pigmented nevus, or dimple (Fig. 4–18*A*). The fact that spina bifida at L5 or S1 is common in newborn infants but significantly rarer in adults suggests that it represents a normal variation in the timing of vertebral arch fusion at these levels. Moreover, genetic studies indicate that causes of this malformation may differ from the causes of more severe forms of spina bifida described later.

In more severe cases of spina bifida, the dura and the arachnoid protrude from the vertebral canal in the affected region, resulting in a **meningocele** (see Fig. 4–18*B*). If neural tissue as well as meninges protrudes, the defect is called a **meningomyelocele** (Fig. 4–19; also see 4–18*C*).

The neural tube defects in this series may not be fatal, but when they are severe, they cause motor and mental impairments that require lifelong management. The spinal cord and spinal nerves involved in a meningomyelocele, for example, often fail to develop normally, resulting in dysfunction of pelvic organs and legs. If the normal flow of CSF through the central nervous system is interrupted, the malformation may cause an increase in the volume and pressure of CSF in the cerebral ventricles. This condition, called **hydrocephaly** (see Fig. 13–10), is now often controlled by implanting a prosthetic shunt.

The most severe defects of neural tube development are those in which the neural folds not only fail to fuse but also fail to differentiate, invaginate, and, finally, separate from the surface ectoderm. Failure of the entire neural tube to close results in an anomaly called **craniorachischisis totalis,** which has been identified only in poorly developed embryos that underwent spontaneous abortion. If the defect involves only the cranial neural tube, a defect results in which the brain is represented by an exposed dorsal mass of undifferentiated neural tissue (Fig. 4–20*A*). This condition is called **exencephaly, anencephaly,** or **craniorachischisis.** Anencephalic embryos often survive to late fetal life or to term but invariably die within a few hours or days of birth. The analogous defect of spinal cord development, **rachischisis** or **myeloschisis,** is not always fatal but presents very difficult clinical problems. Failure of the neural tube to properly differentiate and close in the occipital and upper spinal regions is called an **inionschisis** (see Fig. 4–20*B*). Because the organs of anencephalic infants are often normal and healthy, the option of using these organs in organ transplants has frequently been considered, particularly since infant or child organ donors are always in short supply. Many arguments pro and con have been expressed, and there is reluctance to initiate such programs on a wide scale.

Herniation of the Brain May Also Occur in an Unrelated Spectrum of Anomalies

In a class of anomalies not related to failure of neural tube closure, differentiated brain and meninges may bulge from an unossified gap in the skull. This malformation is called a **meningoencephalocele.** If the ventricular cistern as well as the brain and meninges protrudes from the skull, the condition is called a **meningohydroencephalocele** (Fig. 4–21).

The Causes of Neural Tube Defects Are Variable and Possibly Multifactorial

Neural tube defects (NTDS) have no single genetic or teratogenic cause. The karyotype usually appears normal, although some animal mutants expressing similar defects exhibit chromosomal anomalies.

A genetic basis for some NTDS in humans is postulated, in part, on evidence that the frequency of meningomyelocele appears to be greater in siblings of affected individuals, although familial cases of NTDS may represent only about 3 percent of the total. However, the frequency of NTDS is higher in some populations and racial groups than in others. For example, the frequency of NTDS is approximately 0.1 percent in the United States as a whole, but it is 0.035 percent among African Americans. In contrast, the frequency of NTDS in some parts of India and in Ireland is on the order of 1.1 percent. Moreover, a rare condition called

Figure 4–18. *A,* Spina bifida occulta may involve minor anomalies of neural arch formation and may not result in malformations of the neural tube. This condition often occurs in the midsacral region and may be revealed by a small dimple, tuft of hair, or nevus overlying the defective vertebra. Defective development of neural arches may result in formation of a cyst or cele. This cyst is called a meningocele if it includes dura and arachnoid only (*B*) or a meningomyelocele if it also contains meninges and a portion of the spinal cord and associated spinal nerves (*C*). CSF = cerebrospinal fluid.

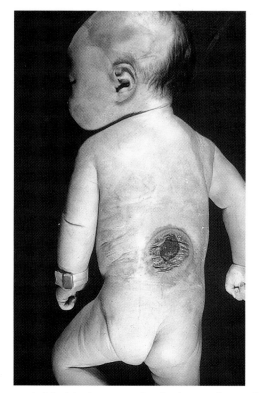

Figure 4–19. Meningomyeolocele in newborn. The spinal cord protrudes into the transparent meningeal sac (cele) in the lumbar region. (Photo courtesy of Children's Hospital Medical Center, Cincinnati, OH.)

Meckel syndrome, which is inherited as an autosomal recessive, may include craniorachischisis (see Fig. 12–29), whereas the autosomal dominant disorder called **brachydactyly syndrome** may also be characterized by exencephaly. In addition, an autosomal dominant spectrum of malformations called **Waardenburg syndrome,** which sometimes includes spina bifida, may result from mutations of the *Pax-3* gene, which also appears to be the basis for NTDS in **splotch** mouse mutants (see the Experimental Principles section). Other forms of Waardenburg syndrome may be caused by mutations of a microphthalmia transcription factor (MiTF), by mutations of endothelin-3 or one of its receptors or by mutations of the SRY-related transcription factor SOX10 (see Experimental Principles section of Ch. 5). In addition, mutation of cytoskeletal components as well as factors in the sonic hedgehog signaling pathway have been implicated in the development of spina bifida.

Teratogens that induce NTDS in animals and humans have also been identified, opening the

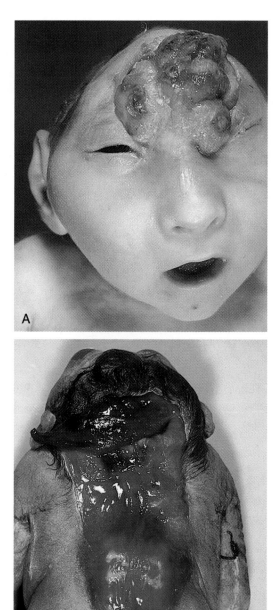

Figure 4–20. Anomalies resulting from failure of neurulation. Although the neural folds may fail to neurulate in almost any region, the most frequent site is the cranial neuropore, resulting in the condition of craniorachischisis or anencephaly (*A*). Occasionally, more caudal regions of the neural tube may fail to form and differentiate, as in this case of inionschisis (*B*). (Photos courtesy of Children's Hospital Medical Center, Cincinnati, OH.)

Figure 4–21. *A, B,* Meningohydroencephalocele. This anomaly may form through defective ossification of the occipital bone and probably is not a consequence of defective closure of the neural tube. (*A,* Photo courtesy of Children's Hospital Medical Center, Cincinnati, OH.)

possibility that some human NTDS may be caused by environmental toxins or nutritional factors. For example, studies on experimental animals have implicated retinoic acid, insulin, high plasma glucose levels, and trypan blue in development of NTDS. Factors implicated in the induction of NTDS in humans include the antiepileptic drug **valproic acid, maternal diabetes,** and **hyperthermia.** It has been suggested that valproic acid may interfere with folate metabolism, and a substantial body of evidence now shows that administration of 0.4 mg of **folic acid** per day during pregnancy significantly reduces the risk of spina bifida and anencephaly, even in the babies of mothers who have previously given birth to infants suffering from NTDS. Indeed, there is now evidence that some families with spina bifida offspring may harbor mutations of genes that regulate folate and vitamin B (cobalamin) metabolism. These include mutations of 5, 10 methyltetrahydrofolate reductase (MTHFR) or of methionine synthase reductase (MTRR). The risk of spina bifida may be especially high in mothers harboring both MTHFR and MTRR homozygous mutant genotypes.

Experimental Principles

SEGMENTATION OF THE PARAXIAL MESODERM

Regulated Coordinate Segmentation of the Paraxial Mesoderm Produces Specific Numbers of Paired Somites

Cells ingressing through the human primitive streak interact with previously formed paraxial mesoderm that then segments into somitomeres. All but the most cranial seven somitomeres sequentially differentiate into somites, giving rise to the distinguishable segmental character of the developing trunk. Initiation of this process of **somitogenesis** in mammals appears to require the action of **fibroblast growth factors** and a secreted protein that associates with the cell surface and extracellular matrix, **Wnt-3a.** Coordination of the segmentation mechanism, however, apparently requires activity of the mammalian gene *Notch-1,* a homolog of the fruitfly gene *Notch*. *Notch-1* is initially expressed within the presomitic paraxial mesoderm, and its role in segmentation of the paraxial mesoderm is inferred from the behavior of paraxial mesoderm in *Notch-1* knockout mice. In these mutants, segmentation is delayed or unequal and is uncoordinated from one side of the embryo to the other. Because *Notch-1* encodes a transmembrane receptor implicated in cell-cell cohesion, it may regulate the cell interactions required to maintain integrity of the somite itself while allowing cell dissociation at somite boundaries. Other regulatory genes such as *Pax-3*, *Pax-7*, and *Pax-1* are also expressed in presomitic mesoderm or at somite borders, but their roles in somite segmentation are unclear (see later).

Somites Produce Vertebrae Characteristic of Specific Regions and Segments of the Trunk

Although somites throughout the trunk are morphologically indistinguishable, they become specified to form structures characteristic of particular body regions. Moreover, the characteristic development of specific vertebrae seems to be related to the intrinsic properties of their particular somitic precursor. Somites transplanted to another region will form structures typical of the region of their origin. Thoracic somites transplanted to the lumbar region, for example, form typical thoracic vertebrae and ribs at the ectopic lumbar site. Based on experiments such as these, it has been suggested that somites acquire their regional specificity during early stages of segmentation.

As noted in the descriptive section of this chapter, specific numbers of presumptive cervical, thoracic, lumbar, sacral, and coccygeal somites are formed in human embryos. However, significant variation in the numbers of somites and vertebrae occur within different vertebrate organisms. The number of cervical vertebrae in amphibians, for example, is only 3 or 4, whereas the number of cervical vertebrae in geese is 17. Mice and even giraffes possess the same number of cervical vertebrae as humans (seven), but mice have 13 (not 12) thoracic vertebrae, 6 (not 5) lumbar vertebrae, and 4 (not 5) sacral vertebrae. Snakes, of course, have hundreds of vertebrae. What factors specify regional differences in the vertebrae, and how is the number of vertebrae in any given region determined?

Territories of *Hox* Gene Expression Regulate Regional Specification of the Vertebrae

Interestingly, the most cranial expression of the vertebrate *Hox* genes as shown by in situ hybridization or use of the *Lacz* reporter gene typically occurs at approximate boundaries between somites (Fig. 4–22). This arrangement results in unique combinations of *Hox* gene expression at virtually every segment of the trunk, an organization consistent with a model of *Homc* arthropod segment specification formulated by Edward Lewis, that states that homeotic genes may specify segment diversity through a **combinatorial code.** Is it possible that *Hox* genes in vertebrates, including humans, regulate differentiation of somites by a mechanism similar to that by which *Homc* genes in *Drosophila* specify development of specific body segments?

Alterations of *Hox* Gene Expression Result in Homeotic Transformations of Vertebral Segments

"Loss-of-function" and "gain-of-function" mutants of *Hox* genes normally expressed in the trunk result in intriguing alterations of the identity of skeletal segments in the mouse. For example, a null mutation of *Hoxc-8* leads to transformation of the first lumbar vertebra into a 14th thoracic vertebra, complete with ribs (Fig. 4–23). Moreover, the eighth rib, not the seventh rib, is now the most inferior rib directly attached to the sternum, which also develops an additional ossification center or sternebra. Other, more subtle transformations of thoracic vertebral segments and ribs occur between T7 and T13 (included within the domain of *Hoxc-8* expression), and, in general, the loss-of-function mutation of *Hoxc-8* results in transformation of these segments into the adjacent cranial segment (see Fig. 4–23). Thus, the null mutation of *Hoxc-8* **"cranializes"** somitic segments of the trunk. Similarly, a loss-of-function null mutant of *Hoxa-4* also cranializes the third cervical vertebra, which develops a small dorsal process similar to that normally

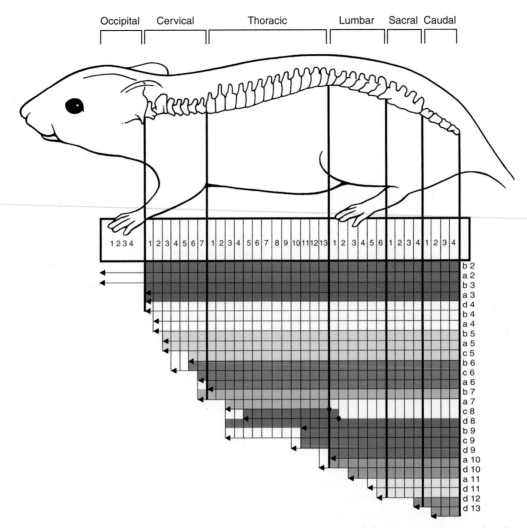

Figure 4–22. Cranial expression boundaries of *Hox* genes in mice parallel their sequence on the chromosomes and sensitivities to retinoic acid (see also Fig. 3–17). The resulting distribution creates specific combinatorial codes that specify development of individual somites or small groups of adjacent somites. It is not possible, however, to determine whether cranial expression boundaries occur precisely between somites or between the recombined caudal and cranial halves of the sclerotomes (prevertebrae) or both, at different times. (From Hunt P, Krumlauf R. 1992. *Hox* codes and positional specification in vertebrate embryonic axes. Annu Rev Cell Biol 8:227.)

associated with the second cervical vertebra. In addition, formation of the small paired rib anlagen that normally forms on the seventh cervical vertebra is suppressed, transforming the seventh cervical vertebra into one more reminiscent of the sixth.

A gain-of-function transgenic mutant of *Hoxa*-7 has the reverse effect. Normally, the cranial expression boundary of *Hoxa*-7 is located at the third thoracic vertebra, but in this gain-of-function mutant, *Hoxa*-7 is ectopically expressed within more cranial regions. In these animals, development of vertebrae is **"caudalized"** so that the

atlas (first cervical vertebra), which normally lacks a vertebral body, now possesses a vertebral body like the second cervical vertebra. The axis (second cervical vertebra), which normally possesses an odontoid process (dens) now lacks a dens and assumes a morphology more reminiscent of the third cervical vertebra. Moreover, an additional cervical vertebra develops in a position just cranial to the former atlas. This **atavistic** vertebra, which normally forms in some reptiles, is called a **proatlas.** Normally, the only rudiments of the proatlas in mammals are small amounts of bone at the base of

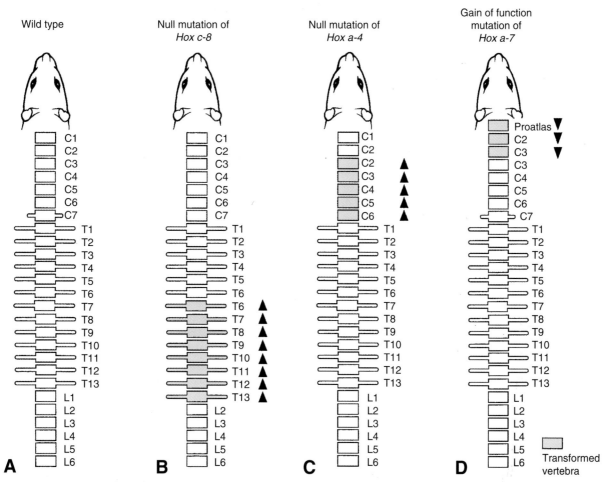

Figure 4–23. Homeotic transformation of vertebral segments in loss-of-function and gain-of-function *Hox* genes in mice. Null mutations of *Hoxc-8* (compare *B* with *A*) and *Hoxa-4* (compare *C* with *A*) cranialize vertebrae within their normal expression domains. A gain-of-function mutation of *Hoxa-7* caudalizes vertebrae outside its normal expression domain (compare *D* with *A*). (Modified from Conlon RA. 1995. Retinoic acid and pattern formation in vertebrates. TIG 11:314.)

the occipital bone (base of the skull) and at the tip of the dens (see Fig. 4–23). Evidence suggests that *Hox* genes may not always regulate segment identity; rather, changes in cell proliferation could mediate changes in shape. This controversy is being intensely investigated.

Disruptions of Retinoic Acid Activity Also Produce Homeotic Transformations of Vertebral Segments

Although it seems possible that regional and segmental specification of the vertebrae is a conse-

quence of the combinatorial expression of *Hox* genes, factors initially responsible for establishing cranial limits of specific *Hox* gene expression are still poorly understood. Nonetheless, some studies have implicated a gradient of **retinoic acid (RA)** along the longitudinal axis of the trunk in this process. First, it is known that more cranially expressed *Hox* genes are more sensitive to induction by RA (see Fig. 3–17). Moreover, it has been suggested that the primitive streak may be the source of the RA gradient in normal vertebrate embryos. It is, therefore, of interest that transgenic knockouts of two or more members of the family of **retinoic acid receptors** results in the **cranialization** of vertebral segments. This effect is similar to that observed in the homeotic null mutations of

Hoxc-8 and *Hoxa-4* described earlier (see Fig. 4–23). Conversely, the **ectopic application of excess retinoic acid** results in the **caudalization** of vertebral segments, similar to that occurring in the *Hoxa-7* "homeotic" gain-of-function mutant (see Fig. 4–23).

The mechanism by which segmental identity is achieved in vertebrates is undoubtedly far more complex than implied by this brief discussion. For example, in contrast to the loss-of-function *Hox* mutations discussed above, a loss-of-function mutation of *Hoxa-6* has been shown to caudalize the seventh cervical vertebra as indicated by its development of a rib. Some other *Hox* gene knockouts simultaneously cranialize one region of the spine and caudalize another region (like *Hox 11* genes discussed in the Experimental Principles section of Ch. 11). Thus, although RA and *Hox* genes appear to play a role in craniocaudal specification of the vertebrae, they may only establish the general pattern of regional specification. Other factors, including other switch genes, may fine-tune the regulation of specific segmental differentiation.

Inductive Mechanisms in Formation of the Neural Tube and Differentiation of the Somite

The Notochord and Neural Tube Induce Development of the Sclerotome.
Recall from the descriptive section of this chapter that somites rapidly split into subunits soon after they are formed. At first they segment into a dorsolateral dermomyotome and a ventromedial sclerotome (see Fig. 4–1). The sclerotomes then split and recombine to form the vertebrae and intervertebral discs (see Descriptive Embryology in this chapter). The dermomyotomes split into a dermatome, which contributes to the formation of the dermis and to the myotome, which forms trunk musculature (see Fig. 4–6).

It now appears that segmentation and differentiation of these somitic subunits are under the control of regulatory genes and growth factors that act through specific **inductive mechanisms.** The process of **induction** is defined as the stimulation of a specific developmental pathway in one group of cells (the **responding tissue**) by a closely approximated group of cells (the **inducing tissue**). The inducing tissue typically produces an **inducing substance** that may require direct cell-cell contact to produce its effect on the responding tissue or that may diffuse and act over short spaces or gaps between the inducing and responding tissues.

Indeed, even though somites contain positional or regional information before their differentiation into sclerotomes and dermomyotomes, the cells within newly formed somites are not specifically committed to any specific tissue lineage. The differentiation of somitic subregions appears to require inductive signals from adjacent tissues. For example, if a notochord or neural tube floor plate tissue (see later) is grafted into a host embryo next to the lateral side of a somite, the dermomyotome fails to form, and, instead, this lateral somitic subregion gives rise to a sclerotome. Conversely, when regions of the notochord are experimentally removed, the entire somite in these regions develops exclusively into a dermomyotome. Similar failure of sclerotome formation occurs in mutant mice with disrupted development of the notochord (such as **truncate, pintail,** and **Danforth's short tail**). Likewise, when ventromedial parts of the somite are grafted to more dorsolateral regions, they develop into dermomyotomes rather than into sclerotomes. Moreover, by performing the grafting experiments at different stages of paraxial mesoderm and somite development, it has been shown that the reprogramming of the somitic mesoderm is only possible at early stages of somite development. As the somite ages, developmental fates of respective somitic subregions quickly become irreversibly restricted.

The primary signal responsible for sclerotome induction appears to be a product of the vertebrate homolog of the *Drosophila* hedgehog genes, a small peptide called **sonic hedgehog (Shh).** In situ hybridization studies show that mRNA of sonic hedgehog is strongly expressed in cells of the notochord and the floor plate of the neural tube, whereas immunocytochemical studies show that the Shh protein is also synthesized within these cells during the period of somite differentiation (Figs. 4–24 and 4–25). It now also seems likely that a **winged-helix** transcription factor, **HNF-3β,** plays a pivotal role in the activation of the Shh gene within the notochord and floor plate.

Figure 4–24. Early expression of Shh mRNA in the 9-day postcoitum (dpc) notochord is shown by blue stain with in situ hybridization technique *B,* whereas immunocytochemistry (light brown stain) shows Shh peptides in notochord and floor plate of neural tube (*A, B*). At later stage (9.5 dpc) the floor plate also transcribes Shh mRNA (*D*) and express Shh peptides (*C, D*). (Modified from Marti E, Takada R, Bumcrot DA, et al. 1995. Distribution of sonic hedgehog peptides in the developing chick and mouse embryo. Development 121:2537.)

The use of an in vitro assay for somitic mesoderm differentiation also reveals that the Shh protein can induce the development of the sclerotome from paraxial mesoderm over relatively long distances. When presomitic mesoderm is cultured alone or in the presence of explanted pieces of ventral neural tube (including the floor plate), notochord, dorsal neural tube, or surface ectoderm, only notochord or ventral neural tube can induce expression of specific sclerotome marker genes (the basic helix-loop-helix transcription factor, the M-twist, and the paired-box containing transcription factor, *Pax-1*). Moreover, these inducing tissues can exert their effect even when located as far as 0.2 mm from the responding tissue. These experiments also demonstrate that this inductive mechanism is mediated by a diffusible fragment of the autoproteolytically cleaved Shh protein, specifically, its N-terminal fragment.

Other regulatory genes have also been demonstrated to play key roles in development of the sclerotome. For example, normal development of the dorsal vertebral arches requires induction of the homeobox gene **Msh,** and **Pax-1** expression is required specifically for development of the vertebral bodies and intervertebral discs (see Fig. 4–25 and see later).

The Dorsal Neural Tube and Surface Ectoderm Induce the Dermomyotome. Not surprisingly, tissues primarily responsible for inducing the dermomyotome are those that develop in the vicinity of the dorsolateral region of the somite; namely, the surface ectoderm and dorsal part of the neural tube. However, in contrast to induction of the sclerotome, induction of the dermomyotome requires a much closer association of paraxial meso-

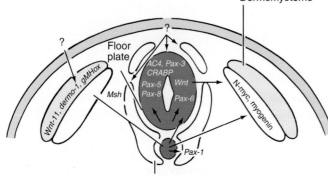

Figure 4–25. Inductive interactions between notochord, neural tube, somites, and surface ectoderm during formation of the vertebrae and development of the spinal cord, trunk musculature, and dermis.

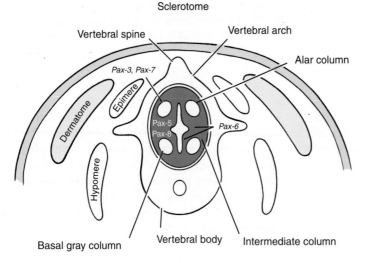

derm (responding tissue) with the surface ectoderm and dorsal neural tube (inducing tissues). In this system, the inductive signal has been identified as cell surface- and extracellular matrix-associated proteins encoded by members of the ***Wnt* gene family** (see Fig. 4–25). Not only are the isoforms *Wnt-1*, *Wnt-3*, and *Wnt-4* expressed within the dorsal neural tube during the period of dermomy-

otome, myotome, and dermatome induction, but exogenous application of Shh and *Wnt-1* or *Wnt-3* is sufficient to induce the expression of muscle-specific markers like **N-*myc*** and **myogenin** within the myotomes (see Fig. 4–25). On the other hand, specific inducers of the dermatome-specific marker **gMHox** have not been identified but appear to be produced by the surface ectoderm. Other dermatome-specific markers including **Wnt-11** and the twist-related basic helix-loop-helix transcriptional factor **dermo-1** are also induced during differentiation of the dermatome (see Fig. 4–25).

Differentiation of the dermomyotomes also requires an inductive Shh signal from the notochord and ventral neural tube. Long-term interaction with Shh is required for differentiation of sclerotomes by the notochord or floor plate. Shh apparently must act only briefly, however, upon the dorsolateral region of the somite at early stages of dermomyotome differentiation, apparently to induce their **competence** to respond to inductive signals from the surface ectoderm. Dorsoventral differentiation of the somite, therefore, seems to require the **synergistic interaction** between dorsal and ventral growth factors and regulatory genes (see Fig. 4–25).

Dorsoventral Differentiation of the Neural Tube: Inducing Tissues May Also Behave as Responding Tissues. Although evidence was discussed supporting a role for the notochord and floor plate together in the induction of the sclerotome, experiments with avian embryos demonstrate that the notochord is also the inducer of the floor plate. Moreover, these experiments imply that induction requires prolonged direct contact between notochord and floor plate. Similar studies have shown that differentiating floor plate tissue itself may also act as an inducer of the floor plate **(self-induction)**. This may be explained by the fact that the notochord's inductive activity is mediated by Shh, which also induces expression of Shh within the floor plate along with floor plate-specific proteins such as FP1, FP2, and SC1 (see Fig. 4–25).

Grafting experiments also show that notochord and/or floor plate, in turn, can induce motor neurons characteristic of the ventral neural tube even when grafted to lateral and dorsal regions of the presumptive spinal cord. The induction of ventral markers in these ectopic locations is accompanied by a decrease in expression of markers typical of the dorsal spinal cord, including the antigen AC4, neural crest cell markers, and cellular retinoic acid binding protein (CRABP), which is normally localized within spinal relay neurons. Conversely, only dorsal neural tube markers are expressed in neural tube when notochord and floor plate are experimentally extirpated from the developing embryo. Finally, evidence that Shh is the prime mediator of differentiation of the ventral neural tube is strongly supported by studies showing that purified Shh by itself is capable of inducing the development of motor neurons in culture. Although the differentiation of neurons within the dorsal neural tube may be under independent control, the experiments discussed earlier support the idea that a ventrodorsal gradient of Shh, generated by the notochord and floor plate, may play a pivotal role in ventrodorsal patterning of the neural tube.

Pax **Genes Are Expressed Within the Neural Tube and Sclerotome.** Nine different *Pax* genes have been identified, *Pax-1* to *Pax-9*, and all appear to behave as transcription factors, capable of binding to specific sequences of DNA. All of these genes contain a specialized paired domain, whereas some contain the paired-type homeodomain and others contain only the first helix of this domain. They are all related to the *Drosophila* **segmentation genes** (see the Experimental Principles section of Ch. 3).

The expression patterns described for the *Pax* genes are consistent with their possible roles in specification of different regions of the central nervous system and the somites. During neural tube induction, for example, *Pax-3* and *Pax-7* are expressed only in the dorsal region of the tube, in the alar (sensory) columns, in the roof plate, and in neural crest derivatives. *Pax-6* is localized within the ventricular zone of the intermediate and basal regions of the neural tube, and *Pax-5* and *Pax-8* are expressed in the longitudinal intermediate gray columns. As noted above, specific regions of the somites also express specific *Pax* genes. Notochord and/or the floor plate or Shh by itself induces the expression of *Pax-1* within the ventromedial region of the somite, the presumptive sclerotomes, whereas induction by surface ectoderm results in the eventual restriction of expression of *Pax-3* and *Pax-7* within the dorsolateral region of the somite (see Fig. 4–25).

Pax **Gene Mutations Appear to Underline Some Anomalies of the Mammalian Axial Skeleton and Neural Tube.** Several well-defined mutations of specific *Pax* genes have now been correlated with anomalies of the vertebral bodies, vertebral discs, spina bifida, and exencephaly. Several **undulated** mouse mutants, for example, that exhibit a spectrum of abnormalities of vertebral body and vertebral disc formation have been shown to harbor mutations of their *Pax-1* loci. However, vertebral arches of the vertebrae that arise from a region of the sclerotome where *Pax-1* is not expressed are normal in these mutants.

Murine **splotch** mutants, however, exhibit the spina bifida and exencephalic spectrum of anomalies described in the Clinical Applications section of this chapter and also display abnormalities of neural crest cell migration and differentiation. Thus, tissues whose embryonic precursors normally express *Pax-3* appear to be specifically affected. Indeed, these mice harbor mutations of *Pax-3*, including splice-site mutations, chromosomal deletions, and amino acid substitutions.

More recently, it has been demonstrated that some humans diagnosed with disorders of neural crest migration and displaying developmental characteristics of splotch mutant mice also possess mutations of *Pax-3*. This autosomal dominant syndrome is called **Waardenburg syndrome type 1** (see the Clinical Applications sections of Chs. 4 and 5). However, although mutations of *Pax-3* have been cited as an underlying cause of spina bifida in some patients with Waardenburg syndrome, it has been difficult to establish linkage between familial **NTDS** and the *Pax-3* gene, suggesting that *Pax-3* is not a major gene for NTDS in humans. The roles of other genes in development of NTDS in mice, including open brain (*opb*) and *patched* and their genetic and metabolic regulation and interactions, are subjects of considerable current interest.

A Homologue of the *Drosophila* Segment Polarity Gene Patched Is Implicated in Regulation of the Shh Signal in Development of Vertebrae and Neural Tube. In situ hybridization studies have shown that mRNA encoding the mouse homologue of the *Drosophila* segment polarity gene patched (*ptc*) is expressed in the ventral neural tube and ventromedial sclerotome in conjunction with Shh expression in the notochord. The likelihood that Shh either directly or indirectly induces patched in mice is implied by the induction of the *ptc* mRNA in the dorsal neural tube when Shh is ectopically expressed in neighboring cells and the induction of *ptc* in the cranial region of the limb buds of Strong's luxoid mice, in the region of an ectopic zone of polarizing activity that expresses Shh (see Experimental Principles section of Ch 11). Studies of patched in *Drosophila* and clinical studies of humans support the idea that patched normally functions to counteract the inductive effects of Shh on other downstream genes such as *Wnt-1* and transforming growth factor-β by repressing their expression.

Mutations of PTCH in Humans Result in Spina Bifida. Messenger RNA encoding *ptc* in mice is expressed in hair and whisker follicles, pharyngeal arches, tongue, and toothbuds. The likelihood that these tissues utilize the Shh-> patched signaling pathway is also supported by the spectrum of malformations exhibited in humans with mutations of the human homologue of patched, PTCH. Mutations of PTCH result in Gorlin syndrome (nevoid basal carcinoma syndrome, NBCCS), which maps to chromosome 9q22.3. Gorlin syndrome is an autosomal dominant disorder occurring in about 1:100,000 individuals. It is characterized by spina bifida, bifid ribs, polydactyly, syndactyly (see Ch. 11), odontogenic keratocysts, craniofacial and brain anomalies, generalized overgrowth, and a predisposition to development of a variety of cancers, including basal cell carcinoma, medulloblastomas, ovarian fibromas, meningiomas, and others (see Ch. 14 for related discussion). PTCH may also be characterized as a human tumor suppressor gene (see discussion in Ch. 14) as is DPC4 of the MAD gene family (Ch. 3) and WT-1 (Ch. 10).

SUGGESTED READING

Descriptive Embryology

Bronner-Fraser M. 1982. Distribution of latex beads and retinal pigment epithelial cells along the ventral neural crest pathway. Dev Biol 91:50

Christ B, Jacob M, Jacob HJ. 1983. On the origin and development of the ventrolateral abdominal muscles in the avian embryo. Anat Embryol 166:87

Christ B, Ordahl CP. 1995. Early stages of chick somite formation. Anat Embryol 191:381

Grasser RF. 1979. Evidence that sclerotomal cells do not migrate medially during normal embryonic development in the rat. Am J Anat 154:509

Jacobson A. 1988. Somitomeres: mesodermal segments of vertebrate embryos. Development 104:209

Jacobson A, Tam PPL. 1982. Cephalic neurulation in

the mouse embryo analyzed by SEM and morphometry. Anat Rec 203:375

Karfunkel P. 1974. Mechanisms of neural tube formation. Int Rev Cytol 38:245

Lash JW, Ostrovsky D. 1986. On the formation of somites. p. 547. In Browder LW (ed): Developmental Biology. A Comprehensive Synthesis. Vol. 2. The Cellular Basis of Morphogenesis. Plenum Press, New York

Le Douarin NM. 1980. The ontogeny of the neural crest in avian embryo chimeras. Nature 286:663

Meier S. 1984. Somite formation and its relationship to metameric patterning of the mesoderm. Cell Differ 14:235

Morriss-Kay GM. 1981. Growth and development of pattern in the cranial neural epithelium of rat embryos during neurulation. J Embryol Exp Morphol 65:225

Müller F, O'Rahilly R. 1980. The early development of the nervous system in staged insectivore and primate embryos. J Comp Neurol 193:741

Müller F, O'Rahilly R. 1987. The development of the human brain, the closure of the cranial neuropore, and the beginning of secondary neurulation at stage 12. Anat Embryol 176:413

Noden DM. 1980. The migration and cytodifferentiation of cranial neural crest cells. p. 3. In Pratt RM, Christiansen RL (eds): Current Research Trends in Prenatal Craniofacial Development. Elsevier/North Holland, New York

O'Rahilly R, Müller F. 1986. The meninges in human development. J Neuropathol Exp Neurol 45:588

O'Rahilly R, Müller F. 1989. Bidirectional closure of the rostral neuropore. Am J Anat 184:259

Robinson V, Smith A, Flenniken AM, Wilkinson DG. 1997. Roles of Eph receptors and ephrins in neural crest pathfinding. Cell Tissue Res 290:265

Sanes JR. 1983. Roles of extracellular matrix in neural development. Annu Rev Physiol 45:581

Schoenwolf G. 1984. Histological and ultrastructural studies of secondary neurulation in mouse embryos. Am J Anat 169:361

Tam PPL. 1984. The histogenetic capacity of tissues in the caudal end of the embryonic axis of the mouse. J Embryol Exp Morphol 82:253

Tamarin A. 1983. Stage 9 macaque embryos studied by scanning electron microscopy. J Anat 137:765

Clinical Applications

Campbell LR, Dayton DH, Sohal GS. 1986. Neural tube defects: a review of human and animal studies on the etiology of neural tube defects. Teratology 34:171

Harris MJ, Juriloff DM. 1999. Mini-review: toward understanding mechanisms of genetic neural tube defects in mice. Teratology 60:292

Lammer EJ, Sever LE, Oakley GP Jr. 1987. Teratogen update: valproic acid. Teratology 35:465

Müller F, O'Rahilly R. 1984. Cerebral dysraphia (future anencephaly) in a human twin embryo at stage 13. Teratology 30:167

Nau H. 1994. Valproic Acid-Induced Neural Tube Defects. Neural Tube Defects. CIBA Symp. 181. John Wiley Sons, New York, p. 144

Shewmon DA, Capron AM, Peacock WJ, Schulman B. 1989. The use of anencephalic infants as organ sources: a critique. JAMA 261:1773

van der Put NM, Thomas CM, Eskes TK, et al. 1997. Altered folate and vitamin B_{12} metabolism in families with spina bifida offspring. QJM 90:505

Wilson A, Platt R, Wu Q, et al. 1999. A common variant in methionine synthase reductase combined with low cobalamin (vitamin B_{12}) increases risk for spina bifida. Mol Genet Metab 67:317

Experimental Principles

Conlon RA. 1995. Retinoic acid and pattern formation in vertebrates. TIG 11:314

Chidabaram A, Goldstein AM, Gailani MR, et al. 1996. Mutations in the human homolog of the *Drosophila* patched gene in Caucasian and African-American nevoid basal cell carcinoma syndrome patients. Cancer Res 56:4599

Gurdon JB, Mohun TJ, Sharpe CR, Taylor MV. 1989. Embryonic induction and muscle gene activation. Trends Genet 5:51

Hamburger V. 1988. The Heritage of Experimental Embryology. Hans Spemann and the Organizer. Oxford University Press, New York

Jacobson AG, Sater A. 1988. Features of embryonic induction. Development 104:341

Jessell TM, Melton DA. 1992. Diffusible factors in vertebrate embryonic induction. Cell 68:257

Fan C-M, Tessier-Lavigne M. 1994. Patterning of mammalian somites by surface ectoderm and notochord: evidence for sclerotome induction by a hedgehog homolog. Cell 79:1175

Fan C-M, Porter JA, Chiang C, et al. 1995. Long-range sclerotome induction by sonic hedgehog: direct role of the amino-terminal cleavage product and modulation by the cyclic AMP signaling pathway. Cell 81:457

Günther T, Struwe M, Aguzzi A, Schughart K. 1994. Open brain, a new mouse mutant with severe neural tube defects, shows altered gene expression patterns in the developing spinal cord. Development 120:3119

Hol FA, Hamel BCJ, Geurds MPA, et al. 1995. A frameshift mutation in the gene for *Pax 3* in a girl with spina bifida and mild signs of Waardenburg syndrome. J Med Genet 32:52

Hunt P, Krumlauf R. 1992. *Hox* codes and positional specification in vertebrate embryonic axes. Annu Rev Cell Biol 8:277

Johnson R, Rothman AL, Xie J, et al. 1996. Human homolog of patched, a candidate gene for basal cell nevus syndrome. Science 272:1668

Kessel M, Balling R, Gruss P. 1990. Variations in cervical vertebrae after expressions of *Hox1.1* transgene in mice. Cell 61:301

Kostic D, Capecchi MR. 1994. Targeted disruptions of the murine *Hoxa-4* and *Hoxa-6* genes result in homeotic transformations of components of the vertebral column. Mech Dev 45:231

Krull CE, Lansford R, Gale NW, et al. 1997. Interactions of Eph-related receptors and ligands confer rostrocaudal pattern to trunk neural crest migration. Curr Biol 7:571

LaBonne C, Bronner-Fraser M. 1999. Molecular mechanisms of neural crest formation. Annu Rev Cell Dev Biol 15:81

LeMouellic H, Lallemand Y, Brûlet P. 1992. Homeosis in the mouse induced by a null mutation in the *HOX-3.1* gene. Cell 69:251

Mansouri A, Stoykova A, Gruss P. 1994. *Pax* genes in development. J Cell Sci Suppl 18:35

Marigo V, Scott MP, Johnson RL, et al. 1996. Conservation in hedgehog signaling: induction of a chicken patched homolog by sonic hedgehog in the developing limb. Development 122:1225

Marti E, Takada R, Bumcrot DA et al. 1995. Distribution of sonic hedgehog peptides in the developing chick and mouse embryo. Development 121:2537

Monsoro-Burg A-H, Bontoux M, Teillet M-A, Le-Douarin N. 1994. Heterogeneity in the development of vertebrae. Proc Natl Acad Sci U S A 591:10435

Münsterberg AE, Kitajewski J, Bumcrot DA, et al. 1995. Combinatorial signaling by sonic hedgehog and Wnt family members induces myogenic *bHIH* gene expression in the somite. Gene Devel 9:2911

Robinson V, Smith A, Flenniken AM, Wilkinson DG. 1997. Roles of Eph receptors and ephrins in neural crest pathfinding. Cell Tissue Res 290:265

Roelink H, Augsburger A, Heemskerk J, et al. 1994. Floor plate and motor neuron induction by Vhh-1, a vertebrate homolog of hedgehog expressed by the notochord. Cell. 76:761

Tam PPL, Trainor PA. 1993. Specification and segmentation of the paraxial mesoderm. Anat Embryol 189:275

Tassabehji M, Newton VE, Leverton K, et al. 1994. *PAX3* gene structure and mutations: close analogies between Waardenburg syndrome and the Splotch mouse. Hum Mol Genet 3:1069

Yamada T, Pfaff SL, Edlund T, Jessell TM. Control of cell pattern in the neural tube: motor neuron induction by diffusible factors from notocord and floor plate. Cell 73:673

5

Development of the Peripheral Nervous System

Summary

The nervous system consists of complex networks of neurons that carry information from the sensory receptors to the central nervous system (CNS); integrate, process, and store it; and return motor impulses to various effector organs in the body. The peripheral nervous system and its central pathways are traditionally divided into two systems. The **somatic nervous system** is responsible for carrying conscious sensations and for innervating the voluntary (striated) muscles of the body. The **autonomic nervous system** is strictly motor and controls most of the involuntary, visceral activities of the body. The autonomic system itself consists of two divisions: the **parasympathetic system,** which, in general, promotes the visceral activities characteristic of periods of peace and relaxation, and the **sympathetic system,** which controls the involuntary activities that occur under stressful "fight or flight" conditions.

Neurons originate from three embryonic tissues: from the neuroepithelium lining the neural canal (see Ch. 4), from the neural crest, and (in the case of some cranial nerve ganglia) from specialized regions of ectoderm in the head and neck called **ectodermal placodes** (see Ch. 13). As described in Chapter 4, all the postcranial peripheral ganglia are formed by migrating neural crest cells. The sensory **dorsal root ganglia** that condense next to the spinal cord to register with each pair of somites house the sensory cells that relay information from receptors in the body to the CNS. The **sympathetic chain ganglia** that also flank the spinal cord and the **prevertebral ganglia** that form next to branches of the abdominal aorta contain the peripheral neurons of the two-neuron sympathetic pathways. Finally, the **parasympathetic ganglia** embedded in the walls of the visceral organs contain the peripheral neurons of the two-neuron parasympathetic system.

While the ganglia are forming, somatic motor axons begin to grow out from the basal columns of the spinal cord (see Ch. 4), forming a pair of **ventral roots** at the level of each somite. These somatic motor fibers are later joined by autonomic motor fibers arising in the interomediolateral cell columns. The somatic motor fibers grow into the myotomes and thus come to innervate the voluntary muscles. The autonomic fibers, in contrast, terminate in the autonomic ganglia, where they synapse with the peripheral autonomic neurons that innervate the appropriate end organs.

The central neurons of the sympathetic system develop in the

Integration of the Developing Nervous System

Innervation of Motor and Sensory End Organs

Week Day

Neural crest cells begin
to migrate away from the
neural tube, starting
in the cervical region

Cranial neuropore
closes

Caudal neuropore
closes

Motor neurons appear in
the ventral column of the
neural tube, starting in the
cervical region

Dorsal root ganglia
are present at
most levels

Ventral roots begin to
form, starting in the
cervical region

Spinal nerves sprout and
grow into the myotomes,
starting in the cervical
region

Sympathetic trunks form,
starting in the cervical
region

Spinal nerves and
sympathetic trunks form in
the thoracic region; limb
buds are innervated as
they form

Vagal parasympathetic
fibers grow from
parasympathetic ganglia;
vagal fibers innervate
heart

Most of spinal ganglia
formed

Outgrowth of sympathetic
and parasympathetic pre-
and postganglionic nerves
has begun at all levels

Timeline. Development of the peripheral nervous
system from the fourth to the eighth week.

intermediolateral cell columns of the **thoracolumbar** spinal cord (T1 through L3). The axons of these cells leave the spinal cord in the ventral root, but immediately branch off to form a **white ramus** that enters the corresponding chain ganglion. Some of these fibers synapse with peripheral sympathetic neurons in the chain ganglion; others pass onward to synapse in another chain ganglion or in one of the prevertebral ganglia. The postganglionic axons of the peripheral sympathetic chain ganglion neurons reenter the spinal nerve via a branch called the **gray ramus.**

The central neurons of the parasympathetic pathways are located in the brain stem and in the sacral spinal cord at levels S2 through S4. The parasympathetic system is thus called a **craniosacral system.** Parasympathetic fibers from the hindbrain reach the parasympathetic ganglia of the neck and trunk viscera via the vagus nerve, whereas the sacral parasympathetic fibers innervate hindgut and pelvic visceral ganglia via the pelvic splanchnic nerves. The parasympathetic innervation of the head is discussed in Chapter 13.

AXONS ARE GUIDED TO THEIR TARGETS BY APICAL GROWTH CONES

As development proceeds, the sensory and motor neurons of the brain become interconnected in functional patterns, and axons grow out of the CNS and ganglia to innervate appropriate **target organs (end organs)** in the body. Axons travel to their target structures through the active locomotion of an apical structure called a **growth cone** (Fig. 5–1; see also Fig. 13–21). The growth cone, which is thought to move by means of filopodia, is believed to guide the axon to its destination by sensing molecular markers that designate the correct route. This activity of the growth cone is called **pathfinding.** Once the growth cone reaches its target, it halts and forms a synapse. Somatic motor and sensory fibers synapse directly with their end organs. The axons of central autonomic neurons, in contrast, terminate in peripheral autonomic ganglia, where they synapse with the peripheral neuron of the two-neuron autonomic pathway.

Numerous mechanisms have been proposed to explain the ability of neurons to establish correct connections with each other and with end organs. Most of these proposals focus on the various mechanisms by which a growth cone may be guided from its origin to its destination in the periphery. It has been suggested, for example, that at the appropriate time during development, the end organ secretes either a **tropic substance** that attracts the correct growth cones or a **trophic substance** that supports the viability of the growth cones that happen to take the right path. Examples of tropic substances are **netrin-1** and **netrin-2.** These laminin-related proteins are implicated in the guidance of spinal cord **commissural axons** along a pathway from the dorsal cord to the ventral floor plate cells. **Netrin** has also been implicated in the guidance of retinal axons. Examples of trophic substances include the brain-derived neurotrophic growth factor (BDNF), the insulin-like growth factor (IGF), and the c-kit ligand, molecules that support the viability of appropriately situated axons or neuronal cell bodies.

According to other theories, the growth cone may be guided by adhering to special guidance structures in the extracellular matrix. According to

Figure 5–1. Axonal growth cone. The nerve cell body is at the left. The actin filaments in the fan-shaped growth cone are stained with rhodamine-labeled phalloidin. Rhodamine is a fluorescent molecule, and phalloidin (the toxin in the poisonous green fungus *Amanita phalloides*) binds strongly to actin filaments. (From Bridgeman PC, Dailey ME. 1989. The organization of myosin and actin in rapid frozen nerve growth cones. J Cell Biol 108:95.)

the **contact guidance theory,** the growing axon tip is guided by the physical orientation of molecules or structures in the extracellular matrix. According to the somewhat different **chemoaffinity hypothesis,** the growth cone exhibits differential adherence to molecules that are specifically distributed in the extracellular matrix, such as fibronectin, laminin, and neural cell adhesion molecule (NCAM).

It is also likely that the first or **"pioneer"** growth cones to traverse a route establish a pathway that is used by later growing axons. This mechanism would account for the formation of nerves, in which many axons travel together. The phenomenon of axonal pathfinding is a very active area of research, with obvious implications for the process of nerve regeneration after injury in children or adults.

VENTRAL COLUMN MOTOR AXONS ARE THE FIRST TO SPROUT FROM THE SPINAL CORD

The first axons to emerge from the spinal cord are produced by somatic motor neurons in the ventral gray columns. These fibers appear in the cervical region on about day 30 (Fig. 5–2) and (like so many other embryonic processes) proceed in a craniocaudal wave down the spinal cord.

The ventral motor axons initially leave the spinal cord as a continuous broad band. As they grow toward the sclerotomes, however, they rapidly condense to form discrete segmental nerves. Although these axons will eventually synapse with muscles derived from the developing myotomes, their initial guidance apparently depends only on the sclerotomes and not on myotomal or dermatomal elements of the somite. Like neural crest cells (see Ch. 4), the ventral column axons prefer to migrate within the cranial portion of each sclerotome. As a result, these growing axons pass close to the dorsal root ganglion at each level.

The pioneer axons that initially sprout from the cord are soon joined by more ventral column motor axons, and the growing bundle is now called a **ventral root** (see Fig. 5–2). At spinal levels T1 through L2, the ventral root is also joined by axons from the sympathetic motor neurons developing in the intermediolateral cell columns at these levels (see Fig. 5–2).

SOMATIC AND AUTONOMIC MOTOR FIBERS COMBINE WITH SENSORY FIBERS TO FORM SPINAL NERVES

As the tip of each ventral root approaches its corresponding dorsal root ganglion, the neurons in

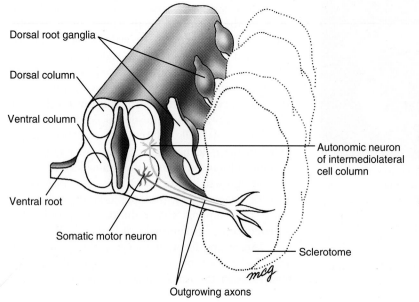

Dorsal root ganglia

Dorsal column

Ventral column

Ventral root

Somatic motor neuron

Autonomic neuron of intermediolateral cell column

Sclerotome

Outgrowing axons

Figure 5–2. Outgrowth of the ventral roots and formation of the dorsal root ganglia. Axons growing from ventral column motor neurons at each segmental level of the spinal cord are guided by the superior part of the sclerotome to form a ventral root. Dorsal root ganglia form in the same plane.

Figure 5–3. *A,* Once the ventral roots are formed, sensory neurons within each dorsal root ganglion sprout processes that grow into the neural tube to synapse with association neurons in the dorsal column. Other processes grow outward from the dorsal root ganglion to join the ventral root, forming a typical spinal nerve. The dorsal root ganglion and its fibers constitute the dorsal root. The axon of the association neuron in this illustration synapses with a motor neuron on the same side of the spinal cord at the same segmental level (axons may also display other patterns of connection; see text). *B,* This double-stained immunochemical preparation shows neuronal cell bodies (green) and neurofilaments within nerve cell processes (red). (*B,* Photo courtesy of Drs. James Weston and Michael Mausich.)

the dorsal root ganglion begin to sprout axons. Each of these neurons has a branch that grows medially toward the dorsal column of the spinal cord and a branch that joins the ventral root and grows toward the periphery to innervate the end organ (Fig. 5–3 appears on page 117). Collectively, the dorsal root ganglion plus the rami (branches) that connect it to the spinal cord and the ventral root are called the **dorsal root.** The medially growing dorsal root fibers penetrate the dorsal columns of the spinal cord and synapse there with the developing **association neurons** (see Fig. 5–3). These association neurons in turn sprout axons that either synapse with autonomic motor neurons in the intermediolateral cell columns or with somatic motor neurons in the ventral columns or else ascend to higher levels in the spinal cord in the form of **tracts.** The axons of some association neurons synapse with motor neurons on the same or **ipsilateral** side of the spinal cord, whereas others cross over to synapse with motor neurons on the opposite or **contralateral** side of the cord.

The mixed motor and sensory trunk formed at each level by the confluence of the dorsal and ventral roots is called a **spinal nerve** (see Fig. 5–3). The sympathetic fibers that exit via the ventral roots at levels T1 through L2 soon branch from the spinal nerve and grow ventrally to enter the corresponding sympathetic chain ganglion (see Ch. 4) (Fig. 5–4). This branch is called a **white ramus.** Some of the sympathetic fibers carried in the white ramus synapse directly with a neuron in the chain ganglion (see Fig. 5–4). This neuron becomes the second (peripheral) neuron in a two-neuron sympathetic pathway and sprouts an axon that grows to innervate the appropriate peripheral end organ. Because the peripheral autonomic neurons reside in ganglia, the axons of the central sympathetic neurons are called **preganglionic fibers,** and the axons of the peripheral sympathetic

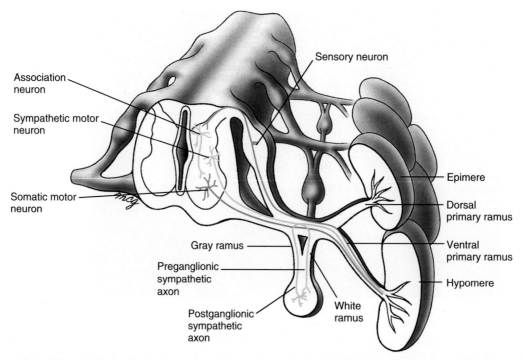

Figure 5–4. Organization of spinal nerves and associated chain ganglia at levels T1–L2 and S2–S4. In this example, the preganglionic fiber growing from the intermediolateral cell column exits the spinal nerve through a white ramus and synapses with a neuron in the chain ganglion at the same level. The postganglionic fiber then exits through the gray ramus and rejoins the same spinal nerve. Each spinal nerve splits into a dorsal primary ramus and a ventral primary ramus, which innervate the segmental epimere and hypomere, respectively. Both rami contain motor, sensory, and autonomic fibers.

gray ramus. As a result, the spinal nerves at levels T1 through L2 have both white and gray rami, whereas all other spinal nerves have just a gray ramus. The motor fibers linking chain ganglia to one another thus are exclusively preganglionic sympathetic fibers. These fibers plus chain ganglia themselves constitute the **sympathetic trunk.**

THE HEAD RECEIVES SYMPATHETIC INNERVATION VIA THE CERVICAL CHAIN GANGLIA, WHEREAS THE HEART, TRACHEA, AND LUNGS RECEIVE SYMPATHETIC INNERVATION FROM CERVICAL AND THORACIC CHAIN GANGLIA

The sympathetic supply to the heart originates at cord levels T1 through T4 (Fig. 5–7). Some of the fibers from T1 travel up the sympathetic trunk to synapse in the three cervical chain ganglia—the **inferior cervical ganglion** (which is sometimes fused with the chain ganglion at T1 to form the **stellate ganglion**), the **middle cervical ganglion,** and the **superior cervical ganglion.** Postgangli-

onic fibers from these ganglia join postganglionic fibers emanating directly from nerves T1 through T4 to form the cardiac nerves, which innervate the heart muscle.

The sympathetic supply to the head originates at cord levels T1 through T4 and reaches the head exclusively via the sympathetic trunk. The preganglionic fibers synapse in the superior cervical ganglion, and the postganglionic fibers arising here follow blood vessels to the various structures in the head that receive sympathetic innervation, such as the lacrimal glands, the dilator pupillae muscles of the iris, and the nasal and oral mucosa.

Postganglionic sympathetic fibers exiting directly from chain ganglia associated with levels T1 through T4 or from cervical ganglia innervated by preganglionic fibers originating at cord levels T1 to T4 also innervate the trachea and lungs.

THE PREGANGLIONIC SYMPATHETIC FIBERS THAT SUPPLY THE GUT TERMINATE IN THE PREVERTEBRAL GANGLIA

The preganglionic sympathetic fibers destined to supply the gut arise from cord levels T5 through

Figure 5–7. Some postganglionic sympathetic fibers do not join with spinal nerves. Postganglionic fibers emanating from cervical and thoracic chain ganglia follow blood vessels to structures in the head and pharynx and to the heart and lungs. The splanchnic nerves are preganglionic fibers that pass directly out of the chain ganglia at levels T5 to L2 to innervate neurons within the celiac, superior, mesenteric, aorticorenal, and inferior mesenteric ganglia. Postganglionic fibers from these ganglia grow out along blood vessels to innervate their visceral end organs.

Superior cervical ganglion

Middle cervical ganglion

Stellate ganglion

Cardiac and lung plexus

Celiac ganglion

Superior mesenteric ganglion

Aorticorenal ganglion

Inferior mesenteric ganglion

―――― Preganglionic fibers

---------- Postganglionic fibers

L2 and enter the corresponding chain ganglia. Instead of synapsing, however, they immediately leave via **splanchnic nerves,** which emerge directly from the chain ganglia (see Fig. 5–7). These splanchnic nerves innervate the various prevertebral ganglia, which in turn send postganglionic fibers to the visceral end organs. The pattern of distribution is as follows:

Fibers from levels T5 through T9 come together to form the **greater splanchnic nerves** serving the **celiac ganglia.**

Fibers from T10 and T11 form the **lesser splanchnic nerves** serving the **aorticorenal ganglia.**

Fibers from T12 alone form the **least splanchnic nerves** serving the superior mesenteric ganglia.

Fibers from L1 and L2 form the **lumbar splanchnic nerves** serving the **inferior mesenteric ganglia.**

Recall from Chapter 4 that the prevertebral ganglia develop next to major branches of the descending aorta. The postganglionic sympathetic axons from the prevertebral ganglia grow out along these arteries and thus come to innervate the same tissues that the arteries supply with blood (see Fig. 5–7). Thus, the postganglionic fibers from the celiac ganglia innervate the distal *foregut* region vascularized by the celiac artery—that is, the portion of the foregut from the abdominal esophagus

through the duodenum to the entrance of the bile duct. Similarly, fibers from the superior mesenteric ganglia innervate the **midgut** (the remainder of the duodenum, the jejunum, and the ileum) plus the ascending colon and about two thirds of the transverse colon. The aorticorenal ganglia innervate the kidney and suprarenal gland, and the inferior mesenteric ganglia innervate the **hindgut,** including the distal one third of the transverse colon, the descending and sigmoid colons, and the upper two thirds of the anorectal canal.

THE PARASYMPATHETIC SYSTEM HAS LONG PREGANGLIONIC FIBERS AND SHORT POSTGANGLIONIC FIBERS

Recall from Chapter 4 that the parasympathetic ganglia, unlike the sympathetic ganglia, form close to the organs they are destined to innervate and therefore produce only short postganglionic fibers. The central neurons of the two-cell parasympathetic pathways reside either in one of four motor nuclei in the brain (associated with cranial nerves III, VII, IX, and X) or in the intermediolateral cell columns of the sacral cord at levels S2 through S4. The cranial nuclei supply the head and the viscera

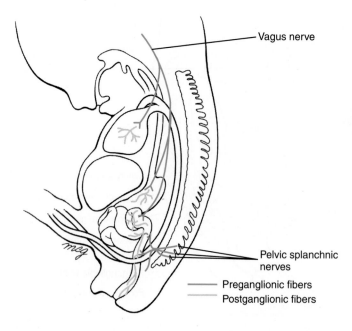

- Vagus nerve

Pelvic splanchnic nerves

—— Preganglionic fibers
—— Postganglionic fibers

Figure 5–8. The vagus nerve and pelvic splanchnic nerves provide preganglionic parasympathetic innervation to ganglia embedded in the walls of visceral organs. The preganglionic fibers originating at cord levels S2 through S4 issue from the cord at those levels and then branch off to form pelvic splanchnic nerves, which innervate the parasympathetic ganglia of the target viscera. The postganglionic parasympathetic fibers are relatively short.

superior to the hindgut, whereas the sacral neurons supply the viscera inferior to this point (Fig. 5–8).

The preganglionic parasympathetic fibers associated with cranial nerves III, VII, and IX travel to parasympathetic ganglia located near the structures to be innervated, where they synapse with the second neuron of the pathway. Organs receiving parasympathetic innervation in this way include the dilator pupillae muscles of the eye, the lacrimal and salivary glands, and glands of the oral and nasal mucosa (see Ch. 13). In contrast, the preganglionic parasympathetic fibers associated with cranial nerve X join with somatic motor and sensory fibers to form the vagus nerve. Some branches of the vagus nerve serve structures in the head and neck, but other parasympathetic and sensory fibers within the nerve continue into the thorax and abdomen, where the parasympathetic fibers synapse

with secondary neurons in numerous small parasympathetic ganglia embedded in the walls of target organs such as the heart, liver, adrenal cortex, kidney, gonads, and gut. The preganglionic vagal fibers, therefore, are very long, whereas the postganglionic fibers that penetrate the target organs are short.

The parasympathetic preganglionic fibers arising in the sacral cord emerge from the ventral rami of the cord and join together to form the **pelvic splanchnic nerves.** These nerves ramify throughout the pelvis and lower abdomen, innervating ganglia embedded in the walls of the descending and sigmoid colons, rectum, ureter, prostate, bladder, urethra, and phallus. The postganglionic fibers from these ganglia innervate smooth muscle or glands in the target organs (see Fig. 5–8).

Clinical Applications

HIRSCHSPRUNG'S DISEASE: A CONGENITAL DEFECT OF NEURAL CREST MIGRATION

The Dilated Colon Characteristic of Hirschsprung's Disease Is Not the Site of the Primary Defect

The most prominent feature of the common (1 in 5000 live births) congenital disorder called Hirschsprung's disease is abnormal dilation of a segment of the colon. The disease was first described by Hirschsprung in 1888, but its cause remained controversial for 60 years. As recently as the 1940s, it was thought that the enlarged bowel segment was the primary site of the defect and that the disease could be cured by resecting it. In 1948, however, Swenson, by using barium enema and x-rays for diagnosis, demonstrated that the enlarged bowel in patients with Hirschsprung's disease was a secondary symptom caused by obstruction and lack of peristalsis in the colon segment distal to the dilation (Fig. 5–9). Swenson devised a procedure for removing this constricted distal segment, and this operation, or a variation of it, remains the only effective treatment for the disease. Untreated patients may eventually die of an infected colon.

The Classic Symptoms of Hirschsprung's Disease Usually Appear Soon After Birth

The first sign of Hirschsprung's disease is usually a delay in the passage of meconium, the material that fills the lower bowel of newborn infants. This sign may be accompanied by symptoms such as constipation, vomiting, abdominal distention, and rupture of the cecum. Most individuals with Hirschsprung's disease are diagnosed during their first year of life. Barium enema examinations show that the nonperistaltic segment always represents the most distal part of the gastrointestinal tract, although it may vary in length from a small portion of the rectum to the entire large intestine and part of the ileum.

The Constriction and Paralysis of the Colonic Segment Appear to Result From Abnormal Migration of Neural Crest Cells

In the late 1940s, it was reported that the constricted, nonperistaltic segment of the colon also lacked parasympathetic enteric ganglia. These gan-

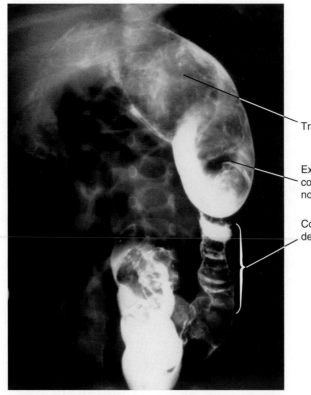

Transverse colon

Expanded segment of colon proximal to constriction (parasympathetic ganglia are normal)

Constricted aganglionic segment of descending colon

Figure 5–9. Radiograph after a barium enema showing the constricted inferior gastrointestinal tract of an individual with Hirschsprung's disease. The adjacent superior region of the tract with normal autonomic innervation is distended. (Photo courtesy of Children's Hospital Medical Center, Cincinnati, OH.)

glia normally are present in the gut wall and innervate the smooth muscle and mucosa. Although the absence of these ganglia was recognized as the cause of the disease, it was only through animal experiments that the defect was shown to result from the failure of neural crest cells to migrate into the gut wall in the affected segment.

Recall from Chapter 4 that the parasympathetic ganglion cells that innervate the gut are derived from the neural crest. The process by which these cells populate the gut was first elucidated by using the quail-chick chimera system described in the following Experimental Principles section. Most of the parasympathetic ganglion cells along the entire length of the gut are derived from the neural crest of the occipitocervical (vagal) region, although a scattering of the ganglion cells in the hindgut are derived from the sacral neural crest. However, it now seems likely that much of the sacral neural crest that invades the terminal gastro-

intestinal tract may give rise to the glia and connective tissue.

In chicks, the terminal region of the gut is populated by neural crest cells as late as 3 days after the foregut. Therefore, it was hypothesized that Hirschsprung's disease could be caused by a failure of neural crest to migrate the full length of the gastrointestinal tract. However, it was later discovered that in mammals the gut primordium is populated by neural crest cells while it is still very short and lies close to the vagal region of the neural tube and that the entire gut tube consequently receives vagal neural crest cells almost simultaneously.

Studies of Mouse and Human Mutants Suggest That Congenital Megacolon May Arise Through Independent Mutations of Several Different Genes. As noted in the preceding discussion, successful development of enteric neurons requires induction of neural crest cells within the neural folds, their detachment from the neural tube, their migration along specific pathways, and their penetration of the gut wall. Finally, they must proliferate and differentiate to produce functional neurons of the enteric nervous system. It is thus possible that defects in any of these developmental mechanisms could result in congenital megacolon. Several studies of mice and humans provide evidence for this suggestion.

One group of proteins that contribute to the development of the enteric nervous system is the **hedgehog** family of signaling molecules. These proteins play diverse morphogenetic roles in both vertebrates and invertebrates. Two proteins in particular, **sonic hedgehog (Shh)** and **Indian hedgehog (Ihh)** are co-expressed in the gut endoderm in patterns that partially overlap. Mice with *Shh* mutations have abnormal innervation of the gut among other abnormalities, whereas mice with targeted *Ihh* mutations have a number of gut-related abnormalities, including features that are typical of Hirschsprung's disease.

The murine **splotch mutant (Sp)** harbors mutations of *Pax-3*, a gene resembling the paired-box *Drosophila* segmentation genes (see Ch. 4). In addition to the neural tube defects these mice exhibit, homozygotes of several well-described mutations of *Pax-3* express severe defects of neural crest migration and/or differentiation including hearing loss, pigmentation defects, and Hirschsprung's disease. Among these, mutations arising from chromosomal deletions are most severe. In the human, the **Waardenburg type 1 syndrome (WS1)** may also include Hirschsprung's disease and has also been shown to result from mutations of the human homologue of *PAX3*, which has been mapped to distal 2q. **Waardenburg type 2 syndrome (WS2)** has also been associated with Hirschsprung's disease and with other neural crest defects.

Another gene implicated in the pathogenesis of human Hirschsprung's disease is the **RET proto-oncogene**. This gene, which has been mapped to chromosome 10q11.2, encodes a protein tyrosine kinase. It has been suggested that disruptions of neural crest cell adhesion and migration in *RET* mutants may occur as a consequence of deletion or disruption of a domain within this gene that encodes a sequence homologous to the **cadherin** family of cell-adhesion molecules. Furthermore, a gene or genes at 9q31 can serve as a modifier of Hirschsprung's disease penetrance.

The **lethal spotted (ls)** and **piebald lethal (sl)** mouse mutants have also served as useful models for the study of Hirschsprung's disease. These mutants are respectively characterized by mutations of the **endothelin-3 ligand** gene (**Edn-3**) and the gene that encodes its receptor, the **endothelin-B receptor** gene (**Ednrb**). It has also been shown that respective transgenic disruptions of either of these genes results in a similar Hirschsprung's phenotype. Coincidentally, some human patients exhibiting the Hirschsprung's phenotype have been shown to carry a mutation in the gene encoding the endothelin-B receptor, which has been mapped to human chromosome 13q22. Disruptions of the endothelin-3/endothelin-B receptor system resulting in Hirschsprung's disease, however, may more directly affect development of the terminal portion of the gut than the migration or development of neural crest cells per se.

Microscopic studies have shown that the nonperistaltic terminal gut in lethal spotted mice lacks enteric ganglia. However, neurons containing the neurotransmitter characteristic of parasympathetic ganglion cells can be found adhering to the outside of the bowel wall in this segment, indicating that the neural crest successfully reached the affected segment but did not penetrate the gut wall. The autonomic axons that normally would synapse with the enteric ganglia are also present and are capable of invading the gut wall. The proximal parts of the gut appear to be completely normal, having enteric ganglia served by preganglionic fibers.

In vitro experiments support the idea that the terminal 2 mm of the bowel in spotted lethal mice is inhospitable to invasion by neural crest cells. Neural crest cells from the mutant *ls/ls* mice invade the explanted colon from wild-type animals in culture, but wild-type neural crest cells fail to invade the explanted terminal segment of the *ls/ls* colon. Studies of mouse **aggregation chimeras** produced by mixing wild-type and *ls/ls* blastomeres and then implanting these aggregates into pseudopregnant mothers also support the likelihood that the quality of the colon in the intact *ls/ls* mouse is responsible for the inability of neural crest cells to invade and differentiate. The strategy used in these studies was a **reporter gene**, specifically, the *DβH-nlacZ* transgene, which was introduced into the *ls/ls* cells.

Figure 5–10. Dorsal and lateral views of transgenic mice that express the bacterial *lacZ* gene in tissues that also produce peripherin (see text). The enzyme encoded by *lacZ* causes the cells producing it to turn blue when appropriately incubated. The blue stain is localized in small neurons of the neural-crest-derived dorsal root ganglia and in the axons of these cells that penetrate the spinal cord in a region overlying the dorsal gray columns of the spinal cord parasagittal stripes). (Photo courtesy of Teri Belecky-Adams and Dr. Linda Parysek.)

The *lacZ* gene encodes the enzyme β-galactosidase, which catalyzes a reaction that produces a blue stain within the *lacZ*-containing cell when the tissue is incubated in solutions containing appropriate substrates (see Fig. 5–10). It was found that aggregation chimeras did not develop congenital megacolon if more than 20 percent of their cells were wild-type cells, and it was also shown that the *ls/ls* cells were capable of populating the entire gut in these animals.

Microscopic studies of the colon of *ls/ls* mice have shown that the extracellular matrix in the affected bowel segment is abnormal; the basal lamina surrounding the smooth muscle cells is overdeveloped and contains an abnormal excess of extracellular matrix molecules, including laminin, collagen type IV, and glycosaminoglycans. It is now thought that the excess laminin within this terminal bowel segment induces the premature differentiation of the neural crest into nonmigrating neurons, resulting in their inability to invade the gut wall. The specific relationship between the endothelin-3/endothelin-B receptor system (see earlier) and the formation of excess laminin in these mice is a question for future studies.

Experimental Principles

EXPERIMENTAL STUDIES OF THE NEURAL CREST

Major Questions About the Neural Crest Remain

The origin and fates of the neural crest were described in Chapter 4. It should be apparent that imaginative, experimental strategies are necessary to investigate the myriad developmental lineages of neural crest cells and the mechanisms underlying this diversity. A number of creative approaches have been devised and have yielded various types of information. We now know much about the origins, migration routes, and developmental fates of neural crest subpopulations. Questions remain, however, including the nature and identity of the signals that guide migrating neural crest cells, the mechanisms by which the cells migrate, and the

nature of the cell-cell interactions that regulate their differentiation.

Various Techniques Are Used to Study the Lineages of Neural Crest Cells

Classic Ablation and Explantation Experiments Are Technically Simple but Present Problems of Interpretation. In a neural crest ablation study, a thin slice of neural tube or neural fold is resected from an experimental animal at the appropriate stage of development, and the question is asked: What does not develop? This approach has provided answers in some cases, but in others the results have been difficult to interpret. One, embryos apparently have some capacity to functionally replace the ablated crest. Two, it is difficult to define precisely the boundaries of presumptive crest cell subpopulations; therefore, the results of different experiments are often hard to compare. Finally, it is very difficult to rule out the possibility that the failure of an expected descendant to develop results not from ablation of the progenitor crest cells but instead from the accidental ablation of other cells essential for their differentiation.

The results of explantation experiments have added fuel to another interesting controversy in this field. In some cases, a single cultured neural crest explant gives rise to several neural crest derivatives. It has, therefore, been argued that neural crest cells may be **pluripotent;** that is, innately able to develop into several or all of the normal neural crest derivatives, and that their developmental fate is determined solely by environmental cues, whether encountered in the culture dish or during their natural migration. An alternative interpretation, however, is that an explant that gives rise to several derivatives actually consists of a heterogeneous population of cells, each of which is **unipotent;** that is, already limited to a single developmental path.

Cell Marking Techniques Make It Possible to Study the Migration and Differentiation of Crest Cells In Vivo.

Early studies of embryonic cell lineages relied on natural markers found in certain cells, such as pigment granules, distinctive nuclear morphologies, or yolk inclusions, which could be used to trace the migration and differentiation of the cells. This approach was not useful in the case of the neural crest, because crest cells have no distinctive natural markers. One technique devised to circumvent this problem was to transplant neural crest cells from an embryo that had been heavily labeled with tritiated thymidine to an unlabeled embryo. The donor crest cells carry radioactive thymidine in their DNA. After the graft heals, the migration of these cells and their descendants can be followed by autoradiography. However, because the radioactive label is diluted each time a cell divides and synthesizes new DNA, the technique can trace a cell line through only a limited number of generations.

The problem of label dilution was solved by the development of the **quail-chick chimera system** (Fig. 5–11). Quail cells develop normally when implanted into chick embryos, and they carry a natural nucleolar marker that is easily visualized in microscopic preparations. A piece of neural tube or neural fold can be transplanted from a quail embryo to a chick embryo, and, after the graft heals, the quail cell lines can be observed by looking for cells with prominent nucleoli.

The question of whether crest cells are pluripotent or unipotent has been partly answered by experiments in which quail cells from one part of the neural crest were transplanted to various locations along the chick neural tube. These investigations showed that neural crest subpopulations have somewhat diverse developmental capabilities: When transplanted to various new locations, they are able to develop into some but not all of the normal derivatives of those locations. Whether this pluripotentiality of neural crest *subpopulations* indicates pluripotentiality of the individual crest cells remains in question, because the explants used in these experiments are relatively large. The possibility cannot be ruled out that an explant is pluripotent because it contains a heterogeneous population of unipotent cells.

Single Cell Labeling Experiments Overcome the Interpretive Problems of Thymidine and Quail-Chick Marking Experiments. The development of individual neural crest cells can be followed in vivo by injecting single cells with highly fluorescent, nontoxic dyes or by infecting cells with retroviruses encoding marker proteins (e.g., *lacZ*). The advantage of dye injection studies is that brightly fluorescent cells can be identified immediately after injection, allowing instantaneous verification that a single cell is labeled. However, as with thymidine labeling experiments, these dyes eventually become diluted beyond the level of detection, although at much later stages. In the case of retroviral labeling experiments, the signal does not become diluted because a gene encoding the label is incorporated into the DNA of the infected cell and its progeny. A drawback to this approach is that one cannot control the area where the retroviral sequences become integrated. Furthermore, it is difficult to verify that only a single cell is infected. Nonetheless, both of these approaches have yielded significant findings about the behavior

Figure 5–11. In the classic quail-chick chimera system pioneered by Le Dourin, a segment of quail neural tube is transplanted to the same position in a chicken embryo of the same age. After the graft has healed, quail neural crest cells migrate to their normal targets, where they are easily distinguished from chicken cells by their distinctive nucleoli. In practice, larger pieces of the neural tube containing presumptive neural crest cells are usually transferred.

and fates of neural crest cells throughout development. These studies have demonstrated that, in some cases, a single neural crest cell injected with lysinated rhodamine dextran (LRD), with the dye DiI, or with replication-incompetent retroviruses before or during migration gives rise to daughters that develop into a variety of neural crest derivatives. Thus, at least some neural crest cells appear to be **multipotent.**

For example, clonal analysis of LRD-injected trunk neural crest cell precursors of the mouse shows that their developmental potential depends, in part, on the time that they emigrate from the neural tube. Single cells injected during early neural crest migration may give rise to neural tube cells as well as neural crest derivatives that migrate along both dorsal pathways and ventral pathways. Derivatives of the dorsal pathway include melanocytes and cells of the dorsal root ganglia, whereas cells of the ventral pathway form sympathetic ganglia and adrenomedullary cells. In contrast, migration of late-emigrating neural crest cells is restricted to the dorsal pathway.

Targeted Migration and Differentiation of Neural Crest Subpopulations Is Also Dependent on Responsiveness to Environmental Signals. The capacity of specific subpopulations of neural crest cells to migrate to specific targets may depend on their ability to recognize specific extracellular matrix molecules. Guidance by **instructive cues** such as laminin, tenascin, and fibronectin, for example, have been implicated in migration of cranial neural crest, whereas specific subregions of cell matrix in the trunk may play only **permissive** roles. The capacity of specific subpopulations to survive and proliferate may also depend on their unique capacities to respond to specific **trophic**

substances expressed along the migratory pathway. For example, **platelet-derived growth factor** and **c-kit ligand** have been implicated in the survival and proliferation of certain non-neuronal neural crest cell precursors (see later), whereas neurotrophic factors such as **neurotrophin-3 (NT-3,** a member of the NGF family of growth factors) and **retinoic acid** may selectively promote the survival of neurogenic precursors of the trunk neural crest.

Some Mutants May Provide Information About the Mechanisms of Neural Crest Migration and Developmental Restriction

Several mouse mutants characterized by defects of neural crest development, in addition to those discussed in the Clinical Applications section, have been described. Some of these mutations affect the proliferative activity of neural crest stem cell populations, whereas others are characterized by regional defects in pigmentation, innervation of the gut, or defects in the development of cranial neural crest.

An interesting series of mouse mutants that affect neural crest cell migration are called **white-spotting (W)** and **Steel (Sl)** mutants. The *W* locus is a proto-oncogene that encodes a c-kit tyrosine kinase receptor **(c-kit receptor),** whereas the *Sl* locus encodes the ligand for this receptor, **c-kit ligand.** Indeed, mutations of either gene produce a similar spectrum of anomalies, specifically involving migrating embryonic stem cells. For example, in severe mutations of either of these loci, primordial germ cells fail to populate the gonads, resulting in sterility (see Ch. 10), whereas hematopoietic stem cells fail to migrate from the yolk sac into the liver, resulting in severe deficiencies of blood formation. Less severe mutations may result in differential male or female sterility and selective loss of specific hematopoietic progenitors (see Ch. 8). In addition to disruptions of germ cell and blood cell development, however, these mutants also display a spectrum of pigmentation defects suggesting an effect on another population of migrating embryonic cells, the neural crest cell precursors of the melanocytes.

It seems likely that c-kit ligand is a trophic factor and that it is required for survival of premelanocytes rather than for their early differentiation and migration. It has been suggested that c-kit ligand may regulate the expression of c-kit receptor by melanocyte precursors of the neural crest and that c-kit ligand and c-kit receptor together then regulate the adhesion of these cells to the extracellular matrix. Thus, it appears that c-kit ligand must be expressed by cells along the melanocyte migration route and at its ultimate target, whereas the c-kit receptor must be expressed by the premelanocytes themselves. A **soluble form** of the c-kit ligand is apparently required for early survival of premelanocytes in a **migration staging area** between the somite, surface ectoderm, and neural tube. In contrast, expression of a **membrane-associated form** of c-kit ligand appears to be required for the later survival of the premelanocytes within the dermis.

A staggering array of additional genes affecting specific mechanisms of neural crest cell differentiation, migration, and survival in mice have been described within the last few years. The Patch mutation (*Ph*) of the alpha subunit of the platelet-derived growth factor ($PDGF_{2\alpha}$) disrupts the development of non-neuronal derivatives of the neural crest. Transgenic knockout of genes encoding retinoic acid receptor proteins results in defects of heart septation (see Ch. 7), whereas homozygotes of the kreisler mutant (*kr*) exhibit wide-ranging craniofacial defects attributed to abnormal expression of several *Hox* genes and consequent disruption of neural crest cell development. These latter genes, therefore, apparently play pivotal roles in the signaling cascades that regulate differentiation and migration of cranial neural crest cells (see Ch. 12). A number of additional genes implicated in neural crest cell differentiation and migration have been identified by screening neural crest and neural tube complementary DNA (cDNA) libraries for genes expressed during early nervous system development. One such gene, *Noelin-1*, is expressed in the open neural plate, then later in the neural folds, neural tube, and in migrating neural crest cells. Interestingly, overexpression of *Noelin-1* prolongs the period during which neural crest cells are generated, producing excess numbers of crest cells. These data indicate that the protein product of *Noelin-1*, shown to be a secreted glycoprotein, can mediate how and when neural tube cells become converted to neural crest cells. The fact that

Noelin-1 is also expressed in migratory crest cells is consistent with the notion that this protein plays a role in later events in neural crest cell differentiation and migration. These findings also demonstrate the power of screening neural crest and neural tube cDNA libraries for novel genes involved in neural crest cell generation, migration, and differentiation. Such research may eventually lead to a better understanding of clinical manifestations of congenital neural crest abnormalities.

SUGGESTED READING

Descriptive Embryology

Altman J, Bayer S. 1985. The development of the rat spinal cord. Adv Anat Embryol Cell Biol 85:1

Bronner-Fraser M. 1993. Environmental influences on neural cell migration. J Neurobiol 24:233

Davies AM. 1990. Ontogeny of the somatosensory system. Annu Rev Neurosci 13:61

Erickson CA. 1988. Control of pathfinding by the avian neural crest. Development (Suppl) 103:63

Fearon ER, Cho KR, Nigro JM, et al. 1990. Identification of a chromosome 18q gene that is altered in colorectal cancers. Science 247:49

Goodman CS. 1996. Mechanisms and molecules that control growth cone guidance. Annu Rev Neurosci 19:341

Henion PD, Weston JA. 1994. Retinoic acid selectively promotes the survival and proliferation of neurogenic precursors in cultured neural crest cell populations. Dev Biol 161:243

Kazuko K-M, Masu M, Hink L, et al. 1996. Deleted in Colorectal Cancer (DCC) encodes a netrin receptor. Cell 87:175

Kennedy TE, Serafini T, de la Torre J, et al. 1994. Netrins are diffusible chemotropic factors for commissural axons in the embryonic spinal cord. Cell 78:425

Keynes R, Cook G, Davies J, et al. 1990. Segmentation and the development of the vertebrate nervous system. J Physiol Paris 84:27

Landmesser L. 1988. Peripheral guidance cues and the formation of specific motor projections in the chick. p. 121. In Easter SS Jr, Barald KF, Carlson BM (eds). Message to Mind. Sinauer Associates, Inc, Publishers, Sunderland, MA

Levi-Montalcini R. 1987. The nerve growth factor: thirty-five years later. EMBO J 6:1145

Tosney KW. 1988. Somites and axon guidance. Scanning Electron Microsc 2:427

Vielmetter J, Kayyem JF, Roman JM, et al. 1994. Neogenin, an avian cell surface protein expressed during terminal neuronal differentiation, is closely related to the human tumor suppressor molecule Deleted in Colorectal Cancer. J Cell Biol 127:2009

Clinical Applications

Baynash AG, Hosoda K, Gia A, et al. 1994. Interaction of endothelin-3 with endothelin-B receptor is essential for development of epidural melanocytes and enteric neurons. Cell 79:1277

Bolk S, Pelet A, Hofstra R, et al. 2000. A human model for multigenic inheritance: phenotypic expression in Hirschsprung's disease requires both the RET gene and a new 9q31 locus. Proc Natl Acad Sci U S A 97:268

Carcassonne M, Guys JM, Monsson-Lacombe G, Kreitman B. 1989. Management of Hirschsprung's disease: curative surgery before 3 months of age. J Pediatr Surg 24:1032

Dow E, Cross S, Wolgemuth J, et al. 1994. Second locus for Hirschsprung's disease/Waardenburg syndrome in a large Mennonite kindred. Am J Med Genet 53:75

Edery P, Lyonnet S, Mulligan L, et al. 1994. Mutations of the RET proto-oncogene in Hirschsprung's disease. Nature 367:378

Hosoda K, Hammer RE, Richardson JA, et al. 1994. Targeted and natural (piebald-lethal) mutations of endothelin-B receptor gene produce megacolon associated with spotted coat color in mice. Cell 79:1267

Kaour RP, Yost C, Palmiter RD. 1993. Aggregation chimeras demonstrate that the primary defect responsible for aganglionic megacolon in 15 thals spotted mice is not neuroblast. Autonomus Dev 117:993

Paran WJ, Liddell RA, Wright A, et al. 1995. A high resolution linkage map of the lethal spotting locus: a mouse model for Hirschsprung's disease. Mammalian Genome 6:1

Payette RP, Tennyson VM, Pomeranz HD, et al. 1988. Accumulation of components of basal laminae: association with the failure of neural crest cells to colonize the presumptive aganglionic bowel of *ls/ls* mutant mice. Dev Biol 125:341

Puffenberger EG, Hosoda K, Washington SS, et al. 1994. A missense mutation of the endothelin-B receptor gene in multigenic Hirschsprung's disease. Cell 79:1259

Ramalho-Santos M, Melton D, McMahon A. 2000. Hedgehog signals regulate multiple aspects of gastrointestinal development. Development 127:2763

Rothman TP, Gershon MD. 1984. Regionally defective colonization of the terminal bowel by precursors of enteric neurons in lethal spotted mutant mice. Neuroscience 12:1293

Swenson O. 1989. My early experience with Hirschsprung's disease. J Pediatr Surg 24:839

Experimental Principles

Barembaum M, Moreno T, LaBonne C, et al. 2000. Noelin-1 is a secreted glycoprotein involved in generation of the neural crest. Nat Cell Biol 2:219

Besmer P, Manova K, Duttlinger R, et al. 1993. The c-kit ligand (steel factor) and its receptor c-kit/w pleiotropic roles in gene to genesis and melanogenesis. Development (Suppl.) 125

Bolk S, Pelet A, Hofstra R, et al. 2000. A human model for multigenic inheritance: phenotypic expression in Hirschsprung's disease requires both the *RET* gene and a new 9q31 locus. Proc Natl Acad Sci U S A 97:268

Bronner-Fraser M. 1995. Origins and developmental potential of the neural crest. Exp Cell Res 218:405

Cable J, Jackson I, Steel K. 1995. Mutations of the *W* locus affect survival of neural crest-derived melanocytes in the mouse. Mech Dev 50:139

Gershon MD, Clalazonitis A, Rothman TP. 1993. From neural crest to bowel: development of the enteric nervous system. J Neurobiol 24:199

Horstadius S. 1950. The Neural Crest. Its Properties and Derivatives in the Light of Experimental Research. Oxford University Press, London

Kinashi T, Springer T. 1994. Steel factor and c-kit regulate cell-matrix adhesion. Blood 83:1033

Le Douarin NM, Smith J. 1988. Development of the peripheral nervous system from the neural crest. Annu Rev Cell Biol 4:375

Morrison-Graham K, Weston JA. 1989. Mouse mutants provide new insights into the role of extracellular matrix in cell migration and differentiation. Trends Genet 5:116

Motro B, vander Kooy D, Rossant J, et al. 1991. Contiguous patterns of c-kit and steel expression: analysis of mutations at the *W* and *Sl* loci. Development 113:120

Ramalho-Santos M, Melton D, McMahon A. 2000. Hedgehog signals regulate multiple aspects of gastrointestinal development. Development 127:2763

Reid K, Nishikawa S-I, Bartlett PF, Murphy M. 1995. Steel factor directs melanocyte development in vitro through selective regulation of the number of c-kit+ progenitors. Dev Biol 169:568

Serbedzija G, Bronner-Fraser M, Fraser S. 1994. Developmental potential of trunk neural crest cells in mouse. Development 120:1709

Vogel K, Marusich M, Weston JA. 1993. Restriction of neurogenic ability during neural crest migration. J Neurobiol 24:162

Wehrle-Haller B, Weston J. 1995. Soluble and cell-bound forms of steel factor activity play distinct roles in melanocyte precursor dispersal and survival on the lateral neural crest migration pathway. Development 121:731

Weston JA. 1970. The migration and differentiation of neural crest cells. Adv Morphog 8:41

Embryonic Folding

Summary

During the brief span of the fourth week, the embryo undergoes a complex process of **embryonic folding** that converts it from a flat germ disc into a three-dimensional structure that is recognizable as a vertebrate. The main force responsible for embryonic folding is the differential growth of different portions of the embryo. The embryonic disc grows vigorously during the fourth week, particularly in length, whereas the growth of the yolk sac stagnates. Because the outer rim of the embryonic endoderm is attached to the yolk sac, the expanding disc is forced to bulge into a convex shape. Folding commences in the cephalic and lateral regions of the embryo on day 22 and in the caudal region on day 23. As a result of folding, the cephalic, lateral, and caudal edges of the germ disc are brought together along the ventral midline. The endodermal, mesodermal, and ectodermal layers of the embryonic disc each fuse to the corresponding layer on the opposite side, thus creating a fish-like three-dimensional body form.

The process of midline fusion transforms the flat embryonic endoderm into a **gut tube.** Initially, the gut consists of cranial and caudal blind-ending tubes—the **foregut** and **hindgut,** respectively—separated by the future **midgut,** which remains open to the yolk sac. As the lateral edges of the various germ disc layers continue to zipper together along the ventral midline, the midgut is progressively converted into a tube, and the yolk sac neck correspondingly is reduced to a slender **vitelline duct.**

When the edges of the ectoderm fuse along the midline, the space formed within the lateral plate mesoderm is enclosed in the embryo and becomes the **intraembryonic coelom.** The lateral plate mesoderm gives rise to the **serosal membranes** that line the coelom—the **somatopleuric mesoderm** coating the inner surface of the body wall and the **splanchnopleuric mesoderm** ensheathing the gut tube. The abdominal portion of the gut becomes suspended in the coelom by a thin, double-layered reflection of serosal membrane, the **dorsal mesentery.**

The fourth week also sees the development of the three partitions that will subdivide the coelom into pericardial, pleural, and peritoneal cavities. The first partition to appear is the **septum transversum,** a blocklike wedge of mesoderm that forms a ventral structure partially dividing the coelom into a thoracic **primitive pericardial cavity** and an abdominal **peritoneal cavity.** Cephalic folding and the differential growth of the head and neck translocate this block of mesoderm from the superior edge of the germ disc caudally to the position of the future diaphragm. Coronal **pleuropericardial folds** meanwhile appear on the lateral body wall of the primitive pericardial cavity and grow medially to fuse with each other and with the ventral surface of the foregut mesoderm, thus subdividing the primitive pericardial cavity into a definitive **pericardial cavity** and two **pleural cavities.** The pleural cavities initially

Folding of the Embryo and Formation of the Body Cavities and Mesenteries

Development of the Lungs

communicate with the peritoneal cavity through a pair of **pericardioperitoneal canals** passing dorsal to the septum transversum. However, a pair of transverse **pleuroperitoneal membranes** grow ventrally from the dorsal body wall to fuse with the transverse septum, thus closing off the pericardioperitoneal canals. The septum transversum and the pleuroperitoneal membranes thus form major parts of the future diaphragm.

On day 22, the foregut produces a ventral evagination called the **respiratory diverticulum** or **lung bud,** which is the primordium of the lungs. As the lung bud grows, it remains ensheathed in a covering of splanchnopleuric mesoderm, which will give rise to the lung vasculature and to the cartilage and muscle tissue within the bronchi. On days 26 to 28, the lengthening lung bud bifurcates into left and right **primary bronchial buds,** which will give rise to the two lungs. In the fifth week, a second generation of branching produces three **secondary bronchial buds** on the right side and two on the left. These are the primordia of the future lung lobes.

The bronchial buds and their splanchnopleuric sheath continue to grow and bifurcate, gradually filling the pleural cavities. By week 28, the 16th round of branching generates **terminal bronchioles,** which subsequently divide into two or more **respiratory bronchioles.** By week 36, these respiratory bronchioles have become invested with capillaries and are called **terminal sacs** or **primitive alveoli.** Between 36 weeks and birth, the alveoli mature. Additional alveoli continue to be produced throughout early childhood, perhaps until the eighth year.

As a result of folding, the amnion, which initially arises from the dorsal margin of the germ disc ectoderm, is carried ventrally to enclose the entire embryo, taking origin from the **umbilical ring** surrounding the roots of the vitelline duct and connecting stalk. The amnion also expands until it fills the chorionic space and fuses with the chorion. As the amnion expands, it encloses the connecting stalk and yolk sac neck in a sheath of amniotic membrane. This composite structure becomes the **umbilical cord.**

THE VERTEBRATE BODY FORM ARISES THROUGH CEPHALOCAUDAL AND LATERAL FLEXION

Differential Growth and Active Reshaping Cause the Embryo to Fold

At the end of the third week, the embryo is a flat, ovoid, trilaminar disc. During the fourth week it grows rapidly, particularly in length, and undergoes a process of folding that generates the recognizable vertebrate body form (Figs. 6–1, 6–2). Although some active remodeling of tissue layers takes place, the main force responsible for embryonic folding is the differential growth of various embryonic structures. During the fourth week, the embryonic disc and amnion grow vigorously, but the yolk sac hardly grows at all. Because the yolk sac is attached to the ventral rim of the embryonic disc, the expanding disc is compelled to balloon into a three-dimensional, somewhat cylindrical shape. The developing notochord, neural tube, and somites stiffen the dorsal axis of the embryo; therefore, most of the folding is concentrated in the thin, flexible outer rim of the disc. The cranial, caudal, and lateral margins of the disc fold completely under the dorsal axis structures and give

rise to the ventral surface of the body. Because the embryo grows faster in length than in width, these reflections are deeper at the caudal and (especially) the cranial ends of the embryo than along the sides.

Cephalic Folding May Occur in Response to the Overgrowth and Flexure of the Cephalic Neural Plate

In preparation for folding, the broad, thick cephalic neural folds become elevated dorsally by proliferation and migration of the underlying head mesenchyme (**mesenchyme** is loose embryonic connective tissue). As the cephalic portion of the embryonic axis overgrows the yolk sac, the cephalic neural plate flexes sharply at specific levels. The first of these flexures to appear is the **mesencephalic** or **cranial flexure,** which occurs in the region of the future mesencephalon (see Chs. 4 and 13). By day 22, the angle between the prosencephalon and the rhombencephalon is approximately 150 degrees; by day 23, it has diminished to 100 degrees.

As described in Chapter 3, the cranial rim of the germ disc—the thin area located cranial to the neural plate—contains the buccopharyngeal mem-

Weeks | Days

21 — At the beginning of the fourth week, the embryo is a trilaminar germ disc

The lung bud appears

4

22 — Embryonic folding commences

24

The lung bud branches into left and right bronchial buds

26 — Folding is complete, yielding a three-dimensional embryo that contains an intraembryonic coelom and is enclosed in the amniotic sac

28

5

Pericardioperitoneal canals

Coronal pleuropericardial folds begin to separate the primitive pericardial cavity into a pericardial cavity and two pleural cavities. The latter are initially continuous with the peritoneal cavity through the pericardioperitoneal canals, but a pair of pleuroperitoneal membranes begin to grow ventrally from the dorsal body wall to close off these canals

Branching yields the secondary bronchial buds (three on the right; two on the left). These represent the future lung lobes

35 —
36 —

6

Branching yields the tertiary bronchial buds (ten on the right; eight on the left). These represent the future bronchopulmonary segments

42 — Expansion of the amnion encloses the yolk sac and connecting stalk in a common sheath, forming the umbilical cord

7

Formation of the pericardial sac is complete. The lungs are growing

Terminal bronchioles form

16 — The pleuroperitoneal membranes have closed off the pericardioperitoneal canals. The diaphragm begins to differentiate

Terminal bronchioles have formed respiratory bronchioles; the surrounding mesenchyme becomes highly vascular; first terminal sacs (primitive alveoli) form

28

36

Terminal sacs begin to differentiate into mature alveoli. Alveoli continue to form through the 8th year

birth

8 years

Timeline. Embryonic folding; development of the pericardial, pleural, and peritoneal cavities; and development of the lungs.

brane, which represents the future mouth of the embryo. Cranial to the buccopharyngeal membrane, a second important structure has begun to appear: the horseshoe-shaped **cardiogenic area,** which will give rise to the heart (see Ch. 7). The overgrowth and flexure of the cephalic neural plate cause the thin cranial rim of the disc to fold under, forming the ventral surface of the future face,

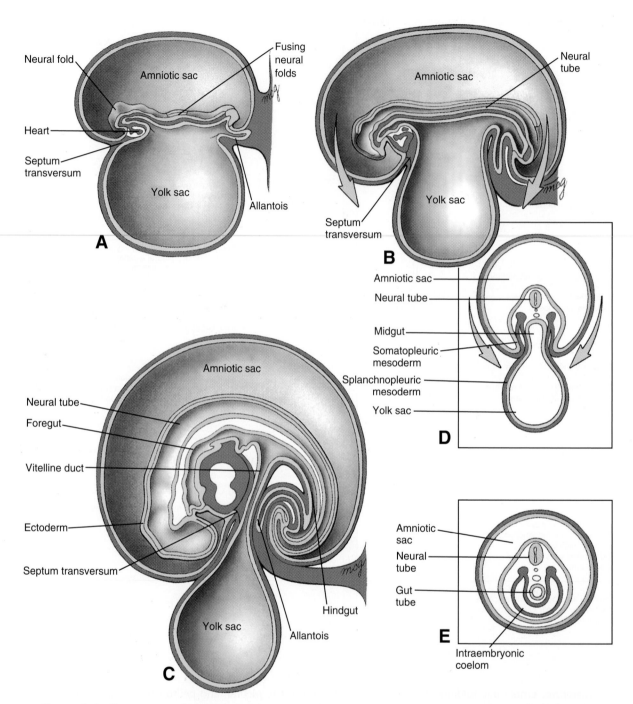

Figure 6–1. The process of cephalocaudal and lateral folding that transforms the embryo from a flat disc to a three-dimensional vertebrate body form. As folding occurs, the embryo grows more rapidly than the yolk sac, the cavity of which remains continuous with the developing gut tube through the narrowing vitelline duct. The septum transversum forms cranial to the cardiogenic area in the germ disc, *A*, and is translocated to the future lower thoracic region through the folding of the cranial end of the embryo, *B*, *C*. The allantois and connecting stalk combine with the yolk sac and vitelline duct through the folding of the caudal end of the embryo, *A–C*. Fusion of the ectoderm, mesoderm, future coelomic cavities, and endoderm from opposite sides is prevented in the immediate vicinity of the vitelline duct, *D*, but not in the more cranial and caudal regions, *E*.

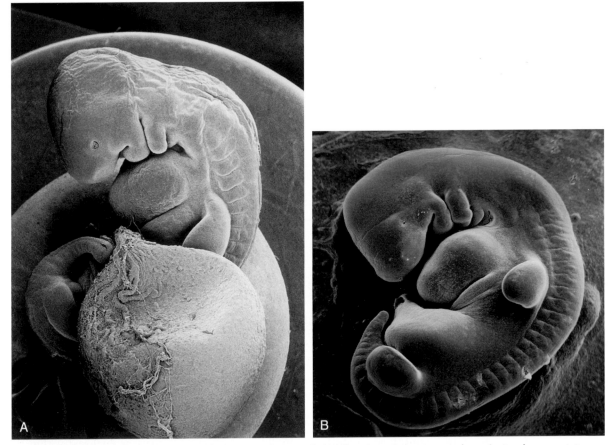

Figure 6–2. *A,* The form of this embryo is characteristic of a 4-week human embryo just subsequent to the folding process. Note the relatively large definitive yolk sac. *B,* A three-dimensional incipient human form is apparent in this 5-week embryo. The yolk sac has been removed. (*A,* Scanning electron micrograph courtesy of Dr. Arnold Tamarin.)

neck, and chest. This process translocates the buccopharyngeal membrane to the region of the future mouth and also carries the cardiogenic area toward the future chest (see Fig. 6–1).

A second important structure that is brought into the future thorax by cephalic folding is the **septum transversum.** This structure appears on day 22 as a thickened bar of mesoderm lying between the cardiogenic area and the cranial margin of the embryonic disc. Cephalic folding carries this bar ventrally and caudally until it is wedged between the cardiogenic region and the neck of the yolk sac (see Fig. 6–1*B, E;* see also Fig. 6–5*A*). As described later in this chapter, the septum transversum forms the initial partition separating the coelom into thoracic and abdominal cavities and gives rise to part of the diaphragm and the ventral

mesentery of the stomach and duodenum (see Ch. 9).

Caudal Folding Places the Connecting Stalk Next to the Yolk Sac

Starting on about day 23, a similar process of folding commences in the caudal region of the embryo as the rapidly lengthening neural tube and somites overgrow the caudal rim of the yolk sac. Because of the relative stiffness of these dorsal axis structures, the thin caudal rim of the germ disc, containing the cloacal membrane, folds under and becomes part of the ventral surface of the embryo (see Fig. 6–1). When the caudal rim of the disc folds under the body, the connecting stalk (which connects the caudal end of the germ disc to the developing placenta) is carried cranially until it merges with the neck of the yolk sac, which has begun to lengthen and constrict (see Fig. 6–1 and Fig. 6–2). The root of the connecting stalk contains a slender endodermal hindgut diverticulum called the **allantois** (see Fig. 6–1E). The fate of this structure is discussed in Chapter 9.

The Lateral Edges of the Germ Disc Fuse Along the Ventral Midline

Simultaneously with cephalocaudal flexion, the right and left sides of the embryonic disc flex sharply ventrally, constricting and narrowing the neck of the yolk sac (see Fig. 6–1C). At the head and tail ends of the embryo, these lateral edges of the germ disc make contact with each other and then zipper toward the umbilicus. When the edges meet, the ectodermal, mesodermal, and endodermal layers on each side fuse with the corresponding layers on the other side (see Fig. 6–1E). As a result, the ectoderm of the original germ disc covers the entire surface of the three-dimensional embryo except for the future **umbilical region,** where the yolk sac and connecting stalk emerge. The ectoderm, along with contributions from the dermatomes, lateral plate mesoderm, and neural crest, will eventually produce the skin (see Ch. 14).

The Fusion of the Lateral Edges of the Endoderm Creates the Gut Tube

The endoderm of the trilaminar germ disc is destined to give rise to the lining of the gastrointestinal tract. When the cranial, caudal, and lateral edges of the embryo meet and fuse, the superior and inferior portions of the endoderm are converted into blind-ending tubes—the future **foregut** and **hindgut.** At first, the central **midgut** region remains broadly open to the yolk sac (see Fig. 6–1A, B). However, as the gut tube forms, the neck of the yolk sac is gradually constricted, reducing its communication with the midgut. By the end of the sixth week, the gut tube is fully formed and the neck of the yolk sac has been reduced to a slim

stalk called the **vitelline duct** (see Fig. 6–1C). The cranial end of the foregut is capped by the buccopharyngeal membrane, which ruptures at the end of the fourth week to form the mouth. The caudal end of the hindgut is capped by the cloacal membrane, which will rupture during the seventh week to form the orifices of the anus and urogenital system (see Ch. 10).

FOLDING OF THE EMBRYO CONVERTS THE INTRAEMBRYONIC COELOM INTO A CLOSED CAVITY

The Intraembryonic Coelom, Its Serosal Lining, and the Mesenteries Are Products of the Lateral Plate Mesoderm

As described in Chapter 3, the lateral plate mesoderm splits into two layers: the **somatopleuric mesoderm,** which adheres to the ectoderm, and the **splanchnopleuric mesoderm,** which adheres to the endoderm. The space between these layers is originally open to the chorionic cavity. When the folds of the embryo fuse along the ventral midline, however, this space is enclosed within the embryo and becomes the **intraembryonic coelom** (Fig. 6–3; see also Fig. 6–1D, E). The two layers of the lateral plate mesoderm become the **serous membranes** lining this cavity: the somatopleuric mesoderm lines the inside of the body wall, and the splanchnopleuric mesoderm invests the visceral organs derived from the gut tube.

The Dorsal Mesentery Suspends the Abdominal Gut Tube Within the Coelom

When the coelom first forms, the gut is broadly attached to the dorsal body wall (see Figs. 6–1E and 6–3A). In the region of the future abdominal viscera (from the abdominal esophagus to the most proximal part of the future rectum), however, mesenchyme within this region of attachment gradually disperses during the fourth week, resulting in formation of a thin, bilayered **dorsal mesentery** that suspends the abdominal viscera in the coelomic cavity (see Fig. 6–3B). Because the abdomi-

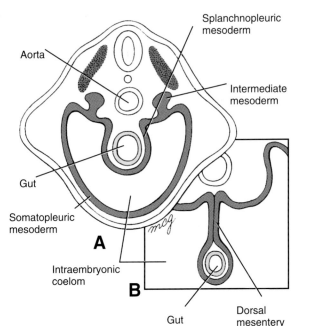

Aorta

Splanchnopleuric
mesoderm

Intermediate
mesoderm

Gut

Somatopleuric
mesoderm

A

Intraembryonic
coelom

B

Gut

Dorsal
mesentery

Figure 6–3. Formation of the dorsal mesentery. *A,* The primitive gut tube initially hangs from the posterior body wall by a broad bar of mesenchyme but, *B,* in regions inferior to the septum transversum this connection thins out to form a membranous dorsal mesentery composed of reflected peritoneum.

nal gut tube and its derivatives are suspended in what will later become the peritoneal cavity, they are referred to as **intraperitoneal** viscera. This term is traditional and rather loose; strictly, there is nothing in the peritoneal cavity itself except serous fluid and, in women, a monthly ovulated oocyte.

Retroperitoneal Organs Are Not Suspended by Mesentery. In contrast to the intraperitoneal location of most of the gut tube and its derivatives, some of the visceral organs develop in the body wall and are separated from the coelom by a covering of serous membrane (Fig. 6–4*A*). These organs are said to be **retroperitoneal.** It is important to realize that the designation *retroperitoneal* means that an organ is located behind the peritoneum from a viewpoint inside the peritoneal cavity—not that it is necessarily located in the posterior body wall. Thus, the kidneys are retroperitoneal, and so is the bladder, which develops in the anterior body wall (see Fig. 6–4*A*).

Parts of the Gut Tube Adhere to the Body Wall During Development and Become Secondarily Retroperitoneal. To complicate the intraperitoneal/retroperitoneal distinction further, some

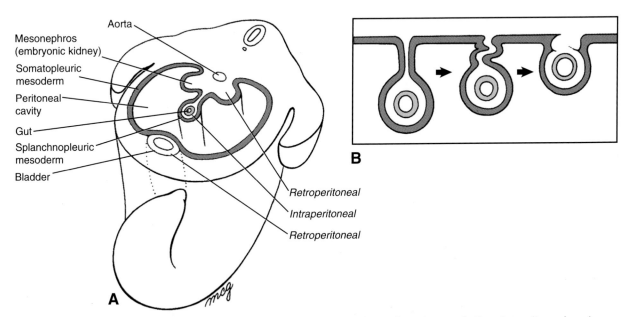

Mesonephros
(embryonic kidney)

Aorta

Somatopleuric
mesoderm

Peritoneal
cavity

Gut

Splanchnopleuric
mesoderm

Bladder

Retroperitoneal

Intraperitoneal

Retroperitoneal

A

B

Figure 6–4. The distinction between intraperitoneal, retroperitoneal, and secondarily retroperitoneal positions of the viscera. *A,* Viscera suspended within the peritoneal cavity by a mesentery are called intraperitoneal, whereas organs embedded in the body wall and covered by peritoneum are called retroperitoneal. *B,* The mesentery suspending some intraperitoneal organs disappears as both mesentery and organ fuse with the body wall. These organs are then called secondarily retroperitoneal.

parts of the gut tube that are initially suspended by mesentery later become fused to the body wall, thus taking on the appearance of retroperitoneal organs (see Fig. 6–4B). These organs, which include the ascending and descending colon, the duodenum, and the pancreas, are said to be **secondarily retroperitoneal.** (The development of the gastrointestinal tract is discussed in detail in Ch. 9.)

THE FORMATION OF THE PERICARDIAL SAC AND DIAPHRAGM BETWEEN 5 AND 7 WEEKS SUBDIVIDES THE COELOM INTO FOUR CAVITIES

The Septum Transversum Partially Separates the Thoracic and Abdominal Cavities

The septum transversum forms a transverse (horizontal) partition that partially separates the coe-

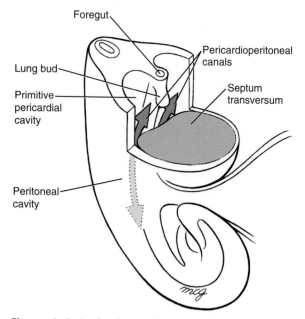

Figure 6–5. In the future thoracic region, the septum transversum forms a ventral partition partially separating the intraembryonic coelomic cavity into a primitive pericardial cavity superiorly and a peritoneal cavity inferiorly. These cavities remain in continuity through the posterior pericardioperitoneal canals (arrows).

lomic cavity into superior (thoracic) and inferior (abdominal) portions (Fig. 6–5; see also Fig. 6–1B, C). The superior portion contains the developing heart and is called the **primitive pericardial cavity,** whereas the inferior portion is the future **peritoneal cavity.** The septum transversum is attached ventrally and laterally to the body wall and dorsally to the mesenchyme associated with the foregut. However, the peritoneal and primitive pericardial cavities communicate through two large dorsolateral openings, the **pericardioperitoneal canals** (see Fig. 6–5).

Caudal Translocation of the Septum Transversum Is Accompanied by Elongation of the Phrenic Nerves

During the fourth and fifth weeks, the continued folding and differential growth of the embryonic axis cause a gradual caudal displacement of the septum transversum. The ventral edge of the septum finally becomes fixed to the anterior body wall at the 7th thoracic level, and the dorsal connection to the esophageal mesenchyme becomes fixed at the 12th thoracic level. Meanwhile, myoblasts (muscle cell precursors) differentiate within the septum transversum. These cells, which will form part of the future diaphragm muscle, are innervated by spinal nerves at a transient, cervical level of the septum transversum—that is, by fibers from the spinal nerves of cervical levels 3, 4, and 5 (C3, C4, C5). These fibers join together to form the paired **phrenic nerves,** which elongate as they follow the migrating septum caudally.

The Pericardial Sac Is Formed by Pleuropericardial Folds That Grow From the Lateral Body Wall in a Coronal Plane

During the fifth week, the pleural and pericardial cavities are divided from each other by **pleuropericardial folds** that originate along the lateral body walls in a coronal plane (Fig. 6–6). These septae appear at the beginning of the fifth week as broad folds of mesenchyme and pleura that grow medially toward each other between the heart and the developing lungs (see Fig. 6–6A, B). At the end of the fifth week, the folds meet and fuse with the foregut mesenchyme, thus subdividing the primitive pericardial cavity into three compartments: a fully enclosed, ventral **definitive pericardial cavity** and two dorsolateral **pleural cavities** (see Fig. 6–6C). The latter are still continuous with the peritoneal cavity through the pericardioperitoneal canals. (The term *pericardioperitoneal canal* is retained, even though the peritoneal canal now provides communication between the pleural cavities and the peritoneal cavity.)

As the tips of the pleuropericardial folds grow medially toward each other, their roots migrate toward the ventral midline (see Fig. 6–6B, C). By the time the tips of the folds meet to seal off the pericardial cavity, their roots take origin from the ventral midline. Thus, the space that originally constituted the lateral portion of the primitive pericardial cavity is converted into the ventrolateral part of the right and left pleural cavities.

The pleuropericardial folds are three-layered, consisting of body wall mesenchyme sandwiched between two layers of somatopleuric mesoderm. The thin definitive pericardial sac retains this threefold composition, consisting of inner and outer serous membranes (the inner **serous pericardium** and the outer **mediastinal pleura**) separated by a delicate filling of mesenchyme-derived connective tissue, the **fibrous pericardium.** The phrenic nerves, which originally run through the portion of the body wall mesenchyme incorporated into the pleuropericardial folds, course through the fibrous pericardium of the adult.

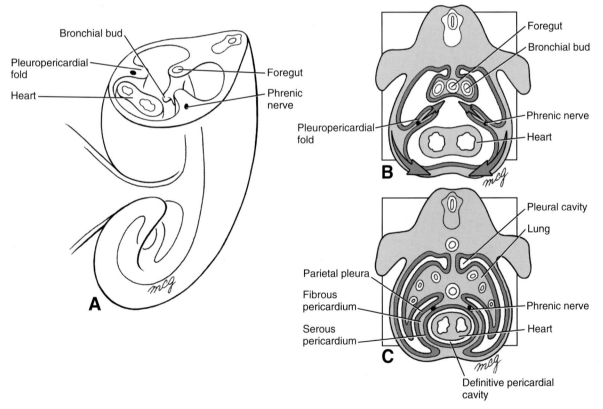

Figure 6–6. Subdivision of the primitive pericardial cavity. *A,* During the fifth week, coronal pleuropericardial folds grow out from the lateral body wall toward the midline, where they fuse with each other and with mesoderm associated with the esophagus. Simultaneously, the roots of these folds migrate ventrally so that they ultimately originate from the ventral body wall. *B,* The phrenic nerves initially embedded in the body wall are swept into these developing partitions. *C,* The pleuropericardial folds with their associated serous membrane form the pericardial sac and transform the primitive pericardial cavity into a definitive pericardial cavity and right and left pleural cavities.

Pleuroperitoneal Membranes Growing From the Posterior and Lateral Body Wall Seal Off the Pericardioperitoneal Canals

At the beginning of the fifth week, a pair of transverse membranes, the **pleuroperitoneal membranes,** arise along an oblique line connecting the root of the 12th rib with the tips of ribs 12 through 7 (Fig. 6–7*A*). These membranes grow ventrally to fuse with the posterior margin of the septum transversum, thus sealing off the pericardioperitoneal canals. Closure of the canals is complete by the seventh week (see Fig. 6–7*B*). The membranes are called *pleuroperitoneal membranes* because they do not contact the septum transversum until after the pericardial sac is formed; thus, they separate the definitive pleural cavities from the peritoneal cavity.

The left pericardioperitoneal canal is larger than the right and closes later. As discussed in the Clinical Applications section of this chapter, this difference may account for the fact that congenital diaphragmatic hernias of the abdominal viscera are more common on the left side than on the right.

THE DIAPHRAGM IS A COMPOSITE OF FOUR EMBRYONIC STRUCTURES

The definitive musculotendinous diaphragm incorporates derivatives of four embryonic structures: (1) the septum transversum, (2) the pleuroperitoneal membranes, (3) paraxial mesoderm of the body wall, and (4) esophageal mesenchyme (Fig 6–8*A*). Some of the myoblasts that arise in the septum transversum emigrate into the pleuroperitoneal membranes, pulling their phrenic nerve branches along with them. Most of the septum transversum then gives rise to the nonmuscular **central tendon** of the diaphragm (see Fig. 6–8*B*).

The bulk of the **diaphragm muscle** within the pleuroperitoneal membranes is innervated by the phrenic nerve. The outer rim of diaphragmatic muscle, however, arises from a ring of body wall paraxial mesoderm (see Fig. 6–7*B*) and is, therefore, innervated by spinal nerves from thoracic spinal levels T7 through T12. Finally, mesenchyme associated with the foregut at vertebral levels L1 through L3 condenses to form two muscular

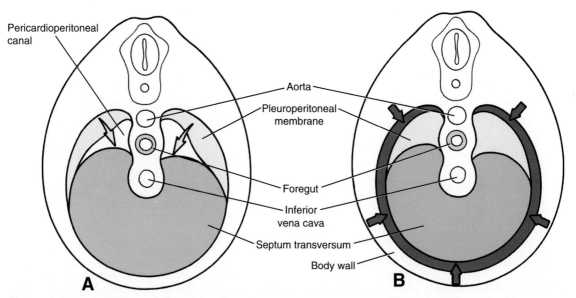

Figure 6–7. *A, B,* Closure of the pericardioperitoneal canals. Between weeks 5 and 7, a pair of horizontal pleuroperitoneal membranes grow from the posterior body wall to meet the posterior edge of the septum transversum, thus closing the pericardioperitoneal canals. These membranes form the posterior portions of the diaphragm and completely seal off the pleural cavities from the peritoneal cavity.

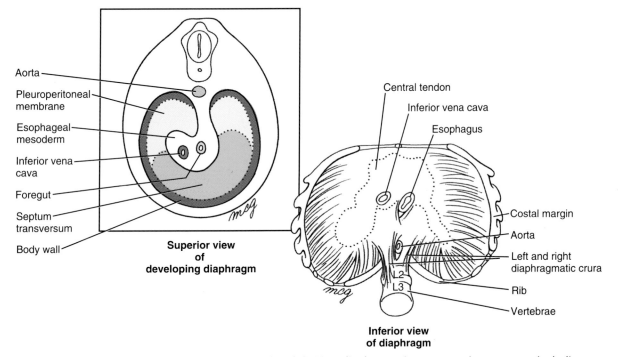

Figure 6–8. Formation of the diaphragm. The definitive diaphragm is a composite structure including elements of the septum transversum, pleuroperitoneal membranes, and esophageal mesenchyme, as well as a rim of body wall mesoderm.

bands, the **right** and **left crura** of the diaphragm, which originate on the vertebral column and insert into the dorsomedial diaphragm (see Fig. 6–8B). The right crus originates on vertebral bodies L1 through L3, and the left crus originates on vertebral bodies L1 and L2.

THE LUNGS BEGIN TO DEVELOP IN THE FOURTH WEEK AND BEGIN TO MATURE JUST BEFORE BIRTH

The Respiratory Tree Originates as a Foregut Diverticulum That Undergoes a Controlled Series of Branchings

The first rudiment of the lung, a keel-shaped ventral outpouching of the endodermal foregut called the **respiratory diverticulum,** or **lung bud,** appears on day 22 (Fig. 6–9). The lung bud begins to grow ventrocaudally through the mesenchyme surrounding the foregut. On days 26 to 28, it undergoes a first bifurcation, splitting into right and left **primary bronchial buds** (see Fig. 6–9). These buds are the rudiments of the two lungs. Between weeks 5 and 28, they branch an additional 16 times to generate the respiratory trees of the lungs. Experiments suggest that the pattern of branching of the lung endoderm is regulated by the surrounding mesenchyme. The stages of development of the lungs are summarized in Table 6–1.

The stem of the respiratory tree proximal to the first bifurcation becomes the trachea and larynx, and the stems of the right and left primary bronchial buds become the right and left primary bronchi. The third round of branching, which occurs early in the fifth week, yields three **secondary bronchial buds** on the right side and two on the left (see Fig. 6–9). These buds give rise to the lung lobes: three in the right lung and two in the left lung. During the sixth week, a fourth round of branching yields 10 tertiary bronchi on both sides; these become the bronchopulmonary segments of the mature lung (see Fig. 6–9).

By week 16, after about 14 more branchings,

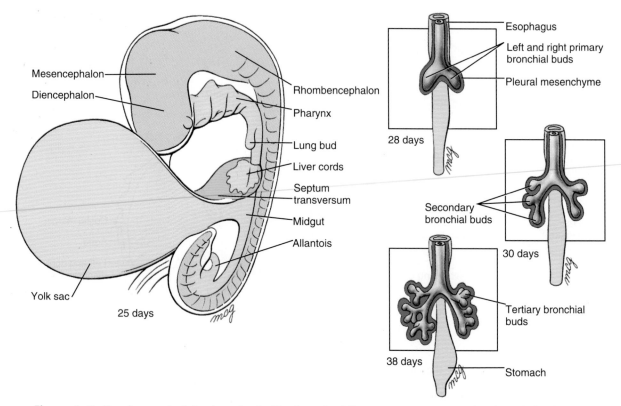

Figure 6–9. Development of the lung buds. The lung bud first appears as an evagination of the foregut on day 22 and bifurcates into two primary bronchial buds between day 26 and day 28. Early in the fifth week, the right bronchial bud branches into three secondary bronchial buds, whereas the left bronchial bud branches into two. By the sixth week, secondary bronchial buds branch into tertiary bronchial buds (usually about 10 on both sides) to form the bronchopulmonary segments.

Table 6–1
Stages of Human Lung Development

STAGE OF DEVELOPMENT	PERIOD	EVENTS
Embryonic	26 days to 6 weeks	The lung bud arises as a ventral outpouching of the foregut endoderm and undergoes three initial rounds of branching, producing the primordia successively of the two lungs, the lung lobes, and the bronchopulmonary segments.
Pseudoglandular	6 to 16 weeks	The respiratory trees of the lungs undergo 14 more generations of branching, resulting in the formation of terminal bronchioles.
Canalicular	16 to 28 weeks	Each terminal bronchiole divides into two or more respiratory bronchioles. The respiratory vasculature begins to develop.
Saccular	28 to 36 weeks	The respiratory bronchioles subdivide to produce terminal sacs (primitive alveoli). Terminal sacs continue to be produced until well into childhood.
Alveolar	36 weeks to term	The alveoli mature.

(Modified from Langston C, Kida K, Reed M, Thurlbeck WM. 1984. Human lung growth in late gestation in the neonate. Am Rev Respir Dis 129:607.)

the respiratory tree produces small branches called **terminal bronchioles** (Fig. 6–10). Between 16 and 28 weeks, each terminal bronchiole divides into two or more **respiratory bronchioles,** and the mesodermal tissue surrounding these structures becomes highly vascularized (see Fig. 6–10). By week 28, the respiratory bronchioles begin to sprout a final generation of stubby branches (see Fig. 6–10). These branches develop in craniocaudal progression, appearing first at more cranial terminal bronchioles. By week 36, the first-formed wave of terminal branches are invested in a dense network of capillaries and are called **terminal sacs (primitive alveoli)** (see Fig. 6–10). Limited respiration is possible at this point, but the alveoli are still so few and immature that infants born at this age may die of respiratory insufficiency without adequate therapy. (This topic is discussed in the Experimental Principles section of this chapter.) Ad-

ditional terminal sacs continue to form and differentiate in craniocaudal progression both before and after birth, possibly until as late as 8 years. About 20 to 70 million terminal sacs are formed in each lung before birth; the total number in the mature lung is 300 to 400 million. Continued thinning of the squamous epithelial lining of the terminal sacs begins just before birth, resulting in the differentiation of these primitive alveoli into mature alveoli (see Fig. 6–10).

The lung is a composite of endodermal and mesodermal tissues. The endoderm of the lung bud gives rise to the mucosal lining of the bronchi and to the epithelial cells of the alveoli. The vasculature of the lung and the muscle and cartilage supporting the bronchi are derived from the foregut splanchnopleuric mesoderm, which covers the bronchi as they grow out from the mediastinum into the pleural space.

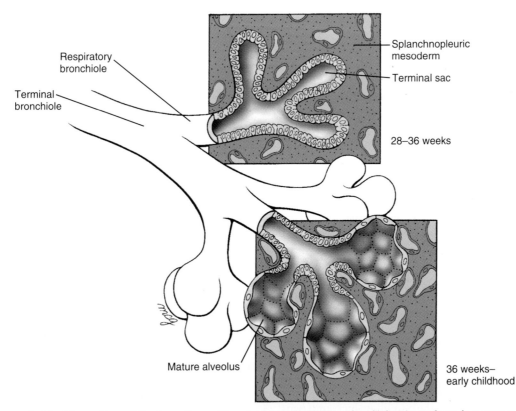

Figure 6–10. Maturation of the lung tissue. Terminal sacs (primitive alveoli) begin to form between weeks 28 and 36 and begin to mature between 36 weeks and birth. Only 5 to 20 percent of all terminal sacs produced by the age of 8 years, however, are formed before birth.

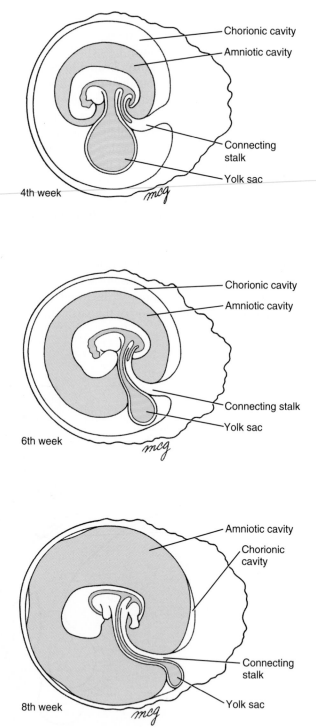

Figure 6–11. Genesis of the umbilical cord. The folding of the embryo and the expansion of the amniotic cavity bring the connecting stalk and yolk sac together to form the umbilical cord. As the amnion continues to grow, a layer of amniotic membrane gradually encloses the umbilical cord.

The Umbilical Cord Is Formed When the Connecting Stalk and Vitelline Duct Are Bound Together by the Expanding Amnion

As the embryo grows and folds, the amnion keeps pace, expanding until it encloses the entire embryo except for the umbilical area where the connecting stalk and yolk sac emerge (Fig. 6–11). Between the fourth and eighth weeks, an increase in the production of amniotic fluid causes the amnion to swell until it completely takes over the chorionic space (Fig. 6–12). When the amnion contacts the chorion, the layers of extraembryonic mesoderm covering the two membranes fuse loosely. The chorionic cavity thus disappears except for a few rudimentary vesicles.

After embryonic folding is complete, the amnion takes origin from the **umbilical ring** surrounding the roots of the vitelline duct and connecting stalk. The progressive expansion of the amnion therefore creates a tube of amniotic mem-

Figure 6–12. The rapidly expanding amniotic cavity fills with fluid and obliterates the chorionic cavity between weeks 4 and 8.

brane that encloses the connecting stalk and the vitelline duct (see Figs. 6–11 and 6–12). This composite structure is now called the **umbilical cord.** As the umbilical cord lengthens, the vitelline duct narrows and the pear-shaped body of the yolk sac remains within the umbilical sheath. Normally, both the yolk sac and the vitelline duct disappear by birth.

The main function of the umbilical cord is to circulate blood between the embryo and the pla-centa. Umbilical arteries and veins develop in the connecting stalk to perform this function (see Ch. 7). The expanded amnion creates a roomy, weight-less chamber in which the fetus can grow and de-velop freely. If the supply of amniotic fluid is inad-equate (the condition known as **oligohydramnios**), the abnormally small amniotic cavity may restrict fetal growth, which may result in severe malforma-tions and pulmonary hypoplasia (see the Clinical Applications section of this chapter).

Clinical Applications

DEVELOPMENTAL ABNORMALITIES OF THE LUNG

Abnormal Differentiation of the Lung Bud or Bronchial Buds Results in Pulmonary Malformations

Many lung anomalies result from a failure of the lung bud or a bronchial bud to branch or differen-tiate correctly. The most severe of these anomalies, **pulmonary agenesis,** results when the lung bud fails to split into right and left bronchi and to continue growing. Errors in the pattern of pulmo-nary branching **(branching morphogenesis)** dur-ing the embryonic and early fetal periods result in defects ranging from an abnormal number of pul-monary lobes or bronchial segments to the com-plete absence of a lung. Finally, defects in the sub-division of the terminal respiratory bronchi can result in an abnormal paucity of alveoli, even if the respiratory tree is otherwise normal. Some of these types of pulmonary anomalies are caused by intrin-sic molecular and cellular defects of branching morphogenesis (see the Experimental Principles section of this chapter). However, the primary cause of **pulmonary hypoplasia**—a reduced num-ber of pulmonary segments or terminal air sacs—often represents a response to some condition that reduces the volume of the pleural cavity and thus restricts growth of the lungs. For ex-ample, pulmonary hypoplasia can be produced in experimental animals by inflating a bal-loon in the pleural cavity while the fetus is in utero.

The Most Common Cause of Pulmonary Hypoplasia in Humans Is Congenital Diaphragmatic Hernia

In **congenital diaphragmatic hernia,** one of the pericardioperitoneal canals fails to close and allows the developing abdominal viscera to bulge into the pleural cavity (Fig. 6–13). If the mass of displaced viscera is large enough, it will stunt the growth of the lung on that side. Congenital diaphragmatic hernia occurs in about 1 of 2500 live births. The left side of the diaphragm is involved four to eight times more often than the right, probably because the left pericardioperitoneal canal is larger and closes later than the right. Diaphragmatic hernias can be surgically corrected at birth and have also rarely been corrected by surgery during fetal life (see Ch. 15). However, if the hernia has resulted in severe pulmonary hypoplasia, the newborn may die of pulmonary insufficiency even if the hernia is repaired. Small congenital hernias sometimes occur in the parasternal region or through the esopha-geal hiatus, but these usually do not have severe clinical consequences.

A Variety of Other Malformations Can Cause Pulmonary Hypoplasia by Reducing the Thoracic Volume

If the development of muscle tissue in the dia-phragm is deficient, the excessively compliant dia-

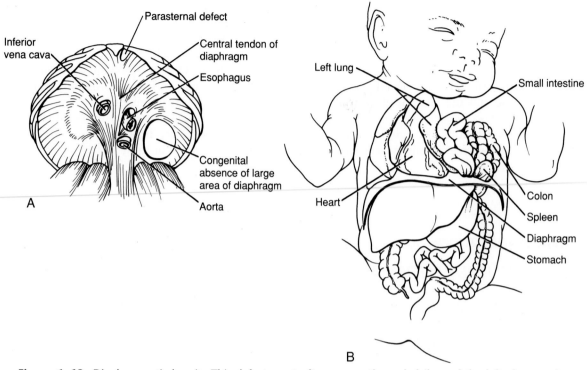

Figure 6–13. Diaphragmatic hernia. This defect most often occurs through failure of the left pleuroperitoneal membrane to seal off the left pleural cavity completely from the peritoneal cavity. *A,* Ventral view. *B,* Abdominal contents may herniate through the patent pericardioperitoneal canal, preventing normal development of the lung on that side.

phragm may allow the underlying abdominal contents to balloon or **eventrate** into the pulmonary cavity (Fig. 6–14). This condition can result in pulmonary hypoplasia, which may be fatal. Another classic cause of pulmonary hypoplasia is **oligohydramnios,** the condition in which there is an insufficient amount of amniotic fluid. Presumably, oligohydramnios causes pulmonary hypoplasia by allowing the uterine wall to compress the fetal thorax. Beginning at about 16 weeks of gestation, a substantial fraction of the amniotic fluid is contributed by the fetal kidneys. Therefore, **bilateral renal agenesis**—failure of both kidneys to form—results in oligohydramnios. Bilateral renal agenesis and pulmonary hypoplasia are characteristic defects in Potter's syndrome (discussed in the Clinical Applications section of Ch. 10). Although it has been suggested that the pulmonary hypoplasia seen in Potter's syndrome may develop before 16 weeks and therefore may not be solely an effect of oligohydramnios, several studies support the idea that oligohydramnios can produce pulmonary hypoplasia by compression of the chest. For example, if a

fetus with bilateral renal agenesis shares the amniotic cavity with a normal twin who produces enough amniotic fluid, lung development is normal in both twins. Oligohydramnios resulting from premature rupture of the amnion can also cause pulmonary hypoplasia. Similarly, oligohydramnios induced in experimental animals by amniocentesis during the third trimester sometimes results in a reduced number of respiratory bronchioles and alveoli as well as structural abnormalities of the alveoli. At critical periods of development, premature rupture of amniotic membranes, with resultant loss of amniotic fluid, is another cause of pulmonary hypoplasia.

The Defects Responsible for Malformations of the Esophagus and Trachea Are Poorly Understood

Esophageal atresia (a blind esophagus) and **esophagotracheal fistula** (an abnormal connection

Figure 6–14. Eventration of the diaphragm. Failure of the pleuroperitoneal membranes to differentiate normally during fetal life may allow abdominal organs to dilate the abnormally thin regions of the diaphragm and eventrate into the pleural cavity. (Photo courtesy of Children's Hospital Medical Center, Cincinnati, OH.)

between tracheal and esophageal lumina) are usually found together, although in about 10 percent of cases one occurs independently (Fig. 6–15). Both defects are dangerous to the newborn because they allow milk or other fluids to be aspirated into the lungs. In addition, esophageal atresia has an effect on the intrauterine environment opposite to that of renal agenesis: the blind-ending esophagus prevents the fetus from swallowing amniotic fluid and returning it to the mother via the placental circulation and thus results in an excess of amniotic fluid **(polyhydramnios)** and consequent distention of the uterus. Surgical correction of both defects is generally successful.

The cause of esophageal atresia is thought to be a failure of the esophageal endoderm to proliferate rapidly enough during the fifth week to keep up with the elongation of the embryo. However, the cause of tracheoesophageal fistula and the rea-

son why the two defects are usually found together are unknown. In experimental mouse models, disruption of the sonic hedgehog pathway or thyroid transcription factor-1 causes tracheoesophageal fistula.

LUNG MATURATION AND THE SURVIVAL OF PREMATURE INFANTS

The Lungs Mature Rapidly Just Before Birth

As parturition approaches, the lungs undergo a rapid and dramatic series of transformations that prepare them for air breathing. The fluid produced by the respiratory epithelium filling the alveoli is absorbed at birth, the defenses that will protect the lungs against invading pathogens and against the oxidative effects of the atmosphere are activated, and the surface area for alveolar gas exchange increases greatly. Changes in the structure of the lung take place during the last 2 months, accelerating in the days just preceding a normal term delivery. If a child is born prematurely, the state of development of the lungs is usually the prime factor determining whether it will live. Infants born between 26 weeks and term—during the phase of accelerated terminal lung maturation—have a good chance of survival. Infants born before 26 weeks (in the canalicular phase of lung development) cannot survive without intensive respiratory assistance and, even then, often die.

Although the total surface area for gas exchange in the lung depends on the number of alveoli and on the density of alveolary capillaries, efficient gas exchange will only occur if the barrier separating air from blood is thin—that is, if the alveoli are thinwalled, properly inflated, and not filled with fluid. The walls of the maturing alveolar sacs thin out during the weeks before birth. In addition, specific alveolar cells (the alveolar type II cells) begin to secrete **pulmonary surfactant,** a mixture of phospholipids and surfactant proteins that reduces the surface tension of the liquid film lining the alveoli and thus facilitates inflation. In the absence of surfactant, the surface tension at the air liquid interface of the alveolar sacs tends to collapse the alveoli during exhalation, and these collapsed alveoli can be inflated only with great effort.

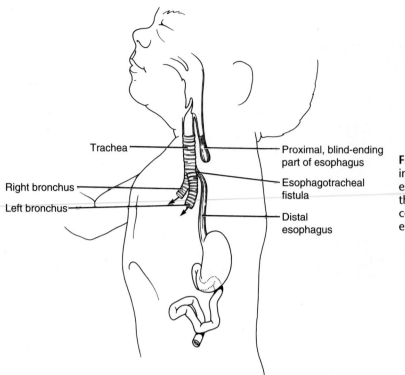

Trachea

Right bronchus

Left bronchus

Proximal, blind-ending part of esophagus

Esophagotracheal fistula

Distal esophagus

Figure 6–15. This diagram of an infant with esophageal atresia and esophagotracheal fistula shows how the first drink of fluid after birth could be diverted into the newly expanded lungs (arrows).

It appears that the primary cause of the **respiratory distress syndrome** of premature infants (pulmonary insufficiency accompanied by gasping and cyanosis) is an inadequate production of surfactant. Respiratory distress syndrome not only threatens the infant with immediate asphyxiation, but the increased rate of breathing and mechanical ventilation required to support the infant's respiration also can damage the delicate alveolar lining, allowing fluid and cellular and serum proteins to exude into the alveolus. Continued injury may lead to detachment of the alveolar lining, a condition called **hyaline membrane disease.** Chronic lung injury associated with preterm infants causes a condition termed bronchopulmonary dysplasia.

Molecular Engineering May Lead to Improved Surfactant Replacement Therapy

Critically ill newborns were first successfully treated by **surfactant replacement therapy**—the administration of exogenous surfactant—in the late 1970s. A variety of surfactant preparations are now used for this purpose, some derived from animal lungs or human amniotic fluid, others synthetic. However, experiments indicate that these phospholipid preparations would be more effective if they also included some of the supplementary proteins found in natural surfactant. For example, it has been found that the addition of small amounts of human surfactant proteins enhances surfactant activity. Two of these proteins (A and B) apparently act by organizing the surfactant phospholipids into tubular structures termed tubular myelin, which is particularly effective at reducing surface tension. Although surfactant protein C is not required for tubular myelin formation, it does enhance the function of surfactant phospholipids. Surfactant proteins A and D apparently play important roles in innate host defense of the lung against viral, bacterial, and fungal pathogens.

Surfactant B Deficiency Causes Respiratory Distress in Term Infants

A fatal disease called **hereditary surfactant protein B deficiency** has been described as an uncommon cause of **respiratory failure** in full-term newborn infants. Alveolar air spaces are filled with granular eosinophilic proteinaceous material and tubular myelin is absent. Even though aggressive medical interventions have been applied in these cases, including surfactant replacement therapy, infants afflicted with this disease typically die within the first year of life. It was found that this disease is an autosomal recessive condition typically characterized by a complete absence or mutation of one of the surfactant proteins, surfactant protein B (SP-B).

The genetic basis for hereditary surfactant B deficiency has been examined, and, in most cases, a **frameshift mutation** in exon 4 of the human surfactant B gene has been found. This mutation results in premature termination of translation of the surfactant B protein. Other mutations of the surfactant B gene have also been identified, resulting in synthesis of defective forms of the surfactant B

protein. It has also been demonstrated that effects of surfactant B deficiency extend beyond the disruption of translation of the surfactant B gene. The results of studies of null mutations of the surfactant B gene in transgenic mice, for example, show that, although the amount of surfactant C or surfactant A mRNA is not affected, precursors of the mature surfactant C protein are not completely processed. In addition, the processing of pulmonary phospholipids is also disrupted. Similar disruptions of surfactant C peptide and phospholipid processing have been described in a human infant with surfactant protein B deficiency. More than 15 different mutations in the SP-B gene have been associated with hereditary SP-B deficiency. Mild mutations can cause chronic pulmonary disease in infants. Although these studies have been useful in diagnosis, it is hoped that they will also lead to effective therapies for this usually fatal disease.

Experimental Principles

MOLECULAR STUDIES OF LUNG DEVELOPMENT

In Situ Hybridization and Immunocytochemical Studies Reveal Patterns of Expression of Lung-Specific Regulatory Factors

As described in earlier sections of this text, the technique of **in situ hybridization** utilizes radiolabeled antisense oligonucleotide or ribonucleotide probes to localize specific messenger RNAs at the cellular level (see the Experimental Principles Section of Ch. 3). An advantage in localizing the specific mRNA produced by a given gene is identification of the cell expressing the particular factor encoded by that gene. One disadvantage of this technique is that evidence of expression of the specific mRNA is not sufficient to demonstrate expression and activity of the factor itself. However, the protein factor may be localized by **immunocytochemical techniques,** but this may provide confusing information regarding its site of expression,

because the factor may be detected in a target cell after its expression and secretion by some other tissue or cell. Thus, a combination of these approaches is often useful in delineating the functional roles of specific factors in interacting tissues. These techniques have been extremely useful in the study of developing lungs, providing a basis for the targeting of **growth factors, growth factor receptors, retinoic acid receptors,** and **transcription factors** in many of the experimental studies of **branching morphogenesis** and **surfactant synthesis** described later.

Branching of the Lung Primordia May Be Studied in Organ Culture

Just after the bifurcation of the lung bud into primary bronchial buds, the lung primordia can be removed from embryonic birds or mice and cul-

Figure 6–16. Dominant-negative mutation of fibroblast growth factor (FGF) receptor specifically expressed in the lungs results in inhibition of branching of the respiratory tree and formation of elongated epithelial tubes. (Modified from Peters K. Werner S. Liao X, et al. 1994. Targeted expression of a dominant negative FGF receptor blocks branching morphogenesis and epithelial differentiation of the mouse lung. EMBO J. 13:3296.)

tured in media free of serum and other exogenous growth factors. Under these conditions, the lung primordia will grow and bifurcate, producing a normal respiratory tree. As a consequence, it is possible to treat these cultured lungs with specific inhibitors to analyze the roles of growth factors and other agents in the branching process. In one such study, a small peptide that served as a competitive inhibitor of ligand binding to **integrin receptors** resulted in abnormal morphology of the developing lung primordium. In another study, incubation with **monoclonal antibodies** to specific sequences of the extracellular matrix protein **laminin** resulted in reduction of terminal buds and segmental dilation of the explanted lung primordia. In

another strategy, lung explants are treated with **antisense oligonucleotides,** which bind with and inactivate the mRNA of the specific factor of interest. Experiments with antisense oligonucleotides against transcription factors such as **thyroid transcription factor-1 (TTF-1)** result in reduction in the number of terminal branches of the lung primordium.

Transgenic Animal Technologies Are Used in Studies of Lung Development

Transgenic strategies, including knockouts and gain-of-function mutants, have been utilized to examine factors involved in lung development. For example, a **surfactant B gene knockout** was described in the Clinical Applications section of this chapter. Similar approaches have implicated the proto-oncogene N-*myc* and the homeobox gene *Gsh-4* in regulation of branching of the lung and the homeodomain containing **TTF-1** and the **winged helix transcription factor hepatic nuclear factor-3 (HNF-3)** in the regulation of surfactant synthesis. A dramatic result was obtained by the targeted disruption of a **fibroblast growth factor (FGF) receptor protein** in a **dominant-negative mutation.** A transgene consisting of the surfactant C promoter element and a mutant form of the FGF receptor that lacked a kinase sequence was constructed and incorporated into ES cells, which were used to create several founder mice. Inclusion of the surfactant C promoter element in the transgene resulted in its expression only in the airway epithelium. Because development of functional FGF receptors requires dimerization of two normal FGF protein monomers, the dimerization of the mutant protein produced by the transgene, with the endogenous wild-type (normal) FGF protein, resulted in formation of inactive receptors only in the lungs. As a consequence, other tissue of the embryos developed normally, but branching of the respiratory tree in these heterozygotes was completely inhibited, resulting in formation of elongated epithelial tubes that were incapable of supporting normal respiratory function at birth (Fig. 6–16). Subsequent gene knockout experiments in mice demonstrated that fibroblast growth factor-10 (FGF-10) and an isoform of its receptor in the respiratory epithelium, the FGF-receptor 2(FGF-R2), were critical for formation of both lungs and limbs. Similarly, ablation of thyroid transcription factor-1 (TTF-1) blocked formation of both thyroid and lung.

Transgenic strategies have also been utilized to create models of human pulmonary disease such as **cystic fibrosis.** Mouse mutants in which the c-AMP-stimulated chloride secretory activity of the cystic fibrosis gene is absent or reduced are created by homologous recombination (see the Experimental Principles Section of Ch. 1). Animals that have incorporated transgene-containing ES cells into the germ line are then bred to produce transgenic animals homozygous for the mutant transgene. Although some phenotypic features of these mice differ somewhat from the human condition, they express many characteristics of the human disease. Other transgenic mice have been created that carry the normal human cystic fibrosis gene to demonstrate that it is nontoxic and therefore probably safe to use in human therapy. Currently, various approaches for human gene therapy of cystic fibrosis are being developed with viral- and DNA-based delivery systems to insert the cystic fibrosis gene directly to the somatic airway epithelial cells of afflicted infants and children.

A Molecular and Cellular Basis for Branching Morphogenesis and Alveolar Differentiation Is Being Rapidly Deciphered

As discussed in the descriptive section of this chapter, the endodermal lung bud and subsequent bronchial branches grow into the mesenchyme surrounding the thoracic gut tube. Moreover, deficiencies or abnormalities in the branching of the respiratory diverticulum are the basis of many forms of **pulmonary hypoplasia** (see the Clinical Applications of this chapter). Studies over the past six decades have demonstrated that the **branching morphogenesis** of the respiratory diverticulum is regulated by the interaction between the diverticulum and surrounding mesoderm. Moreover, based

on recent studies such as those described in the immediately preceding section, several molecular factors produced by the mesenchyme alone or by the mesenchyme in concert with the proliferating endodermal outgrowth have been found to play critical roles in the pattern of branching of distal elements as well as in the subsequent inhibition of branching in proximal regions of the respiratory tree. For example, when mesenchyme in the region of the bifurcating bronchial bud is replaced with tracheal mesenchyme, further branching is inhibited. Conversely, replacement of tracheal mesenchyme with that from the region of the bifurcating bronchial buds stimulates resumption of tracheal branching. Based on experiments such as these, components of the **extracellular matrix** have been implicated in the stimulation and inhibition of branching. Collagens type IV and V, laminin, fibronectin, and tenascin, for example, are thought to play either a permissive or a stimulatory role in branching of the bronchial buds. Likewise, regulation of expression of receptors for these matrix components has also been implicated in control of branching morphogenesis.

Several **growth factors** have also been implicated in the regulation of branching morphogenesis of the lung, including retinoic acid, epithelial growth factor (EGF), platelet-derived growth factor (PDGF), FGF, insulin-like growth factor (IGF), fibroblast pneumocyte factor (FPF), tumor necrosis factor-α (TNF-α), transforming growth factor-α (TGF-α), transforming growth factor-β (TGF-β), and Wnt-2. These growth factors and their receptors are expressed during different phases of lung growth and branching, consistent with their postulated roles in this complex process (see Fig. 6–16). For example, branching during the **pseudoglandular stage** is apparently influenced in part by retinoic acid, sonic hedgehog, FGFs, BMP-4 (bone morphogenetic protein), and TGF-β signaling pathways. The homeodomain-containing factor TTF-1 and FGF-10 are required for normal branching morphogenesis during the embryonic and pseudoglandular stages (see earlier).

On the other hand, both FGF and EGF may play pivotal roles in the formation and maturation of terminal sacs during the **saccular stage** of lung maturation. In addition to the function of TTF-1 and HNF-3 in surfactant synthesis (see earlier), cytokines, glucocorticoids, and thyroxine have also been shown to stimulate surfactant synthesis before birth. It is hoped that these findings will lead to therapeutic manipulations that will result in stimulation of adequate alveolar formation and differentiation and surfactant synthesis within the lungs of premature infants.

SUGGESTED READING

Descriptive Embryology

Bucher U, Reid L. 1961. Development of the intrasegmental bronchial tree: the pattern of branching and development of cartilage at various stages of intrauterine life. Thorax 16:207

Burri PH. 1984. Fetal and postnatal development of the lung. Annu Rev Physiol 46:617

Frank L. 1990. Preparation for birth. p. 1141. In Massaro D (ed): Lung Cell Biology. Marcel Dekker, New York.

Gattone VH, Morse DE. 1984. Pleuroperitoneal canal closure in the rat. Anat Rec 208:445

Heuser CH, Corner GW. 1957. Developmental horizons in human embryos. Description of age group X, 4–12 somites. Contrib Embryol 244:29

Hilfer SR, Rayner RM, Brown JW. 1985. Mesenchymal control of branching in fetal mouse lung. Tissue Cell 17:523

Hislop A, Howard S, Fairweather DVI. 1984. Morphometric studies on the structural development of the lung in Macaca fascicularis during fetal and postnatal life. J Anat 138:95

Langston C, Kida K, Reed M, Thurlbeck WM. 1984. Human lung growth in late gestation and in the neonate. Am Rev Respir Dis 129:607

Müller F, O'Rahilly R. 1983. The first appearance of the major divisions of the human brain at stage 9. Anat Embryol 168:419

O'Rahilly R, Müller F. 1984 Respiratory and alimentary relations in staged human embryos. Ann Otol Rhinol Laryngol 93:421

Pringle KC. 1986. Human fetal lung development and related animal models. Clin Obstet Gynecol 29: 502

Rudnick D. 1933. Developmental capacities of the chick lung in chorioallantoic grafts. J Exp Zool 66:125

Searles RL. 1986. A description of caudal migration during growth leading to the formation of the pericardial and pleural coeloms, the caudal movement of the aortic arches, and the development of the shoulder. Am J Anat 77:271

Tyler WS. 1983. Small airways and terminal units. Comparative subgross anatomy of lungs. Am Rev Respir Dis 128:S32

Wigglesworth JS. 1988. Lung development in the second trimester. Br Med Bull 44:894

Zeltner TB, Burri PH. 1987. The postnatal development and growth of the human lung. II. Morphometry. Respir Physiol 67:269

Clinical Applications

Avery ME, Taeusch HW. 1984. Disorders of the diaphragm. p. 189. In Schaffer AJ (ed): Schaffer's Diseases of the Newborn. WB Saunders, Philadelphia

Clark JC, Wert S, Bachurski C, et al. 1995. Targeted disruption of the surfactant protein B gene disrupts surfactant homeostasis causing respiratory failure in newborn mice. Proc Natl Acad Sci U S A 92:7794

Fujiwara T, Maeta H, Chida S, et al. 1980. Artificial surfactant therapy in hyaline membrane disease. Lancet ii:55

Hislop A, Fairweather DVI, Blackwell RJ, Howard S. 1984. The effect of amniocentesis and drainage of amniotic fluid on lung development in Macaca fascicularis. Br J Obstet Gynaecol 91:835

Lawrence S, Rosenfeld CR. 1986. Fetal pulmonary development and abnormalities of amniotic fluid volume. Semin Perinatol 10:142

Nogee LM, Garnier G, Dietz HC, et al. 1994. A mutation in the surfactant B gene responsible for fatal neonatal respiratory disease in multiple kindreds. J Clin Invest 93:1860

Notter RH. 1988. Biophysical behavior of lung surfactant: implications for respiratory physiology and pathophysiology. Semin Perinatol 12:180

O'Rahilly R, Müller F. 1984. Respiratory and alimentary relations in staged human embryos. Ann Otol Rhinol Laryngol 93:421

Pringle KC. 1986. Human fetal lung development and related animal models. Clin Obstet Gynecol 29: 502

Singer DB. 1984. Morphology of hyaline membrane disease and its pulmonary sequelae. p. 63. In Stern L (ed): Hyaline Membrane Disease, Pathogenesis and Pathophysiology. Grune & Stratton, New York

Zaw-Tun H. 1982. The tracheoesophageal septum—fact or fantasy? J Anat 114:1

Experimental Principles

Cardoso WV. 1995. Transcription factors and pattern formation in the developing lung. Am J Physiol 269:2429

Crump RG, Askew GR, Wert SE, et al. 1995. In situ localization of sodium-potassium ATPase mRNA in developing mouse lung epithelium. Am J Physiol 269:2299

Glasser SW, Korthagen TR, Wert SE, Whitsett JA. 1994. Transgenic models for study of pulmonary development and disease. Am J Physiol 267:2489

Hilfer SR. 1996. Morphogenesis of the lung: control of embryonic and fetal lung branching. Annu Rev Physiol 58:93

Kelly SE, Bachuski CJ, Burhaus MS, Glasser SW. 1996. Transcription of the lung specific surfactant protein C gene is mediated by thyroid transcription factor-1. JBC 271:6881

Kitterman JA. 1984. Fetal lung development. J Dev Physiol 6:67

Litingtung Y, Lei L, Westphal H, Chiang C. 1998. Sonic hedgehog is essential to foregut development. Nat Genet 20:58

Min H, Danilenko DM, Scully SA, et al. 1998. *Fgf-10* is required for both limb and lung development and exhibits striking functional similarity to *Drosophila branchless*. Genes Dev 12:3156

Minoo P, Penn R, DeLennos DM et al. 1993. Tissue inhibitor of metalloproteinase-1 mRNA is specifically induced in lung after birth. Pediatr Res 34:729

Peters SK, Werner S, Liao X, et al. 1994. Targeted expression of a dominant negative FGF receptor blocks branching morphogenesis and epithelial differentiation of the mouse lung. EMBO J 13:3296

Retsch-Bogart GZ, Moats-Staats BM, Howard K, et al. 1996. Cellular localization of messenger RNAs for insulin-like growth factors (IGFs), their receptors and binding proteins during fetal rat lung development. Am J Respir Cell Mol Biol 14:61

Rice W. 1995. Developmental aspects of surfactant. Semin Respir Crit Care Med. 16:11

Whitsett JA. 1991. Pulmonary surfactant and respiratory distress syndrome in the premature infant. p. 1723. In Crystal RG, Est JB, Barren PJ, et al (eds): The Lung. Vol II (Section 6). Raven Press, New York

Whitsett JA, Korfhagen TR. 1996. Regulation of gene transcription in respiratory epithelial cells. Am J Respir Cell Mol Biol 14:118

Whitsett JA, Negee LM, Weaver T, Horowitz AD. 1995. Human surfactant protein B; structure function, regulation and genetic disease. Physiol Rev 75:749

Zhao Y, Young S. 1995. Tenasin in rat lung development: in situ localization and cellular sources. Am J Physiol 269:2482

Development of the Heart

Summary

The heart primordium forms in a horseshoe-shaped region of the splanchnopleuric mesoderm at the cranial end of the germ disc called the **cardiogenic region.** In response to signals from the underlying endoderm, the angioblastic cords in this region coalesce to form a pair of **lateral endocardial tubes.** The cephalic and lateral folding of the embryo during the early fourth week causes these tubes to be brought together along the midline in the future thoracic region, where they fuse to form a single **primitive heart tube.**

Between weeks 5 and 8, the primitive heart tube undergoes a process of looping, remodeling, and septation that transforms its single lumen into the four chambers of the definitive heart, thus laying down the basis for the separation of pulmonary and systemic circulations at birth.

Initially, the primitive heart tube develops a series of expansions and shallow sulci that subdivide it into primordial heart chambers. Starting at the inflow end, these are the left and right horns of the **sinus venosus,** the **primitive atrium,** the **ventricle,** and the **bulbus cordis.** The inferior end of the bulbus cordis then differentiates into the right ventricle, whereas the primitive ventricle gives rise to most of the left ventricle. The superior end of the bulbus cordis (the **conotruncus**) will form the **conus cordis** and the **truncus arteriosus,** which split to become outflow regions of both ventricles (the ascending aorta and the pulmonary trunk).

Venous blood initially enters the sinus horns through paired, symmetrical **common cardinal veins.** As described in Chapter 8, however, changes in the venous system rapidly shift the entire systemic venous return to the right so that all the blood from the body and umbilicus enters the future right atrium through the developing superior and inferior venae cavae. The left sinus horn becomes the **coronary sinus,** which drains the myocardium. A process of intussusception incorporates the right sinus horn and the ostia of the venae cavae into the posterior wall of the future right atrium, displacing the original right half of the atrium as it forms the right auricle. Meanwhile, the future left atrium sprouts a pulmonary vein, the trunk of which is subsequently incorporated by intussusception to form most of the definitive left atrium. In the fifth and sixth weeks, a pair of septa, the **septum primum** and the **septum secundum,** grow to separate the right and left atria. These septa are perforated by a staggered pair of foramina that allow right-to-left shunting of blood throughout gestation. The **bicuspid (mitral)** and **tricuspid atrioventricular valves** also develop during the fifth and sixth weeks. Meanwhile, the

Formation and Folding of the Primitive Heart Tube

Morphogenesis of the Heart Chambers and Valves

Development of the Cardiac Conduction System

Weeks   Days

— 19   Vasculogenesis in the cardiac region forms the lateral endocardial tubes

3

— 20   Embryonic folding brings the endocardial tubes together in the thoracic region

Bulboventricular sulcus

— 21   The endocardial tubes fuse to form the primitive heart tube, which is divided into incipient chambers by sulci

Atrioventricular sulcus

— 22   Splanchnopleuric mesoderm invests the heart tube and forms the myocardium and cardiac jelly; migrating mesothelial cells invest the myocardium and form the epicardium

The heart begins to beat

4

— 23   The heart begins to fold

The septum primum begins to form

The muscular ventricular septum begins to form

— 28   Folding is complete

5

— 33   The atrioventricular valves begin to form (complete by 3 mo)

— 35   Right and left truncoconal ridges begin to form

6

Superior and inferior endocardial cushions fuse to form the septum intermedium

Definitive atria and auricles are present

— 42

7   — 46   The ostium secundum and foramen ovale form as the septum primum meets the septum intermedium

The muscular ventricular septum ceases to grow

8   — 56   The coronary sinus is formed

The aortic and pulmonary outflow tracts and the ventricles are fully separated by growth of the truncoconal ridges

9

— 63   The semilunar valves are complete

10

Timeline. Formation of the heart.

heart undergoes a remodeling that brings the future atria and ventricles into correct alignment and also aligns both ventricles with their respective outflow tracts. The base of the bulbus cordis expands to enlarge the right ventricle, and during the sixth week a **muscular ventricular septum** partially separates the ventricles. Finally, during the seventh and eighth weeks, the outflow tract of the heart—the conotruncus—undergoes a process of septation and division that converts it into the separate, helically arranged ascending aorta and pulmonary trunk. During this process swellings within the truncus arteriosus give rise to the **semilunar valves** of the aorta and pulmonary trunk. The conotruncal septa also grow into the ventricles to complete ventricular septation.

THE LATERAL ENDOCARDIAL TUBES DEVELOP IN THE CARDIOGENIC REGION AND FUSE TO FORM THE PRIMARY HEART TUBE

On day 19, a pair of vascular elements called the **endocardial tubes** begin to develop in the **cardiogenic region,** a horseshoe-shaped zone of splanchnopleuric mesoderm located cranial and lateral to the neural plate on the embryonic disc. These vessels form from splanchnopleuric mesoderm by a process called **in situ vesicle formation and fusion, or vasculogenesis** (Fig. 7–1). This process is described in detail in Chapter 8. Late in the third week, the cephalic and lateral folding of the embryo brings the two lateral endocardial tubes into the thoracic region (see Ch. 6), where they meet along the midline and fuse to form a single tube (Fig. 7–2). The fusion of the two tubes is facilitated by programmed cell death in their contacting surfaces. (Programmed cell death, a common mechanism in embryonic morphogenesis, is discussed in the Experimental Principles section at the end of this chapter.)

The Paired Dorsal Aortae of the Primitive Circulatory System Form Simultaneously With the Lateral Endocardial Tubes

It is important to realize that many of the major vessels of the embryo, including the paired dorsal aortae, develop at the same time as the endocardial tubes. The **inflow** and **outflow** tracts of the future heart make connection with the paired lateral endocardial tubes even before these tubes are translocated into the thorax and fuse to form the heart (Fig. 7–3; see also Fig. 7–1). The paired **dorsal aortae,** which form the primary outflow tract of the heart, develop in the dorsal mesenchyme of the embryonic disc on either side of the notochord and make their connection with the endocardial tubes before folding begins. As the flexion and growth of the cephalic fold carries the endocardial tubes first into the cervical and then into the thoracic region (Fig. 7–4), the cranial ends of the dorsal aortae are pulled ventrally until they form a dorsoventral loop, the **first aortic arch** (see Fig. 7–3D). A series of four more aortic arches will develop during the fourth and fifth weeks in connection with the pharyngeal arches (Fig. 7–5) (see Ch. 8).

The inflow to the heart is initially supplied by six vessels, three on each side (see Fig. 7–5). Venous blood from the body of the embryo enters the heart through a pair of short trunks, the **common cardinal veins,** which are formed by the confluence of the paired **posterior cardinal veins** draining the trunk and the paired **anterior cardinal veins** draining the head region (Fig. 7–5). The yolk sac is drained by a pair of **vitelline veins,** and oxygenated blood from the placenta is delivered to the heart by a pair of **umbilical veins.** The formation and development of the embryonic venous system are discussed in Chapter 8.

A Series of Constrictions and Expansions Subdivide the Primary Heart Tube

By day 21, a series of constrictions **(sulci)** and expansions appear in the presumptive heart tube (Fig. 7–6). Over the next 5 weeks, these expansions contribute to the various heart chambers. Starting at the inferior (inflow) end, the **sinus venosus** consists of the partially confluent left and right **sinus horns** into which the common cardinal veins drain. Cranial to the sinus venosus, the next

A   19 days

Figure 7–1. Formation of the lateral endocardial tubes and more medial dorsal aortae by vasculogenesis during the third week. Splanchnopleuric mesodermal cells aggregate in the horseshoe-shaped cardiogenic area (*A*) and form short cords (*B*), which coalesce into a plexus of vessels (*C*). These vessels will further consolidate into larger channels. Presumptive endothelial cells contributing to vessel formation are stained in parts *B* and *C*, with antibodies specific for these cells. (From Poole TJ, Coffin JD. 1991. Morphogenetic mechanisms in avian vascular development. p. 25. In Feinberg RP, Shiever G, Auerbach R [eds]: International Symposium on Vascular Development. Karger, Basel.)

two chambers are the **primitive atrium** and the **ventricle,** which are separated by the **atrioventricular sulcus.** The primitive atrium will give rise to parts of both atria, and the ventricle will give rise to most of the definitive left ventricle. The ventricle is separated from the next expansion, the **bulbus cordis,** by the **bulboventricular sulcus.** Because the inferior part of the bulbus cordis will form most of the **right ventricle,** this sulcus is also called the **interventricular sulcus.** The superior end of the bulbus cordis is also called the **conotruncus.** This region of the heart will form the distal outflow regions of the left and right ventricles, including the **conus cordis** and the **truncus arteriosus.** The truncus arteriosus eventually splits to form the **ascending aorta** and the

pulmonary trunk and is connected at its superior end to a dilated expansion sometimes called the **aortic sac.** The aortic sac is continuous with the first aortic arch and, eventually, with the other four aortic arches. The aortic arches form major arteries that transport blood to the head and trunk (see Ch. 8).

Four Layers Become Apparent in the Wall of the Primary Heart Tube

The primary heart tube consists initially of endothelium. By day 22, however, a thick mass of splanchnopleuric mesoderm invests the fused endo-

A 20 days

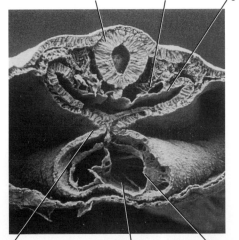

B 21 days

cardial tubes and differentiates into two new layers: the **myocardium,** or heart muscle, and the **cardiac jelly,** a layer of thick acellular matrix secreted by the developing myocardium that separates it from the fused endocardial tubes (Fig. 7–7). This structure, comprised of an endocardial tube and invested by cardiac jelly within a myocardial tube, is called the primitive heart tube. The **serous epicardium (visceral pericardium)** is formed by a population of **mesothelial cells** that are independently derived from splanchnopleuric mesoderm and that migrate onto the surface of the heart from the region of the sinus venosus or septum transversum (see Fig. 7–7B).

The Transverse Pericardial Sinus Is Formed by Rupture of the Dorsal Mesocardium

The primary heart tube is initially suspended in the primitive pericardial cavity by a **dorsal mesocardium (dorsal mesentery of the heart)** formed of foregut splanchnopleuric mesoderm. This dorsal mesocardium promptly ruptures, however, leaving the heart suspended in the primitive pericardial cavity by its attached vasculature. The region of the ruptured dorsal mesocardium becomes the **transverse pericardial sinus** within the pericardial sac of the definitive heart (Fig. 7–8).

The Heart Tube Folds and Loops to Establish the Spatial Relationships of the Future Heart Chambers

On day 23, the heart tube begins to elongate and simultaneously to loop and fold. The bulbus cordis is displaced inferiorly, ventrally, and to the right;

C

Figure 7–2. Cephalocaudal and lateral folding at the end of the third week quickly brings the lateral endocardial tubes into the ventral midline in the upper thoracic region (*A, B*), where they fuse to form the primitive heart tube (*C*). (*C*, From Hurle JM, Icardo JM, Ojeda JL. 1980. Compositional and structural heterogeneity of the cardiac jelly of the chick embryo tubular heart: a TEM, SEM and histochemical study. J Embryol Exp Morphol 56:211.)

Figure 7–3. Formation of embryonic vessels. *A,* Vascular cords in the dorsal body wall form paired dorsal aortae (DA) both cranial and caudal to the embryonic heart tube (EH) developing in the ventral thoracic region. Vitelline veins (VV) are forming just caudal to the primitive heart tube, and the ventral region of the first aortic arch (VA) is forming just superior to the embryonic heart. The first aortic arch itself (AA) loops superiorly and dorsally to connect with the superior ends of the dorsal aortae (DA). *B,* At a slightly later stage, the lateral endocardial tubes have fused and formed a distinct bulbus cordis (BC). The aortic arches (AA) loop dorsally to connect the superior end of the ventrally located heart with the superior ends of the dorsal aortae (DA). The dorsal aortae give off intersomitic arteries (ISA) and finally break up into capillary plexuses (CP). The third arch has begun to sprout internal carotid arteries (ICA). *C,* Ventral view shows the fusing endocardial tubes within the primitive pericardial cavity. *D,* Drawing shows the first aortic arches encircling the superior end of the foregut. Illustrations *A* and *B* were prepared in the same way as *B, C. (A, B,* From Coffin JD, Poole TJ. 1988. Embryonic vascular development: immunohistochemical identification of the origin and subsequent morphogenesis of the major vessel primordia in quail embryos. Development 102:735. *C,* From Icardo JM, Fernandez-Teran MA, Ojeda JL. 1990. Early cardiac structure and developmental biology. p. 3. In Meisami E, Timiras PS [eds]: Handbook of Human Growth and Developmental Biology. Vol. 3. CRC Press, Boca Raton, FL.)

Figure 7–4. Scanning electron micrographs showing how cephalic flexion translocates the developing endocardial tubes from a region just cranial to the neural plates to the thoracic region. (Arrow, cardiogenic region.) (From Kaufman MH. 1981. The role of embryology in teratological research, with particular reference to the development of the neural tube and the heart. J Reprod Fertil 62:607.)

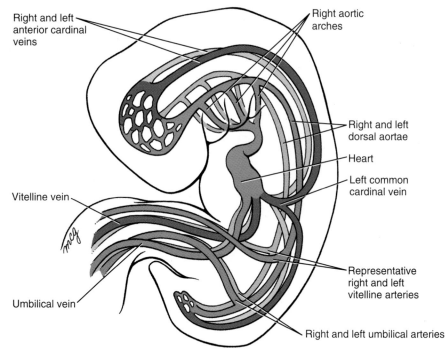

Figure 7–5. Schematic depiction of the embryonic vascular system in the middle of the fourth week. The heart has begun to beat and to circulate blood. The outflow tract of the heart now includes four pairs of aortic arches and the paired dorsal aortae that circulate blood to the head and trunk. Three pairs of veins—umbilical, vitelline, and cardinal—deliver blood to the inflow end of the heart.

the ventricle is displaced to the left; and the primitive atrium is displaced posteriorly and superiorly (Fig. 7–9). Looping is complete by day 28.

Considerable effort has gone into identifying the forces responsible for looping. It was at one time suggested that looping occurs simply because the heart tube outgrows the primitive pericardium;

however, hearts excised from experimental animals and grown in culture demonstrate an intrinsic ability to loop. Some studies have suggested that the state of hydration of the cardiac jelly controls looping, but when the jelly was removed enzymatically, looping was unaffected. Another suggestion is that looping is induced by the hemodynamic

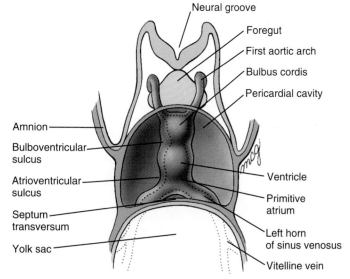

Figure 7–6. As early as day 21, a series of visible constrictions and expansions divide the heart tube into primitive regions that will give rise to chambers of the adult heart.

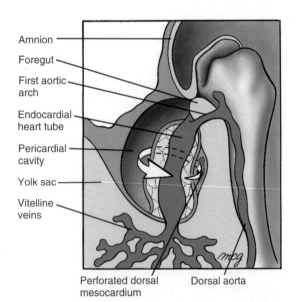

Figure 7–7. Differentiation of the heart wall. *A,* By 22 days, the primitive heart tube (the endocardium of the future heart) is invested by a layer of cardiac jelly, a layer of myocardial cells, and an epicardium. The myocardium is derived from a mass of splanchnopleuric mesoderm that encloses the primitive heart tube. The myocardium then secretes the extracellular cardiac jelly between itself and the primitive heart tube. *B,* The epicardium is derived from a sheet of splanchnopleuric mesoderm that migrates from the region of the sinus venosus to cover the myocardium. (*B,* From Ho E, Shimada Y. 1978. Formation of the epicardium studied with the scanning electron microscope. Dev Biol 66:579.)

forces of circulating blood. Hemodynamic forces are certainly important in heart morphogenesis, but, again, cultured hearts loop correctly in the absence of blood flow. Looping may alternatively be caused by active migration or remodeling of myocytes or by controlled regional proliferation.

The result of looping is to bring the four presumptive chambers of the future heart into their correct spatial relation to each other. The remainder of heart development consists of the remodeling of these chambers and the development of the appropriate septa and valves between them.

COORDINATED REMODELING OF THE BILATERALLY SYMMETRICAL HEART TUBE AND PRIMITIVE VASCULATURE PRODUCES THE SYSTEMIC AND PULMONARY CIRCULATIONS

Figure 7–8. Formation of the transverse pericardial sinuses of the definitive pericardial cavity by rupture of the dorsal mesocardium early in the fourth week.

At day 22, the heart and primitive circulatory system are bilaterally symmetrical: right and left car-

Figure 7–9. Looping of the heart tube. The looping of the heart tube repositions the bulbus cordis anteriorly and to the right and shifts the ventricle to the left and the primitive atrium posteriorly and superiorly. The superior end of the bulbus cordis will form outflow regions of the right and left ventricles, whereas its inferior end will form most of the right ventricle. The ventricle will form most of the definitive left ventricle, and the primitive atrium will give rise to the rudimentary auricles of the heart. (Photographs from Kaufman MH. 1981. The role of embryology in teratological research, with particular reference to the development of the neural tube and the heart. J Reprod Fertil 62:607.)

dinal veins drain the two sides of the body, and blood from the heart is pumped into right and left aortic arches and dorsal aortae. The paired dorsal aortae fuse from T4 to L4 in the fourth week to form a single midline dorsal aorta. The venous system undergoes a complicated remodeling (detailed in Ch. 8), with the result that all the systemic venous blood drains into the right atrium through the newly formed superior and inferior venae cavae.

Starting at birth, the systemic and pulmonary circulations are wholly separate and are arranged in series. This arrangement would be impracticable in the fetus, however, because oxygenated blood enters the fetus via the umbilical vein and because little blood can flow through the collapsed lungs. The fetal heart chambers and outflow tracts therefore contain foramina and ducts that shunt the oxygenated blood entering the right atrium to the left ventricle and aortic arch, thus largely bypassing the pulmonary circulation. These shunts close at birth, abruptly separating the two circulations (see Ch. 8).

Remodeling of the Heart Tube Commences as the Venous Inflow to the Sinus Venosus Shifts to the Right

The heart starts to beat on day 22, and by day 24 blood begins to circulate throughout the embryo. Venous return initially enters the right and left sinus horns via the common cardinals (Fig. 7–10A). Within the next few weeks, however, the venous system is remodeled so that all the systemic venous blood enters the right sinus horn via the **superior** and **inferior venae cavae** (see Fig. 7–10B, C). As venous inflow shifts to the right, the left sinus horn ceases to grow and is transformed into a small venous sac on the posterior wall of the heart (see Fig. 7–10C). This structure gives rise to the **coronary sinus** and the small **oblique vein of the left atrium.** The coronary sinus will receive most of the blood draining from the coronary circulation of the heart muscle.

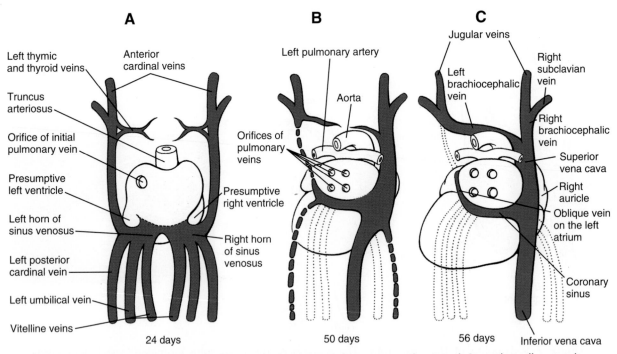

Figure 7–10. Remodeling of the inflow end of the heart between weeks 4 and 8 so that all systemic blood flows into the future right atrium. The left sinus horn is reduced and pulled to the left. It loses its connection with the left anterior cardinal vein and becomes the coronary sinus that drains blood only from the heart wall. The left anterior cardinal vein becomes connected to the right anterior cardinal vein through an anastomosis of thymic and thyroid veins, which form the left brachiocephalic vein. A remnant of the right vitelline vein becomes the terminal segment of the inferior vena cava (see Ch. 8).

THE LEFT AND RIGHT ATRIA UNDERGO EXTENSIVE REMODELING

The Right Sinus Horn Is Incorporated Into the Right Posterior Wall of the Primitive Atrium

As the right sinus horn and the venae cavae enlarge to keep pace with the rapid growth of the rest of the heart, the right side of the sinus venosus is gradually incorporated into the right posterior wall of the developing atrium, displacing the original right half of the primitive atrial wall ventrally and to the right (Fig. 7–11; see also Fig. 7–

10). The differential growth of the right sinus venosus also pulls the vestigial left sinus horn (the future coronary sinus) to the right. The portion of the atrium that consists of incorporated sinus venosus is now called the **sinus venarum,** whereas the original right side of the primitive atrium becomes a diminutive ventral flap of tissue called the **right auricle.** The auricle can be distinguished in the adult heart by the pectinate (comblike) trabeculation of its wall, which contrasts with the smooth wall of the sinus venarum.

Through this process of **intussusception** of the right sinus venosus, the openings or **ostia** of the superior and inferior venae cavae and future coronary sinus (former left horn of the sinus venosus) are pulled into the posterior wall of the definitive right atrium, where they form the **orifices of**

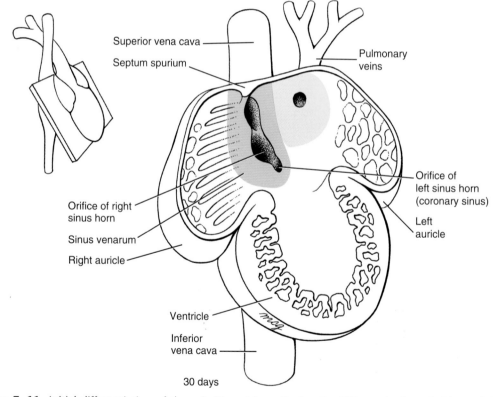

Figure 7–11. Initial differentiation of the primitive atrium. During the fifth week, the primitive atrial tissue on the left and right sides is displaced anteriorly and laterally to form the trabeculated, rudimentary auricles of the adult heart. On the right side, the right sinus horn is incorporated into the posterior wall of the right side of the atrium as the smooth-walled sinus venarum, which will give rise to the definitive right atrium. Meanwhile, a single pulmonary vein sprouts from the left side of the primitive atrium and then branches twice to produce two right and two left pulmonary veins. The sinus venarum continues to expand within the posterior wall of the future right atrium.

the superior and inferior venae cavae and the **orifice of the coronary sinus** (Figs. 7–12 and 7–13). As this occurs, a pair of tissue flaps, the **left** and **right venous valves,** develop on either side of the three ostia. Superior to the sinuatrial orifices, the left and right valves join to form a transient septum called the **septum spurium.** The left valve eventually becomes part of the septum secundum, one of the septa that contributes to the separation of the definitive right and left atria (discussed later). The right venous valve, in contrast, remains intact and forms the **valve of the inferior vena cava** and the **valve of the coronary sinus.**

Superior to the valve of the inferior vena cava, a ridge of tissue called the **crista terminalis** now delimits the trabeculated right auricle from the smooth-walled sinus venarum (see Fig. 7–13). The crista terminalis contains the fibers that carry impulses from the primary pacemaker region of the heart (the **sinoatrial node**) to a secondary pacemaker center, the **atrioventricular node.** This fiber tract is part of the conducting system that channels the spread of depolarizing electrical cur-

rents through the heart and thus organizes the beating of the myocardium.

The Trunk of the Pulmonary Venous System Is Incorporated Into the Posterior Wall of the Left Atrium

While the right atrium is being remodeled during the fourth and fifth weeks, the left atrium undergoes a somewhat similar process. At the beginning of the fourth week, the primitive atrium sprouts a pulmonary vein (see Fig. 7–11). This vein promptly branches into right and left pulmonary branches, which bifurcate again to produce a total of four pulmonary veins. These veins grow toward the lungs, where they anastomose with veins developing in the mesoderm investing the bronchial buds (see Ch. 6).

During the fifth week a process of intussusception incorporates the trunk and first two

Superior vena cava

Sinus venarum

Septum spurium

Pulmonary veins

Orifice of superior
vena cava

Venous valves

Crista terminalis

Orifice of inferior
vena cava

Orifice of coronary
sinus

Right auricle

Left
auricle

Ventricle

Inferior
vena cava

31 days

Figure 7–12. Further differentiation of the atrium. Later in the fifth week, the pulmonary vein system begins to undergo intussusception into the posterior wall of the primitive atrium to form the definitive left atrium.

branchings of the pulmonary vein system into the posterior wall of the left side of the primitive atrium (see Figs. 7–11 and 7–12), where they form the smooth wall of the definitive left atrium. The trabeculated left side of the primitive atrium is displaced ventrally and to the left, where it becomes the vestigial left auricle. As a result of this process of intussusception, the pulmonary venous system opens into the atrium initially through a single large orifice, then transiently through two orifices, and finally through the four orifices of the definitive pulmonary veins (see Fig. 7–13).

SEPTATION OF THE ATRIA AND DIVISION OF THE ATRIOVENTRICULAR CANAL BEGIN IN THE FOURTH WEEK, BUT RIGHT-TO-LEFT SHUNTING OF BLOOD PERSISTS UNTIL BIRTH

The first step in the separation of the systemic and pulmonary circulations is the partial separation of the definitive atria and the division of the common atrioventricular canal into right and left canals. The adult interatrial septum is formed by the fusion of two embryonic partial septa, the septum primum and the septum secundum. These septa both have large openings that allow right-to-left shunting of blood throughout gestation.

At the End of the Fourth Week, the Septum Primum Begins to Grow Down From the Atrial Roof

On about day 26, while atrial remodeling is in progress, the roof of the atrium becomes depressed along the midline by the overlying conotruncus. On day 28, this deepening depression produces a crescent-shaped wedge of tissue called the **septum primum** that begins to extend into the atrium from the superoposterior wall (Fig. 7–14). During the fifth week, the free edge of the septum primum grows caudally toward the atrioventricular canal, thus gradually separating the nascent right and left atria. The diminishing foramen between the atria is called the **ostium primum.**

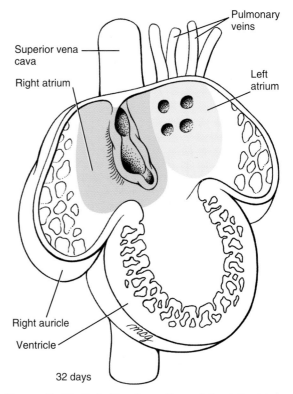

Figure 7–13. Definitive formation of the left atrium. The first four pulmonary branches are incorporated into the posterior wall of the left side of the primitive atrium, completing the formation of the smooth-walled part of the future left atrium.

The Septum Primum Fuses With the Septum Intermedium

As the septum primum is growing downward, four expansions of tissue develop in the endocardium around the periphery of the atrioventricular canal (see Fig. 7–14A). These thickenings are called the **left, right, superior,** and **inferior endocardial cushions.** The endocardium is induced to form the cushions by signals from the adjacent myocardium. At the end of the sixth week, the superior and inferior cushions meet and fuse, forming the **septum intermedium** that divides the common atrioventricular canal into **right** and **left atrioventricular canals** (Figs. 7–15A, 7–16, and 7–17C). At the end of the sixth week, the growing edge of

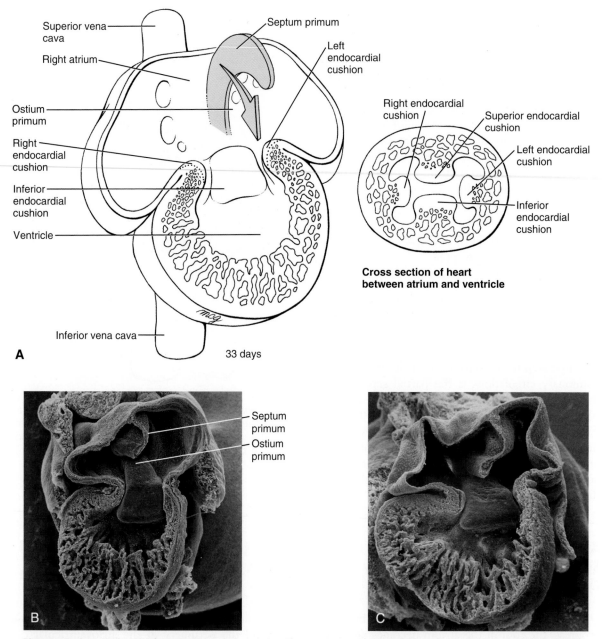

Figure 7–14. *A–C,* Initial septation of the atria. The septum primum forms from the roof of the atrial chamber during the fifth week and grows as a crescent-shaped wedge toward the atrioventricular canal. Simultaneously, the atrioventricular canal is being divided into right and left atrioventricular orifices by the growing superior and inferior endocardial cushions. (*B, C,* From Icardo JM. 1988. Heart anatomy and developmental biology. Experientia 44:910.)

the septum primum fuses with the septum intermedium (see Figs. 7–15*A* and 7–19*D*). This event obliterates the ostium primum.

Before the ostium primum closes, however, programmed cell death in an area near the supe-

rior edge of the septum primum creates small perforations that coalesce to form a new foramen, the **ostium secundum** (see Fig. 7–15*B*). Thus, a new channel for right-to-left shunting opens before the old one closes.

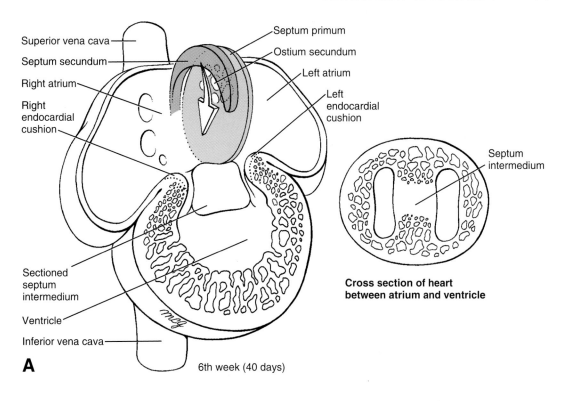

Cross section of heart between atrium and ventricle

A 6th week (40 days)

Figure 7–15. Further septation of the atria. *A,* During the sixth week, the thick septum secundum grows from the roof of the right atrium and the septum primum fuses with the superior and inferior endocardial cushions (septum intermedium). Before the ostium primum is obliterated, however, the ostium secundum forms by the coalescence of small ruptures in the septum primum. *B,* Scanning electron micrograph showing the development of the ostium secundum. (*B,* From Hendrix MJC, Morse DE. 1977. Atrial septation. I. Scanning electron microscopy in the chick. Dev Biol 57:345.)

Mid 6th week (38 days)

An Incomplete Septum Secundum Forms Next to the Septum Primum

While the septum primum is growing, a second crescent-shaped ridge of tissue appears on the ceiling of the right atrium, just adjacent to the septum primum (see Fig. 7–15*A*). This **septum secundum** is thick and muscular, in contrast to the thin, membranous septum primum. The edge of the septum secundum grows posteroinferiorly, but it halts before it reaches the septum intermedium, leaving an opening called the **foramen ovale** near the floor of the right atrium (see Fig. 7–16). Throughout the rest of fetal development, there-

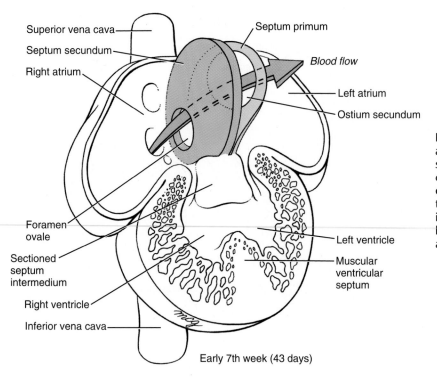

Superior vena cava

Septum secundum

Right atrium

Septum primum

Blood flow

Left atrium

Ostium secundum

Foramen ovale

Left ventricle

Sectioned septum intermedium

Muscular ventricular septum

Right ventricle

Inferior vena cava

Early 7th week (43 days)

Figure 7–16. Definitive fetal separation of the atria. The septum secundum does not completely close, leaving a patent foramen ovale. During embryonic and fetal life, much of the blood entering the right atrium passes to the left atrium via the foramen ovale and the ostium secundum.

fore, the blood that shunts from the right atrium to the left atrium passes through two staggered openings: the foramen ovale near the floor of the right atrium and the foramen secundum near the roof of the left atrium. This shunt closes at birth because the abrupt dilation of the pulmonary vasculature, combined with the cessation of umbilical flow, reverses the pressure difference between the atria and pushes the flexible septum primum against the more rigid septum secundum (see the discussion of changes in circulation at birth at the end of Ch. 8).

future left ventricle (see Fig. 7–17A). Moreover, the superior end of the presumptive right ventricle, but not the presumptive left ventricle, is initially continuous with the conus cordis and truncus arteriosus that will eventually give rise to both the aortic and pulmonary outflow tracts. The heart must therefore undergo a complicated remodeling to bring the developing right atrioventricular canal into line with its atrium and ventricle and simultaneously to provide the left ventricle with a direct outflow path through the conus cordis to the truncus arteriosus. This process is illustrated in Figure 7–17.

EXTENSIVE REMODELING ALIGNS THE RIGHT AND LEFT ATRIOVENTRICULAR CANALS WITH THEIR RESPECTIVE ATRIA AND VENTRICLES AND THE LEFT AND RIGHT VENTRICLES WITH THEIR FUTURE OUTFLOW TRACTS

Even after the heart tube finishes looping and folding, the atrioventricular canal provides a direct pathway only between the future atrium and the

The Atrioventricular Canal Is Repositioned to the Right

The atrioventricular canal initially lies in a coronal plane between the left side of the primitive atrium and the future left ventricle. Two theories have been proposed for the mechanism by which the right side of the canal comes into alignment with the future right atrium and right ventricle. Part of this change may be accomplished by active migra-

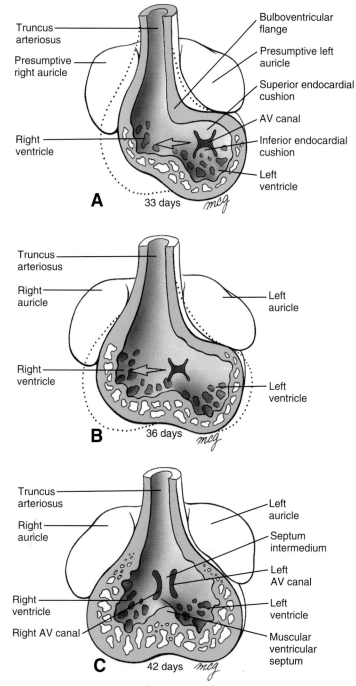

Figure 7–17. *A–C,* Realignment of the heart. As the septum intermedium forms during the fifth and sixth weeks, the heart is remodeled to align the developing left atrioventricular canal with the left atrium and ventricle and the right atrioventricular canal with the right atrium and ventricle.

tion of the common atrioventricular canal during the fifth week. Alternatively, the apparent rightward movement of the canal may result wholly from the obliteration of the superior internal protrusion of the bulboventricular sulcus and the widening of the conotruncus.

In addition, at the same time that the canal is shifting to the right, it is being divided into right and left canals by the growth of the superior and inferior endocardial cushions. Thus, by the time the common canal has split into right and left atrioventricular canals, they are correctly aligned with their respective atria and ventricles (see Fig. 7–17C).

Simultaneously, the Left Ventricle Gains Access to the Truncus Arteriosus

The repositioning that brings the presumptive left ventricle into line with the proximal portion of the truncus arteriosus is apparently due to several factors working in concert. The reduction of the bulboventricular flange by differential growth and the widening of the proximal part of the conus cordis partly effect this shift. A role also seems to be played by the left wall of the proximal end of the conus cordis, which is incorporated into the left ventricle, and by the differential expansion of the right wall of the right ventricle and the left wall of the left ventricle (see Fig. 7–17).

Both ventricles seem thus to be composite structures. The right ventricle is derived mainly from the most inferior part of the bulbus cordis and from the right wall of the conus cordis. In addition, part of the inlet region of the right ventricle, near the tricuspid atrioventricular valve, originates in the primitive ventricle and is carried over to the right ventricle during the repositioning of the atrioventricular canal. The definitive left ventricle is derived from the primitive ventricle and from the left wall of the conus cordis.

SEPTATION OF THE VENTRICLES IS COORDINATED WITH THE FORMATION OF ATRIOVENTRICULAR VALVES AND SEPTATION OF THE OUTFLOW TRACTS

Once the atrioventricular canals, ventricles, and cardiac outflow tract are all correctly aligned, the stage is set for the remaining phases of heart morphogenesis: the septation of the ventricles, the division of the outflow tract into ascending aorta and pulmonary trunk, and the development of the heart valves.

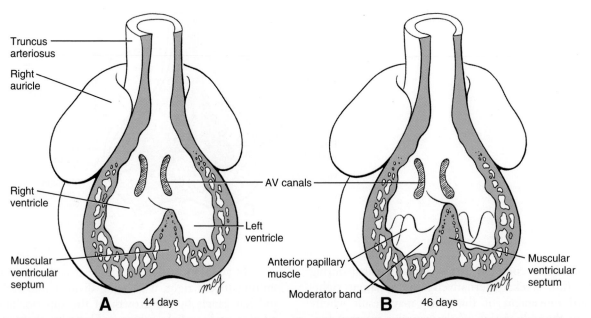

Figure 7–18. *A, B,* Initial septation of the ventricles. The muscular interventricular septum enlarges in the region of the interventricular sulcus between weeks 4 and 7. (See Fig. 7–19 for the completion of ventricular septation.)

Starting at the End of the Fourth Week, a Muscular Ventricular Septum Incompletely Separates the Ventricles

At the end of the fourth week, the inferior part of the bulboventricular sulcus begins to protrude into the cardiac lumen along the interface between the presumptive right and left ventricular chambers (Fig. 7–18; see also Fig. 7–17). This septum apparently forms as the growing walls of the right and left ventricles become more closely apposed to one another. However, the growth of this **muscular ventricular septum** halts in the middle of the seventh week before its leading edge meets the septum intermedium. This arrest of growth is crucial: If fusion occurred too soon, the left ventricle would be shut off from the ventricular outflow tract.

At the same time that the muscular ventricular septum is forming, the myocardium begins to thicken, and myocardial ridges or **trabeculae** appear on the inner wall of both ventricles. The anterior portion of the muscular ventricular septum is trabeculated and is called the **primary ventricular fold** or **septum** (see Fig. 7–18B). The posterior part of the septum is smooth walled and is called the **inlet septum** because of its proximity to the atrioventricular canals. On the right wall of the muscular ventricular septum, the boundary between the trabeculated primary fold and the inlet septum is marked by a constant, prominent trabeculation called the **septomarginal trabecula** or **moderator band** (see Fig. 7–18B). This structure connects the muscular septum with the **anterior papillary muscle** that has begun to form as part of the right atrioventricular valve.

The Atrioventricular Valves Are Formed from the Ventricular Myocardium and Prevent Backflow of Blood During Systole

The atrioventricular valves begin to form between the fifth and eighth weeks. Undermining of the myocardium surrounding the left and right atrioventricular canals forms anterior and posterior **leaflets** or **cusps** on either side of both canals (Fig. 7–19). These valve leaflets are firmly rooted in the

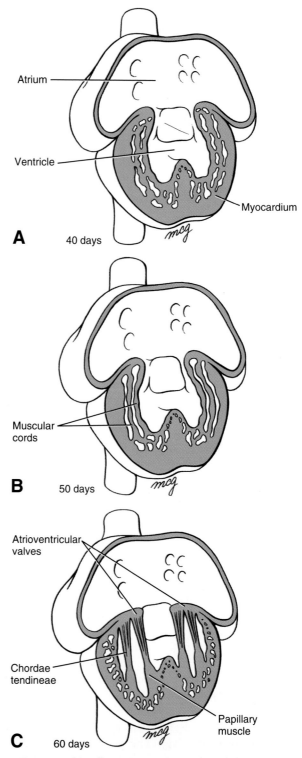

Figure 7–19. *Illustration continued on following page*

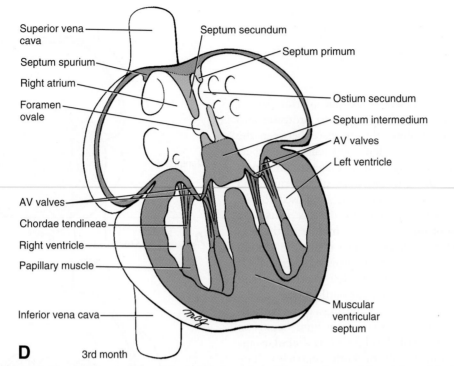

Superior vena cava
Septum spurium
Right atrium
Foramen ovale
Septum secundum
Septum primum
Ostium secundum
Septum intermedium
AV valves
Left ventricle
AV valves
Chordae tendineae
Right ventricle
Papillary muscle
Inferior vena cava
Muscular ventricular septum

D   3rd month

Figure 7–19. *A–D,* Development of the atrioventricular valves. The structures of the atrioventricular valves, including the papillary muscles, chordae tendineae, and cusps, are sculpted from the muscular walls of the ventricles. The definitive tricuspid valve within the right ventricle is not completely formed until the development of a septal cusp in the third month.

rim of the canals but are not thought to arise as differentiations of the adjacent endocardial cushions. The free edge of each leaflet is attached to the anterior and posterior ventricular walls by thin sinews called **chordae tendineae,** which insert into small hillocks of myocardium called **papillary muscles** (see Fig. 7–19C, D). The valve leaflets are designed so that they fold back to allow blood to enter the ventricles from the atria during diastole but shut to prevent backflow when the ventricles contract (see Fig. 7–19D).

The left atrioventricular valve has only anterior and posterior leaflets and is called the **bicuspid valve** (**mitral valve**). The right atrioventricular valve usually (but not always) develops a third, small **septal cusp** during the third month and therefore is called the **tricuspid valve** (see Fig. 7–19D).

The Spiral Growth of the Conotruncal Septa Results in the Helical Arrangement of the Ascending Aorta and Pulmonary Trunk

At the time when the muscular interventricular septum ceases to grow, the two ventricles communicate with each other through the interventricular foramen and also with the expanded base of the conus cordis (Fig. 7–20). Further septation of the ventricles and the outflow tract must occur in tight coordination if the heart is to function properly. Not surprisingly, a large proportion of cardiac defects are due to errors in this complex process (see the Clinical Applications section of this chapter).

The cardiac outflow pathway is divided into

two by swellings or ridges that grow from the opposite walls of the conus cordis and truncus arteriosus and meet in the middle (Fig. 7–21; see also Fig. 7–20A). These ridges are bulbous at first (see Fig. 7–21A) and fill much of the conotruncal lumen, but eventually they thin and fuse to form a septum that completely separates the right and left ventricular outflow pathways. The final division of the truncus arteriosus to form the **ascending aorta** and the **pulmonary trunk** is accomplished by a split that develops within the plane of the septum itself.

It has been suggested that as many as three separate pairs of swellings join to form the final septum. An alternative theory is that septation is accomplished by a single pair of **truncoconal swellings** that grow in both directions. In either case, it is clear that septation commences at the inferior end of the truncus arteriosus and proceeds superiorly and inferiorly.

Separation of the aortic and pulmonary outflow tracts becomes complete when the truncoconal swellings fuse with the inferior endocardial cushion and the muscular interventricular septum, thus completely separating the right and left ventricles. Growth of this **membranous ventricular septum** normally occurs between weeks 5 and 8; however, failure of complete fusion, resulting in a ventricular septal defect, is the most common congenital heart defect (see the Clinical Applications section of this chapter).

The swellings that separate left and right ventricular outflow tracts apparently arise in a spiral along the walls of the truncus arteriosus and the ventricular outflow tracts. As a result, the left and right ventricular outflow tracts and, eventually, the aorta and pulmonary trunk twist around each other in a helical arrangement (see Fig. 7–20).

The Truncus Swellings Also Contribute to the Semilunar Valves in the Aortic and Pulmonary Trunks

By the middle of the fifth week, a small tubercle or bulge appears on the tip of each truncus swelling at the inferior end of the truncus arteriosus (see Fig. 7–21A). At this level, the truncus swellings are rooted in the right and left lateral walls of the truncus. When the swellings fuse together to separate the outflow tracts, these lateral tubercles are split in two, so that half of each is distributed into each of the resulting outflow tracts (see Fig. 7–21B). Meanwhile, a second pair of tubercles develop on the anterior and posterior walls of the truncus at the same level. After septation, the tubercle on the anterior wall lies in the developing pulmonary channel, and the tubercle on the posterior wall lies in the developing aortic channel.

After septation, each outflow tract thus contains three tubercles laid out in a triangle: two formed from the split lateral tubercles and a third growing on the anterior or posterior truncal wall. These tubercles give rise to the cusps of the three-cusped **semilunar valves** that prevent backflow from the aorta and pulmonary trunk into the ventricles. The cup-shaped valve leaflets are formed by the excavation of truncal tissue inferior to the initial site of tubercle formation. As a result of this excavation, the bases of the leaflets migrate inferiorly during the maturation of the valves. This migration follows the spiral course of the outflow vessels, so the valves appear to rotate slightly during development (see Fig. 7–21C). Development of the semilunar valves is complete by 9 weeks.

THE PACEMAKER AND CONDUCTION SYSTEM FORM EARLY TO COORDINATE THE BEATING OF THE HEART

The heart is one of the few organs that has to function almost as soon as it is formed—it begins to beat and to propel blood through the embryo and placenta on day 22. The rhythmic waves of electrical depolarization (action potentials) that trigger the myocardium to contract are **myogenic**—that is, they arise spontaneously in the cardiac muscle itself and spread from cell to cell. The sympathetic and parasympathetic neural input to the heart modifies the heart rate but does not initiate beats. Myocytes removed from the primitive heart tube and grown in tissue culture will begin to beat in unison if they become connected to one another, and studies with voltage-sensitive dyes indicate that cardiac myocytes may begin to produce rhythmic electrical activity even before the lateral endocardial tubes have fused.

In a normally functioning heart, the beat is

Figure 7–20. *See legend on opposite page*

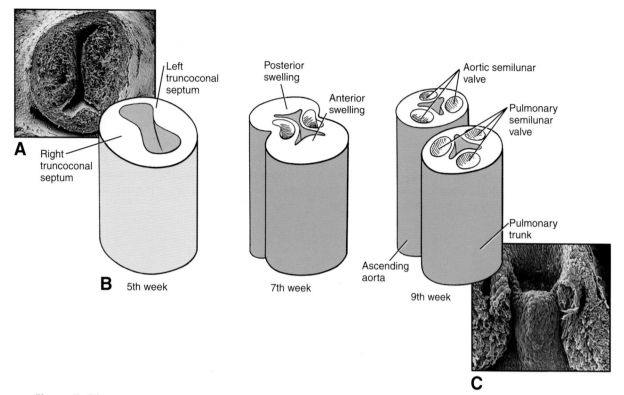

Figure 7–21. *A, B,* Formation of the semilunar valves. The semilunar valves are specializations of the right and left truncoconal swellings and two minor swellings. Note that the left and right truncoconal swellings each form right and left semilunar valves of the aorta and the pulmonary trunk. (*A, C,* From Hurle JM, Colvee E, Blanco AM. 1980. Development of mouse semilunar valves. Anat Embryol 160:83.)

initiated in a **pacemaker region** that has a faster rate of spontaneous depolarization than the rest of the myocardium. Moreover, the depolarization spreads from the pacemaker to the rest of the heart along specialized **conduction pathways** that control the timing of contraction of the various regions of the myocardium and thus ensure that the chambers will contract efficiently and in the right sequence. In the primitive heart tube, the ventricle seems to serve as the initial pacemaker. However, pacemaker activity is rapidly taken over by a cluster of pacemaking cells in the sinoatrial region, which are derived either from the right common cardinal vein or from the right sinus ve-

Figure 7–20. Septation of the cardiac outflow tract and final septation of the ventricles. Right oblique view. The anterolateral wall of the right ventricle has been removed to show the interior of the right ventricular chamber and the presumptive outflow tracts of both ventricles. *A, B,* Starting in the fifth week, the right and left truncoconal swellings grow out from the walls of the common ventricular outflow tract at the junction of the truncus arteriosus and conus cordis. When they meet, they begin to zipper together superiorly and inferiorly. *C, D,* By the ninth week, the inferior regions of the truncoconal swellings have grown down onto the upper ridge of the muscular ventricular septum and onto the inferior endocardial cushion separating the right and left ventricular chambers. The truncoconal swellings have grown in a spiral configuration, separating the aortic and pulmonary outflow tracts from each other. (Modified from Steding G, Seidl W. 1980. Contribution to the development of the heart. Part I. Normal development. Thorac Cardiovasc Surg 28:386.)

nosus. These cells form a distinct ovoid structure called the **sinoatrial node** (SAN) in the left venous valve.

Soon after the development of the SAN, cells in the superior endocardial cushion begin to form a secondary pacemaker center, the **atrioventricular node** (AVN), which receives impulses from the SAN and controls the beating of the two ventricles. The main conduction pathway between the SAN and the AVN runs through the crista terminalis, as mentioned earlier, although other pathways in the interatrial septum have also been found. The development of the AVN is accompanied by the appearance of a bundle of specialized conducting cells, the **bundle of His,** which sends one branch into the right ventricle and the other into the left ventricle within the septomarginal trabeculation or moderator band. This conduction pathway must be carefully avoided during the repair of ventricular septal defects.

The detailed ontogeny of the cardiac conduction system is somewhat controversial. It has been suggested that most of the conduction pathway arises from cardiogenic mesoderm but that the sinus node may originate from the neural crest.

Clinical Applications

Congenital Cardiovascular Disease

CARDIOVASCULAR MALFORMATIONS ARE THE MOST COMMON TYPE OF LIFE-THREATENING CONGENITAL DEFECT

Congenital cardiovascular malformations account for about 20 percent of all congenital defects observed in live-born infants. They occur in about 5 to 8 of every 1000 live births, and the percentage in stillborn infants is probably even higher. Ventricular septal defects are the most common congenital cardiovascular malformation, although defects may involve almost any region of the heart.

The Cause of Most Cardiovascular Malformations Is Not Well Understood

Like other congenital malformations, heart defects presumably result from a disturbance of normal developmental mechanisms. Neither the cause nor the pathogenesis of most heart defects is understood, however. A few can be associated with specific genetic errors or environmental teratogens. Overall, about 4 percent of cardiovascular defects can be ascribed to single-gene mutations, another 6 percent to chromosomal aberrations such as trisomies or monosomies, and 5 percent to exposure to specific teratogens. The teratogens known to induce heart defects include not only drugs such as lithium, alcohol, and retinoic acid but also factors associated with certain maternal diseases such as diabetes and rubella (German measles).

The etiology of most of the remaining 85 percent of cardiac abnormalities appears to be **multifactorial**—that is, they stem from the interaction of environmental or outside influences with a poorly defined constellation of the individual's own genetic determinants. Thus, individuals may show very different genetic susceptibilities to the action of a given teratogen. If two embryos of the same age are exposed to the same dose of the teratogen, for example, one may develop severe cardiac malformations, whereas the other may remain unaffected. The molecular basis for this difference in susceptibility might, for instance, be a genetic difference in the rate at which the enzyme systems of the two embryos detoxify the teratogen. It must be borne in mind when such findings are interpreted that an embryonic structure (such as the interventricular septum) is usually susceptible to teratogens only during very specific **critical sensitive periods,** which usually correspond to periods of active differentiation and morphogenesis. Thus, a potent teratogen may have no effect on the development of an embryonic structure if it is administered before or after the critical period during which that structure is susceptible to its action.

Figure 7–22. Acardia. Surprisingly complete development of the human fetus may occur in the absence of a heart. (Photograph courtesy of Children's Hospital Medical Center, Cincinnati, OH.)

Several Human Congenital Cardiac Conditions Are Linked to Single-Gene Mutations

Based on genetic studies of family histories, many cardiac malformations may be ascribed to single-gene mutations. However, such specific mutations have been shown to cause only a handful of human cardiac malformations, including familial hypertrophic cardiomyopathy, laterality disruptions of heart development, and congenital long QT syndrome.

Familial hypertrophic cardiomyopathy (FHC) is a well-studied human cardiac malformation that is caused by one of several single-gene mutations. This disease, first definitively described in 1958, is an autosomal dominant disease with variable phenotype. In Finland, where autopsies are routine, it is estimated to affect 4 in 100,000 people. However, this estimate may be conservative, because a large proportion of individuals who carry the gene are asymptomatic.

The FHC phenotype includes gradual thickening of the ventricular walls and interventricular septum, disorganization of the muscle fibrils, and formation of loose connective tissue. In many cases, these conditions result in arrhythmias (irregularity of heartbeat) and pumping inefficiency, leading to cardiac failure and sudden death in early adulthood. The genetic basis for the disease appears to be mutation of the **β-cardiac myosin heavy chain gene** on human chromosome 14. Since 1990, well over a dozen **missense mutations** of the β-cardiac myosin heavy chain gene have been detected in patients who exhibit symptoms of FHC. Moreover, patients suffering from FHC have also been shown to possess mutations of genes encoding other cardiac contractile proteins such as **troponin T** and **α-tropomyosin,** suggesting that FHC is a **disease of the sarcomere.**

Another spectrum of human cardiac malformations that includes anomalies of folding and laterality of the heart has been related to an apparent autosomal recessive disease characterized by mutations of the **gap junction protein connexin 43.** The mutation of the connexin 43 gene in most of the affected individuals studied so far results in a substitution of proline for serine at amino acid residue 364. This region of the protein is thought to bind phosphate, which may regulate the intracellular trafficking or function of connexin 43.

Most of the 250,000 individuals who suffer sudden death each year in the United States die of **cardiac arrhythmias.** One variant of this syndrome, **congenital long QT syndrome,** is characterized by prolongation of the electrocardiogram (ECG or EKG), fainting, and sudden death. Not surprisingly, genetic disruptions underlying this autosomal dominant disease include mutations of the *SCN5A, HERG,* and *KVLQT1* genes, which encode **cardiac ion channels.**

Perturbation of Any Normal Process of Cardiac Development May Result in a Malformation

An error in almost any step of heart formation, from the initial formation of the primary heart tube (Fig. 7–22) to the septation of the outflow tracts, may result in a cardiac defect. This section describes some of the more common malformations arising during various steps of cardiogenesis.

The malformation called **dextrocardia** is caused when the primitive heart tube folds to the right instead of to the left (Fig. 7–23). Most individuals with dextrocardia exhibit a general reversal in the handedness of many organs, a condition known as **situs inversus** (see the Experimental Principles section of Ch. 9 for a thorough discus-

Figure 7–24. Infant heart with atrial septal defect. The ostium secundum and foramen ovale in this heart overlap abnormally and therefore could not close at birth, resulting in continued mixing of right and left atrial blood after birth. (Photograph courtesy of Children's Hospital Medical Center, Cincinnati, OH.)

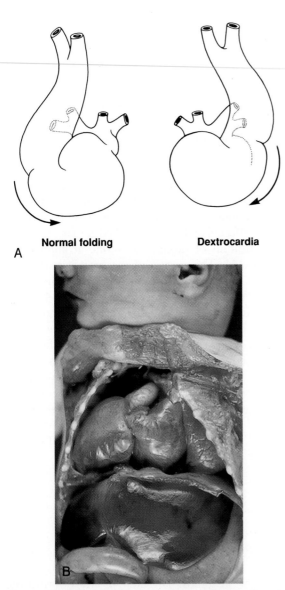

Normal folding   Dextrocardia

Figure 7–23. Dextrocardia. *A,* In dextrocardia, the folding of the heart tube is reversed from the normal sinistral folding, producing a heart that is normal in form but is a mirror image of the normal heart. *B,* Infant with dextrocardia. (*B,* Photograph courtesy of Children's Hospital Medical Center, Cincinnati, OH.)

sion of situs inversus). Research suggests that situs inversus is caused by the absence or defective function of a single protein that is critical to the body's ability to adopt the correct handedness. This hypothesis arose from studies on mice homozygous for a particular mutation on chromosome 12. Half of these mice exhibit more or less normal folding, whereas half exhibit reversed folding, although there is usually some incoordination among the viscera. Presumably, this finding indicates that the viscera of the mutant mice adopt correct or reversed handedness at random during embryogenesis, or, in other words, that they lack a factor necessary to impose the correct handedness. In humans, as in this mouse model, the reversal of heart tube looping is not always precise or complete, and errors in the alignment of the heart chambers often result in additional cardiac anomalies.

In about 6 of 10,000 live-born infants, the

septum secundum is too short to cover the ostium secundum completely, so an **atrial septal defect** persists after the septum primum and septum secundum are pressed together at birth (Fig. 7–24). The hemodynamic forces that cause these **septum secundum defects** (see the Experimental Principles section of this chapter) also cause massive shunting of blood from the left atrium to the right atrium in the newborn. Infants with this abnormality are generally asymptomatic, but the persistent increase in flow to the right atrium may lead to enlargement of the right ventricle and pulmonary trunk, and cardiac failure may ensue in later life. Atrial septal defects can now be detected by echocardiography in childhood and may warrant surgical closure (see Ch. 15 for a discussion of echocardiography). Atrial septal defect is associated with almost all documented autosomal and sex chromosome aberrations and is a common accompaniment of several partial and complete trisomies, including trisomy 21 (Down syndrome).

Atrioventricular septal defect (endocardial cushion defect) arises from failure of the superior and inferior endocardial cushions to fuse. This defect is one of the most common, if not the most common, cardiac malformation in Down syndrome. The failure of the superior and inferior endocardial cushions to fuse can lead to a variety of secondary abnormalities, including incomplete closure of the septum primum or interventricular septum and malformation of the atrioventricular valves. One physiologic consequence of the defect is persistent left-to-right shunting of blood after birth, the magnitude of which depends on the severity of the defect. **Congestive heart failure** in infancy is not unlikely if the defect is severe, but individuals in whom only the ostium primum is patent may be asymptomatic. Surgical correction of the atrial septal defect, malformed mitral valve, and absent interventricular septum are all possible.

In **double-outlet left ventricle malformation,** the aortic and pulmonary outflow tracts both connect to the left ventricle. The right ventricle becomes hypoplastic because it has no outflow tract, whereas the left ventricle expands to become the dominant ventricle. The pathogenesis of this defect is not well understood; most likely it is caused by some error in the remodeling of the conotruncus that results in normal alignment of the right half of the outflow tract with the right ventricle.

Ventricular septal defects are the most common of all congenital heart malformations, accounting for 25 percent of all cardiac abnormalities documented in live-born infants and occurring as isolated defects in 12 of 10,000 births. The prevalence of this defect appears to be increasing, a statistic that may represent an actual increase in incidence or may simply reflect the application of better diagnostic methods. A ventricular septal defect can arise from several causes: (1) deficient development of the proximal truncoconal swellings, (2) failure of the muscular and membranous ventricular septa to fuse, (3) failure of the superior and inferior endocardial cushions to fuse (atrioventricular septal defect), and (4) excessive perforation of the interventricular muscular septum during development (Fig. 7–25). Whatever the origin of a ventricular septal defect, its most serious consequence is massive left-to-right shunting of blood and consequent pulmonary hypertension after birth. Surgical repair of the defect in children usually results in rapid correction of the pulmonary blood pressure and reduction of the heart to normal size.

Tricuspid and mitral valve defects arise from errors in the process by which the valve leaflets, chordae tendineae, and papillary muscles are sculpted from the ventricular wall. The endocardial cushions do not seem to be directly involved in pathogenesis, any more than they are involved in normal valve formation. The pathogenesis of valve **atresia,** in which the valve orifice is completely obliterated, is not understood. In one type of tricuspid valve anomaly, **Ebstein's disease,** the valve is displaced downward into the right ventricle, and the leaflets have an abnormal ballooned shape. The dysfunctional valve allows blood to regurgitate into the right atrium and also blocks access to the pulmonary trunk. As a result, right atrial blood shunts to the left atrium through a persistent foramen ovale. Moreover, most of the blood that reaches the pulmonary arteries does so by taking a roundabout route through the left ventricle, aorta, and persistent ductus arteriosus. (The ductus arteriosus is a connection between the aorta and the pulmonary trunk that normally closes soon after birth; see Ch. 8.) The uneven distribution of blood between the ventricles causes the left ventricle to enlarge, whereas the right becomes hypoplastic. Tricuspid valve atresia has the same effect on ventricle size. Both conditions tend to cause **cyanosis**

Ventricular septal defect

Pin holding ventricle open

Muscular ventricular septum

Figure 7–25. Typical ventricular septal defect in a mouse fetus with trisomy 12. Failure of the membranous ventricular septum to fuse with the upper ridge of the muscular septum in this heart has resulted in a ventricular septal defect. (From Pexieder T. 1978. Development of the outflow tract of the embryonic heart. Birth Defects XIV:29.)

(inadequate oxygenation of the blood) in the newborn. Both can be corrected surgically.

A variety of outflow tract malformations result from errors in the septation of the conotruncus. Errors in this process may in turn be caused by abnormal neural crest migration (see the Experimental Principles section of this chapter). In about 1 of 10,000 live-born infants, the truncoconal septa do not form at all, resulting in a **persistent truncus arteriosus** (Fig. 7–26A). This malformation necessarily includes a ventricular septal defect. The result is that blood from the two sides of the heart mixes thoroughly in the common outflow tract, and both the body and the lungs receive partially deoxygenated blood. Untreated infants usually die within the first 2 years. Surgical correction is possible but difficult, involving repair of the ventricular septal defect and implantation of a valved prosthetic shunt between the right ventricle and the pulmonary arteries.

In about 5 of 10,000 live-born infants, the truncoconal septa develop but do not display the usual spiral pattern (see Fig. 7–26B, C). The result is **transposition of the great vessels,** in which the left ventricle empties into the pulmonary circulation and the right ventricle empties into the systemic circulation. This condition is not immediately fatal because the deoxygenated systemic blood and the oxygenated pulmonary blood can mix through a patent foramen ovale or ductus arteriosus. Nevertheless, it is the leading cause of death in infants younger than 1 year old with cyanotic heart disease.

Tetralogy of Fallot Represents a Group of Cardiac Malformations That Arise Through a Pathogenetic Cascade

Many cardiac defects occur together more often than in isolation. In some cases, such associated defects are actually components of the same malformation—in the way that a ventricular septal defect is a necessary consequence of persistent truncus arteriosus. In other cases, a primary malformation sets off a cascade of effects that leads to other malformations. An example is the pathogenesis of **tetralogy of Fallot,** a syndrome described by Steno of Denmark in 1673 and referred to as *maladie bleue* by Etienne-Louis Arthur Fallot in 1888 (Fig. 7–27). Fallot used the term **tetralogy** to refer to the four classic malformations in this syndrome: (1) **pulmonary stenosis,** (2) **ventricular septal defect,** (3) rightward displacement of the aorta (sometimes called **overriding aorta**), and (4) **right ventricular hypertrophy.** The primary defect is a malalignment of the muscular outlet sep-

A   **Persistent truncus arteriosus**

B   **Transposition of the vessels**

Figure 7–26. *A,* Persistent truncus arteriosus. Incomplete separation of aortic and pulmonary outflow tracts may accompany a ventricular septal defect when the right and left truncoconal septa fail to form. *B, C,* Transposition of the great arteries results from failure of the truncoconal septa to spiral as they separate the aortic and pulmonary outflow tracts. (*C,* Photograph courtesy of Children's Hospital Medical Center, Cincinnati, OH.)

tum between the subpulmonary and subaortic outlets. Pulmonary stenosis results from the narrowing of the subpulmonary orifice by the muscular and fibrous tissues of this abnormal outlet septum and by misplaced ventricular trabeculae. These malformations are caused in turn by the failure of the orifices of the developing aorta and pulmonary

trunk to align normally with the outflow regions of the two ventricles. The malalignment of the outlet septum also interferes with the normal fusion of the muscular and membranous ventricular septa, resulting in a ventricular septal defect. In addition, it contributes both to the rightward displacement of the overriding aorta and to the development of

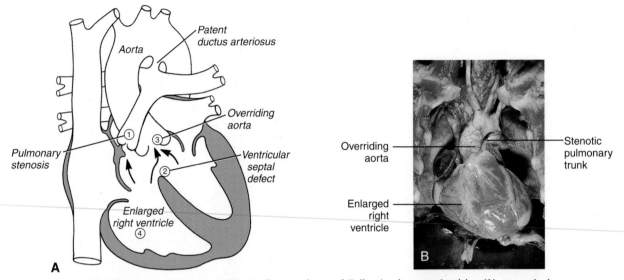

Figure 7–27. Tetralogy of Fallot. *A,* Classically, tetralogy of Fallot is characterized by (1) stenosis (narrowing) of the pulmonary trunk, (2) ventricular septal defect, (3) overriding aorta, and (4) an enlarged right ventricle. A patent ductus arteriosus is also present, however. *B,* The enlarged right ventricle and overriding aorta are obvious in this case of tetralogy of Fallot. (*B,* Photograph courtesy of Children's Hospital Medical Center, Cincinnati, OH.)

a fifth characteristic defect—the **abnormal origin of part of the mitral valve from the right ventricle.** All these defects conspire to raise the blood pressure in the right ventricle, resulting in progressive right ventricular hypertrophy. Tetralogy of Fallot is the most common cyanotic congenital heart malformation, occurring in approximately 10 of 10,000 live-born infants. The condition may be corrected surgically by relieving the obstruction of the pulmonary trunk and repairing the ventricular septal defect. Care must be exercised, however, in avoidance of postoperative **complete right bundle branch block,** which may lead to fatal ventricular dysrhythmia.

Hemodynamic Forces Are Important in the Morphogenesis of Several Regions of the Heart

It seems clear that the pressure of intracardiac blood is important in the development of the heart and that perturbations in the pressure relationships among the heart chambers and outflow tracts can result in malformations. Such perturbations can be brought about by several kinds of primary defect—by abnormal compliance or deformability of the atrial, ventricular, or outflow tract walls or by abnormal expansion or constriction of the ductus venosus or ductus arteriosus (see Ch. 8).

If the normal shunting of blood from the right to the left atrium during gestation is restricted, the left side of the heart will be underdeveloped, a syndrome known as **hypoplastic left heart.** The hypoplasia may involve the left atrium, left ventricle, mitral valve, and aorta. The syndrome usually has a multifactorial etiology, although it can also be inherited as an autosomal recessive trait and is associated with the genetic disease phenylketonuria. Alternatively, excessive interatrial flow can cause a septum secundum defect by enlarging the foramen ovale and eroding septal structures. As previously noted, the resulting increased inflow through the left side of the heart may interfere with the normal growth of the truncoconal septa and prevent normal closure of the ventricular membranous septum.

The role of hemodynamics in heart morphogenesis has been investigated experimentally in animals. Constriction or obstruction of the aortic arches, for example, has been found to result in ventricular membranous septal defects, whereas experimental obstruction of the left atrioventricular canal can cause hypoplastic left heart.

Errors in Programmed Cell Death Can Lead to Several Anomalies

A number of remodeling events in the heart involve **programmed cell death (apoptosis),** a process in which well-defined necrotic zones called **cell death foci** appear at specific stages and locations, resulting in the reshaping of existing structures. The timing and location of these foci are thought to be under genetic control.

In the heart, programmed cell death is thought to play a role in (1) the fusion of the endocardial tubes to form a single primitive heart tube, (2) the effacement of the bulboventricular flange and the remodeling of the conotruncus, (3) the remodeling of the ventricular muscular septum, (4) the fusion of the superior and inferior endocardial cushions, (5) the sculpting of the atrioventricular valves, (6) the remodeling of the conus and truncus swellings during the development of the outflow tracts, and (7) the sculpting of the semilunar valves.

Both exposure to teratogens and altered hemodynamics have been implicated in the abnormal development of cell death foci. Abnormal patterns of programmed cell death may play a role in anomalous remodeling of the truncoconal swellings and the ensuing malformations of the outflow tracts, in the maldevelopment of the tricuspid valve in Ebstein's disease, and in excessive erosion of the muscular ventricular septum leading to ventricular septal defect.

Experimental Principles

Molecular Mechanisms of Cardiac Development and Pathogenesis

Ultimately, an understanding of normal and abnormal development of the human heart will require knowledge of the **morphogenetic, cellular,** and **molecular processes** that underlie formation of the cardiogenic mesoderm at gastrulation and the regional differentiation, folding, and septation of the developing heart. Because of the paucity of human specimens, most of our knowledge of the very early stages of heart morphogenesis is derived from the study of chicken or mouse embryos. Clearly, care must be exercised in application of this information to human heart development. In other cases, however, inferences about normal mechanisms can be drawn from studies of the clinical manifestations of human malformations. This approach is often productive but has also led to erroneous interpretations. In spite of these difficulties, however, novel genetic approaches using experimental animals have rapidly expanded our understanding of heart development and have also provided a basis for extension of some of this information to humans. Three particular problems have been a focus of active research: (1) the cranio-caudal specification of intrinsic heart regions, (2) transgenic models of cardiac development and malformation, and (3) the role of neural crest cells in septation of the ventricles and outflow tracts.

Subregions of the Heart Are Specified Early in Development, but Developmental Regulatory Mechanisms Remain Enigmatic

The atrial myosin heavy chain **AMHC1** is selectively expressed within atrial cells of the chick embryo heart. Indeed, restriction of AMHC1 expression occurs as early as the heart initially differentiates, because the technique of in situ hybridization shows that mRNA encoding this protein is only found within the caudal end of the heart tube (Fig. 7–28*A*). Following formation of the primitive heart chambers, expression of AMHC1 is restricted to the primitive atrium (see Fig. 7–28*B*). In contrast, another myosin heavy

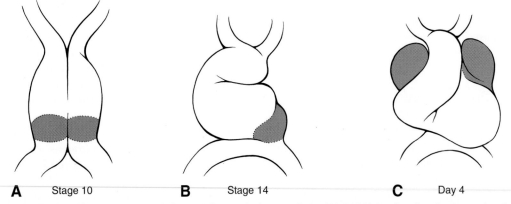

Figure 7–28. Specific expression of the atrial myosin heavy chain (AMHC1) in the developing avian heart. *A,* As the primitive heart tube forms (stage 10), AMHC1 mRNA is expressed only at its caudal end (tinted area). *B,* As the atrial chamber differentiates (stage 14) and the heart tube folds, AMHC1 mRNA expression remains restricted to the primitive atrium. *C,* By day 4, the primitive atrium forms the auricles that maintain expression of AMHC1 mRNA. (Drawn from Yutzey KE, Rhee JT, Bader D. 1994. Expression of the atrial-specific myosin heavy chain AMHC1 and the establishment of anteroposterior polarity in the developing chicken heart. Development 120:871.)

chain, **VMHC1** (ventricular myosin heavy chain-1), is expressed by all cells of the differentiating cardiogenic mesoderm. However, its expression is finally restricted to the presumptive ventricles of the developing heart. Early restriction of expression of a myosin regulatory light chain gene specific to the atrium (*Mlc-2a*) and an isoform specific to the ventricle (*Mlc-2v*) has also been demonstrated in mice.

Studies, however, have shown that application of excess **retinoic acid** to the embryonic chicken heart causes an "atrialization" or "caudalization" of the primitive heart tube, as indicated by ubiquitous expression of AMHC1 throughout the retinoic acid-treated heart tube. Atrial gene expression in mice is similarly expanded throughout the heart with retinoic acid treatments in utero. A potential mechanism for localization of retinoid signaling in the embryos is the restricted expression of retinaldehyde dehydrogenenase-2 (RALDH-2), a limiting enzyme in retinoic acid biosythesis. Restriction of RALDH-2 expression to the posterior area of heart has been associated with atrial gene expression in both chicken and mouse embryos. These results implicate vitamin A in developmental regulation of the myocardium per se.

Several transcription factors have been identified in developing mouse and chicken hearts that play pivotal roles in cardiac morphogenesis. For example, the paired-related homeobox genes *Prx-1* and *Prx-2* are specifically expressed in heart and forebrain as early as gastrulation. Later in heart development, *Prx-1* is localized in the endocardial cushions and heart valves, whereas *Prx-2* is localized in the muscular ventricular septum and ductus arteriosus. *Nkx-2.3* and *Nkx-2.5* are vertebrate homologues of the *Drosophila* homeobox gene **tinman,** which is required for heart formation in the fruitfly. *Nkx-2.5* is apparently first induced in chick embryo cardiac primordia by cranial endoderm. A human homologue of this gene has also been mapped to chromosome 5q34, and mutations in *NKX-2.5* have been associated with human congenital heart disease. *NKX-2.5* is near another homeobox gene, **MSX2,** which is expressed by cells of the developing cardiac conduction system. Irx4, an Iroquois homeoprotein, and Tbx5, a T-box family member, have been linked to ventricular and atrial lineage determination, respectively. Mutations in human *TBX5* have been identified in families with Holt-Oram syndrome, which includes heart chamber malformations. "Downstream" transcription factors that act much later during differentiation of the myocardium include transcription factors such as **MEF-2C** and **GATA4** which are necessary for cardiac development even before looping. These cardiac muscle transcription factors may differ from those expressed in striated and smooth muscle.

Transgenic Mouse Models May Mimic Human Cardiac Congenital Disease or Reveal Functions of Pivotal Regulatory Factors in Cardiac Development

In mice, transgenic **mutants** expressing proteins with partial function, completely lacking function **(knockouts),** or **overexpressing** specific genes are now widely utilized to study the roles of cardiac-specific regulatory genes. For example, transgenic mice that express a mutant form of a **myosin heavy chain** develop a phenotype similar to that seen in humans with familial hypertrophic myopathy. Because expression of the mutant gene is much lower than endogenous expression of the wild-type myosin heavy chain gene, its capacity to interfere with normal development has been explained by its possible behavior as a **dominant-negative mutation** (recall the dominant-negative FGF receptor of the lung in Ch. 6). The mutant form of MHC1 may interact with wild-type MHC1 within the sarcomere, thereby disrupting its normal function.

Likewise, transgenic mice have been created that express the *ras* **oncogene** within the developing ventricles. These animals also exhibit a phenotype similar to that of familial hypertropic cardiomyopathy in humans, suggesting a function for a *ras*-dependent signaling pathway in the etiology of this disease.

Transgenic knockouts of the gap junction protein **connexin 43** result in mice that are viable through gestation but die at birth. In spite of the wide distribution of connexin 43 in normal animals, however, the knockouts are virtually normal except for swelling and blockage of the right ventricular outflow tract. This suggests that the lack of connexin 43 in many tissues may be compensated for by other gap junction proteins, but that connexin 43 is required for normal cardiac morphogenesis.

Knockouts of the *Rxr-α* (**retinoid x receptor alpha)** gene result in an atrial-like phenotype in the ventricles. In situ hybridization shows that cranial regions of the primitive heart tube, normally destined to differentiate into ventricular tissue, express the atrial-specific isoform of myosin light chain-2. Moreover, the walls of these presumptive ventricles never thicken, again supporting the hypothesis that retinoic acid plays a direct role in normal differentiation of ventricular myocardium from its more primitive atrium-like condition.

Finally, transgenic mice that are homozygous for a mutant form of the **Sox-4** gene die of cardiac failure during embryonic development. Defects of the semilunar valves in these animals have been ascribed to failure of the truncoconal septa to fuse, which also results in disruption of the aorticopulmonary septum. Thus, the phenotype of this knockout is similar to the phenotype of **persistent truncus arteriosus** in humans. It should be noted, however, that persistent truncus arteriosus in humans may often be a consequence of failure of migration and invasion of neural crest cells that contribute directly to formation of the truncoconal septa (see later). In contrast, in the *Sox-4* knockout, it seems likely that the established truncoconal septa fail to fuse or that the incoming neural crest cells are not appropriately induced to differentiate.

The Neural Crest Contributes to the Truncoconal Septum

It is now clear that critical components of the truncoconal septum are derived from the neural crest of a specific area of the future myelencephalon (Fig. 7–29). Both cell tracing experiments and, more recently, the quail-chick chimera system (discussed in the Experimental Principles section of Ch. 5) have revealed that these cardiac neural crest cells differentiate as **ectomesenchymal cells** (mesenchymal cells derived from the ectodermal neural crest) and invade the truncoconal swellings after migrating through pharyngeal arches 3, 4, and 6. In addition to forming connective tissue and smooth muscle of the truncoconal septa, these cells give rise to the parasympathetic postganglionic neurons of the heart (the cardiac ganglia).

The role of the cardiac neural crest in normal and aberrant septation of the cardiac outflow channels has been confirmed by neural crest abla-

5–6 weeks

Migrating neural crest cells

Neural tube

Truncus arteriosus

Bulbus cordis

Descending aorta

Vitelline artery

Umbilical artery

Figure 7–29. Formation of the truncoconal septa from neural crest cells. Neural crest cells migrate from the hindbrain through pharyngeal arches 3, 4, and 6 and then invade the truncus arteriosus to form the truncoconal septa. (Modified from Kirby ML. 1988. Role of extracardiac factors in heart development. Experientia 44:944.)

tion experiments. If the cardiac neural crest is removed from experimental animals before it begins to migrate, the truncoconal septa completely fail to develop, and blood leaves both ventricles through a persistent truncus arteriosus. Ablation of part or all of the cardiac neural crest may also cause other anomalies, including dextroposed aorta, tricuspid stenosis, right fourth aortic arch hypoplasia, ventricular septal defects related to the absence or hypoplasia of the truncoconal swellings, and tetralogy of Fallot. Further evidence for the role of altered neural crest migration is the frequent association of these cardiac anomalies with defects of the pharyngeal arches through which the cardiac neural crest cells normally migrate. The CHARGE (*c*oloboma of the eye, *h*eart anomaly, choanal *a*tresia, *r*etardation, and *g*enital and *e*ar anomalies), CATCH-22 (*c*ardiac defects, *a*bnormal facies, *t*hymic hypoplasia, *c*left palate, *h*ypocalcemia, and a variable deletion on chromosome *22*q11) and Di-

George syndromes are examples of this type of association (see the Clinical Applications section of Ch. 12).

Retinoic Acid, *Hox* Genes, *Nf-1,* and *Pax-3* Are Implicated in Regulation of Cardiac Neural Crest Cell Migration and Differentiation

As discussed earlier, ablation of neural crest associated with the third to sixth pharyngeal arches results in anomalies of the heart characterized by defects of the outflow tracts and ventricular septation. The role of **Hox** genes in the regulation of migration and differentiation of cardiac neural crest cells is implied by the spectrum of craniofacial and cardiac anomalies characteristic of the DiGeorge syndrome. However, transgenic animals possessing null mutations of *Hox* genes expressed in the head and neck regions (e.g., *Hoxa-3*) exhibit expected craniofacial anomalies but possess normal hearts. Nonetheless, there is still reason to think that *Hox* gene expression is relevant to normal development of cardiac neural crest. **Double retinoic acid receptor** knockout animals, for example, display intrinsic defects of the myocardium such as those described in the *RXR-α* knockouts (see earlier), but they also exhibit anomalies of heart development similar to those produced by neural crest ablation such as persistent truncus arteriosus, transposition of the great vessels, and double-outlet right ventricle. Thus, although these data are indirect, the documented sensitivity of *Hox* gene expression to retinoic acid (see Chs. 4 and 12) implicates these regulatory genes in development of the cardiac neural crest.

The paired domain-paired homeodomain transcription factor *Pax-3* has also been implicated in the regulation of cardiac neural crest. Recall that the Splotch mice characterized by mutation of *Pax-3*, described in Chapter 4, exhibit defects of neural crest cells. It has also been demonstrated that these mice exhibit persistent truncus arteriosus and ventricular septal defect. Moreover, transgenic disruption of the **neurofibromatosis gene *Nf-1*** is shown to produce cardiac defects resulting from disruption of cardiac neural crest. Interestingly, this gene possesses a sequence that may be able to bind the *Pax-3* transcription factor.

Detailed Dissection of Epigenetic Cascades Regulating Heart Morphogenesis Is Now on the Horizon

When the first edition of this text was written, virtually nothing was known about the molecular regulation of cardiac development or the molecular basis of cardiac disease. Clearly, the void in this area of developmental biology is rapidly being filled. Among the greatest challenges to scientists working in this exciting and rapidly moving area are to relate the activities of relevant regulatory factors specifically to mechanisms such as looping, septation, differentiation of the valves, and differentiation of myocardial function and to describe in sufficient detail epigenetic sequences that may be amenable to therapeutic modifications in human cardiac disease. There is every reason to be optimistic that these challenges will be successfully met.

SUGGESTED READING

Descriptive Embryology

Anderson RH, Becker AE, Tranum-Jensen J, Janse MJ. 1981. Anatomico-electrophysiological correlations in the conduction system—a review. Br Heart J 45:67

Anderson RH, Wilkinson JL, Becker AE. 1978. The bulbus cordis—a misunderstood region of the developing human heart: its significance to the classification of congenital cardiac malformations. Birth Defects XIV:1

Arguello C, Alanis J, Valenzuela B. 1988. The early development of the atrioventricular node and bundle of His in the embryonic chicken heart. An electrophysiological and morphological study. Development 102:623

Baldwin HS, Solursh M. 1989. Degradation of hyaluronic acid does not prevent looping of the mammalian heart in situ. Dev Biol 136:555

Bartelings MM, Gittenberger-de Groot AC. 1989. The outflow tract of the heart—embryologic and morphologic correlations. Int J Cardiol 22:289

Cooper MH, O'Rahilly R. 1971. The human heart at seven postovulatory weeks. Acta Anat 79:280

De Haan RL. 1965. Morphogenesis of the vertebrate heart, p. 377. In De Haan RL, Ursprung H (eds): Organogenesis. Holt Rinehart and Winston, New York

Dieterlen-Lieve F, Pardanaud L, Yassine F, Cormier F. 1988. Early haemopoietic stem cells in the avian embryo. J Cell Sci Suppl 10:29

Gorza L, Schiaffino S, Vitadello M. 1988. Heart conduction system: a neural crest derivative? Brain Res 457:360

Harvey RP, Rosenthal N. 1999. Heart Development. Academic Press, San Diego.

Hay DA. 1978. Development and fusion of the endocardial cushions. Birth Defects XIV:69

Hirota A, Kamino K, Komuro H, Sakai T. 1987. Mapping of early development of electrical activity in the embryonic chick heart using multiple-site optical recording. J Physiol 383:711

Hiruma T, Hirakow R. 1989. Epicardial formation in embryonic chick heart: computer-aided reconstruction, scanning, and transmission electron microscopy studies. Am J Anat 184:129

Kirby ML. 1988. Role of extracardiac factors in heart development. Experientia 44:944

Linask KK, Lash JW. 1986. Precardiac cell migration: fibronectin localization at the mesoderm-endoderm interface during directional movement. Dev Biol 114:87

Manasek FJ. 1969. Embryonic development of the heart. II, Formation of the epicardium. J Embryol Exp Morphol 22:333

Manasek FJ. 1972. Early cardiac morphogenesis is independent of function. Dev Biol 27:584

Maron BJ, Hutchins GM. 1974. The development of the semilunar valves in the human heart. Am J Pathol 74:331

Netter FH. 1969. Heart. p. 112. In Yonkman FF (ed): The CIBA Collection of Medical Illustrations. Vol. 5 CIBA, New York

O'Rahilly R. 1971. The timing and sequence of events in human cardiogenesis. Acta Anat 79:70

Pexieder T. 1978. Development of the outflow tract of the embryonic heart. Birth Defects XIV:29

Pexieder T, Janecek P. 1984. Organogenesis of the human embryonic and early fetal heart as studied by microdissection and SEM. p. 401. In Nora JJ, Takao A (eds): Congenital Heart Disease: Causes and Processes. Futura Publishing Co, Mount Kisco, NY

Satin J, Fujii S, DeHaan RL. 1988. Development of the cardiac beat rate in early chick embryos is regulated by regional cues. Dev Biol 129:103

Shimada Y, Ho E, Toyota N. 1981. Epicardial covering over myocardial wall in the chicken embryo as seen with the scanning electron microscope. Scanning Microsc 11:275

Steding G, Seidl W. 1984. Cardiac septation in normal development. p. 481. In Nora JJ, Takao A (eds): Congenital Heart Disease: Causes and Processes. Futura Publishing Co, Mount Kisco, NY

Teal SI, Moore W, Hutchins GM. 1986. Development of aortic and mitral valve continuity in the human embryonic heart. Am J Anat 176:447

Viragh SZ, Challice CE. 1981. The origin of the epicardium and the embryonic myocardial circulation of the mouse. Anat Rec 201:157

Viragh SZ, Challice CE. 1983. The development of the early atrioventricular conduction system in the embryonic heart. Can J Physiol Pharmacol 61:775

Vuillemin M, Pexieder T. 1989. Normal stages of cardiac organogenesis in the mouse. II. Development of internal relief of the heart. Am J Anat 184:114

Wenink ACG. 1976. Development of the human cardiac conducting system. J Anat 121:617

Wenink ACG, Gittenberger-de Groot AC. 1986. Embryology of the mitral valve. Int J Cardiol 11:75

insights into cardiovascular disease. Science 272: 681

Layton WM, Manasek FJ. 1980. Cardiac looping in early iv/iv mouse embryos, p. 109. In Van Praagh R, Takao A (eds): Etiology and Morphogenesis of Congenital Heart Disease. Futura Publishing Co, Mt. Kisco, NY

McKenna WJ. 1993. Hypertrophic cardiomyopathy: an update. Cardiologia 38:277

Payne RM, Johnson MC, Grant JW, Strauss AW. 1995. Toward a molecular understanding of congenital heart disease. Circulation 91:494

Pierpont MEM, Moller JH. 1987. Congenital cardiac malformations, p. 13. In Pierpont MEM, Moller JH (eds): Genetics of Cardiovascular Disease. Martinus Nijhoff Publishing, Boston

Roden DM, George AL Jr, Bennett PB. 1995. Recent advances in understanding the molecular mechanisms of the long QT syndrome. J Cardiovasc Electron Physiol 6:1023

Tanigawa G, Jarcho JA, Kass S, et al. 1990. A molecular basis for familial hypertrophic cardiomyopathy: an a/B cardiac myosin heavy chain hybrid gene. Cell 62:991

Wenink ACG, Gittenberger-de Groot AC, Brom AG. 1986. Developmental considerations of mitral valve anomalies. Int J Cardiol 11:85

Clinical Applications

Anderson RH, Tynan. 1988. Tetralogy of Fallot—a centennial review. Int J Cardiol 21:219

Anderson RH, Wenink ACG. 1988. Thoughts on concepts of development of the heart in relation to the morphology of congenital malformations. Experientia 44:951

Ando M, Takao A, Yutani C, et al. 1984. What is cardiac looping? Consideration based on morphologic data. p. 553. In Nora JJ, Takao A (eds): Congenital Heart Disease: Causes and Processes. Futura Publishing, Mt. Kisco, NY

Behrman RE, Vaughan VC III. 1983. Congenital heart disease, p. 1121. In Nelson W (ed): Nelson Textbook of Pediatrics. 12th Ed. WB Saunders, Philadelphia

Britz-Cunningham SH, Shah MM, Zuppan CW, Fletcher WH. 1995. Mutations of the connexin 43 gap-junction gene in patients with heart malformations and defects of laterality. N Engl J Med 332:1323

Brueckner M, D'Eustachio P, Horwich AL. 1989. Linkage mapping of a mouse gene, iv, that controls left-right asymmetry of the heart and viscera. Proc Natl Acad Sci U S A 86:5035

Clark EB. 1987. Mechanisms in the pathogenesis of congenital cardiac malformations, p. 3. In Pierpont MEM, Moller JH (eds): Genetics of Cardiovascular Disease. Martinus Nijhoff Publishing, Boston

Hooper C. 1991. Decoding the secrets of the heart. J NIH Res 3:69

Keating MT, Sanguinetti MC. 1996. Molecular genetic

Experimental Principles

Chultheiss TM, Xydas S, Lassar AB. 1995. Induction of avian cardiac myogenesis by anterior endoderm. Development 121:4203

Clark EB. 1987. Mechanisms in the pathogenesis of cardiac malformations, p. 3. In Pierpont MEM, Moller JH (eds): Genetics of Cardiovascular Disease. Martinus Nijhoff Publishing, Boston

Dyson E, Sucov HM, Kubalak SW, et al. 1995. Atrial-like phenotype is associated with embryonic ventricular failure in retinoid x receptor 2 −/− mice. Proc Natl Acad Sci U S A 92:7386

Eisenberg LM, Markwald RR. 1995. Molecular regulation of atrioventricular valvuloseptal morphogenesis. Circ Res 77:1

Evans SM, O'Brien T. 1993. Expression of the helix-loop-helix factor ID during mouse embryonic development. Dev Biol 159:485

Evans SM, Yan W, Murillo MP, et al. 1995. Tinman, a Drosophila homeobox gene required for heart and represented by a family of genes in vertebrates: XNKx-2.3, a second vertebrate homolog of tinman. Development 121:3889

Fuller SJ, Chien KR. 1994. Genetic engineering of cardiac muscle cells: in vitro and in vivo. Genet Eng 16:17

Geisterfer-Lowrance AAT, Christe M, Corner DA, et al. 1996. A mouse model of familial hypertrophic cardiomyopathy. Science 272:731

Gorza L, Schiaffino S, Vitadello M. 1988. Heart conduction system: a neural crest derivative? Brain Res 457:360

Grace AA, Chien KR. 1995. Congenital long QT syndromes. Toward molecular dissection of arrhythmia substrates. Circulation 92:2786

Hunter JJ, Tanaka N, Rockman HA, et al. 1995. Ventricular expression of a *MLC-2v-ras* fusion gene induces cardiac hypertrophy and selective diastolic dysfunction in transgenic mice. J Biol Chem 270:23173

Kirby ML. 1987. Cardiac morphogenesis—recent research advances. Pediatr Res 21:219

Kirby ML. 1989. Plasticity and predetermination of mesencephalic and trunk neural crest transplanted into the region of the cardiac neural crest. Dev Biol 134:402

Kirby ML, Cheng G, Stadt H, Hunter G. 1995. Differential expression of the 110 ribosomal protein during heart development. Biochem Biophys Res Commun 212:461

Krug EL, Mjaavedt CH, Markwald RR. 1987. Extracellular matrix from embryonic myocardium elicits an early morphogenetic event in cardiac endothelial differentiation. Dev Biol 120:348

Kubalak SW, Miller-Hance WC, O'Brien T, et al. 1994. Chamber specification of atrial myosin light chain-2 expression precedes septation during murine cardiogenesis. J Biol Chem 269:16961

Leussink B, Brouwer A, el Kattabi M, et al. 1995. Expression patterns of the paired related homeobox genes *Mhox/Prxl* and *S8/Prx2* suggest roles in development of the heart and forebrain. Mech Dev 52:51

Lints TJ, Parsons LM, Hartley L, et al. 1993. *Nkx-2.5:* a novel murine homeobox gene expressed in early heart progenitor cells and their myogene descendants. Development 119:419

Mendelson C, Lohnes D, Decimo D, et al. 1994. Function of the retinoic acid receptors (RARs) during development (II). Multiple abnormalities at various stages of organogenesis in RAR double mutants. Development 120:2749

Morrison-Graham K, Schattman GC, Bork T, et al. 1992. A PDGF receptor mutation in the mouse (patch) perturbs the development of a non-neuronal subset of neural crest-derived cells. Development 115:113

Ojeda JL, Hurle JM. 1981. Establishment of the tubular heart. Role of cell death, p. 101. In Pexieder T (ed): Mechanisms of Cardiac Morphogenesis and Teratogenesis. Perspectives in Cardiovascular Research. Vol. 5. Raven Press, New York

Olson EN, Srivastava D. 1996. Molecular pathways controlling heart development. Science 272:671

Pexieder T. 1981. Introduction. p. 93. In Pexieder T (ed): Mechanisms of Cardiac Morphogenesis and Teratogenesis. Perspectives in Cardiovascular Research. Vol. 5. Raven Press, New York

Pyeritz RE, Murphy EA. 1989. Genetics and congenital heart disease: perspectives and prospects. J Am Coll Cardiol 13:1458

Rindt H, Subamaniam A, Robbins J. 1995. An in vivo analysis of transcription elements in the mouse of myosin heavy chain gene promoter. Transgenic Res 4:397

Rindt H, Knotts S, Robbins J. 1995. Segregation of cardiac and skeletal muscle-specific regulatory elements of the β-myosin heavy chain gene. Proc Natl Acad Sci U S A 92:1540

Reanne AG, deSousa PA, Kulkarni S, et al. 1995. Cardiac malformation in neonatal mice lacking connexin 43. Science 267:1831

Rosenquist TH, McCoy JR, Waldo KL, Kirby ML. 1988. Origin and propagation of elastogenesis in the developing cardiovascular system. Anat Rec 221:860

Sweeny LJ. 1988. A molecular view of cardiogenesis. Experientia 44:930

Schilhaur MW, Oosterwegel MA, Moerer P, et al. 1996. Defects in cardiac outflow tract formation and pro-B-lymphocyte expansion in mice lacking *Sox-4*. Nature 380:711

Shiojima I, Komuro I, Inazawa J, et al. 1995. Assignment of cardiac homeobox gene *csx* to human chromosome 5q3r. Genomics 27:204

Wenink ACG, Zevallos JC. 1988. Developmental aspects of atrioventricular septal defects. Int J Cardiol 18:65

Yutzey KE, Rhee JT, Bader D. 1994. Expression of the atrial-specific myosin heavy chain AMHC1 and the establishment of anteroposterior polarity in the developing chick heart. Development 120:871

Yutzey KE, Bader D. 1995. Diversification of cardiomyogenic cell lineages during early heart development. Circ Res 77:216

8

Development of the Vasculature

Summary

Starting on day 17, vessels begin to arise in the splanchnopleuric meso-derm of the yolk sac wall from aggregations of cells called **blood islands.** On day 18, **vasculogenesis** (blood vessel formation) commences in the splanchnopleuric mesoderm of the embryonic disc, where it occurs by a somewhat different process. In the embryonic disc, splanchnopleuric mesoderm differentiates into endothelial cell precursors that ag-gregate and grow to form networks of **angioblastic cords.** These then coalesce, grow, and invade other tissues to form the embryonic vas-culature.

As embryonic folding carries the endocardial tubes into the ventral thorax during the fourth week, the paired dorsal aortae attached to the cranial ends of the tubes are pulled ventrally to form a pair of dorsoven-tral loops, the **first aortic arches.** During the fourth and fifth weeks, four additional pairs of aortic arches develop in craniocaudal suc-cession, connecting the aortic sac at the superior end of the truncus arteriosus to the dorsal aortae. This aortic arch system is subsequently remodeled to form the system of great arteries in the upper thorax and neck.

The paired dorsal aortae remain separate in the region of the aortic arches but fuse below the level of the fourth thoracic segment to form a single median dorsal aorta. The dorsal aorta develops three sets of branches: (1) a series of ventral branches, which supply the gut and gut derivatives; (2) lateral branches, which supply retroperitoneal structures such as the suprarenal glands, kidneys, and gonads; and (3) dorsolateral intersegmental branches called **intersegmental arteries,** which penetrate between the somite derivatives and give rise to part of the vasculature of the head, neck, body wall, limbs, and vertebral column. The ventral branches, which supply the gastrointestinal tract, are derived from remnants of a network of **vitelline arteries,** which develop in the yolk sac and vitelline duct and anastomose with the paired dorsal aortae. The paired dorsal aortae become connected to the **umbilical arteries** that develop in the connecting stalk and carry blood to the placenta.

The primitive venous system consists of three major components, all of which are initially bilaterally symmetrical: the **cardinal system,** which drains the head, neck, body wall, and limbs; the **vitelline veins,** which initially drain the yolk sac; and the **umbilical veins,** which develop in the connecting stalk and carry oxygenated blood from the placenta to the embryo. All three systems initially drain into both sinus horns, but all three undergo extensive modification during development as the systemic venous return is shifted to the right atrium.

Vasculogenesis

Development of the Aortic Arches and Great Arteries

Development of the Vitelline, Umbilical, and Cardinal Venous Systems

Development of the Coronary Circulation

Circulatory Changes at Birth

Veins   Weeks Days   **Arteries**

Cardinal system   *Portal system*

Blood islands form in yolk sac (day 17)

R. umbilical v.

Vitelline veins

Intersegmental arteries sprout from dorsal aorta

Posterior cardinal veins develop (28 days)

Aortic arches form (days 24-29); vitelline network is present (day 26)

Hepatic sinusoids develop

Upper limb: 41 days

Coronary vessels form

Subcardinal veins develop

Upper limb: 46 days

Lower limb: 49 days

Supracardinal veins develop

Definitive arteries to the gut, viscera, and body wall differentiate

Ductus venosus

Portal v.

Superior mesenteric v.

Splenic v.

L. umbilical v.

Inferior mesenteric v.

Definitive aortic arch system differentiates

Lower limb: 60 days

SVC
Azygos v.
Hemiazygos v.
IVC

Definitive system

Definitive system

Timeline. Development of the arterial and venous systems.

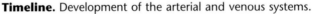

The cardinal system initially consists of paired **anterior (superior)** and **posterior (inferior) cardinal veins,** which meet to form short **common cardinal veins** draining into the right and left sinus horns. However, the posterior cardinals are supplemented and later replaced by two subsidiary venous systems, the **subcardinal** and **supracardinal** systems, which grow caudally from the base of the posterior cardinals in the medial dorsal body wall. All three of these cardinal systems, along with a small region of the right vitelline vein, give rise to portions of the inferior vena cava and its major branches. The supracardinals also form the azygous and hemiazygous systems draining the thoracic body wall. The vitelline venous system also gives rise to the liver sinusoids and to the portal system, which carries venous blood from the gastrointestinal tract to the liver. Within the substance of the liver, the **vitelline system** also forms the **ductus venosus,** a channel that shunts blood from the umbilical vein directly to the inferior vena cava during gestation.

All three systems undergo extensive modification during development. In the cardinal and vitelline systems, the longitudinal veins on the *left* side of the body tend to regress, whereas those on the *right* side persist and give rise to the great veins. Thus, a bilateral system that drains into both sinus horns becomes a right-sided system that drains into the right atrium. In contrast, the *right* umbilical vein disappears, whereas the *left* umbilical vein persists. The left umbilical vein loses its original connection to the left sinus horn, however, and secondarily empties into the ductus venosus.

The **coronary arteries** that supply blood to the heart muscle develop, in part, as branches from the base of the aorta, and the **coronary veins** sprout from the coronary sinus.

A dramatic and rapid change in the pattern of circulation occurs at birth as the newborn begins to breathe and the pulmonary vasculature expands. Much of the development described in this chapter is focused on the problem of producing a circulation that will effectively distribute the oxygenated blood arriving from the placenta via the umbilical vein to the tissues of the embryo and fetus, yet will be able to convert rapidly at birth to the adult pattern of circulation required by the air-breathing infant.

THE VASCULATURE BEGINS TO FORM EARLY IN THE THIRD WEEK

Vasculogenesis Commences With the Formation of Blood Islands in the Extraembryonic Mesoderm of the Yolk Sac, Chorion, and Connecting Stalk

The first evidence of blood vessel formation can be detected in the splanchnopleuric mesoderm of the yolk sac on day 17, as mesodermal aggregations called **blood islands** develop next to the endoderm. Each blood island segregates into a core of embryonic **hemoblasts** surrounded by flattened **endothelial cells.** The hemoblasts differentiate into the first blood cells of the embryo, and the endothelial cells develop into blood vessel endothelium. These vessel precursors lengthen and interconnect, establishing an initial vascular network. By the end of the third week, this network completely vascularizes the yolk sac, the connecting stalk, and the chorionic villi (see Ch. 2).

Vasculogenesis in the Embryo Commences in the Splanchnopleuric Mesoderm and Does Not Involve the Formation of Blood Cells

On day 18, blood vessels begin to develop in the splanchnopleuric mesoderm of the embryonic disc, where they form by a process somewhat different than that in the yolk sac. Inducing substances secreted by the underlying endoderm cause some cells of the splanchnopleuric mesoderm to differentiate into **angioblasts,** which develop into flattened endothelial cells that join together to form small vesicular structures called **angiocysts** (see the Experimental Principles section of this chapter). These angiocysts in turn coalesce into long tubes or vessels called **angioblastic cords** (Fig. 8–1*A, D*; see also Fig. 7–1*B, C*). The entire process is referred to as **in situ vesicle formation and fusion** or **vasculogenesis.** Angioblastic cords develop throughout the germ disc and coalesce to form a pervasive network of **angioblastic plexuses** that

Figure 8–1. A sampling of the methods used to study embryonic blood vessels. *A,* Immunocytochemical staining vascular precursors with antibodies that bind to antigens of presumptive endothelial cells. *B,* Microangiography (a radiologic technique). *C,* Plastic casting of the vasculature. *D,* Scanning electron microscopy. (*A,* From Coffin D, Poole TJ. 1988. Embryonic vascular development: immunohistochemical identification of the origin and subsequent morphogenesis of the major vessel primordia of quail embryos. Development 102:735. *B,* From Effman E. 1982. Development of the right and left pulmonary arteries: a microangiographic study in the mouse. Invest Radiol 17:529. *C,* From Bockman DE, Redman ME, Kirby ML. 1989. Alteration of early vascular development after ablation of cranial neural crest. Anat Rec 225:209. *D,* From Hirakow R, Hiruma T. 1981. Scanning electron microscopic study in the development of primitive blood vessels in chick embryos at the early somite stage. Anat Embryol 163:299.)

establish the initial configuration of the circulatory system of the embryo (see Fig. 8–1). This network grows and spreads throughout the embryo by three processes: (1) the continued formation and fusion of angiocysts; (2) **angiogenesis,** the budding and sprouting of new vessels from existing angioblastic cords; and (3) the intercalation of new mesodermal cells into the walls of existing vessels. Nonsprouting angiogenesis is also known to be a further mechanism for growth of the vascular network. This process is thought to involve the *Tie* receptor tyrosine kinase pathway and has also been termed intussusception.

All types of embryonic mesoderm except the prechordal plate have been shown to be capable of vasculogenesis. The mesoderm-like ectomesenchyme derived from the neural crest also cannot form blood vessels.

The Origin of the Stem Cells That Populate the Embryonic Hematopoietic Organs Is Unclear

The yolk sac is the first supplier of blood cells to the embryonic circulation. Starting in the fifth week, however, the task of **hematopoiesis** (blood cell production) is taken over by a sequence of embryonic organs, including the liver, spleen, thymus, and, finally, the bone marrow. The source of the hematopoietic stem cells that populate these organs, however, remains an enigma. Cell tracing and immunochemical studies suggest that blood cells form in the splanchnopleuric mesoderm near the dorsal aorta at an early somite stage. It is possible that these are the ancestral blood cells of the embryo (see the Experimental Principles section of this chapter).

Almost All Splanchnopleuric Mesoderm Can Form Blood Vessels

Because blood vessels appear in the yolk sac on about day 17 but not in the embryonic disc until day 18, it was originally thought that intraembryonic vessels arose primarily as a result of centripetal extension of the yolk sac vasculature into the embryo proper. Recently, however, quail-chick chimera experiments have provided evidence that almost all the intraembryonic splanchnopleuric mesoderm has the ability to form blood vessels. Furthermore, experiments in which mesoderm is transplanted from one region in the quail to another region in the chick show that the characteristic branching pattern of the blood vessels in each region is determined by cues from the underlying endoderm and its extracellular matrix. These studies have been facilitated by the availability of antibodies that recognize quail vessels specifically, making it possible to visualize their branching patterns (see Fig. 8–1*A*).

Classic approaches to the study of vasculogenesis include the infiltration of the vasculature with stains such as India ink as well as serial sectioning and three-dimensional reconstruction. A modern variant of the former technique, **microangiography,** involves the radiologic visualization of injected contrast medium (see Fig. 8–1*B*). Alternatively, the vasculature can be perfused with a soluble plastic that is then polymerized to form a solid cast of the vasculature that can be isolated and examined by scanning electron microscopy (see Fig. 8–1*C*). Scanning electron microscopy has also been useful in directly examining development of the vasculature. For this technique, fixed specimens are broken open, and then the exposed vascular structures are coated with metal (see Fig. 8–1*D*).

THE HUMAN AORTIC ARCHES ARE REMNANTS OF THE GILL VASCULATURE OF FISHES

The respiratory apparatus of the jawless fishes that gave rise to higher vertebrates consisted of a variable number of gill bars separated by gill slits (Fig. 8–2). Water flows in through the mouth and out through the gill slits. Each of the gill bars or **branchial arches** is vascularized by an **aortic arch artery,** which arises as a branch of the ventral aorta (aortic sac). Gas exchange takes place in the gill capillaries, and the dorsal half of each aortic arch conveys the oxygenated blood to the paired dorsal aortae.

In the human embryo, five pairs of mesen-

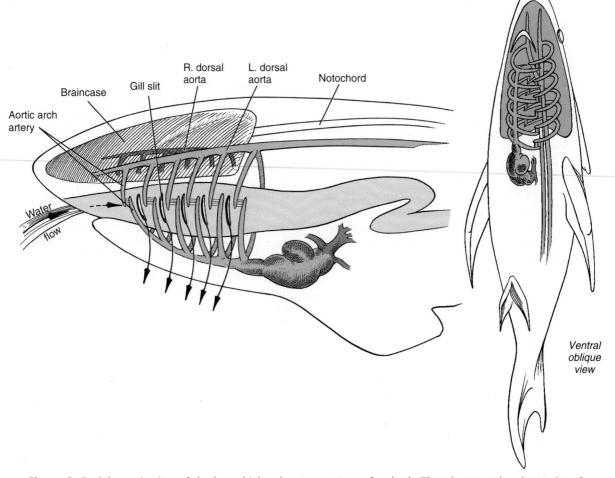

Figure 8–2. Schematic view of the branchial arch artery system of a shark. The pharyngeal arch arteries of humans evolved from the branchial arch arteries of protochordates and fishes. The branchial arch arteries occupy the gill bars and thus enclose the pharynx like a basket. The arteries supply blood to the gills, which extract oxygen from water flowing through the gill slits.

chymal condensations develop on either side of the pharynx, corresponding to branchial arches 1, 2, 3, 4, and 6 of the early fish. The fifth arch never develops at all or appears briefly and then regresses. The mesodermal and endodermal components of the arches have been modified through evolution so that, in humans, they form structures of the lower face and neck and derivatives of the pharyngeal foregut. These structures are thus more appropriately called **pharyngeal arches** than branchial arches. The development of the pharyngeal arches is detailed in Chapter 12; the following discussion is limited to the development of the aortic arch arteries.

The Human Aortic Arches Arise in Craniocaudal Sequence and Form a Basket of Arteries Around the Pharynx

As described in Chapter 7, the first pair of aortic arches is formed between day 22 and day 24, when the process of embryonic folding that carries the endocardial tubes into the future thorax also draws the cranial ends of the attached aortae into a dorsoventral loop (see Fig. 7–3). The resulting first pair of aortic arches lies in the thickened mesenchyme of the first pair of pharyngeal arches on either side of the developing pharynx (Fig. 8–3*A*). Ventrally, the aortic arch arteries arise from the **aortic sac,** an expansion at the cranial end of the truncus arteriosus. Dorsally, they connect to the left and right dorsal aortae. The dorsal aortae remain separate in the region of the aortic arches, but during the fourth week they fuse together from the fourth thoracic segment to the fourth lumbar segment to form a midline **dorsal aorta** (see Fig. 8–5*A*, later).

Between days 26 and 29, aortic arches 2, 3, 4, and 6 develop by vasculogenesis and angiogenesis within their respective pharyngeal arches, incorporating angioblasts that migrate from the surrounding splanchnopleuric mesoderm. The migration of neural crest-derived ectomesenchymal cells into the arches plays a significant role in the normal development of the arch arteries, although neural crest cells do not contribute directly to the endothelium of these vessels (see the Experimental Principles section of Ch. 7).

The first two arches regress as the later arches form. The second aortic arch arises in the second pharyngeal arch by day 26 and grows to connect the aortic sac to the dorsal aortae. Simultaneously, the first pair of aortic arches regresses completely (except, possibly, for small remnants that may give rise to portions of the **maxillary arteries**) (see Fig. 8–3*A*). On day 28, while the first arch is regressing, the third and fourth aortic arches appear. Finally, on day 29, the sixth arch forms, and the second arch regresses except for a small remnant that gives rise to part of the **stapedial artery** (see Fig. 8–3*B*, *C*), which supplies blood to the primordium of the stapes bone in the developing ear (see Ch. 12).

Arches 3, 4, and 6 Give Rise to Important Vessels of the Head, Neck, and Upper Thorax

The Third Aortic Arch Becomes the Common Carotid and Internal Carotid Arteries. By day 35, the segments of dorsal aorta connecting the third and fourth arch arteries disappear on both sides of the body, so that the cranial extensions of the dorsal aortae that supply the head receive blood entirely through the third aortic arches (see Fig. 8–3*B*). The third arch arteries give rise to the

right and left **common carotid arteries** (Fig. 8–4*A*) and also to the proximal portion of the right and left **internal carotid arteries.** The distal portion of the internal carotid arteries is derived from the cranial extensions of the dorsal aortae, and the right and left **external carotid arteries** sprout from the common carotids (see Fig. 8–3*C*).

The Fourth and Sixth Arches Undergo Asymmetric Remodeling to Supply Blood to the Upper Extremities, Dorsal Aorta, and Lungs. By the seventh week, the right dorsal aorta loses its connections with both the fused midline dorsal aorta and the right sixth arch, while remaining connected to the right fourth arch (see Fig. 8–3*C*). Meanwhile, it also acquires a branch, the **right seventh cervical intersegmental artery,** which grows into the right upper limb bud. The definitive **right subclavian artery** supplying the upper limb, therefore, is derived from (1) the right fourth arch, (2) a short segment of the right dorsal aorta, and (3) the right seventh intersegmental artery. The region of the aortic sac connected to the right fourth artery is modified to form the branch of the developing aorta called the **brachiocephalic artery** (see Fig. 8–3*C*).

The left fourth aortic arch retains its connection to the fused dorsal aorta and with a small segment of the aortic sac becomes the **aortic arch** and the most cranial portion of the **descending aorta.** The remainder of the descending aorta, from the fourth thoracic level caudally, is derived from the fused dorsal aortae. The **left seventh intersegmental artery** sprouts directly from the left dorsal aorta and gives rise to the **left subclavian artery** supplying the left upper extremity (see Fig. 8–3*C*).

The right and left sixth arches arise from the proximal end of the aortic sac, but further development is then asymmetrical (see Figs. 8–3*C* and 8–4*B*). By the seventh week, the distal connection of the right sixth arch with the right dorsal aorta disappears. The left sixth arch, in contrast, remains complete, and its distal portion forms the **ductus arteriosus** that allows blood to shunt from the pulmonary trunk to the descending aorta throughout gestation. This bypass closes at birth and is later transformed into the **ligamentum arteriosum** that attaches the pulmonary trunk to the aorta (see Fig. 8–3*B*, *C*). (The changes in the cir-

Stapedial a. (remnant of 2nd arch)

Aortic arches 3, 4, 6

Part of maxillary a. (remnant of 1st arch)

7th intersegmental a.

Descending aorta

1st arch
2nd
3rd
4th
6th
Aortic sac
Truncus arteriosus
Dorsal aorta
Pulmonary a.
7th intersegmental a.
External carotid a.

Part of maxillary a.

Stapedial a.

1
2
3
4
6

L. dorsal aorta

7th intersegmental a.

A 29 days

Internal carotid a.

External carotid a. (sprout of 3rd arch)

Stapedial a.

Part of maxillary a.

Common carotid a.

R. vagus n.

7th intersegmental a.

Pulmonary a.

Lung bud

2 3
1

L. recurrent laryngeal n.

L. vagus n.

Ductus arteriosus

4
6

1
2
3
4
6

B 7 weeks

Figure 8–3. *See legend on opposite page*

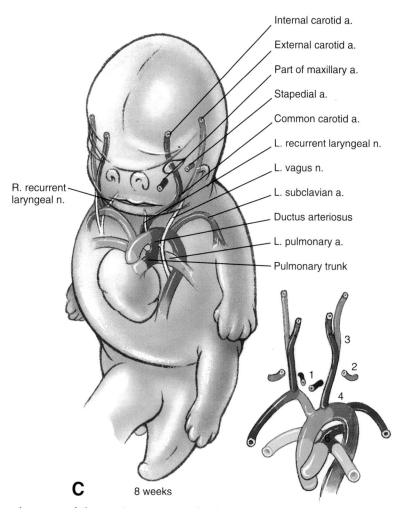

Internal carotid a.

External carotid a.

Part of maxillary a.

Stapedial a.

Common carotid a.

L. recurrent laryngeal n.

L. vagus n.

L. subclavian a.

Ductus arteriosus

L. pulmonary a.

Pulmonary trunk

R. recurrent laryngeal n.

C   8 weeks

Figure 8–3. Development of the aortic system. *A,* The five pairs of aortic arch arches that form in humans correspond to arches 1, 2, 3, 4, and 6 of evolutionary predecessors. The first arch is complete by day 24 but regresses as the second arch forms on day 26. The third and fourth arches form on day 28; the second arch degenerates as the sixth arch forms on day 29. *B,* Development of the arches in the second month. Note that the structures arising from the first three pairs of aortic arches are bilateral, whereas arches 4 and 6 develop asymmetrically. The pulmonary arteries initially sprout from arch 4 and become secondarily reconnected to the roots of the sixth arches. *C,* 8 weeks. Note the asymmetric development of the recurrent laryngeal branches of the vagus nerve, which innervate the laryngeal muscles. As the larynx is displaced superiorly relative to the arch system, the recurrent laryngeal nerves are caught under the most inferior remaining arch on each side. The right recurrent laryngeal nerve therefore loops under the right subclavian artery, while the left recurrent laryngeal nerve loops under the ductus arteriosus.

culation that take place at birth are discussed in detail at the end of this chapter.)

As shown in Figure 8–3*B, C,* the asymmetrical development of the left and right sixth arches is responsible for the curious asymmetry of the **left and right recurrent laryngeal nerves,** which branch from the vagus. These nerves originally arise below the level of the sixth arch and cross under them to innervate intrinsic muscles of the larynx. During development, the larynx is translocated cranially relative to the aortic arches. The left recurrent laryngeal nerve becomes caught under the sixth arch on the left side and remains looped under the ligamentum arteriosum. Because the distal right sixth aortic arch disappears (and because no fifth arch develops), the right recurrent

Figure 8–4. *A,* Frontal view of a cast of the aortic arch system. The left and right common carotid arteries (C) are growing toward the viewer from the dorsal segments of the third arches. The third and fourth arches arise from the aortic sac (arrow). V, ventricle; A, primitive atrium. *B,* Inferolateral view of a cast of the aortic arch system. Arches 2, 3, and 4 are fully developed, and the sixth pair is beginning to form. The truncus arteriosus is marked by an arrow. (From Bockman DE, Redman ME, Kirby ML. 1989. Alteration of early vascular development after ablation of cranial neural crest. Anat Rec 225:209.)

laryngeal nerve becomes caught under the fourth arch, which becomes the right subclavian artery.

The pulmonary arteries may initially arise from the fourth rather than the sixth aortic arch. Although the pulmonary arteries become connected to the sixth arch arteries and finally to the pulmonary trunk, several classic observations, as well as more recent quail-chick chimera experiments, suggest that these arteries initially sprout from the fourth aortic arches. As these pulmonary artery sprouts grow toward the lungs, their roots make secondary contact with the sixth arches as they lose their connection to the fourth arches. In the lungs, their distal ends anastomose with the vasculature developing in the mesenchyme surrounding the bronchial buds (see Ch. 6).

THE DORSAL AORTA DEVELOPS VENTRAL, LATERAL, AND POSTEROLATERAL BRANCHES

The Vitelline Arteries to the Yolk Sac Give Rise to the Arterial Supply of the Gastrointestinal Tract

The blood vessels that arise in the yolk sac wall differentiate to form the arteries and veins of the **vitelline system** (Fig. 8–5). As the yolk sac shrinks relative to the folding embryo, the right and left vitelline plexuses coalesce to form a number of major arteries that anastomose both with the vascular plexuses of the future gut and with the

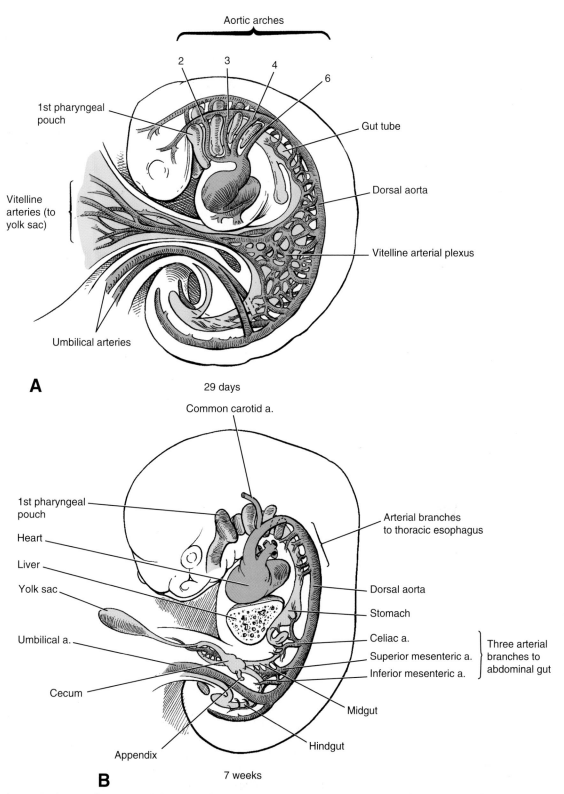

Figure 8–5. Development of the ventral aortic branches supplying the gut tube and derivatives. *A,* In the fourth week, a multitude of vitelline arteries emerge from the ventral surfaces of the dorsal aortae to supply the yolk sac. *B,* After the paired dorsal aortae fuse at the end of the fourth week, many of the vitelline channels disappear, reducing the final number to about five in the thoracic region and to three (the celiac, superior mesenteric, and inferior mesenteric arteries) in the abdominal region.

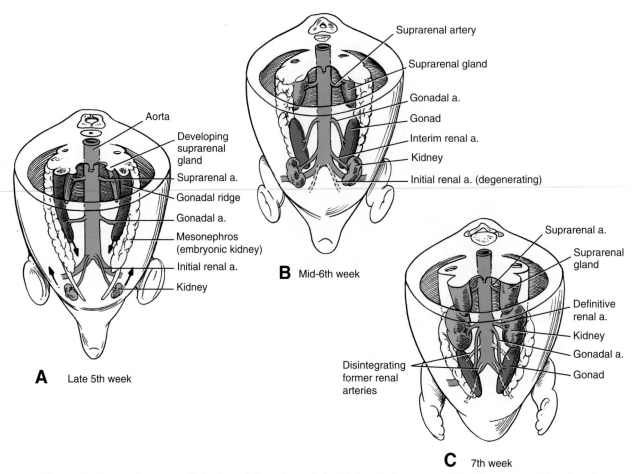

Figure 8–6. Development of the lateral branches of the abdominal aorta. *A,* Lateral sprouts of the dorsal aorta vascularize the suprarenal glands, the gonads, and the kidneys. During the sixth week, the gonads begin to descend while the kidneys ascend. *B, C,* The gonadal artery lengthens during the migration of the gonad, but the ascending kidney is vascularized by a succession of new, more superior aortic sprouts. The suprarenal arteries remain in place.

ventral surface of the dorsal aorta. These vessels eventually lose their connection with the yolk sac, becoming the arteries that supply blood from the dorsal aorta to the gastrointestinal tract.

Cranial to the diaphragm, about five pairs of these arteries usually develop and anastomose with the dorsal aorta at variable levels to supply the thoracic esophagus. Caudal to the diaphragm, three pairs of major arteries develop to supply specific regions of the developing abdominal gut. The fields of vascularization of these three arteries constitute the basis for dividing the abdominal gastrointestinal tract into three embryologic regions: the **abdominal foregut,** the **midgut,** and the **hindgut.**

The most superior of the three abdominal

vitelline arteries, the **celiac artery,** initially joins the dorsal aorta at the seventh cervical level. This connection subsequently descends to the twelfth thoracic level, and the celiac artery develops branches that vascularize not only the abdominal part of the foregut from the abdominal esophagus to the descending segment of the duodenum, but also the several embryologic outgrowths of the foregut—the liver, pancreas, and gallbladder. The celiac artery also produces a large branch that vascularizes the spleen, which is a mesodermal derivative of the dorsal mesogastrium (see Ch. 9). (The dorsal mesogastrium is the portion of the dorsal mesentery that suspends the stomach.)

The second abdominal vitelline artery, the

Developing dorsal aorta

Intersegmental arteries developing between somites

Figure 8–7. Intersegmental arteries sprout from the dorsal aortae and penetrate between the somites as they grow toward the midline. (From Coffin D, Poole TJ. 1988. Embryonic vascular development: immunohistochemical identification of the origin and subsequent morphogenesis of the major vessel primordia of quail embryos. Development 102:735.)

superior mesenteric artery, initially joins the dorsal aorta at the second thoracic level; this connection later migrates to the first lumbar level. This artery supplies the developing midgut—the intestine from the descending segment of the duodenum to a region of the transverse colon near the left colic flexure.

The third and final abdominal vitelline artery, the **inferior mesenteric artery,** initially joins the dorsal aorta at the twelfth thoracic level and later descends to the third lumbar level. It supplies the hindgut: the distal portion of the transverse colon, the descending and sigmoid colon, and the rectum. (As described in Ch. 9, the inferior end of the anorectal canal is vascularized by branches of the iliac arteries.)

Lateral Sprouts of the Descending Aorta Vascularize the Suprarenal Glands, the Gonads, and the Kidneys

The suprarenal (adrenal) glands, gonads, and kidneys are all vascularized by lateral branches of the descending aorta. As shown in Fig. 8–6, however, these three organs and their arteries have different developmental histories. The suprarenal glands form in the posterior body wall between the sixth and twelfth thoracic segments and become vascularized mainly by a pair of lateral aortic sprouts that arise at an upper lumbar level. The suprarenal glands also acquire branches from the renal artery and inferior phrenic artery, but the **suprarenal arteries** developing from these aortic sprouts remain the major supply to the glands. These glands and their aortic branches develop in place. The presumptive gonads become vascularized by **gonadal arteries** that arise initially at the tenth thoracic level. The gonads descend during development, but the origin of the gonadal arteries becomes fixed at the third or fourth lumbar level. As the gonads (especially the testes) descend further, the gonadal arteries elongate. The definitive kidneys, in contrast, arise in the sacral region and migrate upward to a lumbar site just below the suprarenal glands. As they migrate, they are vascularized by a succession of transient aortic sprouts that arise at progressively higher levels. These arteries do not elongate to follow the ascending kidneys but instead degenerate and are replaced. The final pair of arteries in this series form in the upper lumbar region and become the definitive **renal arteries.** Occasionally, a more inferior pair of renal arteries persist as accessory renal arteries.

Intersegmental Sprouts Arise From the Posterolateral Surface of the Descending Aorta and Vascularize the Somite Derivatives

At the end of the third week, small posterolateral sprouts arise from the dorsal aorta at the cervical through sacral levels and grow into the spaces between the developing somites (Fig. 8–7). In the **cervical, thoracic,** and **lumbar** regions, a dorsal branch of each of these intersegmental sprouts vascularizes both the developing neural tube and the epimeres that will form the deep muscles of the neck and back (Fig. 8–8A). Cutaneous branches of these arteries also supply the dorsal skin. The ventral branch of each of these intersegmental sprouts supplies the developing hypomeric muscles and associated skin. In the **thoracic** region, these ventral branches become the **intercostal arteries** and their cutaneous branches, whereas in the lumbar

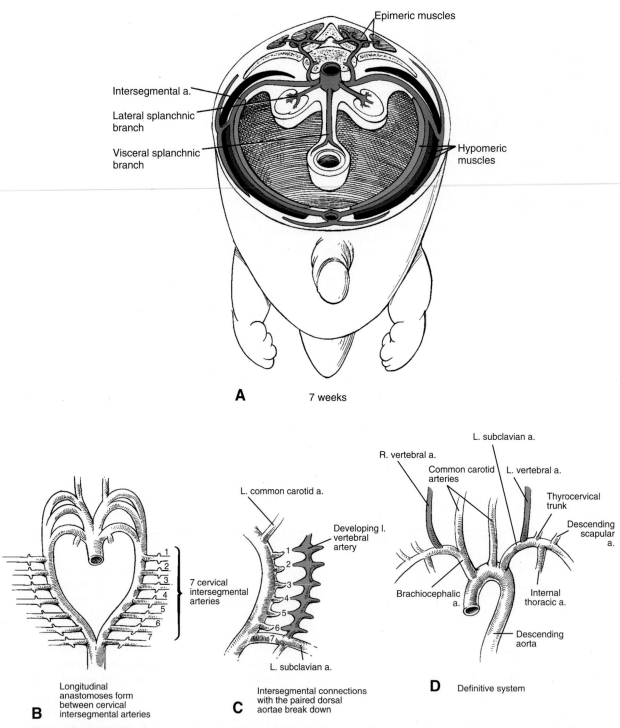

Figure 8–8. Development of the arterial supply to the body wall. *A,* Intersegmental artery system in the trunk region. Branches of the paired intersegmental arteries supply the posterior, lateral, and anterior body wall and musculature, the vertebral column, and the spinal cord. *B–D,* The vertebral artery is formed from longitudinal anastomoses of the first through seventh cervical intersegmental arteries.

and sacral regions, they become the **lumbar** and **lateral sacral arteries.** The short continuation of the dorsal aorta beyond its bifurcation into the common iliac arteries is called the **median sacral artery.**

In the cervical region, the intersegmental sprouts anastomose with each other to form a more complex pattern of vascularization (see Fig. 8–8B). The paired **vertebral arteries** arise from longitudinal branches that link together to form a longitudinal vessel and secondarily lose their intersegmental connections to the aorta. The **deep cervical, ascending cervical, superior intercostal, internal thoracic,** and **superior** and **inferior epigastric arteries** also develop from anastomoses of intersegmental arteries.

The Umbilical Arteries Initially Join the Dorsal Aortae but Shift Their Origin to the Internal Iliac Arteries

The right and left **umbilical arteries** develop in the connecting stalk in the early fourth week and are thus among the earliest embryonic arteries to arise. These arteries form an initial connection with the paired dorsal aortae in the sacral region (see Fig. 8–5A). During the fifth week, however, these connections are obliterated, and the umbilical arteries develop a new junction with a pair of fifth lumbar intersegmental artery branches called the **internal iliac arteries.** The internal iliac arteries vascularize pelvic organs and (initially) the lower extremity limb bud. As discussed later, the fifth intersegmental arteries also give rise to the **external iliac arteries.** Proximal to these branches, the root of the fifth intersegmental artery is called the **common iliac artery** (see Fig. 8–10).

The Arteries to the Limbs Are Formed by Remodeling of Intersegmental Artery Branches

As indicated above, the arteries to the developing upper and lower limbs are derived mainly from the seventh cervical intersegmental artery and the fifth lumbar intersegmental artery, respectively. These arteries initially supply each limb bud by joining an **axial** or **axis artery** that develops along the central axis of the limb bud (Figs. 8–9 and 8–10).

In the upper limb, the axis artery develops into the **brachial artery** of the upper arm and the **anterior interosseous artery** of the forearm and thus continues to be the main source of blood for the limb. In the hand, a small portion of the axis artery persists as the **deep palmar arch.** The other arteries of the upper limb, including the **radial, median,** and **ulnar arteries,** develop partly as sprouts of the axis artery.

In the lower limb, in contrast, the axis artery—which arises as the distal continuation of the internal iliac artery—largely degenerates, and the definitive supply is provided almost entirely by the **external iliac artery,** which, as mentioned above, arises as a new branch of the fifth lumbar intersegmental artery (see Fig. 8–10). The axis artery persists as three remnants: the small **sciatic (ischiatic) artery,** which serves the sciatic nerve in the posterior thigh; a segment of the **popliteal artery;** and a section of the **peroneal artery** in the leg. Virtually all the other arteries of the lower limb develop as sprouts of the external iliac artery.

THE PRIMITIVE EMBRYONIC VENOUS SYSTEM IS DIVIDED INTO VITELLINE, UMBILICAL, AND CARDINAL SYSTEMS

The embryo has three major venous systems that fulfill different functions. The **vitelline system** drains the gastrointestinal tract and gut derivatives; the **umbilical system** carries oxygenated blood from the placenta; and the **cardinal system** drains the head, neck, and body wall. All three systems are initially bilaterally symmetric and converge on the right and left sinus horns of the sinus venosus (Figs. 8–11A and 8–12; see also Fig. 7–5). However, the shift of the systemic venous return to the right atrium (see Ch. 7) initiates a radical remodeling that reshapes these systems to yield the adult pattern.

The Vitelline System Gives Rise to the Liver Sinusoids, the Portal System, and a Portion of the Inferior Vena Cava

Like the vitelline arteries, the vitelline veins arise from the capillary plexuses of the yolk sac and

Primary axial a.

30 days

Interosseous a.

41 days

Brachial a.

Radial a.

Interosseous a.

Brachial a.

Ulnar a.

Circumflex humeral a.

Subclavian a.

Brachial a.

46 days

Radial recurrent a.

Profunda branchii a.

Ulnar collateral a.

Radial a.

Anterior interosseous a.

Median a.

Deep palmar arch

Ulnar a.

Superficial palmar arch

Definitive system

Figure 8–9. Development of the arterial system of the upper limb. The seventh cervical intersegmental arteries grow into the limb buds to form the axis arteries of the developing upper limbs. The axis artery gives rise to the subclavian, axillary, brachial, and anterior interosseous arteries and to the deep palmar arch. Other arteries of the upper extremity develop as sprouts of the axis artery.

form part of the vasculature of the developing gut and gut derivatives. Initially, the vitelline system empties into the sinus horns of the heart via a pair of symmetrical **vitelline veins** (see Fig. 8–11*A*). Right and left vitelline plexuses also develop in the septum transversum and connect to the vitelline veins (see Fig. 8–11*B*). The vessels of these plexuses become surrounded by the growing liver cords and give rise to the **liver sinusoids,** a dense network of anastomosing venous spaces. As the left sinus horn regresses to form the coronary sinus, the left vitelline vein also diminishes. By the third month, the left vitelline vein has completely disappeared in the region of the sinus venosus, and the blood from the left side of the abdominal viscera drains across to the right vitelline vein via a series of transverse anastomoses that have formed both

within the substance of the liver and around the abdominal portion of the foregut (see Fig. 8–11*C*).

After the left vitelline vein loses its connection with the heart, the blood from the entire vitelline system drains into the heart via the enlarged right vitelline vein (see Fig. 8–11*C*). The *superior* portion of this vein (the portion between the liver and the heart) becomes the **terminal portion of the inferior vena cava** (IVC) (see Fig. 8–12*E*). Meanwhile, a single oblique channel among the hepatic anastomoses becomes dominant and drains directly into the nascent IVC. As described below, this channel, the **ductus venosus,** is crucial during fetal life because it receives oxygenated blood from the umbilical system and shunts it directly to the right atrium.

The vitelline veins inferior to the liver re-

Figure 8–10. Development of the arterial system of the lower limb. The fifth lumbar intersegmental artery forms the axis artery of the lower extremity. The only remnants of this vessel in the lower limb of the adult are the ischiatic artery, a small portion of the popliteal artery, and the peroneal artery.

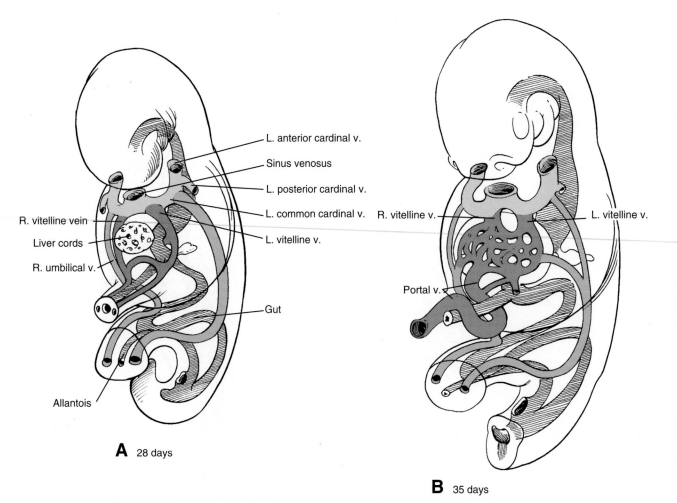

Figure 8–11. *A–D,* Fate of the vitelline and umbilical veins. The right and left vitelline veins form a portal system that drains blood from the abdominal foregut, the midgut, and the upper part of the anorectal canal. (*Figure continues.*)

gress during the second and third months, with the exception of the portion of the right vitelline vein just inferior to the developing liver and a few of the proximal ventral left-to-right vitelline anastomoses (see Fig. 8–11*B*). These veins become the main channels of the **portal system,** which drain blood from the gastrointestinal tract to the liver sinusoids. The segment of the right vitelline vein inferior to the liver becomes the **portal vein and the superior mesenteric vein** (see Fig. 8–11*C, D*). Persisting branches collect blood from the abdominal foregut (including the abdominal esophagus, stomach, gallbladder, duodenum, and pancreas) and the midgut. Prominent left-to-right vitelline anastomoses are remodeled to deliver blood to the distal end of the portal vein through

two veins: the **splenic vein,** which drains the spleen, part of the stomach, and the greater omentum (see Ch. 9), and the **inferior mesenteric vein,** which drains the hindgut.

The Right Umbilical Vein Disappears and the Left Umbilical Vein Anastomoses With the Ductus Venosus

In contrast to the regression of the left vitelline vein, the *right* umbilical vein becomes completely obliterated during the second month, whereas the *left* umbilical vein persists (see Fig. 8–11). Concur-

R. vitelline v.

Ductus venosus

Portal v.

L. umbilical v.

C 8 weeks

Ductus venosus

L. gastric v.

Gastroepiploic v.

Portal v.

Gastroduodenal v.

Splenic v.

Inferior mesenteric v.

L. umbilical v.

Superior mesenteric v.

D 12 weeks

Figure 8–11 (*Continued*). The right umbilical vein disappears, but the left umbilical vein anastomoses with the ductus venosus in the liver, thus shunting oxygenated placental blood into the inferior vena cava and to the right side of the heart. IVC = inferior vena cava.

rently, however, the left umbilical vein loses its connection with the left sinus horn and forms a new anastomosis with the ductus venosus. Oxygenated blood from the placenta thus reaches the heart via the single umbilical vein and the ductus venosus. As described at the end of this chapter, the ductus venosus constricts shortly after birth, eliminating this venous shunt through the liver.

The Posterior Cardinal System Is Augmented and Then Superseded by Paired Subcardinal and Supracardinal Veins

As shown in Figure 8–12*A*, the bilaterally symmetrical cardinal vein system that develops in the third and fourth weeks to drain the head, neck,

and body wall initially consists of paired **posterior (inferior)** and **anterior (superior) cardinal veins,** which join near the heart to form the short **common cardinals** that empty into the sinus horns. The posterior cardinal veins are supplemented and later largely replaced by two additional pairs of veins, the **subcardinal** and **supracardinal** veins, which develop in the body wall medial to the posterior cardinal veins. Like the posterior and anterior cardinals, these two systems are bilaterally symmetrical at first but undergo extensive remodeling during development.

The Subcardinal System Drains Structures of the Median Dorsal Body Wall, Principally the Kidneys and Gonads. The left and right subcardinal veins sprout from the base of the posterior cardinals by the end of the sixth week and grow caudally in the median dorsal body wall (see Fig.

A 28 days

L. anterior cardinal v.
L. vitelline v.
L. umbilical v.
L. posterior cardinal v.

B 35 days

L. subcardinal v.
L. posterior cardinal v.

C 50 days

L. anterior cardinal v.

Thyroid and thymic veins growing toward each other to form a median anastomosis

Sinus venosus

R. vitelline v.
R. supracardinal v.
Subcardinal portion of IVC

L. posterior cardinal v.

Iliac anastomosis connecting the posterior cardinal veins

L. internal iliac v.
L. external iliac v.
Middle sacral v.

Figure 8-12. *See legend on opposite page*

Figure 8–12. Development of the systemic venous system from the four bilaterally symmetrical cardinal vein systems. These systems are remodeled to drain blood from both sides of the head, neck, and body into the right atrium. The head and neck are initially drained by an anterior cardinal system, and the trunk is drained by a posterior cardinal system. The posterior cardinals are replaced by a set of subcardinal and a set of supracardinal veins.

SVC

L. brachiocephalic v.

L. sinus horn

Subclavian v.

R. vitelline portion of IVC

Hepatic v.

Subcardinal portion of IVC

Degenerating posterior cardinal v.

Supracardinal portion of IVC

I. thoracic supracardinal v.

Posterior cardinal portion of IVC

Internal iliac v.

External iliac v.

D   56 days

R. brachiocephalic v.

SVC

R. subclavian v.

R. vitelline segment of IVC

Subcardinal segment of IVC

Supracardinal segment of IVC

Posterior cardinal segment of IVC

Internal jugular v.

External jugular v.

L. brachiocephalic v.

L. subclavian v.

Superior intercostal v.

Coronary sinus

Intercostal v.

Azygos v.

Hemiazygos v.

Renal v.

Gonadal v.

Common iliac v.

Internal iliac v.

External iliac v.

Femoral v.

E   Definitive system

8–12B). By the seventh and eighth weeks, these subcardinal veins become connected to each other by numerous median anastomoses and also form some lateral anastomoses with the posterior cardinals. However, the longitudinal segments of the left subcardinal vein soon regress, so that by the ninth week the structures on the left side of the body served by the subcardinal system drain solely through transverse anastomotic channels to the right subcardinal vein. Meanwhile, the right subcardinal vein loses its original connection with the posterior cardinal vein and develops a new anastomosis with the segment of the right vitelline vein just inferior to the heart to form the portion of the inferior vena cava between the liver and the kidneys (see Fig. 8–12C–E). Through this remodeling process, the organs originally drained by the right and left subcardinal veins ultimately empty into the right heart via the IVC.

The Supracardinal System Gives Rise to a Portion of the IVC and to the Azygos System Draining the Thoracic Body Wall.

While the subcardinal system is being remodeled, a new pair of veins, the supracardinal veins, sprout from the base of the posterior cardinals and grow caudally just medial to the posterior cardinal veins (see Fig. 8–12C). These veins drain the body wall via the segmental **intercostal veins,** thus taking over the function of the posterior cardinals. The abdominal and thoracic portions of the supracardinal veins give rise to separate venous components in the adult and therefore will be described separately.

While the supracardinals are developing, the posterior cardinals become obliterated over most of their length (see Fig. 8–12C, D). The most caudal portions of the posterior cardinals (including a large median anastomosis) do persist, but lose their original connection to the heart and form a new anastomosis with the supracardinal veins. This caudal remnant of the posterior cardinals develops into the common iliac veins and the caudal-most, sacral portion of the IVC. The common iliac veins in turn sprout the internal and external iliac veins, which grow to drain the lower extremities and pelvic organs.

In the abdominal region, the remodeling of the supracardinal system commences with the obliteration of the inferior portion of the left supracardinal vein (see Fig. 8–12D, E). The remaining abdominal segment of the right supracardinal vein

then anastomoses with the right subcardinal vein to form a segment of the IVC just inferior to the kidneys.

The thoracic part of the supracardinal system drains the thoracic body wall via a series of **intercostal veins.** The thoracic portions of the supracardinals originally empty into the left and right posterior cardinals and are connected to each other by median anastomoses. However, the left thoracic supracardinal vein, called the **hemiazygos vein,** soon loses its connection with the left posterior cardinal vein and left sinus horn and subsequently drains into the right supracardinal system (see Fig. 8–12E). The remaining portion of the inferior right supracardinal vein also loses its original connection with the posterior cardinal vein and makes a new anastomosis with the segment of the superior vena cava derived from the anterior cardinal vein (which, in turn, drains into the heart via a segment representing a small remnant of the right common cardinal vein). The right supracardinal vein is now called the **azygos vein.** Both the hemiazygos and the azygos veins now drain into the right atrium via the superior vena cava (see Fig. 8–12E).

The Definitive IVC Is Constructed From Remnants of Four Separate Systems.

Figure 8–12E shows the sources of the four portions of the IVC. From superior to inferior, (1) the right vitelline vein gives rise to the terminal segment of the IVC; (2) the right subcardinal vein gives rise to a segment between the liver and the kidneys; (3) the right supracardinal vein gives rise to an abdominal segment inferior to the kidneys of the IVC; and (4) the right and left posterior cardinal veins plus the median anastomosis connecting them give rise to the sacral segment of the IVC.

Blood Is Drained From the Head and Neck by the Anterior Cardinal Veins

The left and right anterior cardinal veins originally drain blood into the sinus horns via the right and left common cardinal veins (see Fig. 8–12A–D). However, the proximal connection of the left anterior cardinal vein with the left sinus horn soon regresses, leaving only a small remnant lying directly on the heart, called the **oblique vein of the** left atrium (see Fig. 8–12E, Ch. 7, and Fig. 7–10). This small remnant collects blood from the left atrial region of the heart and returns it directly to the coronary sinus, which is a vestige of the left sinus horn.

The cranial portions of the anterior cardinal veins in the developing cervical region give rise to the internal jugular veins, whereas capillary plexuses in the face become connected with these vessels to form the external jugular veins. Simultaneously, a median anastomosis connecting the left and right anterior cardinals develops from thymic and thyroid veins (see Fig. 8–12C–E). Once the left anterior cardinal vein loses its connection with the heart, all the blood from the left side of the head and neck shunts over to the right anterior cardinal through this anastomosis. The subclavian vein, which coalesces from the venous plexus of the left upper limb bud, also empties into the proximal left anterior cardinal vein. The intercardinal anastomosis thus carries the blood from the left upper limb as well as the left side of the head and is called the left brachiocephalic vein (see Fig. 8–12C–E). The left brachiocephalic vein enters the right anterior cardinal at its junction with the right brachiocephalic vein draining the right upper limb bud. The small segment of right anterior cardinal vein between the junction of the right and left brachiocephalic veins and the right atrium becomes the superior vena cava (see Fig 8–12E). Thus, by the end of the eighth week, the definitive superior vena cava drains blood from (1) both sides of the head, (2) both upper limbs, and (3) the thoracic body wall (via the azygos vein).

THE CORONARY VESSELS DEVELOP FROM BLOOD ISLANDS DEEP TO THE EPICARDIUM

The first evidence of coronary vessel development is the appearance at the beginning of the fifth week of structures such as blood islands just under the epicardium in the sulci of the developing heart. During the late fifth and sixth weeks, the capillary plexuses developing from these foci form connections both with coronary veins sprouting from the coronary sinus and with coronary arteries growing from the aorta. In fact, the coronary arteries actually sprout not directly from the aorta but rather from a pair of special aortic branches, the left and right aortic sinuses, that emerge from the aorta just above the two cusps of the semilunar valve (Fig. 8–13). It has been suggested that the developing capillary plexuses in the sulci induce the sprouting of the coronary veins and arteries.

THE LYMPHATIC SYSTEM DEVELOPS BY MECHANISMS SIMILAR TO THOSE THAT PRODUCE THE BLOOD VESSELS

Like blood vessels, lymphatic channels arise by vasculogenesis and angiogenesis from splanchnopleuric mesodermal precursors. Lymphatics do not begin to appear until about the fifth week, however. By the end of the fifth week, a pair of enlargements, the jugular lymph sacs, develop and collect fluid from the lymphatics of the upper limbs, upper trunk, head, and neck (Fig. 8–14). In the sixth week, four additional lymph sacs develop to collect lymph from the trunk and lower extremities: the retroperitoneal lymph sac, the cysterna chyli, and the paired posterior lymph sacs associated with the junctions of the external and internal iliac veins.

The cysterna chyli initially drains into a symmetrical pair of thoracic lymphatic ducts that empty into the venous circulation at the junctions of the internal jugular and subclavian veins. During development, however, portions of both of these ducts are obliterated, and the definitive thoracic duct is derived from the caudal portion of the right duct, the cranial portion of the left duct, and a median anastomosis.

DRAMATIC CHANGES OCCUR IN THE CIRCULATORY SYSTEM AT BIRTH

The transition from fetal dependence on maternal support via the placenta to the relatively independent existence of the infant in the outside world at birth brings about dramatic changes in the pattern of blood circulation within the newborn. In the fetal circulation (Fig. 8–15A), oxygenated blood enters the body through the left umbilical vein. In the ductus venosus, this blood mixes with a small volume of deoxygenated portal blood and then

Figure 8–13. Cast of the embryonic aorta, showing the coronary arteries sprouting from the aortic sinuses. (From Aikawa E, Kawano J. 1982. Formation of coronary arteries sprouting from the primitive aortic sinus wall of the chick embryo. Experientia 38:816.)

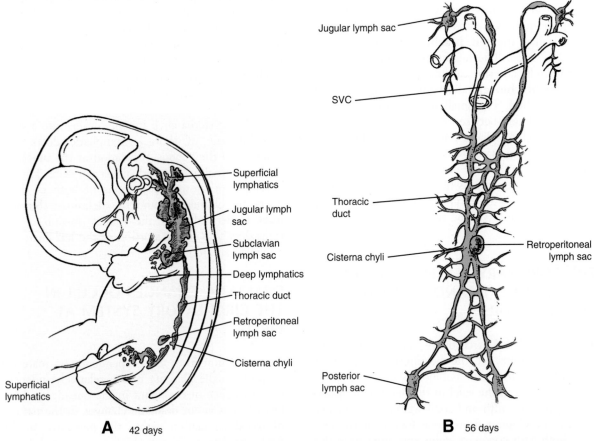

Figure 8–14. Development of the lymphatic system. *A,* Several lymph sacs and ducts develop by vasculogenesis and eventually drain fluid from tissue spaces throughout the entire body. *B–D,* The single thoracic duct that drains the cisterna chyli and the posterior thoracic wall is derived from parts of the right and left thoracic ducts and their anastomoses. SVC = superior vena cava.

Figure 8–14. *Continued*

SVC

Foramen ovale

Ductus arteriosus

Aorta

Placenta

Ductus venosus

Portal sinus

Portal v.

R. umbilical a.

Umbilical v.

Umbilical arteries

Bladder

A

Approximate O₂ saturation

80%

62–67%

57%

52%

25–30%

Figure 8–15. Conversion of the circulation from the fetal to the air-breathing pattern. At birth, the single circuit of the fetal circulation is rapidly converted to two circuits (pulmonary and systemic), arranged in a series. *A,* Pattern of blood flow in the fetus and placenta just before birth. *B,* Pattern of blood flow just after birth. IVC = inferior vena cava; SVC = superior vena cava.

enters the IVC, where it mixes with deoxygenated blood returning from the trunk and legs. In the right atrium, this stream of blood, still highly oxygenated, is largely shunted through the foramen ovale to the left atrium. The oxygenated blood entering the fetal right atrium from the inferior vena cava and the deoxygenated blood entering from the superior vena cava form hemodynamically distinct streams and undergo very little mixing in the atrium. This separation of streams is accomplished partly by the shape and placement of the valve of the IVC.

Figure 8–15. *Continued*

In the left atrium, oxygenated blood from the right atrium mixes with the very small amount of blood returning from the lungs via the pulmonary veins. Little blood flows through the pulmonary circulation during fetal life because the vascular resistance of the collapsed fetal lungs is very high. The oxygenated blood in the left ventricle is then propelled into the aorta for distribution first to the head, neck, and arms and then, via the descending aorta, to the trunk and limbs. As blood enters the descending aorta, it mixes with the deoxygenated blood shunted through the ductus arteriosus. This blood consists mainly of the blood entering the right atrium from the superior vena cava and expelled via the right ventricle and pulmonary trunk. Thus, the blood delivered to the head, neck, and arms by the fetal circulation is more highly oxygenated than the blood delivered to the trunk and lower limbs. After the descending aorta has distributed blood to the trunk and lower limbs, the remaining blood enters the umbilical arteries and returns to the placenta for oxygenation.

The fetal circulatory pattern functions throughout the birth process. As soon as the newborn infant takes its first breath, however, major changes convert the circulation to the adult configuration, in which the pulmonary and systemic circuits are separate and are arranged in series (see Fig. 8–15B). As the alveoli fill with air, the constricted pulmonary vessels open and the resistance of the pulmonary vasculature drops precipitously. The opening of the pulmonary vessels is thought to be a direct response to oxygen, because hypoxia in newborns can cause the pulmonary vessels to constrict. At the same time, spontaneous constriction (or obstetrical clamping) of the umbilical vessels cuts off the flow from the placenta.

The opening of the pulmonary circulation and the cessation of umbilical flow create changes in pressure and flow that cause the ductus arteriosus to constrict and the foramen ovale to close. When the pulmonary circulation opens, the resulting drop in pressure in the pulmonary trunk is thought to cause a slight reverse flow of oxygenated aortic blood through the ductus arteriosus. This increase in local oxygen tension apparently induces the ductus arteriosus to constrict. Constriction of the ductus arteriosus normally occurs within 10 to 15 hours after birth in infants born at term.

The initial closing of the foramen ovale, in contrast, is a strictly mechanical effect of the reversal in pressure between the two atria. The opening of the pulmonary vasculature and the cessation of umbilical flow reduce the pressure in the right atrium, whereas the sudden increase in pulmonary venous return raises the pressure in the left atrium. The resulting pressure change forces the flexible septum primum against the more rigid septum secundum, functionally closing the foramen ovale. The septum primum and septum secundum normally fuse by about 3 months after birth.

In some individuals, the ductus venosus also closes soon after birth. Rapid constriction of the ductus venosus is not essential to the infant, however, because blood is no longer flowing through the umbilical vein.

Prostaglandins appear to play a role in maintaining the patency of the ductus venosus during fetal life, but the signal that brings about the apparently active constriction of this channel after birth is not understood. Nevertheless, the hepatic blood flow from the placenta is supplanted by a normal portal circulation within a few days of birth.

The fact that the patency of the ductus arteriosus is under hormonal control has important clinical consequences. In term infants, as mentioned above, the ductus arteriosus apparently constricts in response to a rise in oxygen tension. During fetal life, however, the ductus is apparently kept patent by circulating prostaglandins. Infants who have cardiovascular malformations in which a patent ductus is essential to life (see the Clinical Applications section of this chapter) may be treated with injections of prostaglandins to keep the ductus open until the malformation can be corrected surgically. Conversely, premature infants in whom the ductus arteriosus does not constrict spontaneously are sometimes treated with prostaglandin inhibitors such as indomethacin.

Clinical Applications

Malformations of the Vasculature

MANY VASCULAR ANOMALIES CAN ARISE FROM ERROR IN THE REMODELING OF THE GREAT VESSELS

As described in this chapter, the bilaterally symmetrical vascular system of the early embryo undergoes an intricate sequence of regressions, remodelings, and anastomoses to produce the adult pattern of great veins and arteries. Regression affects mainly the *left* side of the venous system but the *right* side of the aortic arch system. As a result, systemic venous return is channeled to the right atrium, whereas the original left fourth aortic arch becomes the arch of the definitive aorta. Congenital vascular malformations can arise at many stages of this process. Most vascular malformations result from the failure of some primitive element to undergo regression.

Elements of the Left Supracardinal and Anterior Cardinal Veins May Persist

A relatively rare anomaly called **double inferior vena cava** arises when the caudal portion of the left supracardinal system fails to regress and gives rise to an abnormal left IVC (Fig. 8–16A). The blood entering this vessel ultimately drains either into the right IVC via the left renal vein or into the hemiazygos vein arising from the thoracic part of the supracardinal system.

If the left anterior cardinal vein persists and maintains its connection with the left sinus venosus, the result is a **double superior vena cava** (see Fig. 8–16B). Blood from the left side of the head and neck and from the left upper extremity drains through the abnormal left superior vena cava into the coronary sinus. The coronary sinus may open normally into the right atrium, or it may fail to complete its normal migration to the right and open abnormally into the left atrium. Occasionally, the coronary sinus does not fully shift to the right even though the left anterior cardinal vein undergoes normal regression, with the result that the venous blood from the heart wall drains into the left atrium.

In the condition of generalized left-right reversal of visceral handedness called **situs inversus** (see the Experimental Principles section of Ch. 9 and the Clinical Applications section of Ch. 7), the left anterior cardinal vein persists and the right is obliterated. The left anterior cardinal vein then gives rise to a single superior vena cava that collects blood from the head, neck, and both upper extremities as well as from a left-sided azygos system and drains into the left atrium of a heart that has undergone reversed folding.

Persistence of Portions of the Right Dorsal Aorta May Result in "Vascular Rings" That Constrict the Esophagus and Trachea

The aortic arches and dorsal aorta initially form a vascular basket that completely encircles the pha-ryngeal foregut (see Fig. 8–5A). In normal development, the regression of the right dorsal aorta opens this basket on the right side so that the esophagus is not encircled by aortic arch derivatives. Occasionally, however, the right dorsal aorta persists and maintains its connection with the dorsal aorta, resulting in a **vascular ring** that encloses the trachea and esophagus (Fig. 8–17). This ring may constrict the trachea and esophagus, interfering with both breathing and swallowing.

Another malformation that can cause difficulties in swallowing (**dysphagia**) results from the abnormal disappearance of the right fourth aortic arch. If the right fourth arch regresses, the seventh intersegmental artery (future right subclavian artery), which normally connects to the right fourth aortic arch, forms a connection with the descending aorta instead and therefore crosses over the midline posterior to the esophagus (Fig. 8–18). After the great arteries mature, the esophagus is pinched between the arch of the definitive aorta and the abnormal right subclavian artery. Compression of the esophagus causes dysphagia, and the esophagus may reciprocally compress the right subclavian artery, reducing the blood pressure in the right upper extremity.

Coarctation of the Aorta Results From a Localized Thickening of the Aortic Wall Next to the Ductus Arteriosus

Coarctation of the aorta is a congenital malformation in which an abnormal thickening of the aortic wall severely constricts the aorta in the region of the ductus arteriosus. This malformation occurs in approximately 0.3 percent of all live-born infants. It is more common in males than females and is the most common cardiac anomaly in Turner syndrome (see later in this chapter and the Clinical Applications section of Ch. 10). The pathogenesis of aortic coarctation is not understood, although the malformation may be triggered by genetic factors or by teratogens. It has been suggested that insufficient cardiac blood flow during gestation causes altered hemodynamics that inhibit the normal growth of the left fourth aortic arch or encourage abnormal proliferation of ectopic ductus-like tissue in the aorta.

In infants with aortic coarctation proximal to

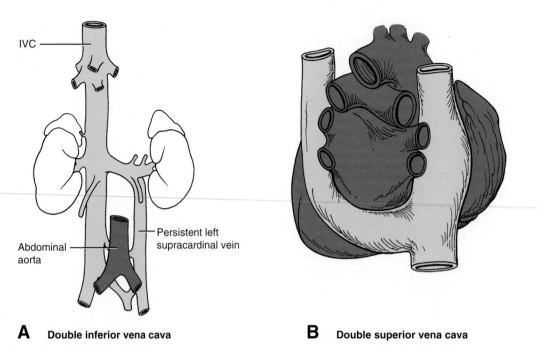

A   Double inferior vena cava   **B**   Double superior vena cava

Figure 8–16. Venous anomalies caused by failure of cardinal veins on the left to undergo normal regression. *A,* Preservation of the left supracardinal vein inferior to the kidney may result in double inferior vena cava. *B,* Preservation of the left anterior cardinal at the level of the heart may result in double superior vena cava. The anomalous left superior vena cava empties into the coronary sinus.

Figure 8–17. A double aortic arch results from failure of the right dorsal aorta to regress in the region of the heart. Both the esophagus and trachea are enclosed in the resulting double arch.

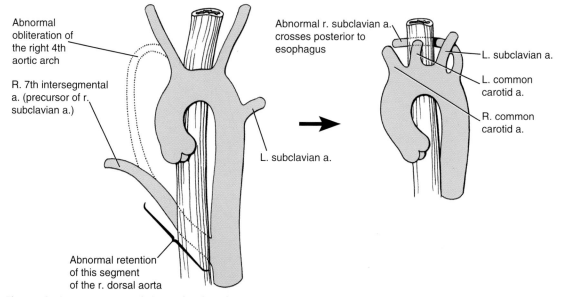

Figure 8–18. Retention of the right dorsal aorta at the level of the seventh intersegmental artery coupled with abnormal regression of the right fourth aortic arch may result in an anomalous right subclavian artery that passes posterior to the esophagus.

a patent ductus arteriosus most or all of the blood expelled from the left ventricle is distributed to the head, neck, and upper extremities, whereas the blood reaching the lower trunk and legs is derived almost entirely from the right ventricle via the pulmonary trunk and a patent ductus arteriosus. Following normal constriction of the ductus in these individuals or when coarctation occurs distal to the ductus, this alternate route to the lower trunk and legs is blocked. This condition may not always be fatal, however, because an adequate collateral circulation to the trunk and lower limbs may develop during childhood from the subclavian, internal thoracic, transverse cervical, suprascapular, superior epigastric, intercostal, and lumbar arteries (Fig. 8–19).

Abnormalities of the Coronary Circulation May Result in Myocardial Ischemia and Heart Failure

As described earlier, the coronary arteries usually originate from the right and left aortic sinuses. In

30 to 50 percent of individuals, however, the conal artery may branch directly from the aorta rather than from the right coronary artery. More rarely, the two major branches of the left coronary artery, the **anterior descending branch** and the **circumflex branch,** also arise directly from the aorta near the left coronary sinus. These variations are considered normal.

Rarely, the coronary arteries show a truly abnormal configuration. Vessels that normally arise from the right or left coronary artery may originate from the opposite coronary artery, from abnormal positions on the aorta, or from the pulmonary trunk. Occasionally, coronary arteries arise from extracardiac vessels such as the internal thoracic, carotid, or subclavian arteries or even directly from a ventricle. Blood may be diverted from the capillary beds of the myocardium either by the presence of an abnormal number of coronary artery branches that return their blood directly to the cardiac lumen or by extensive arteriovenous fistulas. The ostium of a coronary artery may be occluded, or the entire right or left coronary artery may be stenotic or absent.

Coronary artery defects that compromise the delivery of oxygenated blood to the myocardium can cause sudden death in children and young

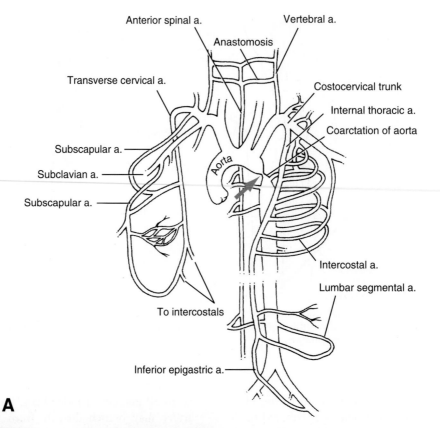

Anterior spinal a.

Vertebral a.

Anastomosis

Transverse cervical a.

Costocervical trunk

Internal thoracic a.

Coarctation of aorta

Subscapular a.

Subclavian a.

Aorta

Subscapular a.

Intercostal a.

Lumbar segmental a.

To intercostals

Inferior epigastric a.

A

B

Figure 8–19. Coarctation of the aorta. The aortic constriction partly or completely blocks the flow of blood into the descending aorta. The trunk and lower extremities receive blood through enlarged collaterals that develop in response to the block. *A,* Diagram showing the constriction in the aorta (red arrow). Collateral circulation developing in postductal coarctation prior to birth may utilize internal thoracic arteries or the thyrocervical trunk to deliver blood to the descending aorta via segmental arteries of the trunk. *B,* Sagittal magnetic resonance imaging scan in lateral view showing the site of coarctation (red arrow) and a major collateral entering the descending aorta (white arrow). (Photograph courtesy of Children's Hospital Medical Center, Cincinnati, OH.)

adults. Moreover, the importance of understanding the normal and abnormal patterns of coronary artery development is made clear by the statistics on coronary angiography: In the United States, this procedure is performed on nearly one million individuals a year, and 300,000 individuals undergo coronary angioplasty or coronary bypass surgery.

Lymphedema May Result From Lymphatic Hypoplasia

A major hereditary congenital disorder of the lymphatic system is **hereditary lymphedema** (swelling of the lymphatic vasculature) caused by hypoplasia of the lymphatic system. This condition may or may not be associated with other abnormalities. The swelling generally occurs in the legs, but, in the case of lymphedema associated with Turner syndrome, blockage of lymphatic ducts in the neck and upper trunk may result in the development of lymph-filled cysts (Fig. 8-20). These cysts may disappear if lymphatic drainage improves during subsequent development.

Excessive Local Angiogenic Vessel Growth May Produce Angiomas

Blood and lymph vessels are stimulated to grow into developing organs by **angiogenic factors.** If vessel growth is not inhibited at the appropriate time or if it is stimulated again later in life, blood or lymph vessels may proliferate until they form a tangled mass that may have clinical consequences. Excessive growth of small capillary networks is called a **capillary hemangioma** or **nevus vascularis,** whereas a proliferation of larger venous sinuses is called a **cavernous hemangioma.**

Many of these abnormalities have a genetic basis, and some are associated with developmental syndromes resulting from chromosomal anomalies. They range in clinical significance from the physically harmless **nevus flammeus,** or **birthmark,** to very dangerous cases in which a vascular tumor growing in the skull or vertebral canal compresses the central nervous system, leading to nervous system dysfunction and potentially to death. Some vascular malformations in humans have recently been shown to have a genetic basis in disruptions in the *Tie-2* pathway, whereas others may be related to disruptions in an as yet unidentified novel gene.

Angiogenesis Inhibitors or Stimulators May Serve as Therapeutic Agents

In addition to the excessive growth of vessels in angiomas, **neovascularization** also occurs in several diseases of the child and adult. For example, the growth and enlargement of solid tumors of many types require the ingrowth of vessels to provide the tumor with oxygen and nutritional support. Neovascularization of the retina, particularly in **diabetes,** is a cause of blindness. Neovascularization also contributes to the pathology of nasopharyngeal angiofibromas, atherosclerotic plaques in coronary arteries, joints affected by rheumatoid arthritis, and pathology of the dermis in psoriasis. Thus, **inhibitors of angiogenesis** have been considered for use as therapeutic agents to inhibit excessive neovascularization. In contrast, it has been suggested that the repair of myocardium after myocardial infarct or of the ulcerated gastrointestinal tract requires the development of new vasculature and so might benefit from treatment with **stimulators of angiogenesis.**

Several techniques have been used to test the **angiogenic** or **antiangiogenic** potential of specific factors. Typically, the capacity of a substance to stimulate or inhibit blood vessel formation can be assayed by applying the test substance to (1) the cornea of a rabbit, mouse, or rat; (2) the chorioallantoic membrane of a chicken embryo (the CAM technique); or (3) a layer of cultured endothelial cells. Activity of the substance is assessed by gauging the degree of growth or regression of blood vessels of the cornea or chorioallantoic membrane. The endothelial culture system is useful for studying the behavior of endothelial cells during vasculogenesis and angiogenesis, including their migration, proliferation, and fusion.

Stimulators of angiogenesis defined by these approaches include growth factors such as angiogenin, basic fibroblast growth factor (bFGF), and transforming growth factor-β (TGF-β). Components of the extracellular matrix such as small hyaluronan polymers consisting of 4 to 16 disaccharide units and heparin (in the absence of corticosteroids) are also angiogenic.

Potent antiangiogenic factors characterized by the cornea system and CAM include low sulfated oligosaccharides derived from heparan sulfate, staurosporine, a large trimeric modular glycoprotein, a 16 kD N-terminal fragment of the hormone prolactin, the triterpene acids ursolic acid and oleanolic acid, as well as the potent antitumor agents titanocene dichloride and AGM-1470, an agent derived from the fungal product fumagillin. AGM-1470 has also been shown to effectively re-

Figure 8–20. Lymphedema in a fetus with Turner syndrome. Blockage of lymphatic channels in many parts of the body has resulted in the formation of distended lymphatic cysts, which are visible as swellings, especially in the limbs and cervical region. The huge, pillow-like swellings at the fetus's nape are formed by the grossly enlarged jugular lymph sacs. Distended jugular lymph sacs are readily identified by ultrasonography (see Fig. 15–5). (Photo courtesy of Children's Hospital Medical Center, Cincinnati, OH.)

circulating angiogenesis inhibitor **angiostatin.** Thrombospondin and glioma-derived angiogenesis inhibitory factor are antiangiogenic factors also produced in association with growth of neovascularized tumors. A potent endothelial cell **mitogen** and **angiogenic factor** produced by tumors is the **vascular endothelial growth factor** (VEGF; see the Experimental Principles section in this chapter). Thus, the neovascularization of tumors may be regulated by the balanced production of angiogenic and antiangiogenic factors.

Genetic and pharmacologic **perturbation studies** provide insight into a possible mechanism by which tumors may regulate expression of VEGF. Typically, expression of **mutant ras oncogenes** is correlated with development of many solid tumors that in turn is associated with increased expression of VEGF. A causal relationship between these two factors is implied by the finding that VEGF production by human colon carcinoma cells is significantly reduced by genetic disruption of the K-*ras* oncogene. Likewise, VEGF synthesis is also suppressed in a transformed intestinal epithelial line by the pharmacologic inhibition of the mutant RAS protein. These studies thus provide possible models for therapies and treatments of solid rumors in humans.

Interferon-α—an Antiangiogenic Factor—May Be Effective in Regression of Corticosteroid-Resistant Hemangiomas in Humans

A clinical application of these current studies is development of a therapy for treatment of **life-threatening** or **vision-threatening hemagiomas.** Approximately one third of these endothelial tumors regress in response to corticosteroid therapy, but the remainder are insensitive, resulting in a 60% mortality. In a recent clinical trial, however, **interferon-α_{2a}** was injected subcutaneously into afflicted neonates or infants, resulting in a 50 percent (or greater) regression of the tumors within 7.8 months (in 18 of 20 patients) and within 3 years after treatment resulted in significant decrease in expected mortality.

duce tumor volume and prolong survival in experimental animals with hemangioendothelioma. The spasmolytic **thalidomide** has also been demonstrated to exhibit antiangiogenic activity, possibly providing some insight into the mechanism by which it inhibits development of human limbs between the fourth and eighth weeks (see the Clinical Applications section of Ch. 11).

It has also been found that tumors themselves may be a useful source of specific angiogenic and antiangiogenic factors. For example, growth of the Lewis lung tumor results in production of the

Experimental Principles

Molecular Studies of Vasculogenesis and Angiogenesis

The use of molecular techniques has vastly increased our understanding of factors that regulate endothelial cell migration, proliferation, and differentiation. For example, the techniques of **in situ hybridization** and **Northern analysis** of mRNA expression have identified factors expressed by presumptive endothelial cells or associated tissues that can then be tested for their angiogenic or antiangiogenic properties. Suspected factors may be tested directly in the corneal, CAM, or endothelial culture systems described in the Clinical Applications section earlier or in a dispersed quail epiblast culture system that generates blood vessels under appropriate conditions. **Transgenic mice** may also be generated that overexpress the factor of interest **(gain-of-function mutant)** or that do not express the factor at all **(knockout** or **null mutation).** Effects of these genetic manipulations upon the vasculature of the experimental animal may then be assessed with appropriate **vascular imaging techniques.** In addition to the techniques described earlier in the Descriptive Embryology section of this chapter, a new technique involving injection of a contrast agent followed by **magnetic resonance imaging** has been shown to be useful in the study of embryonic murine vasculature. Another new approach is to introduce transgenes into mice consisting of an endothelium-specific promoter gene and a reporter gene such as *lacZ* (recall the use of this gene to trace neural crest cells in Ch. 5). In this case, the blue stain specifically colors the developing vasculature.

CELL ADHESION MOLECULES AND GROWTH FACTORS ARE IMPLICATED IN REGULATION OF BLOOD VESSEL FORMATION

In mouse embryos, the **extracellular matrix molecule vascular endothelial cadherin** is expressed predominantly by presumptive endothelial cells in the yolk sac and then in the regions of cell-cell junctions in the endothelium, implicating this molecule in endothelial cell adhesion. Moreover, when the vascular endothelial cadherin gene is transfected into mouse L cells, its expression is correlated with a stimulation of adhesion. **Fibronectin** has also been implicated in vasculogenesis, because knockout of the gene encoding this extracellular matrix molecule results in disruption of migration of mesodermal precursors of the vasculature.

Acidic and **basic fibroblast growth factors** and **TGF-β** and their receptors have been demonstrated to play critical roles in angiogenesis, possibly, in part, by stimulating the upregulation of **endothelial integrin receptors,** which enhance the ability of endothelial cells to migrate within the extracellular matrix. As noted earlier, tumors produce the powerful endothelial mitogen **VEGF.** Indeed, it seems clear that VEGF and its receptors also play a role in normal vasculogenesis in mouse embryos, because in situ hybridization experiments demonstrate *VegF* transcripts within the endoderm and transcripts of **Flt-1,** a VEGF **receptor tyrosine kinase** within the adjacent vessel-producing mesoderm, just before and during blood vessel formation. Moreover, if VEGF is injected into embryos at the outset of vasculogenesis, neovascularization occurs in typically avascular areas, and vessels fuse excessively, giving rise to abnormal patterns of blood vessel formation. **Hypervascularization** is also observed in transgenic gain-of-function quail embryos in which *VegF* is overexpressed. In contrast, null mutations of another VEGF receptor tyrosine kinase, *Flk-1,* fail to form organized blood vessels within the yolk sac or embryo. Similarly, homozygotes with a targeted mutation of the *Flt-1* locus form abnormally organized vascular channels in extraembryonic and embryonic tissues. Finally, it has been shown that the loss of a single *VegF* allele in a transgenic mouse results in disruption of the vasculature and lethality. It therefore seems likely that VEGF and its receptors, among many other factors, are critical elements of an endothelial cell-signaling pathway that regulates the proliferation and organization of endothelial precursors into functional vessels. Current studies are exploring relevant upstream and downstream factors comprising this presumptive epigenetic cascade. The angiopoietins (ang) are recently described cytokines that signal through the TIE1 and TIE2 receptor tyrosine kinase molecules on the surface of endothelial cells. Targeted inactivation and transgenesis experiments in mice have demonstrated that the ang/TIE pathways are important for vascular remodeling during development and for maintaining the integrity of the vasculature.

Studies of the Embryonic Origin of Blood

Human Hematopoietic Stem Cells May First Form in the Yolk Sac and Then Migrate to the Embryo. The origin of the **hematopoietic stem cells (HSCs)** that populate the hematopoietic organs of the embryo, fetus, child, and adult has long been a subject of interest and controversy. The first recognizable blood cells appear within the wall of the **yolk sac** at about day 17 in human embryos. However, the numbers of erythroid burst-forming units (BFU-E) and granulomacrophage progenitors (CFU-GM) within the yolk sac decline between the fourth and fifth weeks as they reciprocally increase within the **liver.** This suggests that HSCs of the yolk sac migrate to the liver, where they establish nests of proliferating cells that may eventually seed other hematopoietic organs of the embryo, including the spleen, lymph nodes, thymus, and bone marrow. This view is further supported by the concomitant "switching" from embryonic to fetal hemoglobin isoforms, which occurs with the establishment of hepatic HSC proliferation.

The idea that hepatic HSCs originate from the yolk sac is also supported by in vitro studies that show that the explanted yolk sac is able to seed liver primordia lacking HSCs (before the 28-somite stage in mice) placed on the other side of a filter with pores large enough to allow cell migration. In addition, although the liver primordia lacking HSCs could not be seeded by a yolk sac placed on the other side of a filter with pores too small to allow cell migration, these embryonic livers were able to induce the switch from embryonic to fetal hemoglobin within the blood cells of the yolk sac. This latter result suggests that some factor made in the liver was able to induce HSCs within the yolk sac to mature even though they

had failed to migrate into the liver. One such factor appears to be absolutely required for normal HSC migration and differentiation. Specifically, a series of weak to strong alleles of the *Sl* (Steel) and *W* (White spotting) genes in mice result in disruptions of germ cell development and neural crest cell migration (see the Experimental Principles section of Ch. 5). In addition, however, homozygous and heterozygous *Sl* mutants and homozygous *W* mutants exhibit pronounced anemia. As discussed in Chapter 5, the *Sl* locus encodes a trophic factor called *c-kit* **ligand,** whereas the **W** locus encodes its receptor, *c-kit* **receptor.** It is thought that *c-kit* ligand is expressed by cells along the migratory pathway or the homing site for migrating HSCs, whereas the *c-kit* receptor must be expressed by the HSCs themselves to ensure their survival and proliferation within the embryonic liver and other sites within the embryo.

The ultimate embryonic origin of blood cell progenitors, of course, is the epiblast or primitive ectoderm. In a series of skillful studies, single cells of the 6.0- and 6.5-day-old mouse primitive ectoderm were injected with the cell lineage tracers horseradish peroxidase or rhodamine-labeled dextran beads. After the injection, the embryos were cultured and allowed to develop. Tracer-positive descendants were then identified. The blood cells of the blood islands of the yolk sac were found to originate from cells at the caudal end of the primitive streak. Other descendants of these injected cells also developed into extraembryonic mesoderm and primordial germ cells. Therefore, all of these studies taken together support the possibility that presumptive blood cells formed within the primitive ectoderm migrate out into the wall of the yolk sac, where they begin to differentiate into hematopoietic stem cells and blood cells of the blood islands. Some of these cells then migrate or circulate to the embryonic liver, where they continue to proliferate, forming blood cells of the embryo that ultimately give rise to the HSCs that migrate to the spleen, lymph nodes, and bone marrow.

However, an alternate hypothesis for the origin of the definitive HSCs of the adult hematopoietic organs has also been proposed. It has been suggested that definitive blood cells of the adult arise from the intraembryonic splanchnopleuric mesoderm in the region of the aorta, gonad, mesonephros (the **AGM**), a site also called the **paraor-**

tic splanchnopleura (P-Sp) which is also characterized by an abundance of primordial germ cells. Moreover, this hematopoietic center has been described in amphibians, birds, mice, and humans. Although it seems likely that this region contains cells with hematopoietic capacity, the developmental relationship of HSCs in the P-Sp with other populations of blood cells in yolk sac, liver, and primary ectoderm remains to be determined. For example, it would be interesting to understand the developmental relationship between these hematopoietic stem cells and the stem cells that also give rise to primordial germ cells, because primordial germ cells may give rise to primitive hematopoietic stem cells under the appropriate culture conditions. Moreover, if adult HSCs are derived from the P-Sp, do they migrate as a separate population of extraembryonic mesoderm, via the yolk sac and/or liver to the region of the aorta, or do they arise from a small subpopulation of HSCs of the yolk sac? Alternatively, do subpopulations of cells within the P-Sp populate the liver? Do HSCs of the P-Sp express the *c-kit receptor*, and do cells along their pathway of migration and their target site in the vicinity of the aorta express *c-kit ligand?* Alternatively, this specialized population of HSCs may arise directly from the intraembryonic mesoderm by gastrulation. Studies would seem to support the possibility that definitive erythrocytes arise from a stem cell population different from the embryonic erythrocytes present before the switch from yolk sac to liver hematopoiesis. Surely, future studies will provide answers to many of these intriguing questions.

SUGGESTED READING

Descriptive Embryology

Aikawa E, Kawano J. 1982. Formation of coronary arteries sprouting from the primitive aortic sinus wall of the chick embryo. Experientia 38:816

Anderson RH, Ashley GT. 1974. Growth and development of the cardiovascular system—anatomical development. p. 165. In Davis JA, Dobbing J (eds): Scientific Foundations of Pediatrics. WB Saunders, Philadelphia

Coceani F, Olley PM. 1988. The control of cardiovascular shunts in the fetal and neonatal period. Am J Physiol Pharmacol 66:1129

Coffin D, Poole TJ. 1988. Embryonic vascular development: immunohistochemical identification of the origin and subsequent morphogenesis of the major vessel primordia of quail embryos. Development 102:735

Congdon ED. 1922. Transformation of the aortic arch system during the development of the human embryo. Carnegie Contrib Embryol 14:46

Dollinger RK, Armstrong PB. 1974. Scanning electron microscopy of injected replicas of the chick embryo circulatory system. J Microsc 102:179

Effmann E. 1982. Development of the right and left pulmonary arteries: a microangiographic study in the mouse. Invest Radiol 17:529

Evans HM. 1909. On the development of the aortae, cardinal and umbilical veins, and the other blood vessels of vertebrate embryos from capillaries. Anat Rec 3:498

Hirakow R. 1983. Development of the cardiac blood vessels in staged human embryos. Acta Anat 115:220

Hirakow R, Hiruma T. 1981. Scanning electron microscopic study on the development of primitive blood vessels in chick embryos at the early somite-stage. Anat Embryol 163:299

Hutchins GM, Kessler-Hanna A, Moore GW. 1988. Development of the coronary arteries in the embryonic human heart. Circulation 77:1250

Netter FH. 1969. Embryology. p. 112. In Yonkman FF (ed): The CIBA Collection of Medical Illustrations. CIBA, Summit, NJ

Noden DM. 1989. Embryonic origins and assembly of blood vessels. Annu Rev Respir Dis 140:1097

Noden DM. 1990. Origins and assembly of avian embryonic blood vessels. Ann N Y Acad Sci 588:236

Pardanaud L, Altmann C, Kitos P, et al. 1987. Vasculogenesis in the early quail blastodisc as studied with a monoclonal antibody recognizing endothelial cells. Development 100:339

Patan S. 1998. TIE1 and TIE2 receptor tyrosine kinases inversely regulate embryonic angiogenesis by the mechanism of intussusceptive microvascular growth. Microvasc Res 56:1

Poole TJ, Coffin JD. 1989. Vasculogenesis and angiogenesis: two distinct mechanisms establish embryonic vascular pattern. J Exp Zool 251:224

Risau W. 1997. Mechanisms of angiogenesis. Nature 386:671

Sato TN, Tozawa Y, Deutsch U, et al. 1995. Distinct roles of the receptor tyrosine kinases Tie-1 and Tie-2 in blood vessel formation. Nature 376:70

Sissman NJ. 1970. Developmental landmarks in cardiac morphogenesis: comparative chronology. Am J Cardiol 25:141

Wilson JG, Warkany J. 1949. Aortic arch and cardiac

anomalies in the offspring of vitamin A deficient rats. Am J Anat 85:113

Clinical Applications

Adkins RB, Maples MD, Graham BS, et al. 1986. Dysphagia associated with aortic arch anomaly in adults. Am Surg 52:238

Anderson RH, Ashley GT. 1974. Growth and development of the cardiovascular system. p. 165. In Davis JA, Dobbing J (eds): Scientific Foundations of Paediatrics. WB Saunders, Philadelphia

Angelini P. 1989. Normal and anomalous coronary arteries: definitions and classifications. Am Heart J 117:418

Boon LM, Brouillard P, Irrthum A, et al. 1999. A gene for inherited cutaneous venous anomalies ("glomangiomas") localizes to chromosome 1p21–22. Am J Hum Genet 65:125

Chen C, Parangi S, Tolentino MJ, Folkman J. 1995. A strategy to discover circulating angiogenesis inhibitors generated by human tumors. Cancer Res 55:4230

Clark EB. 1987. Mechanisms in the pathogenesis of congenital cardiac malformations. p. 3. In Pierpont MEM, Moller JH (eds): The Genetics of Cardiovascular Disease. Martinus Nijhoff Publishing, Boston

Conte G, Pellegrini A. 1984. On the development of the coronary arteries in human embryos stages 14–19. Anat Embryol 169:209

Freedom RM, Cullam JAG, Moss CAF. 1984. Angiocardiography of Congenital Heart Disease. Macmillan, New York

D'Amato RJ, Loughnan MS, Flynn E, Folkman J. 1994. Thalidomide is an inhibitor of angiogenesis. Proc Natl Acad Sci U S A 91:4082

Ezekowitz RA, Mulliken JB, Folkman J. 1992. Interferon α-2a therapy for life-threatening hemangiomas of infancy. N Engl J Med 326:1456

Fan TP, Jaggar R, Bicknell R. 1995. Controlling the vasculature: angiogenesis, antiangiogenesis and vascular targeting of gene therapy. Trends Pharmacol Sci 16:57

Folkman J. 1995. Angiogenesis in cancer, vascular, rheumatoid and other disease. Nature Med 1:27

Folkman J. 1995. The influence of angiogenesis research on management of patients with breast cancer. Breast Cancer Res Treat 36:109

Hartman AF, Goldring D, Strauss AW, et al. 1977. Coarctation of the aorta. p. 199. In Moss AJ, Adams FH, Emmanouilides GC (eds): Heart Diseases in Infants, Children, and Adolescents. Williams & Wilkins, Baltimore

Haywood GA, Ward DE. 1989. Anomalous origins of left anterior descending and circumflex coronary arteries from separate orifices in the right coronary sinus. Int J Cardiol 24:373

Kolch W, Martiny-Baron G, Kieser A, Marme D. 1995. Regulation of the expression of the VEGF/VPS and its receptors: role in tumor angiogenesis. Breast Cancer Res Treat 36:139

Maisonpierre PC, Suri C, Jones PF, et al. 1997. Angiopoietin-2, a natural antagonist for Tie2 that disrupts in vivo angiogenesis. Science 277:55

Moller JH. 1987. Vascular abnormalities. p. 339. In Pierpont MEM, Moller JH (eds): The Genetics of Cardiovascular Disease. Martinus Nijhoff Publishing, Boston

Oppenheimer-Dekker A, Moene RJ, Moulart AJ, Gittenbergerde Groot AC. 1981. Teratogenic considerations regarding aortic arch anomalies associated with cardiovascular malformations. Perspect Cardiovasc Res 5:485

O'Reilly MS, Brem H, Folkman J. 1995. Treatment of murine hemangioendotheliomas with the angiogenesis inhibitor AGM-1470. J Pediatr Surg 30:325

O'Reilly MS, Holmgren L, Shing Y, et al. 1994. Angiostatin: a novel angiogenesis inhibitor that mediates the suppression of metastases by a Lewis lung carcinoma. Cell 79:315

Pierpont MEM, Moller JH. 1987. Congenital cardiac malformations. p. 13. In Pierpont MEM, Moller JH (eds): The Genetics of the Cardiovascular System. Martinus Nijhoff Publishing, Boston

Plate KH, Risau W. 1995. Angiogenesis in malignant gliomas. Glia 15:339

Soto B, Pacifico AD. 1990. Angiocardiography in Congenital Heart Malformations. Futura Publishing Company, Inc, Mount Kisco, NY

Vikkula M, Boon LM, Carraway KL 3rd, et al. 1996. Vascular dysmorphogenesis caused by an activating mutation in the receptor tyrosine kinase TIE2. Cell 87:1181

Experimental Principles

Bennet D. 1956. Developmental analysis of a mutation with pleiotropic effects in the mouse. J Morphol 98:199

Breier G, Breviario F, Caveda L, et al. 1996. Molecular cloning and expression of murine vascular endothelial-cadherin in early stage development of the cardiovascular system. Blood 87:630

Carmeliet P, Ferreira V, Breier G, et al. 1996. Abnormal blood vessel development and lethality in embryos lacking a single VEGF allele. Nature 380:435

Cudennec CA, Thiery J-P, Le Dourarin NM. 1981. In vitro induction of adult erythropoiesis in early mouse yolk sac. Proc Natl Acad Sci U S A 78:2410

D'Amore PA, Thompson RW. 1987. Mechanisms of angiogenesis. Annu Rev Physiol 49:453

Drake CJ, Little CD. 1995. Exogenous vascular endothelial growth factor induces malformed and hyperfused vessels during embryonic neovascularization. Proc Natl Acad Sci U S A 92:7657

Dumont DJ, Fong GH, Puri MC, et al. 1995. Vascularization of the mouse embryo: a study of flk-1, tek, tie, and vascular endothelial growth factor expression during development. Dev Dynam 203:80

Dumont DJ, Gradwohl G, Fong GH, et al. 1994. Dominant-negative and targeted null mutations in the endothelial receptor tyrosine kinase, tek, reveal a critical role in vasculogenesis of the embryo. Genes Dev 8:1897

Dumont DJ, Yamaguchi TP, Conlon RA, et al. 1992. tek, a novel tyrosine kinase gene located on mouse chromosome 4, is expressed in endothelial cells and their presumptive precursors. Oncogene 7:1471

Dzierzak E, Medvinsky A. 1995. Mouse embryonic hematopoiesis. Trends Genet 11:359

Enebstein J, Waleh NS, Kramer RH. 1992. Basic FGF and TGF-β differentially modulate integrin expression of human microvascular endothelial cells. Exp Cell Res 203:499

Fennie C, Cheng J, Dowbenko D, et al. 1995. CD34+ endothelial cell lines derived from murine yolk sac induce the proliferation and differentiation of yolk sac CD34+ hematopoietic progenitors. Blood 86:4454

Ferrar N, Carver-Moore K, Chen H, et al. 1996. Heterozygous embryonic lethality induced by targeted inactivation of the VEGF gene. Nature 380:439

Flamme I, Breier G, Risau W. 1995. Vascular endothelial growth factor (VEGF) and VEGF receptor 2 (flk-1) are expressed during vasculogenesis and vascular differentiation of the quail embryo. Dev Biol 169:699

Flamme I, von Reutern M, Drexler HC, et al. 1995. Overexpression of vascular endothelial growth factor in the avian embryo induced hypervascularization and increased vascular permeability without alterations of embryonic pattern formation. Dev Biol 171:399

Flamme I, Risau W. 1992. Induction of vasculogenesis and hematopoiesis in vitro. Development 116:435

Folkman J. 1986. How is blood vessel growth regulated in normal and neoplastic tissue? GHA Clowes Memorial Award Lecture. Can Res 46:467

Folkman J, Klagsbrun M. 1987. Angiogenic factors. Science 235:442

Fong GH, Rossant J, Gertsenstein M, Breitman ML. 1995. Role of the Flt-1 receptor tyrosine kinase in regulating the assembly of vascular endothelium. Nature 376:66

Friesel RE, Maciag T. 1995. Molecular mechanisms of angiogenesis: fibroblast growth factor signal transduction. FASEB J 9:919

George EL, Georges-Labouesse EN, Patel-King RS, et al. 1993. Defects in mesoderm, neural tube and vascular development in mouse embryos lacking fibronectin. Development 119:1079

Huang E, Nocka K, Beier DR, et al. 1990. The hematopoietic growth factor KL is encoded by the Sl locus and is the ligand of the c-kit receptor, the gene product of the W locus. Cell 63:225

Huang H, Zettergren LD, Auerbach R. 1994. In vitro differentiation of B cells and myeloid cells from the early mouse embryo and its extraembryonic yolk sac. Exp Hematol 22:19

Huang L, Turck CW, Rao P, Peters KG, 1995. GRB2 and SH-PTP2: potentially important endothelial signalling molecules downstream of the TEK/TIE2 receptor tyrosine kinase. Oncogene 11:2097

Huyhn A, Dommergues M, Izac B, et al. 1995. Characterization of hematopoietic progenitors from human yolk sacs and embryos. Blood 86:4474

Jakeman LB, Armanini M, Phillips HS, Ferrara N. 1993. Developmental expression of binding sites and messenger ribonucleic acid for vascular growth factor suggests role for this protein in vasculogenesis and angiogenesis. Endocrinology 133:848

Kallianpur AR, Jordan JE, Brandt SJ. 1994. The SCL/TAL-1 gene is expressed in progenitors of both hematopoietic and vascular systems during embryogenesis. Blood 83:1200

Knochel W, Grunz H, Loppnow-Blinde B, et al. 1989. Mesoderm induction and blood island formation by angiogenic growth factors and embryonic inducing factors. Blut 59:207

Korhonen J, Polvi A, Partanen J, Alitalo K. 1994. The mouse tie receptor tyrosine kinase gene: expression during embryonic angiogenesis. Oncogene 9:395

Lawson KA, Pedersen R. 1992. Clonal analysis of cell fate during gastrulation and early neurulation in the mouse. CIBA Symp. 165. Postimplantation Development in the Mouse. John Wiley & Sons, New York

Lawson KA, Hage WJ. 1994 Clonal analysis of the origin of primordial germ cells in the mouse. CIBA Symp. 182. Germline Development. John Wiley & Sons, New York

Matsui Y, Zsebo KM, Hogan BLM. 1990. Embryonic expression of a hematopoietic growth factor encoded by the Sl locus and the ligand for c-kit. Nature 347:667

Millauer B, Wizigmann-Voos S, Schnurch H. 1993. High affinity VEGF binding and developmental expression suggest Flk-1 as a major regulator of vasculogenesis and angiogenesis. Cell 72:835

Muller AM, Medvinsky A, Strouboulis J, et al. 1994. Development of hematopoietic stem cell activity in the mouse embryo. Immunity 1:291

Nakano T, Kodama H, Honjio T. 1996. In vitro development of primitive and definitive erythrocytes from different precursors. Science 272:722

Peschle C, Mavilio F, Care A, et al. 1985. Haemoglobin switching in human embryos. Nature 313:235

Rak J, Mitsuhashi Y, Bayko L, et al. 1995. Mutant ras oncogenes upregulate VEGF/VPF expression: implications for induction and inhibition of tumor angiogenesis. Cancer Res 55:4575

Rich IN. 1995. Primordial germ cells are capable of producing cells of the hematopoietic system in vitro. Blood 86:463

Sato TN, Qin Y, Kozak CA, Audus KL. 1993. Tie-1 and tie-2 define another class of putative receptor tyrosine kinase genes expressed in early embryonic vascular system. Proc Natl Acad Sci U S A 90:9355

Shalaby F, Rossant J, Yamaguchi TP, et al. 1995. Failure

of blood-island formation and vasculogenesis in Klk-1-deficient mice. Nature 376:62

Smith BR, Johnson GA, Groman EV, Linney E. 1994. Magnetic resonance microscopy of mouse embryos. Proc Natl Acad Sci U S A 91:3530

Suri C, Jones PF, Patan S, et al: Requisite role of angiopoietin-1, a ligand for the TIE2 receptor, during embryonic angiogenesis.

Tavian M, Coulombel L, Luton D, et al. 1996. Aorta-associated CD34+ hematopoietic cells in the early human embryo. Blood 87:67

Wagner EF, Risau W. 1994. Oncogenes in the study of endothelial cell growth and differentiation. Semin Can Biol 5:137

West DC, Kumar S. 1989. Hyaluronan and angiogenesis. CIBA Found Symp 143:187

Yamaguchi TP, Dumont DJ, Conlon RA, et al. 1993. flk-1, an flt-related receptor tyrosine kinase is an early marker for endothelial cell precursors. Development 118:489

Zetter BR. 1988. Angiogenesis state of the art. Chest 93:159s

Development of the Gastrointestinal Tract

Summary

The endodermal gut tube created by embryonic folding during the fourth week (see Ch. 6) consists of a blind-ended cranial foregut, a blind-ended caudal hindgut, and a midgut open to the yolk sac through the vitelline duct. As discussed in Chapter 8, the arterial supply to the gut develops through consolidation and reduction of the ventral branches of the dorsal aortae that anastomose with the vessel plexuses that originally supply blood to the yolk sac. About five of these vitelline artery derivatives vascularize the thoracic foregut, and three—the **celiac, superior mesenteric,** and **inferior mesenteric arteries**—vascularize the abdominal gut. By convention, the boundaries of the foregut, midgut, and hindgut portions of the abdominal gut tube are determined by the respective territories of these three arteries.

By the fifth week, the abdominal portion of the foregut is visibly divided into the esophagus, stomach, and proximal duodenum. The stomach is initially fusiform, and differential growth of its dorsal and ventral walls produces the **greater** and **lesser curvatures.** Meanwhile, **hepatic, cystic,** and **dorsal** and **ventral pancreatic diverticula** bud from the proximal duodenum into the mesogastrium and give rise respectively to the liver, the gallbladder and cystic duct, and the pancreas. In addition, the **spleen** condenses from mesenchyme in the dorsal mesogastrium.

During the sixth and seventh weeks, the stomach rotates around longitudinal and dorsoventral axes so that the greater curvature is finally directed to the left and slightly caudally. This rotation shifts the liver to the right in the abdominal cavity and also brings the duodenum and pancreas into contact with the posterior body wall, where they become fixed (i.e., secondarily retroperitoneal). This event converts the space dorsal to the rotated stomach and dorsal mesogastrium into a recess called the **lesser sac of the peritoneum.** The pouch of dorsal mesogastrium forming the left lateral boundary of the lesser sac subsequently undergoes voluminous expansion, giving rise to the curtain-like greater omentum that drapes over the inferior abdominal viscera.

The midgut differentiates into the distal duodenum, jejunum, ileum, cecum, ascending colon, and proximal two thirds of the transverse colon. The future ileum elongates more rapidly than the peritoneal cavity, so that by the fifth week the midgut is thrown into an anteroposterior hairpin fold, the **primary intestinal loop,** which herniates into the umbilicus during the sixth week. As the primary intestinal loop herniates, it rotates around its long axis by 90 degrees counterclockwise (as viewed from the anterior side) so that the future ileum lies to the left and the

Development of the Stomach, Liver, Digestive Glands, and Spleen

Organization of the Mesenteries

Folding and Rotation of the Midgut

Septation of the Cloaca and Formation of the Anus

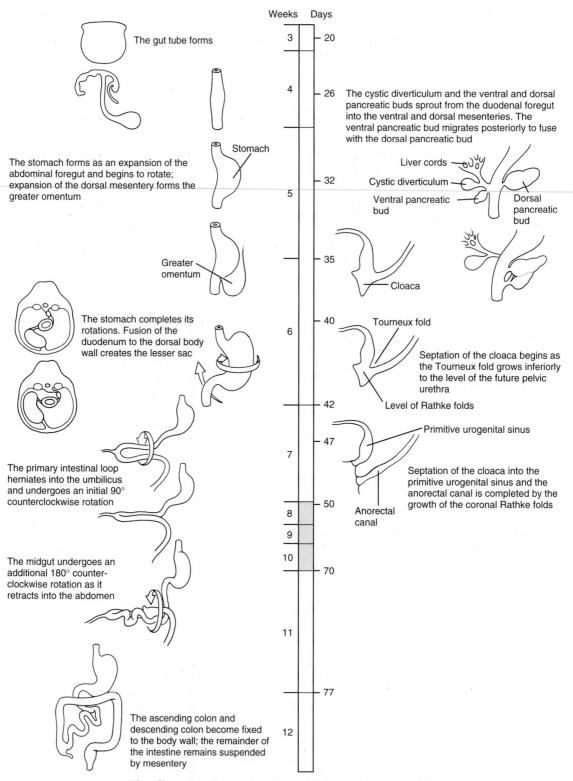

Weeks Days

3 — 20

The gut tube forms

4 — 26   The cystic diverticulum and the ventral and dorsal pancreatic buds sprout from the duodenal foregut into the ventral and dorsal mesenteries. The ventral pancreatic bud migrates posteriorly to fuse with the dorsal pancreatic bud

Stomach

The stomach forms as an expansion of the abdominal foregut and begins to rotate; expansion of the dorsal mesentery forms the greater omentum

5 — 32   Liver cords
Cystic diverticulum
Ventral pancreatic bud
Dorsal pancreatic bud

Greater omentum

— 35   Cloaca

The stomach completes its rotations. Fusion of the duodenum to the dorsal body wall creates the lesser sac

6 — 40   Tourneux fold
Septation of the cloaca begins as the Tourneux fold grows inferiorly to the level of the future pelvic urethra
— 42   Level of Rathke folds

— 47   Primitive urogenital sinus
7
Septation of the cloaca into the primitive urogenital sinus and the anorectal canal is completed by the growth of the coronal Rathke folds

The primary intestinal loop herniates into the umbilicus and undergoes an initial 90° counterclockwise rotation

8 — 50   Anorectal canal
9
The midgut undergoes an additional 180° counter-clockwise rotation as it retracts into the abdomen
10 — 70

11

— 77

The ascending colon and descending colon become fixed to the body wall; the remainder of the intestine remains suspended by mesentery
12

Timeline. Development of the gut tube and its derivatives.

future large intestine to the right. Meanwhile, the cecum and appendix differentiate, and the jejunum and ileum continue to elongate. During the 10th through 12th weeks, the intestinal loop is retracted into the abdominal cavity and rotates through an additional 180 degrees counterclockwise to produce the definitive configuration of the small and large intestines.

The hindgut gives rise to the distal one third of the transverse colon, the descending and sigmoid colon, and the rectum. Just superior to the cloacal membrane, the primitive gut tube forms an expansion called the **cloaca.** During the fourth to sixth weeks, a coronal **urorectal septum** partitions the cloaca into an anterior **primitive urogenital sinus,** which will give rise to urogenital structures, and a posterior rectum. The distal one third of the anorectal canal forms from an ectodermal invagination called the **anal pit.**

Between the sixth and eighth weeks, the lumen of the gut tube becomes solidly filled by proliferating epithelium and then is gradually recanalized.

EMBRYONIC FOLDING CONVERTS THE TRILAMINAR GERM DISC INTO A NESTED SET OF THREE-DIMENSIONAL TUBES

As described in Chapter 6, the cephalocaudal and lateral folding of the embryo in the third and fourth weeks converts the flat trilaminar germ disc into an elongated cylinder (Fig. 9–1). This cylinder consists of three concentric nested tubes. The outer tube is the ectoderm, which now covers the entire outer surface of the embryo, except in the umbilical region, where the yolk sac and connecting stalk emerge. The central tube is the endodermal **primary gut tube.** Separating these two layers is a tube of mesoderm, which contains the coelom. Thus, the three germ layers bear the same funda-

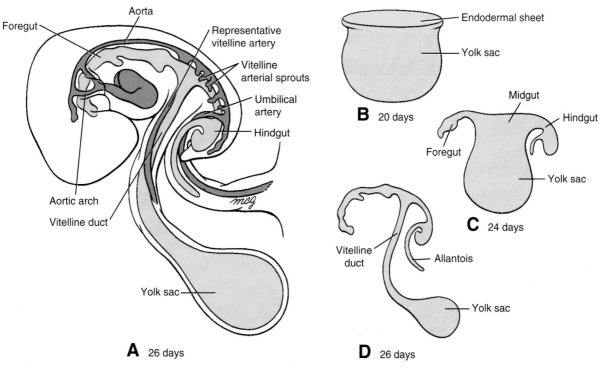

Figure 9–1. *A,* The foregut, midgut, and hindgut of the primitive gut tube are formed by the combined action of differential growth and lateral and cephalocaudal folding. The foregut and hindgut are blindending tubes that terminate at the buccopharyngeal and cloacal membranes, respectively. The midgut is at first completely open to the cavity of the yolk sac *B, C,* As folding proceeds, however, this connection is constricted to form the narrow vitelline duct (*D*).

mental topologic relation to each other after folding as they did in the flat germ disc.

The Foregut, Midgut, and Hindgut Are Distinguished on the Basis of Arterial Supply

When folding first forms the three-dimensional embryo, the gut tube consists of cranial and caudal blind-ending tubes, the presumptive **foregut** and **hindgut,** and a central **midgut,** which still opens ventrally to the yolk sac. Cranially, the foregut terminates in the **buccopharyngeal membrane;** caudally, the hindgut terminates in the **cloacal membrane.** Because the embryo and gut tube lengthen relative to the yolk sac and because folding continues to convert the open midgut into a tube, the neck of the yolk sac narrows until it becomes the slender vitelline duct. As described in Chapter 6, the vitelline duct and yolk sac ulti-

mately are incorporated in the umbilical cord. Table 9–1 shows the organs and structures that are ultimately derived from the three portions of the gut tube.

By convention, the boundaries of the foregut, midgut, and hindgut correspond to the territories of the three arteries that supply the abdominal gut tube. As described in Chapter 8, the gut tube and its derivatives are vascularized by unpaired ventral branches of the descending aorta. These branches develop by a process of consolidation and reduction from the left and right vitelline artery plexuses that arise on the yolk sac, spread to vascularize the gut tube, and anastomose with the dorsal aortae (see Fig. 8–5). About five definitive aortic branches supply the thoracic part of the foregut (the pharynx and thoracic esophagus). Development of the pharyngeal part of the foregut is discussed in Chapter 12. The remainder of the gut tube is served by three arteries: the **celiac trunk,** which supplies the abdominal foregut (the abdominal esophagus, stomach, and superior half of the

Table 9–1	
The Derivatives of the Primitive Gut Tube	
REGIONS OF THE DIFFERENTIATED GUT TUBE	**ACCESSORY ORGANS DERIVED FROM THE GUT TUBE ENDODERM**
Foregut	
Pharynx	Pharyngeal pouch derivatives (see Ch. 12)
Thoracic esophagus	Lungs
Abdominal esophagus	
Stomach	
Superior half of duodenum (superior to the ampulla of Vater)	Liver parenchyma and hepatic duct epithelium
	Gallbladder, cystic duct, and common bile duct
	Dorsal and ventral pancreatic buds (exocrine cells and pancreatic duct epithelium; probably also pancreatic endocrine cells)
Midgut	
Inferior half of duodenum	
Jejunum	
Ileum	
Cecum	
Appendix	
Ascending colon	
Right two thirds of transverse colon	
Hindgut	
Left one third of transverse colon	
Descending colon	
Sigmoid colon	
Rectum	Urogenital sinus and derivatives (see Ch. 10)

duodenum and its derivatives); the **superior mesenteric trunk,** which supplies the midgut; and the **inferior mesenteric artery,** which supplies the hindgut (see Fig. 8–5).

The Primitive Abdominal Gut Is Initially a Straight Tube Suspended in the Peritoneal Cavity by a Dorsal Mesentery

At the end of the fourth week, almost the entire abdominal gut tube—the portion within the peritoneal cavity from the abdominal esophagus to the superior end of the developing cloaca—hangs suspended by the dorsal mesentery (see Ch. 6). Except in the region of the developing stomach, the coelomic cavities in the lateral plate mesoderm on either side of the germ disc coalesce during folding to form a single, continuous peritoneal cavity. In the stomach region, the gut tube remains connected to the ventral body wall by the thick septum transversum (see Ch. 6). By the fifth week, the caudal portion of the septum transversum thins to form the **ventral mesentery** connecting the stomach and developing liver to the ventral body wall (Fig. 9–2).

THE ABDOMINAL FOREGUT GIVES RISE TO THE STOMACH, DUODENUM, LIVER, PANCREAS, AND GALLBLADDER

The Presumptive Stomach Expands and Rotates Around Two Axes

The stomach first becomes apparent during the early part of the fourth week, as the foregut just inferior to the septum transversum expands slightly. On about day 26, the thoracic foregut begins to elongate rapidly. Over the next 2 days, the presumptive stomach, now much farther removed from the lung buds, expands further into a *fusiform* (Latin, spindle-shaped) structure that is readily distinguished from the adjacent regions of the gut tube (Fig. 9–3). During the fifth week, the dorsal wall of the stomach grows faster than the ventral wall, resulting in the formation of the **greater**

curvature of the stomach. Concurrently, deformation of the ventral stomach wall forms the **lesser curvature of the stomach.** Continued differential expansion of the superior part of the greater curvature results in the formation of the **fundus** and **cardiac incisure** by the end of the seventh week.

The Stomach Rotates During the Seventh and Eighth Weeks. The developing stomach undergoes a 90-degree rotation around a craniocaudal axis so that the greater curvature lies to the left and the lesser curvature lies to the right (see Fig. 9–3D). As shown in Figure 9–4, differential thinning of the right side of the **dorsal mesogastrium** (the portion of the dorsal mesentery attached to the stomach) is thought to play a role in this rotation. The right and left vagus plexuses, which originally run through the mesoderm on either side of the gut tube thus rotate to become posterior and anterior vagal trunks in the region of the stomach. Fibers of the left and right vagal plexuses, however, mix to some degree so that the more caudal anterior and posterior vagal trunks contain fibers from each of these more superior plexuses. The stomach also rotates slightly around a ventrodorsal axis so that the greater curvature faces slightly caudally and the lesser curvature slightly cranially (see Fig. 9–3D).

The Rotation of the Stomach and the Secondary Fusion of the Duodenum to the Dorsal Body Wall Create the Lesser Sac of the Peritoneal Cavity. The rotations of the stomach bend the presumptive duodenum into a C shape and also displace it to the right until it lies against the dorsal body wall, to which it adheres, thus becoming secondarily retroperitoneal (Fig. 9–5). The rotation of the stomach and the fusion of the duodenum create an alcove dorsal to the stomach called the **lesser sac of the peritoneal cavity** (see Fig. 9–5). The rest of the peritoneal cavity is now called the **greater sac.**

The lesser sac enlarges as a result of progressive expansion of the dorsal mesogastrium connecting the stomach to the posterior body wall. The resulting large, suspended fold of mesogastrium, called the **greater omentum,** hangs from the dorsal body wall and the greater curvature of the stomach and drapes over more inferior organs of the abdominal cavity (see Fig. 9–5C). The portion of the lesser sac directly dorsal to the stomach is

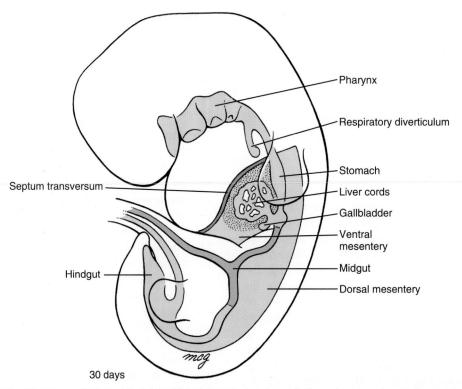

Figure 9–2. Structure of the gut tube. The foregut consists of the pharynx, located superior to the respiratory diverticulum, the thoracic esophagus, and the abdominal foregut. The abdominal foregut forms the abdominal esophagus, stomach, and about half of the duodenum and gives rise to the liver, the gallbladder, the pancreas, and their associated ducts. The midgut forms half of the duodenum, the jejunum and ileum, the ascending colon, and about two thirds of the transverse colon. The hindgut forms one third of the transverse colon, the descending colon and sigmoid colon, and the upper two thirds of the anorectal canal. The abdominal esophagus, stomach, and superior part of the duodenum are suspended by dorsal and ventral mesenteries; the abdominal gut tube excluding the rectum is suspended in the abdominal cavity by a dorsal mesentery only.

now called the **upper recess of the lesser sac,** and the cavity within the greater omentum is called the **lower recess of the lesser sac.** The lower recess, however, is obliterated during fetal life as the anterior and posterior folds of the greater omentum fuse together.

A System of Digestive Glands Develops From Endodermal Buds of the Duodenum

The Liver Parenchyma, the Gallbladder, and Their Ducts Bud From the Duodenal Endoderm and Grow Into the Septum Transversum. On about day 22, a small endodermal thick-

ening, the **hepatic plate,** appears on the ventral side of the duodenum. Over the next few days, cells in this plate proliferate and form a **hepatic diverticulum,** which grows into the inferior region of the septum transversum (Fig. 9–6). The hepatic diverticulum gives rise to the ramifying **liver cords,** which become the hepatocytes (parenchyma); to the **bile canaliculi** of the liver; and to the **hepatic ducts.** The mesoblastic **supporting stroma** of the liver, in contrast, develops from splanchnopleuric mesoderm originating near the cardiac region of the stomach.

The liver is a major early **hematopoietic organ** of the embryo. Even as soon as the fourth week, blood cells begin to be produced by foci of hematopoietic cells derived from the mesenchyme of the septum transversum. Fetal liver cells have

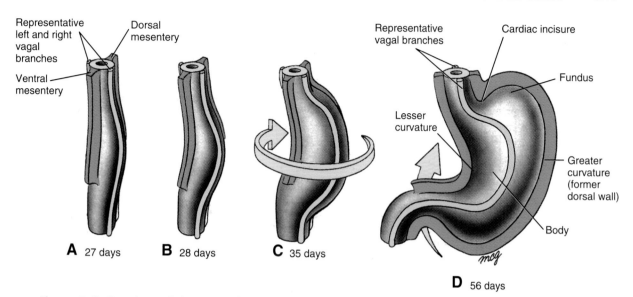

Figure 9–3. Rotations of the stomach. *A–C,* Oblique frontal views; *D,* direct frontal view. The posterior wall of the stomach expands during the fourth and fifth weeks to form the greater curvature. During the seventh week, the stomach rotates clockwise on its longitudinal axis (when viewed from above).

been injected into fetuses suffering from immuno-deficiency disorders and other disorders of the hematopoietic system to repopulate this system with normal stem cells (see Ch. 15).

By day 26, a distinct endodermal thickening appears on the ventral side of the duodenum just caudal to the base of the hepatic diverticulum and buds into the ventral mesentery (see Fig. 9–6). This **cystic diverticulum** will form the **gall-bladder** and **cystic duct.** As shown in Figure 9–6, no sooner does the cystic diverticulum appear than cells at the junction of the hepatic and cystic ducts

proliferate and form the **common bile duct.** As a result, the developing cystic duct is carried away from the duodenum. The gallbladder and cystic duct develop from histologically distinct populations of duodenal cells.

The Pancreas Forms Through the Fusion of Dorsal and Ventral Pancreatic Buds. On day 26, another duodenal bud begins to grow into the dorsal mesentery just opposite to the hepatic diverticulum. This endodermal diverticulum is the **dorsal pancreatic bud** (see Fig. 9–6). Over the next

Figure 9–4. The rotation of the stomach around its longitudinal axis commences with vacuolization of the right side of the thick mesenchymal bar that initially suspends the stomach from the posterior body wall.

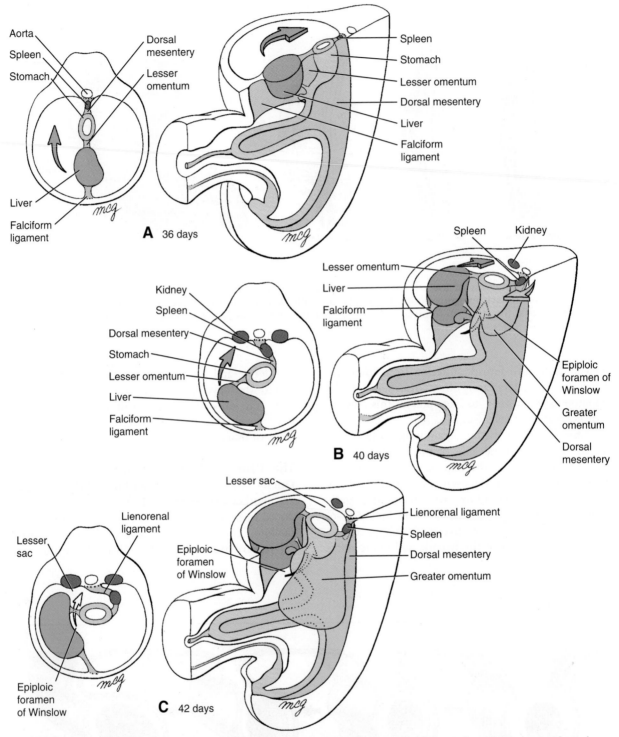

Figure 9–5. Development of the greater omentum and lesser sac. *A, B,* The rotation of the stomach and growth of the dorsal mesogastrium create a sac (the greater omentum) that dangles from the greater curvature of the stomach. *B, C,* When the duodenum swings to the right, it becomes secondarily fused to the body wall, enclosing the space posterior to the stomach and within the expanding cavity of the greater omentum. This space is the lesser sac of the peritoneal cavity. The remainder of the peritoneal cavity is now called the greater sac. The principal passageway between the greater and lesser sacs is the epiploic foramen of Winslow.

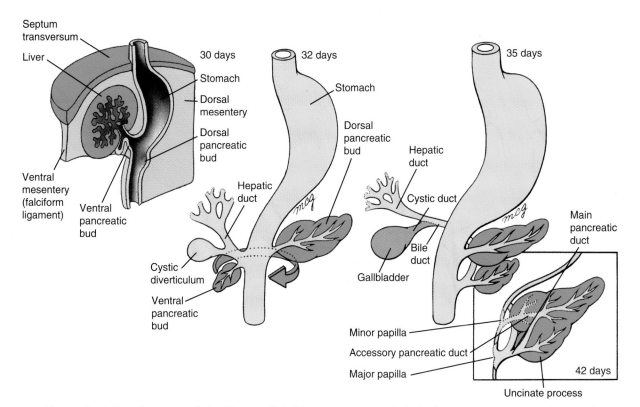

Figure 9–6. Development of the liver, gallbladder, pancreas, and their duct systems from endodermal diverticula of the duodenum. The liver bud sprouts during the fourth week and expands in the ventral mesentery. The cystic diverticulum and ventral pancreatic bud also grow into the ventral mesentery, whereas the dorsal pancreatic bud grows into the dorsal mesentery. During the fifth week, the ventral pancreatic bud migrates around the posterior side (former right side) of the duodenum to fuse with the dorsal pancreatic bud. The main duct of the ventral bud ultimately becomes the major pancreatic duct, which drains the entire pancreas.

few days, as the dorsal pancreatic bud elongates into the dorsal mesentery, another endodermal diverticulum, the **ventral pancreatic bud,** sprouts into the ventral mesentery just caudal to the developing gallbladder (see Fig. 9–6). By day 32, the main duct of the ventral pancreatic bud becomes connected to the proximal end of the common bile duct.

During the fifth week, the mouth of the common bile duct and the ventral pancreatic bud migrate posteriorly around the duodenum to the dorsal mesentery (see Fig. 9–6). By the early sixth week, the ventral and dorsal pancreatic buds lie adjacent in the plane of the dorsal mesentery, and late in the sixth week, the two pancreatic buds fuse to form the definitive pancreas. The dorsal pancreatic bud gives rise to the **head, body,** and **tail** of the pancreas, whereas the ventral pancreatic bud

gives rise to the hooklike **uncinate process.** Like the duodenum, the pancreas fuses to the dorsal body wall and becomes secondarily retroperitoneal.

Occasionally, the pancreas forms a complete ring encircling the duodenum, a condition known as **annular pancreas.** As shown in Figure 9–7, this abnormality probably arises when the two lobes of a bilobed ventral pancreatic bud (a normal variation) migrate in opposite directions around the duodenum to fuse with the dorsal pancreatic bud. An annular pancreas compresses the duodenum and may cause gastrointestinal obstruction.

When the ventral and dorsal pancreatic buds fuse, their ductal systems also become interconnected (see Fig. 9–6). The duct from the dorsal bud to the duodenum usually degenerates, leaving the ventral pancreatic duct, now called the **main pancreatic duct,** as the only conduit to the duode-

Bilobed ventral
pancreatic bud

Annular
pancreas

Figure 9–7. The ventral pancreas may consist of two lobes. If the lobes migrate around the duodenum in opposite directions to fuse with the dorsal pancreatic bud, an annular pancreas is formed.

num. The main pancreatic duct and the common bile duct meet and empty their secretions into the duodenum at the **major duodenal papilla** or **ampulla of Vater.** In some individuals, the dorsal pancreatic duct persists as an **accessory pancreatic duct** that empties into the duodenum at a **minor duodenal papilla** (see Fig. 9–6).

The **exocrine cells** of the pancreas, which produce digestive enzymes, differentiate from the endoderm of the pancreatic buds. The origin of the **pancreatic endocrine cells** in the islets of Langerhans, however, is controversial. It has been suggested that they arise from neural crest. Evidence from cell-tracing experiments (some involving the quail-chick chimera system) and from transgenic animals, however, suggests that these cells arise from gut tube endoderm.

THE SPLEEN IS DERIVED FROM THE DORSAL MESOGASTRIUM, NOT FROM THE GUT TUBE ENDODERM

As the dorsal mesogastrium of the lesser sac begins its expansive growth at the end of the fourth week,

a mesenchymal condensation develops in it near the body wall. This condensation differentiates during the fifth week to form the **spleen,** a vascular lymphatic organ (see Fig. 9–5). Smaller splenic condensations called **accessory spleens** may develop near the hilum of the primary spleen. It is important to remember that the spleen is a *mesodermal* derivative, not a product of the gut tube endoderm like most of the intra-abdominal viscera. The rotation of the stomach and growth of the dorsal mesogastrium translocate the spleen to the left side of the abdominal cavity. The rotation of the dorsal mesogastrium also establishes a mesenteric connection called the **renal-splenic ligament** between the spleen and the left kidney. The portion of the dorsal mesentery between the spleen and the stomach is called the **gastrosplenic ligament.**

The spleen initially functions as a hematopoietic organ and only later acquires its definitive lymphoid character. During the **preliminary stage** of its development, until 14 weeks, the spleen is strictly hematopoietic. From 15 to 18 weeks (the **transformation stage**) the organ develops its characteristic lobular architecture, and the **stage of lymphoid colonization** then commences as T-lymphocyte precursor cells begin to enter the spleen. Starting at 23 weeks, B-cell precursors arrive and form the **B-cell regions** of the definitive spleen.

THE VENTRAL MESENTERY GIVES RISE TO A MULTITUDE OF STRUCTURES AS IT IS INVADED BY THE LIVER

As the liver enlarges, the caudal portion of the septum transversum (the ventral mesentery) is modified to form a number of membranous structures, including the serous coverings of the liver and the membranes that attach the liver to the stomach and to the ventral body wall (Table 9–2). As described in Chapter 6, the central tendon of the diaphragm forms from the superior region of the septum transversum. By the sixth week, the enlarging liver makes contact with the superior and inferior coverings of the septum transversum and begins to split them apart (Fig. 9–8). The inferior serosal membrane of the septum becomes the **visceral peritoneum,** which covers almost the entire surface of the liver. At its superior pole, however, the liver tissue makes direct contact with the developing central tendon of the diaphragm and therefore has no peritoneal covering. This zone becomes the **bare area of the liver** (see Fig. 9–8). Around the margins of the bare area, the peritoneum covering the inferior surface of the peripheral diaphragm makes a fold or *reflection* onto the surface of the liver. Because this reflection encircles the bare area like a crown, it is called the **coronary ligament.** The direct contact between the liver and the diaphragm in the bare area results in the formation of anastomoses between hepatic portal vessels and the systemic veins of the diaphragm.

The narrow sickle-shaped flap of ventral mesentery that attaches the liver to the ventral body wall differentiates into the membranous **falciform ligament** (see Fig. 9–8). The free caudal margin of this membrane carries the umbilical vein from the body wall to the liver. The portion of the ventral mesentery between the liver and the stomach thins out to form a translucent membrane called the **lesser omentum.** The caudal border of the lesser omentum, connecting the liver to the developing duodenum, is called the **hepatoduodenal ligament** and contains the portal vein, the proper hepatic artery and branches, and the hepatic, cystic, and common bile ducts. The region of the lesser omentum between the liver and the stomach is called the **hepatogastric ligament.**

When the stomach rotates to the left and the liver shifts into the right side of the peritoneal cavity, the lesser omentum rotates from a sagittal into a coronal (frontal) plane. This repositioning reduces the communication between the greater and lesser sacs of the peritoneal cavity to a narrow canal lying just posterior to the lesser omentum. This canal is called the **epiploic foramen of Winslow** (see Fig. 9–5).

ROTATIONS OF THE MIDGUT PRODUCE THE DEFINITIVE CONFIGURATION OF THE SMALL AND LARGE INTESTINES

Rapid Elongation of the Ileum Produces a Primary Intestinal Loop That Herniates Into the Umbilicus

By the fifth week, the presumptive ileum, which can be distinguished from the presumptive colon by the presence of a cecal primordium at the junction between the two, begins to elongate rapidly. The growing ileum lengthens much more rapidly than the abdominal cavity itself, and the midgut is therefore thrown into a dorsoventral hairpin fold called the **primary intestinal loop** (Fig. 9–9A). The cranial limb of this loop will give rise to most of the ileum, whereas the caudal limb will become the ascending colon and transverse colon. At its apex, the primary intestinal loop is attached to the umbilicus by the vitelline duct, and the superior mesenteric artery runs down the long axis of the loop. By the early sixth week, the continuing elongation of the midgut, combined with the pressure due to the dramatic growth of other abdominal organs (particularly the liver), forces the primary intestinal loop to herniate into the umbilicus (see Fig. 9–9B).

The Herniated Primary Intestinal Loop Undergoes an Initial 90-Degree Counterclockwise Rotation

As the primary intestinal loop herniates into the umbilicus, it also rotates around the axis of the

Table 9-2
Derivatives of the Septum Transversum

REGIONS OF SEPTUM TRANSVERSUM	DERIVATIVES
Cranial region	Central tendon of the diaphragm
	Myocytes of the pleuroperitoneal membranes
Central mesenchyme	Hematopoietic cells of liver
Caudal region (ventral mesentery)	Falciform ligament
	Visceral peritoneum of the liver, including the coronary ligament
	Visceral peritoneum of the gallbladder
	Lesser omentum, including the hepatoduodenal and hepatogastric ligaments

superior mesenteric artery (i.e., around a dorsoventral axis) by 90 degrees counterclockwise as viewed from in front, so that the cranial limb moves caudally and to the embryo's right, and the caudal limb moves cranially and to the embryo's left (see Fig. 9–9B). This rotation is complete by the early eighth week. Meanwhile, the midgut continues to differentiate. The lengthening jejunum and ileum are thrown into a series of folds called the **jejunal-ileal loops,** and the expanding cecum sprouts a wormlike **vermiform appendix** (see Fig. 9–9C).

During the 10th Week, the Midgut Retracts into the Abdomen and Rotates an Additional 180 Degrees

The mechanism responsible for the rapid retraction of the midgut into the abdominal cavity during the 10th week is not understood but may involve an increase in the size of the abdominal cavity relative to the other abdominal organs. As the intestinal loop reenters the abdomen, it rotates

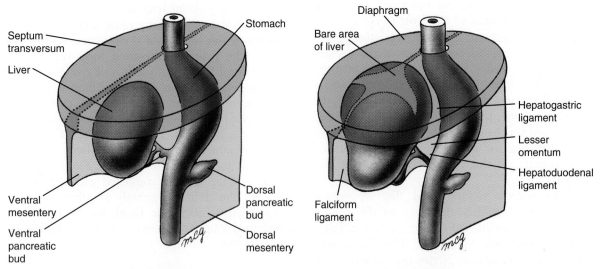

Mid 5th week   Mid 6th week

Figure 9-8. Formation of the liver and associated membranes. As the liver bud grows into the ventral mesentery, its expanding crown makes direct contact with the developing diaphragm. The ventral mesentery that encloses the growing liver bud differentiates into the visceral peritoneum of the liver, which is reflected onto the diaphragm. This zone of reflection, which encircles the area where the liver directly contacts the diaphragm (the bare area), becomes the coronary ligament. The remnant of ventral mesentery connecting the liver with the anterior body wall becomes the falciform ligament, whereas the ventral mesentery between the liver and lesser curvature of the stomach forms the lesser omentum.

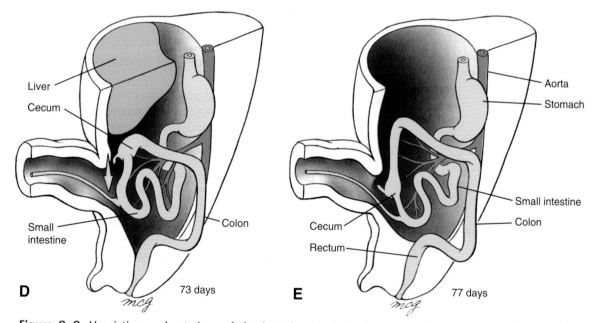

Figure 9–9. Herniation and rotations of the intestine. *A, B,* At the end of the sixth week, the primary intestinal loop herniates into the umbilicus, rotating through 90 degrees counterclockwise (in frontal view). *C,* The small intestine elongates to form jejunal-ileal loops, the cecum and appendix grow, and, at the end of the 10th week, the primary intestinal loop retracts into the abdominal cavity, rotating an additional 180 degrees counterclockwise. *D, E,* During the 11th week, the retracting midgut completes this rotation as the cecum is positioned just inferior to the liver. The cecum is then displaced inferiorly, pulling down the proximal hindgut to form the ascending colon. The descending colon is simultaneously fixed on the left side of the posterior abdominal wall. The jejunum, ileum, and transverse colon and sigmoid colon remain suspended by mesentery.

counterclockwise through an additional 180 degrees, so that now the retracting colon has traveled a 270-degree circuit relative to the posterior wall of the abdominal cavity (see Fig. 9–9C–E). The cecum consequently rotates to a position just inferior to the liver in the region of the right iliac crest. The intestines have completely returned to the abdominal cavity by the 11th week.

The Ascending and Descending Colon Becomes Secondarily Retroperitoneal

After the large intestine returns to the abdominal cavity, the dorsal mesenteries of the ascending colon and descending colon shorten and fold, bringing these organs into contact with the dorsal body wall, where they adhere and become secondarily retroperitoneal (see Ch. 6). The cecum is suspended from the dorsal body wall by a shortened mesentery soon after it returns to the abdominal cavity. In the case of ascending and descending colons, the shortening and folding of the mesenteries is probably related to the relative lengthening of the lumbar region of the dorsal body wall. The transverse colon does not become fixed to the body wall but remains an intraperitoneal organ suspended by mesentery. Pressure from this organ may help to fix the underlying duodenum to the body wall, however. The most inferior portion of the colon, the sigmoid colon, also remains suspended by mesentery. Figure 9–10 summarizes the final disposition of the gastrointestinal organs with respect to the body wall.

THE DISTAL HINDGUT GIVES RISE TO THE RECTUM AND THE UROGENITAL SINUS

The Cloaca is Partitioned Into an Anterior Primitive Urogenital Sinus and a Posterior Rectum

The portion of the primitive gut tube lying just deep to the cloacal membrane forms an expansion called the **cloaca** (Latin, sewer). A slim superoventral diverticulum of the cloaca called the **allantois** extends into the connecting stalk. The develop-

mental fate of this vestigial structure is covered in the Clinical Applications section of this chapter. Between the fourth and sixth weeks, the cloaca is partitioned into a posterior rectum and an anterior **primitive urogenital sinus** by the growth of a coronal partition called the **urorectal septum.** As described in Chapter 10, the urogenital sinus gives rise to the bladder, the pelvic urethra, and a lower expansion, the **definitive urogenital sinus.** In the male, the pelvic urethra becomes the membranous and prostatic urethra, and the definitive urogenital sinus becomes the penile urethra; in the female, the pelvic urethra becomes the membranous urethra, and the definitive urogenital sinus becomes the vestibule of the vagina. All of these urogenital structures are thus derived from the hindgut endoderm.

The distal edge of the urorectal septum fuses with the cloacal membrane, dividing the membrane into an anterior **urogenital membrane** and a posterior **anal membrane.** The zone of fusion between the urorectal septum and the cloacal membrane becomes the **perineum.**

Evidence Suggests That the Urorectal Septum Is a Composite of Two Mesodermal Septal Systems

The urorectal septum was originally considered to form as a single bar of mesoderm growing down from the cloacal roof to meet the cloacal membrane. Evidence suggests, however, that the urorectal septum is actually a composite structure formed by two integrated mesodermal septal systems: a superior fold called the **Tourneux fold** and a pair of lateral folds called the **Rathke folds** (Fig. 9–11). The Clinical Applications section of Chapter 10 describes some urorectal anomalies that seem to arise from errors in the integration of these two septal systems.

The Tourneux fold first appears in the fourth week as a crescentic wedge of mesoderm growing inferiorly between the allantois and the cranial end of the cloaca. This coronal partition ceases to grow when it reaches the level of the future pelvic urethra. The Rathke folds arise as a pair of mesodermal bars located on either side of the cloacal cavity near the cloacal membrane and grow toward the midline, where they fuse with each other and with the Tourneux fold to complete the urorectal septum.

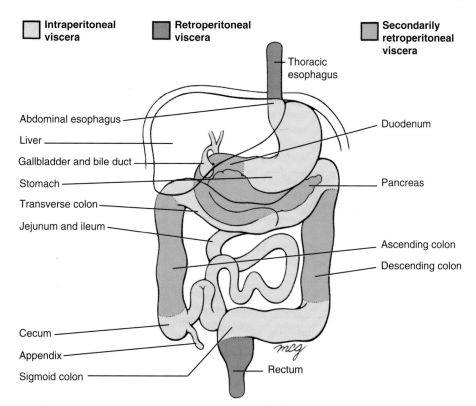

Figure 9–10. Intraperitoneal, retroperitoneal, and secondarily retroperitoneal organs of the abdominal gastrointestinal tract.

Figure 9–11. Subdivision of the cloaca into an anterior primitive urogenital sinus and a posterior rectum between 4 and 6 weeks. The urorectal septum that divides the cloaca is composed of three distinct septa. Initially, a superior Tourneaux fold grows inferiorly to the level of the future pelvic urethra. Separation is then completed by left and right Rathke folds that grow in a coronal plane.

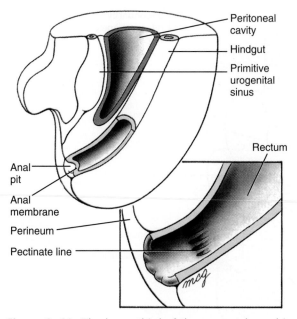

Figure 9-12. The lower third of the anorectal canal is formed by an ectodermal invagination called the anal pit. The border between the superior end of the anal pit and the inferior end of the rectum is demarcated by mucosal folds called the pectinate line in the adult.

The Inferior One Third of the Anorectal Canal Forms From an Ectodermal Pit

The superior two thirds of the anorectal canal forms from the distal part of the hindgut. The inferior one third of the anorectal canal, in contrast, is derived from an ectodermal pit called the **anal pit** or **proctodeum** (Fig. 9–12). This pit is created when the mesenchyme around the anal membrane proliferates to form a raised border. The anal membrane, which thus separates the endodermal and ectodermal portions of the anorectal canal, breaks down in the eighth week. The former location of this membrane is marked in the adult by an irregular folding of mucosa within the anorectal canal, called the **pectinate line.** The vasculature of the anorectal canal is consistent with this dual origin: superior to the pectinate line the canal is supplied by branches of the inferior mesenteric arteries and veins serving the hindgut, whereas inferior to the pectinate line it is supplied by branches of the internal iliac arteries and veins.

Figure 9-13. Formation of the definitive gut lumen. Proliferation of the endodermal lining completely occludes the gut tube during the sixth week. Recanalization is completed by week 9. Incomplete or abnormal recanalization may result in duplication of the lumen or stenosis of the gut tube.

Anastomoses between tributaries of the superior rectal vein and tributaries of the inferior rectal vein within the mucosa of the anorectal canal may later swell into hemorrhoids if the normal portal blood flow into the inferior vena cava is blocked.

The Digestive Tube Becomes Transiently Solid and Then Undergoes Recanalization

During the sixth week, the endodermal epithelium of the gut tube proliferates until it completely oc-cludes the gut tube lumen (Fig. 9–13). Over the next 2 weeks, vacuoles develop in this tissue and coalesce until the gut tube is fully **recanalized.** Finally, in the ninth week, the definitive mucosal epithelium differentiates from the endodermal lin-ing of the new gut lumen. *Stenosis* or *duplication* of the digestive tract may result from incomplete re-canalization.

The mesodermal coating of the primitive gut tube gives rise to the submucosal connective tissue and smooth muscle layers of the definitive gastro-intestinal tract.

Clinical Applications

Anomalies of Gastrointestinal Development

DEFECTS OF THE ANTERIOR ABDOMINAL WALL CAN RESULT IN A WIDE RANGE OF MIDGUT AND HINDGUT ANOMALIES

Omphalocele Results From Failure of the Um-bilicus to Close Completely. Occasionally, an in-fant is born with abdominal organs protruding from the anterior abdominal wall. In the condition called **omphalocele,** the gastrointestinal structures protrude through an unclosed **umbilical ring.** Omphalocele occurs in about 2.5 of 10,000 births.

In one type of omphalocele, the organs pro-trude into a thin, often ruptured sac composed of amniotic membrane alone (Fig. 9–14*A*). In these individuals, the physiologic herniation of the mid-gut in the sixth week apparently occurs normally, but the herniated organs do not fully retract into the abdominal cavity during the tenth week. In a somewhat different type of omphalocele, the ab-dominal organs protrude through the unclosed umbilicus into a sac composed of peritoneum and subserous fascia as well as amniotic membrane. The presence of peritoneum in the sac indicates that the gut tube retracted normally during the tenth week and then herniated again secondarily because the ventral abdominal wall failed to close

in the region of the umbilicus. There is some de-bate about the cause of this kind of midventral abdominal wall defect. It has been attributed to incomplete lateral folding of the embryo from the fourth to the eighth weeks; alternatively, it may be due to incomplete migration and differentiation of the somitic mesoderm that normally forms connec-tive tissue of the skin and hypaxial musculature of the ventral body wall.

The abdominal wall defect in an omphalocele is not always limited to the umbilicus, and the location of the defect determines which organs will eventrate. A defect cranial to the umbilicus may result in evagination of the liver or even, in the condition called **ectopia cordis,** the heart (see Fig. 9–14*B*). Defects below the level of the liver may involve the midgut alone.

An omphalocele may occur in conjunction with a variety of cardiac and renal defects, often as part of the constellation of abnormalities associated with a chromosomal anomaly. An example is **pen-talogy of Cantrell,** which includes an omphalo-cele, diaphragmatic hernia, sternal cleft, ectopia cordis, and intracardiac anomaly.

In Gastroschisis, the Abdominal Wall Defect Does Not Involve the Umbilicus. Gastroschisis is a defect or splitting of the ventral abdominal

Figure 9–14. Congenital defects of anterior abdominal wall closure. *A,* Omphalocele. An omphalocele may be forced back into the abdominal cavity by compressing a Dacron silo. *B,* Ectopia cordis caused by failure of abdominal wall closure more superiorly. (Photographs courtesy of Children's Hospital Medical Center, Cincinnati, OH.)

wall between the developing rectus muscles just lateral to the umbilicus (Fig. 9–15). The umbilical ring closes normally. This defect usually occurs on the right side, supporting the idea that it usually arises through an abnormality in the involution of the right umbilical vein during the fifth and sixth weeks, with a consequent maldevelopment of associated mesodermal elements in that region of the ventral body wall. Visceral organs rarely eventrate through this defect, but when they do, they are not enclosed in an amnioperitoneal sac as in an omphalocele. Gastroschisis also differs from omphalocele in being less often associated with other abnormalities and not correlated with chromo-

somal anomalies. The incidence of this defect is about 1 in 10,000 births.

Bladder Exstrophy, Epispadias, and Similar Hindgut Abnormalities Are Also Associated With Abdominal Wall Defects. In a series of abnormalities ranging from **epispadias** to **exstrophy of the bladder or cloaca,** hindgut structures are exposed through a defect in the mesodermal structures of the ventral body wall. In epispadias, the left and right halves of the penile tubercle do not fuse completely (see Ch. 10), so that the penile urethra has an abnormal opening. In exstrophy of the bladder, the bladder is revealed by an abdomi-

Figure 9–16. In this case of cloacal exstrophy, the undivided cloaca evaginates from an anterior wall defect at the site of the former cloacal membrane. (Photograph courtesy of Children's Hospital Medical Center, Cincinnati, OH.)

Figure 9–15. Severe gastroschisis. As is typical, the visceral organs evaginate to the right of the umbilicus. (Photograph courtesy of Children's Hospital Medical Center, Cincinnati, OH.)

nal wall defect; in exstrophy of the cloaca, the lumina of both the bladder and the anorectal canal are exposed (Fig. 9–16).

The abdominal wall defect in these conditions seems to be a secondary effect of anomalous development of the **cloacal membrane.** According to one theory, the primary defect is that the cloacal membrane is abnormally large, so that when it breaks down it produces an opening that is too wide to permit normal midline fusion of the mesodermal structures on either side of it. A cloacal membrane that was only slightly enlarged might affect only the penile tubercles, resulting in epispadias; severely enlarged cloacal membranes would result in more radical malformations. An alternative theory attributes maldevelopment of the abdominal wall in this complex of abnormalities to precocious disruption of the cloacal membrane.

Exstrophy of the bladder with epispadias is the most common anomaly in this morphologic series, occurring in approximately 1 of 40,000 births. Exstrophy of the cloaca is much less frequent, occurring in about 1 of 200,000 births. All these malformations are about twice as common in males as in females.

Abnormal Rotation and Fixation of the Midgut Can Cause a Variety of Malformations

As described in this chapter, the normal handed asymmetry of the midgut is based on a relatively intricate series of *rotations* and *fixations*. Not surprisingly, errors in one or more of these steps lead to a varied spectrum of anomalies (see the Experimental Principles section of this chapter).

Rotational Defects of the Midgut Can Be Classified as Nonrotations, Reversed Rotations, and Mixed Rotations (Malrotations). The anomaly called **nonrotation of the midgut** arises when the primary intestinal loop fails to undergo the normal 180-degree counterclockwise rotation as it is retracted into the abdominal cavity (Fig. 9–17). The earlier 90-degree rotation may occur normally. The result of this error is that the original cranial limb of the primary intestinal loop (consisting of presumptive ileum and jejunum) ends up on

Figure 9–17. Nonrotation of the gut (also called left-sided colon).

the right side of the body and the original caudal limb of the primary intestinal loop (consisting mainly of presumptive colon) ends up on the left side of the body. This condition is therefore sometimes called **left-sided colon** (see Fig. 9–17). The cecum and the most proximal region of the large intestine may or may not fuse to the dorsal body wall to become secondarily retroperitoneal.

In **reversed rotation of the midgut,** the primary intestinal loop undergoes the initial 90-degree counterclockwise rotation normally, but the second 180-degree rotation occurs *clockwise* instead

of counterclockwise, so the net rotation of the midgut is 90 degrees clockwise (Fig. 9–18). This rotation brings the regions of the midgut and hindgut into their normal spatial relationships, with one important exception: the duodenum lies ventral to the transverse colon instead of dorsal to it. The duodenum thus does not become secondarily retroperitoneal, whereas the region of the transverse colon underlying it does.

In **mixed rotations of the midgut** (also called **malrotations**), the cephalic limb of the primary intestinal loop undergoes only the initial 90-

Figure 9–18. Reversed rotation of the gut. The net rotation is 90 degrees clockwise, so the midgut viscera are brought to their normal locations in the abdominal cavity but the duodenum lies anterior to the transverse colon.

degree rotation, whereas the caudal limb undergoes only the later 180-degree rotation (Fig. 9–19). The result of this mixed or uncoordinated behavior of the two limbs is that the distal end of the duodenum becomes fixed on the right side of the abdominal cavity, and the cecum becomes fixed near the midline just inferior to the pylorus of the stomach. This abnormal position of the cecum may cause the duodenum to be enclosed by a band of thickened peritoneum.

Abnormal Midgut Rotation or Fixation May Lead to Compression or Volvulus of the Intestines. A significant fraction of all cases of intestinal obstruction are caused by abnormal rotation or fixation of the midgut. Specific regions of the intestine, such as the duodenum, may be pinned against the dorsal body wall by bands of abnormal mesentery, resulting in constriction and obstruction. Alternatively, malrotation may leave much of the midgut suspended from a single point of attachment on the dorsal body wall. Such freely suspended coils are prone to torsion or **volvulus,** which can lead to acute obstruction (Fig. 9–20). **Bilious vomiting** is a common symptom of intestinal volvulus.

Intestinal volvulus may also compress part of the intestinal vasculature, resulting in local vascular compromise. If the arterial supply to part of the gut is cut off, the result may be intestinal ischemia or **infarction.** A volvulus may also compress lymphatic vessels, inhibiting lymphatic drainage and leading to **venous mucosal engorgement** and consequent **gastrointestinal bleeding.**

The presence of a rotational abnormality is usually signaled during childhood by abdominal pain, vomiting, gastrointestinal bleeding, or failure to thrive, although occasionally such an abnormality remains clinically silent until adulthood. Definitive diagnosis often involves barium enema or bar-

Cephalic limb (limb *a*) of intestinal
loop undergoes normal 90° counterclockwise rotation; caudal limb (limb
b) does not rotate

a   90°

b

Caudal limb (*b*) undergoes
normal 180° counterclockwise
rotation; cephalic limb (*a*) does
not rotate

Resulting gut anomaly

Aorta

Stomach

Cecum

Transverse
colon

Small intestine

Descending
colon

91 days

Figure 9–19. Mixed rotation of the gut. In this malformation, the cranial and caudal limbs of the primary intestinal loop rotate independently.

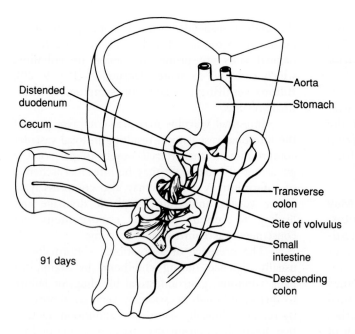

Distended
duodenum

Cecum

Aorta

Stomach

Transverse
colon

Site of volvulus

Small
intestine

Descending
colon

91 days

Figure 9–20. Volvulus. Volvulus may occur as suspended regions of the gut twist around themselves, constricting the intestine and/or compromising its blood supply.

ium swallow. These defects can be repaired surgically.

Abnormalities of the Vitelline Duct and the Allantois Both Affect the Umbilicus

Meckel's Diverticulum Is an Anomaly of the Vitelline Duct. The vitelline duct normally regresses between the fifth and eighth weeks (see Ch. 10), but in about 2 percent of live-born infants it persists as a remnant of variable length and loca-

tion (Fig. 9–21). Most often it is observed as a 1- to 5-cm intestinal diverticulum projecting from the antimesenteric wall of the ileum within 100 cm of the cecum (see Fig. 9–21A). In other cases, part of the vitelline duct within the abdominal wall persists, forming an open **omphalomesenteric fistula,** an **enterocyst,** or a **fibrous band** connecting the small bowel to the umbilicus (see Fig. 9–21B–D). These conditions are known collectively as **Meckel's diverticulum** in honor of J.F. Meckel, who first discussed the embryologic basis of the abnormality in the early 19th century. Meckel's diverticulum is about twice as common in males as in females.

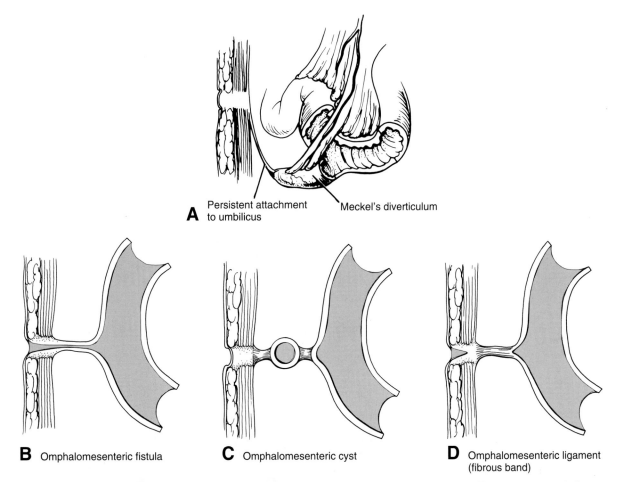

A Persistent attachment to umbilicus   Meckel's diverticulum

B Omphalomesenteric fistula

C Omphalomesenteric cyst

D Omphalomesenteric ligament (fibrous band)

Figure 9–21. Meckel's diverticulum. *A,* A typical Meckel's diverticulum is a finger-like projection of the ileum located about 100 cm proximal to the cecum. A Meckel's diverticulum may form (*B*) a patent fistula connecting the umbilicus with the ileum, (*C*) an isolated cyst suspended by ligaments, or (*D*) a fibrous band connecting the ileum and anterior body wall at the level of the umbilicus. (Drawings courtesy of Children's Hospital Medical Center, Cincinnati, OH.)

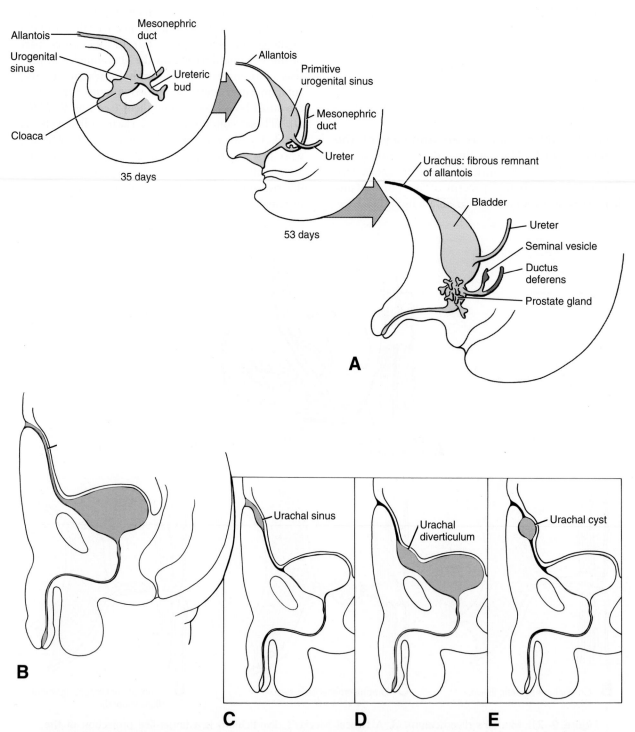

Figure 9–22. Fate of the allantois. *A,* Normally, the allantois becomes occluded to form the urachus or median umbilical ligament of the adult. Very rarely, parts of the allantois may remain patent, producing (*B*) a urachal fistula, (*C*) a urachal sinus, (*D*) a urachal diverticulum, or (*E*) a urachal cyst.

It is estimated that 15 to 35 percent of individuals who have Meckel's diverticulum develop symptoms of intestinal obstruction, gastrointestinal bleeding, or bowel sepsis. Bowel obstruction may be caused by the trapping of part of the small bowel by a fibrous band that represents a remnant of the vitelline vessels connecting the diverticulum to the umbilicus. Symptoms may closely mimic appendicitis, involving periumbilical pain that later localizes to the right lower quadrant. Mortality in untreated cases is estimated to be 2.5 to 15 percent.

Incomplete Obliteration of the Lumen of the Allantois and Bladder Apex Results in Urachal Anomalies. Normally, the allantois and the superior end of the presumptive bladder undergo regression between the fourth and sixth weeks, at the same time that the urorectal septum is partitioning the cloaca into an anterior urogenital sinus and a posterior rectum. The allantois and the constricted bladder apex are transformed into a ligamentous band, the **urachus** or **median umbilical ligament,** that runs through the subperitoneal fat from the bladder to the umbilicus. This band is about 5 cm long and 1 cm wide in the adult (Fig. 9–22A).

In a very small number of individuals (only a few hundred have ever been reported), part or all of the allantois and bladder apex remains patent, resulting in a **patent urachus, umbilical urachal sinus, vesicourachal diverticulum,** or **urachal cyst** (see Fig. 9–22B–E). Symptoms include leakage of urine from the umbilicus, urinary tract infections, and peritonitis resulting from perforation of the patent urachus. These conditions may be life-threatening. The initial symptoms of infection, as with Meckel's diverticulum, are easily confused with those of appendicitis.

Experimental Principles

The Molecular Basis of Handed Asymmetry

THE THIRD AXIS OF DEVELOPMENT IN THE EMBRYO IS THE LEFT-RIGHT AXIS

Mechanisms that underlie craniocaudal and dorsoventral differentiation of the early embryo are discussed in Chapters 3 and 4. As described in Chapters 6 through 9, however, the definitive lungs, heart, vasculature, and gastrointestinal tract exhibit significant differences between the right and left sides of the body. These structures are said to display **handed asymmetry,** because they lack **mirror symmetry** with respect to more than one plane of symmetry. The molecular mechanisms regulating development of the left-right axis are beginning to be understood.

The *iv/iv* Mouse Mutant Provides an Animal Model of Human Situs Inversus

In the rare human disorder **situs inversus viscerum totalis,** the handedness of all of the viscera is reversed. However, the reversal is rarely complete or exact, and errors in folding and rotation often produce subsidiary malformations such as the **malrotations of the midgut** described in the Clinical Applications section of this chapter. More often, the different organ systems exhibit a discordance of sidedness, or **heterotaxia.** For example, the folding of the heart may be reversed (**dextrocardia;** Ch. 7), although lobulation of the lungs is normal (three lobes on the right and two lobes on the left; Ch. 6). In 1959, a mouse mutant, the *iv/iv* mouse, was discovered, which exhibits situs inversus (*iv* means *inversus viscerum*). The phenotype is inherited as an autosomal recessive single-gene trait and has been mapped to chromosome 12, but only half the mice homozygous for the mutant *iv* allele exhibit situs inversus; the other half show normal left/right asymmetry **(situs solitus).** Thus, the gene product of the wild-type locus appears to be an essential component of the mechanism that **biases** the development of handed asymmetry in the correct direction and thus determines the correct handedness or **situs** of the viscera. If this gene product is absent or defective (as in the *iv/iv* mouse), normal or inverted situs is apparently adopted at random.

The cloning of the *iv* mutation provided interesting clues that led to better understanding of the early stages of left-right development. The *iv* mutation was found to occur in a dynein gene designated *left-right dynein*, or *lrd*. Dyneins are molecular motors that use the energy from ATP hydrolysis to generate unidirectional motive force along microtubules, which have plus and minus ends. There are two categories of dyneins, cytoplasmic and axonemal. Cytoplasmic dyneins move cargoes inside of cells, and axonemal dyneins create the sliding force between microtubules that results in the movement of cilia. The sequence of the *lrd* gene suggested it encoded an axonemal dynein.

This connection between dynein and laterality in mice was reminiscent of a previous connection between dynein and laterality made in humans. Patients with Kartegener's syndrome have randomized laterality as well as immotile respiratory cilia and sperm flagella. They often exhibit male infertility and chronic respiratory tract infections. Ultrastructural analysis showed the cilia of Kartegener's patients to have absent or altered dynein.

The Nodal Flow Model

In early mouse embryos, at around E7.5, expression of the *lrd* gene is restricted to the node, an important organizer region. Of interest, the outer cells of the node each contain a single cilium. A breakthrough in understanding came when the cilia of the node were shown to move in a manner that generated a leftward flow of fluid. A **nodal flow model** of left-right development was proposed (Fig. 9–23). According to this model, the leftward movement of fluid across the node generates an asymmetric distribution of a **morphogen,** which has not yet been identified. The resulting left-right morphogen gradient breaks symmetry and initiates a genetic cascade of left-right development.

Although the nodal flow model cannot be considered firmly established, there is some important evidence supporting it. Mice mutant for either the kinesin gene *Kif3A* or *Kif3B* have nodal cells without cilia and altered left-fight development. Kinesins are functionally similar to dyneins in that

they generate motive force along microtubules (although generally in the opposite direction). These results indicate the *Kif3A* and *Kif3B* genes are required for node cilia assembly and suggest the cilia are in turn necessary for normal left-right development.

In addition, mice with a mutation in the *lrd* gene were found to have immotile nodal cilia. This argued that not just the presence but the movement of the nodal cilia is critically important for normal left-right development, again consistent with the nodal flow model. Alternative models have proposed as yet unproved intracellular functions for the *Kif3A*, *Kif3B*, and *lrd* genes in generating a left-right morphogen gradient. Polarized arrays of microtubules within the cells of the node

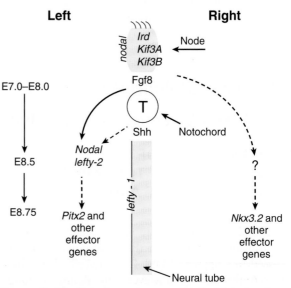

Figure 9–23. Genetic program of left-right development in mammals. The cilia of the node generate a leftward flow, creating an asymmetrical distribution of a morphogen, which may be Fgf8. The *lrd, Kif3A,* and *Kif3B* genes are all required for formation or function of the nodal cilia. T represents the *brachyury* gene, which is also required for normal left-sided expression of *nodal, lefty-1,* and *lefty-2.* Expression of *lefty-1* is restricted to the left side of the floor plate of the neural tube, whereas *nodal, lefty-2,* and *Pitx2* are expressed in the left lateral plate mesoderm. The homeobox gene, *Nkx3.2,* is expressed in the right lateral plate mesoderm. Approximate developmental time course is shown in days of gestation for the mouse at the left. (Modified from Supp DM, Potter SS, Brueckner M. 2000. Molecular motors: the driving force behind mammalian left-right development. Trends Cell Biol 10:43.)

could, for example, direct the asymmetric movement of morphogen through the node rather than across it.

Dozens of genes have now been implicated in the genetic program of left-right development in a variety of species. Here the focus is on genes shown to be of key importance in left-right axis formation in mammals.

Immediately following the onset of nodal flow, two Tgfβ growth factor family member genes, *nodal* and *lefty-1*, show asymmetric expression in the nodal region. The **nodal** gene is initially expressed throughout the node, but after the cilia establish a leftward fluid flow, expression of the *nodal* gene becomes restricted to the left side of the node in one of the first molecular manifestations of left-right asymmetry. The expression of *nodal* then extends to the left lateral plate mesoderm. Following asymmetric expression of **lefty-1** in the nodal region, its expression extends to the left side of the floor plate of the neural tube. A closely related gene, **lefty-2,** shows asymmetric expression in the left lateral plate mesoderm. The growth factor **Fgf8** has been shown to activate *nodal* and *lefty-2* expression, suggesting it might represent the morphogen the cilia move to the left.

Pitx2, a homeobox gene, is downstream of *nodal* and *lefty-2* in the genetic program of left-right development. *Pitx2* is also expressed on the left side, and it appears to be an effector gene, with its expression persisting later in development, during organogenesis. Haploinsufficiency (one wild type and one mutant allele) of the *Pitx2* gene in humans results in **Rieger syndrome,** with defects in eyes and teeth. There is abundant evidence from animal models, however, including mice homozygous for targeted null *Pitx2* mutations, indicating that there is an important function for *Pitx2* in the late phases of the laterality genetic cascade. One striking defect observed in *Pitx2* mutant mice, for example, is right lung isomerism (two right lungs). Normally, the two lungs of the mouse are quite distinct, with the left lung having a single lobe, and the right lung having four lobes. In the *Pitx2* mutant, however, both lungs have four lobes. On the left side, in the absence of *Pitx2* expression, a right lung develops.

The order of genes in a genetic program is often determined by examining gene expression patterns in mutants. For example, if gene A activates gene B, which activates gene C in a program,

then mutation of gene B would alter the expression of gene C but not gene A. In this manner, the *lrd* gene was shown to occupy a high-level position in the genetic hierarchy of left-right development. In the *lrd* gene mutants, the expression patterns of *nodal*, *lefty-1*, *lefty-2*, and *Pitx2* are all altered, indicating they are downstream of *lrd*. The expression of *nodal*, for example, is randomized in *lrd/lrd* mutants. One fourth of *lrd/lrd* mutant embryos show normal nodal expression only on the left, and one fourth show reversed expression only on the right. Interestingly, one fourth show expression on both sides and one fourth show expression on neither side.

Additional Genetic Components of the Left-Right Pathway

Early groundbreaking work in the chicken embryo system provided the first genetic insight into left-right development. It was shown that an activin (Tgfβ family)-like activity restricted to the right side of the primitive streak suppresses sonic hedgehog (SHH) expression on the right and induces expression of an activin receptor **cAct-RIIa.** The remaining SHH expression on the left was shown to induce downstream left-side expression of the chicken *nodal* gene. Although the precise pathways of left-right development may be distinct in chickens and mammals, there is genetic evidence for an important role for these genes in mammals as well. SHH, for example, has not been observed to be expressed asymmetrically in mammals, yet the *SHH* mutant mouse shows a number of laterality defects, including left lungs on both sides (pulmonary left isomerism), altered embryonic turning, and absence of expression of the *lefty-1* gene, which is apparently, therefore, downstream of SHH.

In summary, the left-right axis is the last to show asymmetry. Molecular motor proteins of the node are required for normal left-right development. The vortical motion of the nodal cilia appears to create an asymmetrical left-right morphogen distribution in the fluid surrounding the embryo. This results in the left-specific expression of *nodal*, *lefty-1*, and *lefty-2*, which in turn activates left specific expression of further downstream genes such as *Pitx2*. Many other genes are of known importance in establishing correct laterality in mammals, including *Nkx3.2*, *Smad5*, *inv*, *SIL*, *Activin βB*, and *brachyury*. Indeed, the genetic regulatory interactions driving correct left-right development are being discovered at a remarkable pace.

The Molecular Mechanism That Regulates Asymmetric Expression of Nodal May Explain Patterns of Situs in Conjoined Twins

Twinning experiments on newt embryos also support the idea that the biasing mechanism is set very early. If a newt morula is constricted in the middle, it develops into a pair of conjoined twins. Interestingly, the twin developing from the left half of the embryo always exhibits normal situs, whereas half of the twins on the right side exhibit situs inversus. Remarkably, the situs patterns of these experimental newt twins appear to be shared by human conjoined dicephalic twins (conjoined twins joined in the thoracic region with separate heads), although data are limited because the condition is exceedingly rare. Situs of the left twin is always normal, whereas situs of the right twin may be normal or reversed. Because the primitive streaks of these conjoined embryos develop in close proximity, Tabin has suggested that disturbance of situs in the right-hand twin may result from suppression of its left-sided hedgehog (and/or nodal) expression by an activin-like activity expressed on the right side of the left twin's primi-

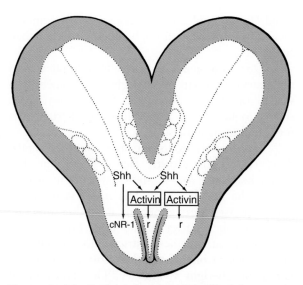

Figure 9–24. Conjoined twins. (Modified from Levin M, Johnson RL, Stern CD et al. 1995. A molecular pathway determining left-right asymmetry in chick embryogenesis. Cell 82:803. Modification based on personal communication from Dr. Clifford Tabin.)

tive streak (Fig. 9–24). Expression of hedgehog (and/or nodal) would then be absent on both sides of the right twin's streak, leading to randomization of situs. Hedgehog and/or nodal and activin expression would still occur in the normal asymmetric pattern in the vicinity of the left embryo's streak, resulting in normal situs 100 percent of the time.

SUGGESTED READING

Descriptive Embryology

Alpert S, Hanahan D, Teitelman G. 1988. Hybrid insulin genes reveal a developmental lineage for pancreatic endocrine cells and imply a relationship with neurons. Cell 53:295

Gordon JI. 1989. Intestinal epithelial differentiation: new insights from chimeric and transgenic mice. J Cell Biol 108:1187

Kanagasuntherum R. 1957. Development of the human lesser sac. J Anat 91:188

Le Douarin NM. 1988. On the origin of pancreatic exocrine cells. Cell 53:169

Moutsouris C. 1966. The "solid stage" and congenital intestinal atresia. J Pediatr Surg 1:446

O'Rahilly R. 1978. The timing and sequence of events in the development of the human digestive system and associated structures during the embryonic period proper. Anat Embryol 153:123

O'Rahilly R, Müller F. 1987. Developmental stages in human embryos. Carnegie Inst Wash Publ 637:1

Reddy S, Elliot RB. 1988. Ontogenic development of peptide hormones in the mammalian fetal pancreas. Experientia 44:1

Severn CB. 1972. A morphological study of the development of the human liver. I. Development of the hepatic diverticulum. Am J Anat 131:133

Severn CB. 1972. A morphological study of the human liver. II. Establishment of liver parenchyma, extrahepatic ducts, and associated venous channels. Am J Anat 133:85

Stephens FD. 1988. Embryology of the cloaca and anorectal malformations. Birth Defects Orig Artic Ser 24:177

Vellguth S, van Gaudecker B, Muller-Hermelink H-K. 1985. The development of the human spleen. Cell Tissue Res 242:579

Yassine F, Fedecka-Bruner B, Dieterlen-Lievre F. 1989. Ontogeny of the chick embryo spleen. Cell Differ Dev 27:29

Yokoh Y. 1970. Differentiation of the dorsal mesentery in man. Acta Anat 76:56

Clinical Applications

Agatstein E, Stabile B. 1984. Peritonitis due to intraperitoneal perforation of infected urachal cysts. Arch Surg 119:1269

Akintan B, Adekunle A. 1985. A fatal case of ruptured infected urachal cyst. Int Urol Nephrol 17:133

Brown CK, Olshaker JS. 1988. Meckel's diverticulum. Am J Emerg Med 6:157

de Vries PA. 1980. The pathogenesis of gastroschisis and omphalocele. J Pediatr Surg 15:245

Dott NM. 1923. Anomalies of intestinal rotation and fixation: their embryology and surgical aspects; with report of five cases. Br J Surg 2:251

Estrada RL. 1958. Anomalies of Intestinal Rotation and Fixation. p. 1. Charles C Thomas, Springfield, IL

Frazer JE, Robbins RH. 1915. On the factors concerned in causing rotation of the intestine in man. J Anat Physiol 50:75

Lodeiro JG, Byers JW, Chuipek S, Feinstein SJ. 1989. Prenatal diagnosis and prenatal management of the Beckwith-Wiedeman syndrome: a case and review. Am J Perinatol 6:446

Mall FP. 1898. Development of the human intestine and its position in the adult. Bull Johns Hopkins Hosp 9:197

Marshall VF, Muecke EC. 1962. Variations in exstrophy of the bladder. J Urol 88:766

Muecke EC. 1964. The role of the cloacal membrane in exstrophy: the first successful experimental study. J Urol 92:659

Pringle KC. 1988. Abdominal wall defects and obstructive uropathies. Fetal Ther 3:67

Reyes HM, Meller JL, Loeff D. 1989. Neonatal intestinal obstruction. Clin Perinatol 16:85

Synder WH, Chaffin L. 1954. Embryology and pathology of the intestinal tract: presentation of 40 cases of malrotation. Ann Surg 140:368

Thomalla JV, Rudolph RA, Rink R, Mitchell ME. 1985. Induction of cloacal exstrophy in the chick embryo using the CO_2 laser. J Urol 134:991

Torfs C, Curry C, Roeper P. 1990. Gastroschisis. J Pediatr 116:1

Vane DW, West KW, Grosfeld JL. 1987. Vitelline duct anomalies. Arch Surg 122:542

Experimental Principles

Afzelius BA. 1976. A human syndrome caused by immotile cilia. Science 193:317

Almirantis Y. 1995. Left-right asymmetry in vertebrates. Bioessays 17:79

Britz-Cunningham SH, Shah MM, Zuppan CW, Fletcher WH. 1995. Mutations of the connexin 43 gap junction gene in patients with heart malformation and defects of laterality. N Engl J Med 332:1323

Brown NA, Hoyle C, McCarthy A, Wolpert L. 1989. The development of asymmetry: the sidedness of drug induced limb abnormalities is reversed in situs inversus mice. Development 107:637

Brown NA, Lander A. 1993. On the other hand. . . . Nature 363:303

Brown NA, Wolpert L. 1990. The development of handedness in left/right symmetry. Development 109:1

Brueckner M, D'Eustachio P, Horwich AL. 1989. Linkage mapping of a mouse gene, iv, that controls left-right asymmetry of the heart and viscera. Proc Natl Acad Sci U S A 86:5035

Capdevila J, Vogan KJ, Tabin CJ, Izpisua Belmonte JC. 2000. Mechanisms of left-right determination in vertebrates. Cell 101:9

Collignon J, Varlet I, Robertson EJ. 1996. Relationship between asymmetric nodal expression and the direction of embryonic turning. Nature 381:155

Collins RL. 1975. When left-handed mice live in right-handed worlds. Science 187:181

Cooke, J. 1995. Vertebrate embryo handedness. Nature 374:681

Danos MC, Jost HJ. 1995. Linkage of cardiac left-right asymmetry and dorsal-anterior development in Xenopus. Development 121:1467

Ewing T. 1993. Genetic "master switch" for left-right asymmetry found. Science 260:624

Galloway J. 1990. A handle on handedness. Nature (London) 346:223

Gurdon JB. 1992. The generation of diversity and pattern in animal development. Cell 68:185

Hoyle C, Brown NA, Wolpert L. 1992. Development of left/right handedness in the chick heart. Development 115:1071

Hummel KP, Chapman DB. 1959. Visceral inversion and associated anomalies in the mouse. J Hered 50:10

Klar AJS. 1994. A model for specification of the left-right axis in vertebrates. TIG 10:392

Layton WM. 1976. Random determination of a developmental process. J Hered 67:336

Levin M, Johnson RL, Stern CD, et al. 1995. A molecular pathway determining left-right asymmetry in chick embryogenesis. Cell 82:803

Lowe L, Supp DM, Sampath K, et al. 1996. Conserved

left-right asymmetry of nodal expression and alterations in murine situs inversus. Nature 381:158

Meno C, Saijoh Y, Fujii H, et al. 1996. Left-right asymmetric expression of the TGFβ-family member lefty in mouse embryos. Nature 381:151

Morgan M. 1977. Embryology and inheritance of asymmetry. p. 173. In Harnad S, Doty RW, Jaynes J, et al. (eds): Lateralization in the Nervous System. Academic Press, San Diego

Nonaka S, Tanaka Y, Okada Y, et al. 1998. Randomization of left-right asymmetry due to loss of nodal cilia generating leftward flow of extraembryonic fluid in mice lacking KIF3B motor protein. Cell 95:829

Roush W. 1995. Embryos travel forking path as they tell left from right. Science 269:1514

Ryan AK, Blumberg B, Rodriguez-Esteban C, et al. 1998. *Pitx2* determines left-right asymmetry of internal organs in vertebrates. Nature 394:545

Siebert JR, Machin GA, Sperber GH. 1989. Anatomic findings in dicephalic conjoined twins: implications for morphogenesis. Teratology 40:305

Stalsburg H. 1969. The origin of heart asymmetry: right and left contributions to the early chick embryo heart. Dev Biol 19:100

Stalsberg H. 1970. Mechanism of dextral looping of the embryonic heart. Am J Cardiol 25:265

Supp DM, Brueckner M, Kuehn MR, et al. 1999 Targeted deletion of the ATP binding domain of left-right dynein confirms its role in specifying development of left-right asymmetries. Development 126:5495

Supp DM, Potter SS, Brueckner M. 2000. Molecular motors: the driving force behind mammalian left-right development. Trends Cell Biol 10:41

Supp D, Witte DP, Potter SS, Brueckner M. 1997. Mutation of an axonemal dynein affects left-right asymmetry in *inversus viscerum* mice. Nature 389:963

Wolpert L, Brown NA. 1995. Hedgehog keeps to the left. Nature 377:103

Yokoyama T, Copeland N, Jenkins NA, et al. 1993. Reversal of left-right asymmetry: a situs inversus mutation. Science 260:679

Yost HJ. 1992. Regulation of vertebrate left-right asymmetries by extracellular matrix. Nature 357:158

10

Development of the Urogenital System

Summary

As important to survival on dry land as the lungs, the **urinary system** maintains the electrolyte and water balance of the body fluids that bathe the tissues in a salty, aqueous environment. The development of this system, as in the case of the pharyngeal arches discussed in other chapters, involves the transient formation and subsequent regression or remodeling of vestigial primitive systems, thereby providing a glimpse of evolutionary history. The development of the **genital system** is closely integrated with these primitive urinary organs in both males and females. This chapter therefore describes the development of the urinary system before turning to the genital system.

The intermediate mesoderm on either side of the dorsal body wall gives rise to three successive nephric structures of increasingly advanced design. The first is a small group of transitory, nonfunctional, segmental **nephrotomes,** which develop in the cervical region. These structures presumably represent a vestige of the **pronephroi** or primitive kidneys, which develop in some lower vertebrates. As these cranial nephrotomes regress in the fourth week, they are succeeded by a pair of elongated **mesonephroi,** which develop in the thoracic and lumbar regions. The mesonephroi are functional, having complete although simple nephrons. The mesonephroi are drained by a pair of **mesonephric (Wolffian) ducts,** which grow caudally to open into the posterior wall of the primitive urogenital sinus. By the fifth week, a pair of **ureteric buds** sprout from the distal mesonephric ducts and induce the overlying sacral intermediate mesoderm to develop into the **metanephroi** or definitive kidneys.

As described in the preceding chapter, the cloaca (the distal expansion of the hindgut) is partitioned into a posterior rectum and an anterior primitive urogenital sinus, the latter continuous superiorly with the allantois. The expanded superior portion of the primitive urogenital sinus becomes the bladder, whereas its inferior portion gives rise (in males) to the **pelvic urethra** and to the **penile urethra** and (in females) to the pelvic urethra and **vestibule of the vagina.** During this period, the openings of the mesonephric ducts are translocated down onto the pelvic urethra by a process that also emplaces the openings of ureters on the bladder wall.

By the sixth week, the germ cells migrating from the yolk sac begin to arrive in the mesenchyme of the posterior body wall. The arrival of germ cells in the area just medial to the mesonephroi at the 10th thoracic segment induces cells of the mesonephros and adjacent coelomic epithelium to aggregate into **somatic sex cords** that invest the germ cells. Cells

Development of the Cervical Nephrotomes, Mesonephric and Metanephric Kidneys, and Urogenital Duct Systems

Development of the Gonads and Genitalia

Intermediate mesoderm

Weeks   Days

— 19

3 —

— 24

By 28 days, the metanephric
blastemas and ureteric buds
appear

— 26

4 —   — 28

At 24 days, cervical
nephrotomes begin to appear;
at 26 days, mesonephros
and mesonephric duct
begin to differentiate

— 32

Ureteric bud enters
metanephric blastema
and bifurcates

5 —   — 35

Major calyces form

Kidneys ascend

6 —   — 42

Metanephric tissue caps on
terminal collecting ducts
begin to form nephric vesicles

Minor calyces form

7 —   — 50

Nephric vesicles differentiate to form
nephrons; each nephron becomes
functional as its distal convoluted tubule
joins with the collecting duct

10 —

12 —

Surface of kidney exhibits lobes

16 —

Mesonephric ducts exstrophy into
the posterior wall of the bladder.
Exstrophy emplaces the ureters
into the bladder wall, while the
mesonephric ducts are carried down
to the pelvic urethra. The region of
exstrophied duct becomes the
bladder trigone

20 —

Collecting duct system complete

32 —

38 —

Timeline. Development of the urinary system.

Weeks

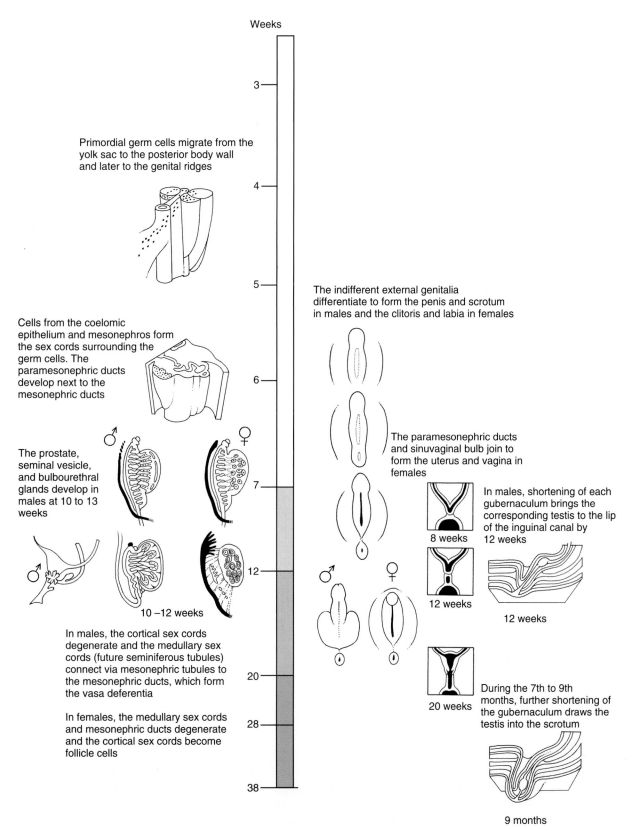

Primordial germ cells migrate from the yolk sac to the posterior body wall and later to the genital ridges

Cells from the coelomic epithelium and mesonephros form the sex cords surrounding the germ cells. The paramesonephric ducts develop next to the mesonephric ducts

The prostate, seminal vesicle, and bulbourethral glands develop in males at 10 to 13 weeks

10 –12 weeks

In males, the cortical sex cords degenerate and the medullary sex cords (future seminiferous tubules) connect via mesonephric tubules to the mesonephric ducts, which form the vasa deferentia

In females, the medullary sex cords and mesonephric ducts degenerate and the cortical sex cords become follicle cells

The indifferent external genitalia differentiate to form the penis and scrotum in males and the clitoris and labia in females

The paramesonephric ducts and sinuvaginal bulb join to form the uterus and vagina in females

In males, shortening of each gubernaculum brings the corresponding testis to the lip of the inguinal canal by 12 weeks

8 weeks

12 weeks

12 weeks

20 weeks

During the 7th to 9th months, further shortening of the gubernaculum draws the testis into the scrotum

9 months

Timeline. Development of the genital system.

of these sex cords will differentiate into Sertoli cells in the male and into follicle cells in the female. During the same period, a new pair of ducts, the **paramesonephric (müllerian) ducts,** form in the dorsal body wall just lateral to the mesonephric ducts.

The sexual differentiation of genetic males begins at the end of the sixth week, when a specific gene on the Y chromosome (SRY) is expressed in the sex cord cells. Embryos in which this gene is not expressed develop as females, even if a Y chromosome is present. The product of this gene, called the **SRY protein,** initiates a **developmental cascade** that leads to the formation of the testes, the male genital ducts and associated glands, the male external genitalia, and the entire constellation of male secondary sex characteristics. The SRY protein exerts autonomous control of sex cord cell development. The cortical (peripheral) portions of the sex cords degenerate, whereas the medullary (deep) portions differentiate into pre-Sertoli cells, which will form the seminiferous tubules. The deepest portions of the sex cords, which do not contain germ cells, differentiate into the rete testis. The rete testis connects with a limited number of mesonephric tubules and canalizes at puberty to form conduits connecting the seminiferous tubules to the mesonephric duct. These nephric tubules become the efferent ductules of the testes, and the mesonephric ducts become the vasa deferentia (singular, vas deferens). The paramesonephric ducts degenerate. During the third month, the distal vas deferens sprouts the seminal vesicle, and the prostate and bulbourethral glands grow from the adjacent pelvic urethra. Simultaneously, the indifferent external genitalia (consisting of paired **urogenital** and **labioscrotal folds** on either side of the urogenital membrane and an anterior **genital tubercle**) differentiate into the penis and scrotum. Late in fetal development, the testes descend into the scrotum through the **inguinal canals.**

In genetic females who lack a Y chromosome and therefore do not produce the SRY protein, the primitive sex cords degenerate, whereas secondary cortical cords proliferate to form the follicles of the ovary. The mesonephric ducts also degenerate, and the paramesonephric ducts become the genital ducts. The proximal portions of these ducts become the oviducts (fallopian tubes). Fusion of the distal portions of the ducts gives rise to the uterus and superior vagina; the inferior portion of the vagina develops from a pair of endodermal **sinuvaginal bulbs** that develop on the posterior wall of the primitive urogenital sinus. The indifferent external genitalia develop into the female external genitals: the clitoris and the paired labia majora and minora.

THREE NEPHRIC SYSTEMS DEVELOP IN CRANIOCAUDAL SEQUENCE

Recall from Chapter 3 that the mesoderm deposited on either side of the midline during gastrulation differentiates into three subdivisions: the paraxial, intermediate, and lateral plate mesoderm (Fig. 10–1). The fates of the paraxial and lateral plate mesoderm are discussed in other chapters. The intermediate mesoderm gives rise to the nephric structures of the embryo, to portions of the gonads, and to the male genital duct system. During embryonic development, three sets of nephric structures develop in craniocaudal succession from the intermediate mesoderm. These are called the **cervical nephrotomes,** the **mesonephroi,** and the **metanephroi** or definitive kidneys.

The Cervical Nephrotomes Are Transient and Nonfunctional

Early in the fourth week, each of five to seven paired cervical segments of intermediate mesoderm gives rise to a small, hollow ball of epithelium called a **nephric vesicle** or **nephrotome** (Fig. 10–2A). Many authors refer to the series of cervical nephrotomes on each side as a **pronephros** (plural, pronephroi; derived from the Greek for first kidney) because they resemble the functional embryonic pronephroi of some lower vertebrates. In humans, however, these units do not differentiate into the primitive but functional excretory structures of a true pronephros, but instead cease developing at the nephrotome stage and therefore seem to be nonfunctional and vestigial. They disappear by day 24 or 25.

The Mesonephroi May Function as Embryonic Kidneys and Also Contribute to the Male Genital System

The next structures to form in the intermediate mesoderm are the **mesonephroi** (singular, mesonephros) and associated **mesonephric ducts.** Early in the fourth week, **nephric tubules** begin to develop within a pair of elongated swellings of intermediate mesoderm located on either side of the

Figure 10–1. The intermediate mesoderm gives rise to paired, segmentally organized nephrotomes from the cervical to the sacral region. Cervical nephrotomes are initially formed early in the fourth week and are sometimes referred to collectively as the pronephros.

vertebral column from the upper thoracic region to the third lumbar level (see Fig. 10–2B–D). These swellings are called the mesonephroi or mesonephric ridges. About 40 mesonephric tubules are produced in craniocaudal succession; thus, several form in each segment. As the more caudal tubules differentiate, however, the more cranial ones regress, so there are never more than about 30 pairs in the mesonephroi. By the end of the fifth week, the cranial regions of the mesonephroi undergo massive regression, leaving only about 20 pairs of tubules occupying the first three lumbar levels.

The mesonephric tubules differentiate into

excretory units that resemble an abbreviated version of the adult nephron (see Fig. 10–2D). The medial end of the tubule forms a cup-shaped sac, called a **Bowman's capsule,** which wraps around a knot of capillaries called a **glomerulus** to form a **renal corpuscle.** The glomeruli are produced on branches of arteries sprouting from the dorsal aorta. Each renal corpuscle and nephric tubule is collectively called a **mesonephric excretory unit.**

The **mesonephric ducts** first appear at about 24 days in the form of a pair of solid longitudinal rods that condense in the intermediate mesoderm of the thoracic region dorsolateral to the developing mesonephric tubules (Fig. 10–3; see also Fig. 10–2A). These rods grow caudally through the proliferation and migration of the cells at their caudal tips. (The growth of the rods may be induced and guided by an adhesion gradient within the extracellular matrix between the ectoderm and endoderm.) As the rods grow into the lower lumbar region, they diverge from the intermediate mesoderm and then grow to and fuse with the ventrolateral walls of the cloaca on day 26 (Fig. 10–4; see also Fig. 10–2 and Ch. 9 and later in this chapter). This region of fusion will become a part of the posterior wall of the future bladder. As the rods fuse with the cloaca, they begin to cavitate at their distal ends to form a lumen. This process of canalization progresses cranially, transforming the rods into the mesonephric ducts.

The lateral tip of each mesonephric tubule fuses with the mesonephric duct, thus opening a passage from the excretory units to the cloaca. The mesonephric excretory units are functional between about 6 and 10 weeks and produce small amounts of urine. After 10 weeks, they cease to function and then regress. As discussed later, the mesonephric ducts also regress in the female. In the male, however, the mesonephric ducts plus a few modified mesonephric tubules persist and form important elements of the male genital duct system.

The Definitive Metanephroi Are Induced Early in the Fifth Week by Ureteric Buds That Sprout From the Mesonephric Ducts

The definitive kidneys or **metanephroi** are induced to form in the intermediate mesoderm of the sacral region by a pair of new structures, the

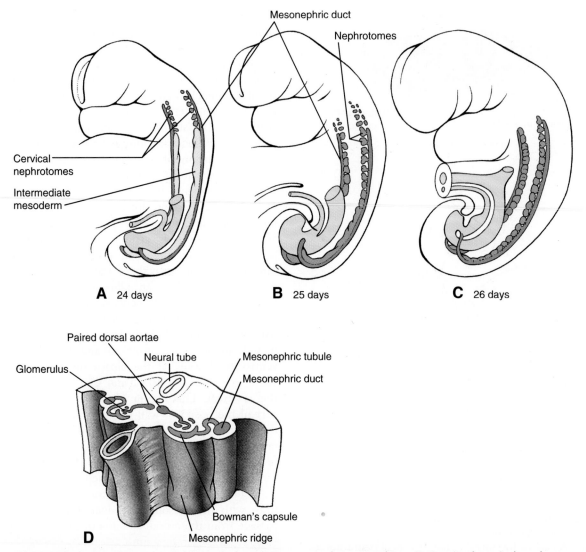

Figure 10–2. Development of the cervical nephrotomes and mesonephros. *A*, A pair of cervical nephrotomes forms in each of five to seven cervical segments, but these quickly degenerate during the fourth week. The mesonephric ducts first appear on day 24. *B, C,* Mesonephric nephrotomes and tubules form in craniocaudal sequence throughout the thoracic and lumbar regions. The more cranial pairs regress as caudal pairs form, and the definitive mesonephroi contain about 20 pairs confined to the first three lumbar segments. *D*, The mesonephroi contain functional nephric units consisting of glomeruli, Bowman's capsules, mesonephric tubules, and mesonephric ducts.

ureteric buds, which sprout from the distal portion of the mesonephric ducts on about day 28 (see Fig. 10–4*A*). On about day 32, each ureteric bud penetrates a portion of the sacral intermediate mesoderm called the **metanephric blastema** and begins to bifurcate (see Fig. 10–4*B*). As the ureteric bud branches, each new growing tip (called

an **ampulla**) acquires a caplike aggregate of metanephric blastema tissue, giving the metanephros a lobulated appearance. By the middle of the sixth week, the developing metanephros consists of two lobes separated by a sulcus, and, by the end of the 16th week, 14 to 16 lobes have formed (see Fig. 10–4*C, D*). The evidence of these initial

Figure 10–3. Scanning electron micrograph showing a growing mesonephric duct just adjacent to the somites (S) on one side of an embryo (arrows). The duct is elongating in a craniocaudal direction. (Photo courtesy of Dr. Thomas J. Poole.)

branchings of the ureteric bud are eventually obscured as the sulci between the lobes are filled in.

The Ureteric Bud and Metanephric Blastema Exert Reciprocal Inductive Effects. The ureters and the collecting duct system of the kidneys differentiate from the ureteric bud, whereas the **nephrons** (the definitive urine-forming units of the kidneys) differentiate from the metanephric blastema. The differentiation of each of these primordia depends on inductive signals from the other. In fact, the interaction between the ureteric bud and the metanephric blastema is one of the classic models of induction. Several hours of direct contact with a ureteric bud ampulla are required to induce nephron differentiation in blastema tissue. If the ureteric bud is abnormal or missing, the kidney does not develop. Conversely, reciprocal inductive signals from the metanephric blastema regulate the orderly branching and growth of the bifurcating tips of the ureteric buds. (Molecular elements of this inductive system are described in the Experimental Principles section of this chapter.)

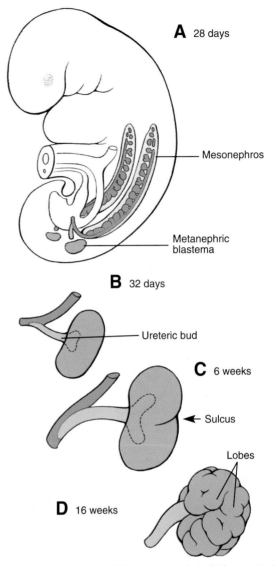

Figure 10–4. Origin of the metanephric kidneys. *A,* A metanephric blastema develops from intermediate mesoderm on each side of the body axis early in the fifth week. *B,* Simultaneously, the metanephric ducts sprout ureteric buds that grow into each metanephric blastema. *C,* By the sixth week, the ureteric bud bifurcates and the two growing tips (ampullae) induce superior and inferior lobes in the metanephros. *D,* Additional lobules form during the next 10 weeks in response to further bifurcation of the ureteric buds.

The Collecting Duct System Is Produced by Sequential Bifurcation of the Ureteric Bud. In the mature kidney, the urine produced by the nephrons flows through a collecting duct system consisting of collecting tubules, minor calyces, major calyces, the renal pelvis, and, finally, the ureter. This system is entirely the product of the ureteric bud. The ureteric bud undergoes an exact sequence of bifurcations (Fig. 10–5), and the expanded major and minor calyces arise through phases of intussusception in which previously formed branches coalesce.

When the ureteric bud first contacts the metanephric blastema, its tip expands to form an initial ampulla that will give rise to the **renal pelvis.** During the sixth week, the ureteric bud bifurcates four times, yielding 16 branches. These branches then coalesce to form two to four **major calyces** extending from the renal pelvis. By the seventh week, the next four generations of branches also coalesce, forming the **minor calyces.** By 32 weeks, approximately 11 additional generations of bifurcation have formed one to three mil-

Figure 10–5. Development of the renal pelvis and calyces. *A–C,* The first bifurcation of the ureteric bud forms the renal pelvis, and the collapse of the next four generations of bifurcations produces the major calyces. *D, E,* The next four generations of bifurcation collapse to form the minor calyces of the renal collecting system.

lion branches, which will become the future **collecting tubules (collecting ducts)** of the kidney (Fig. 10–6*A*). The definitive morphology of the collecting ducts is created by variations in the pattern of branching and by a tendency for distal branches to elongate.

Each nephron originates as a vesicle within the blastemic cap surrounding the ampulla of a collecting duct (see Fig. 10–6*B*). As this vesicle elongates into a tubule, a capillary glomerulus forms near one end of it. The tubule epithelium near the differentiating glomerulus thins and then invaginates to form a Bowman's capsule that surrounds the glomerulus. As in the mesonephros, the unit consisting of the Bowman's capsule and the glomerulus is called a **renal corpuscle.** While the renal corpuscle is forming, the lengthening nephric

tubule differentiates to form the remaining elements of the nephron: the proximal convoluted tubule, the descending and ascending limbs of the loop of Henle, and the distal convoluted tubule. The definitive nephron with its renal corpuscle is also called a **metanephric excretory unit.**

During the 10th week, the tips of the distal convoluted tubules connect to the collecting ducts, and the metanephroi become functional. Blood plasma from the glomerular capillaries is filtered by the renal corpuscle to produce a dilute glomerular filtrate, which is concentrated and converted to urine by the activities of the convoluted tubules and the loop of Henle. The urine passes down the collecting system into the ureters and thence into the bladder. Even though the fetal kidneys produce urine throughout the remainder of gestation, their

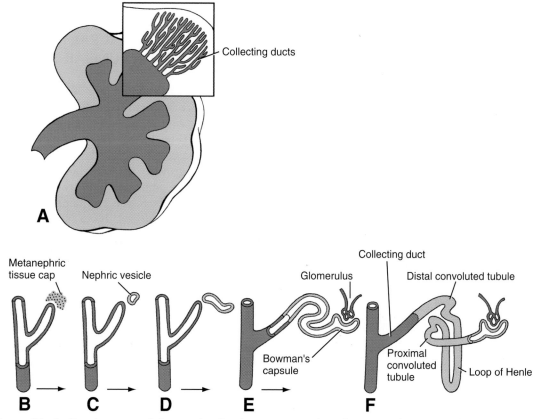

Figure 10–6. Development of the renal collecting system and nephrons. *A,* The ureteric buds continue to bifurcate until the 32nd week, producing 1 to 3 million collecting ducts. *B–F,* The tip of each collecting duct induces the development of a metanephric tissue cap, which differentiates into a renal vesicle. This vesicle ultimately forms a Bowman's capsule and the proximal and distal convoluted tubules and loops of Henle. Functional nephric units (of the type shown in 10–6*E*) first appear in distal regions of the metanephros at 10 weeks.

main function is not to clear waste products out of the blood—that task is handled principally by the placenta. Instead, fetal urine is important because it supplements the production of amniotic fluid. Fetuses with bilateral renal agenesis (complete absence of both kidneys) do not make enough amniotic fluid and hence are confined in an abnormally small amniotic space. The consequences of this condition of **oligohydramnios** were described in the Clinical Applications section of Chapter 6 and are discussed again in Chapter 15.

The Definitive Kidney Architecture Is Created Between Weeks 5 and 15.

Figure 10–7 shows the structure of the definitive fetal kidney. This architecture reflects the events of the first 10 weeks of renal development, that is, weeks 5 to 15 of development. The kidney is divided into an inner medulla and an outer cortex. The cortical tissue contains the nephrons, whereas the medulla contains collecting ducts and loops of Henle. Each minor calyx drains a tree of collecting ducts within

a **renal pyramid,** which converge to form the **renal papilla** (see Fig. 10–7). The renal pyramids of the kidney are separated by zones of nephron-containing cortical tissue called **renal columns** or **columns of Bertin.** In the definitive kidney, the cortical tissue thus not only covers the outside of the kidney but also forms piers projecting toward the pelvis. The nephrons in the cortical tissue nevertheless all arise from the cortical regions of the primary lobes of the metanephric blastema.

The neurons of the kidney, which regulate blood flow and secretory function, arise from neural crest cells that invade the metanephroi early in their development. These neurons can be found at the tips of the metanephric tissue caps during the phase of nephron induction; in vitro experiments suggest that they play a role in this induction process.

THE KIDNEYS ASCEND FROM THEIR ORIGINAL SACRAL LOCATION TO A LUMBAR SITE

Between the sixth and ninth weeks, the kidneys ascend to a lumbar site just below the suprarenal glands, following a path just on either side of the dorsal aorta (Fig. 10–8). The mechanism responsible for this ascent is not understood, although the differential growth of the lumbar and sacral regions of the embryo may play a role. As described in Chapter 8, the ascending kidney is progressively revascularized by a series of arterial sprouts from the dorsal aorta, and the original renal artery in the sacral region disappears (see Fig. 8–6).

Several anomalies can arise from variations in this process of ascent. Occasionally, one or more of the transient inferior renal arteries fail to regress, resulting in the presence of **accessory renal arteries.** Rarely, a kidney completely fails to ascend, remaining as a **pelvic kidney** (see Fig. 10–8C). The inferior poles of the two metanephroi may fuse during the ascent, forming a U-shaped **horseshoe kidney** that crosses over the ventral side of the aorta. During ascent, this kidney becomes caught under the inferior mesenteric artery and therefore does not reach its normal site (see Fig. 10–8D). The right kidney usually does not

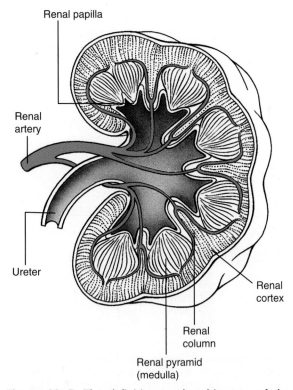

Renal papilla

Renal artery

Ureter

Renal cortex

Renal column

Renal pyramid (medulla)

Figure 10–7. The definitive renal architecture of the metanephros is apparent by the 10th week.

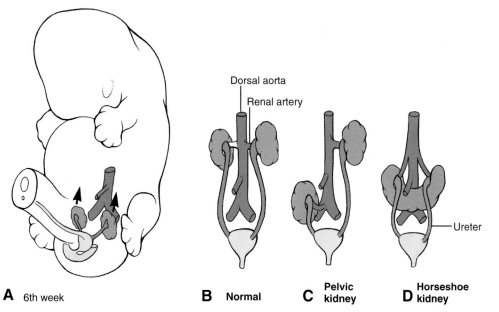

Figure 10–8. Normal and abnormal ascent of the kidneys. *A, B,* The metanephroi normally ascend from the sacral region to their definitive lumbar position between the sixth and ninth weeks. *C,* Infrequently, a kidney may fail to ascend, resulting in a pelvic kidney. *D,* If the inferior poles of the metanephroi make contact and fuse before ascent, the resulting horseshoe kidney catches under the inferior mesenteric artery.

rise as high as the left kidney because of the presence of the liver on the right side, although this is not always the case.

The Remainder of the Urinary Tract Differentiates From the Hindgut Endoderm

Recall from Chapter 9 that the cloacal expansion of the hindgut is partitioned by the urorectal septum into an anterior **primitive urogenital sinus** and a posterior rectum (Fig. 10–9). The primitive urogenital sinus is continuous superiorly with the **allantois** (a hindgut diverticulum that extends into the umbilicus) and is bounded inferiorly by the **urogenital membrane.** It consists of an expanded superior presumptive **bladder,** a narrow neck that becomes the **pelvic urethra,** and an inferior expanded **definitive urogenital sinus.** In males, the pelvic urethra becomes the **membranous** and **prostatic urethra** and the definitive urogenital sinus becomes the **penile urethra.** In females, the

pelvic urethra becomes the **membranous urethra,** and the definitive urogenital sinus becomes the **vestibule of the vagina.**

While the Primitive Urogenital Sinus Is Forming, the Mesonephric Ducts and Ureteric Buds Intercalate Into Its Posterior Wall

Concurrently with the septation of the cloaca by the growth of the urorectal septum, the distal portions of the mesonephric ducts and attached ureteric ducts become incorporated into the posterior wall of the presumptive bladder by a process called **exstrophy** (Fig. 10–10). (*Exstrophy* refers to the eversion of a hollow organ.) Exstrophy begins as the mouths of the mesonephric ducts flare into a pair of trumpet-shaped structures that begin to expand, flatten, and blend into the bladder wall. The superior portion of this trumpet expands and flattens more rapidly than the inferior part, so the mouth of the narrow portion of the mesonephric

Figure 10–9. Development of the primitive urogenital sinus. Between weeks 4 and 6, the urorectal septum splits the cloaca into an anterior primitive urogenital sinus and a posterior rectum. The superior part of the primitive urogenital sinus, continuous with the allantois, forms the bladder. The constricted pelvic urethra at the base of the future bladder forms the membranous urethra in females and the membranous and prostatic urethra in males. The distal expansion of the primitive urogenital sinus, the definitive urogenital sinus, forms the vestibule of the vagina in females and the penile urethra in males.

duct appears to migrate inferiorly along the posterior bladder wall. This process incorporates the distal ureters into the wall of the bladder and causes the mouths of the narrow part of the mesonephric ducts to migrate inferiorly until they open into the pelvic urethra just below the neck of the bladder. The triangular area of exstrophied mesonephric duct wall on the posteroinferior wall of the bladder is called the **trigone** of the bladder. The mesodermal tissue of the trigone is later overgrown by endoderm from the surrounding bladder wall, but the structure remains visible in the adult bladder as a smooth triangular region lying between the openings of the ureters laterally and superiorly and the opening of the pelvic urethra inferiorly. Splanchnopleuric mesoderm associated with the hindgut forms the smooth muscle of the bladder wall in the 12th week.

Several malformations can arise if the ureteric bud sprouts from an incorrect site along the mesonephric duct and therefore is incorrectly emplaced into the posterior wall of the bladder. The consequences of abnormal connection of the ureters are discussed in the Clinical Applications section of this chapter.

THE GENITAL SYSTEM ARISES IN CLOSE CONJUNCTION WITH THE URINARY SYSTEM

Gonadal development is limited in the absence of primordial germ cells that normally migrate from the yolk sac via the dorsal mesentery to populate the mesenchyme of the posterior body wall in the fifth week (Fig. 10–11*A*; see also Fig. 1–1). In both sexes, upon arrival of the primordial germ cells in the area of the future gonads at about the 10th thoracic level, cells in the mesonephros and adjacent coelomic epithelium proliferate and form a pair of **genital ridges** just medial to the developing mesonephroi (Fig. 10–12; see also Fig. 10–11*B, C*).

The Primitive Sex Cords Develop From Cells of the Mesonephros and Coelomic Epithelium

During the sixth week, cells from the mesonephros and coelomic epithelium invade the mesenchyme in the region of the presumptive gonads to form aggregates of supporting cells, the **primitive sex cords,** which completely invest the germ cells (see Fig. 10–11*C*). The genital ridge mesenchyme con-

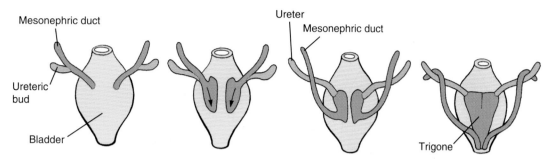

Figure 10–10. Exstrophy of the mesonephric ducts and ureters into the bladder wall. Between weeks 4 and 6, the root of the mesonephric duct exstrophies into the posterior wall of the developing bladder. This process brings the openings of the ureteric buds into the bladder wall, whereas the opening of the mesonephric duct is carried inferiorly to the level of the pelvic urethra. The triangular region of exstrophied mesonephric duct incorporated into the posterior bladder wall forms the trigone of the bladder.

taining the primitive sex cords is regarded as consisting of **cortical** and **medullary regions.** Both regions develop in all normal embryos, but after the sixth week, they pursue different fates in the male and female.

The Paramesonephric Ducts Form by Invagination of the Coelomic Epithelium

Also during the sixth week, a new pair of ducts, the **paramesonephric (müllerian) ducts,** begin to form just lateral to the mesonephric ducts in both male and female embryos (see Fig. 10–11*B, C*). These ducts arise by the craniocaudal invagination of a ribbon of thickened coelomic epithelium extending from the third thoracic segment caudally to the posterior wall of the urogenital sinus. For most of their length, these ducts are enclosed in the basement membrane of the adjacent mesonephric ducts. The caudal tips of the paramesonephric ducts then grow to connect with the pelvic urethra just medial to the openings of the right and left mesonephric ducts. The tips of the two paramesonephric ducts adhere to each other just before they contact the pelvic urethra. The superior ends of the paramesonephric ducts form funnel-shaped openings into the coelom. The further development of the paramesonephric ducts in the female is discussed later.

The Male and Female Genital Systems Are Virtually Identical Until the End of the Sixth Week

At the end of the sixth week, the male and female genital systems are indistinguishable in appearance, although subtle cellular differences may already be present. In both sexes, germ cells and sex cords are present in both the cortical and medullary regions of the presumptive gonads, and complete mesonephric and paramesonephric ducts lie side by side. The **ambisexual** or **indifferent phase** of genital development ends at this point and, from the seventh week on, the male and female systems pursue diverging pathways.

MALE DEVELOPMENT IS INSTIGATED BY A SINGLE FACTOR ENCODED ON THE Y CHROMOSOME; FEMALE DEVELOPMENT OCCURS IN ITS ABSENCE

The genetic basis of sex differentiation is now beginning to be understood (Fig. 10–13). As detailed in Chapter 1, genetic females have two X sex chromosomes, whereas genetic males have an X and a Y sex chromosome. Although the pattern of sex chromosomes determines the choice between male and female developmental paths, the subse-

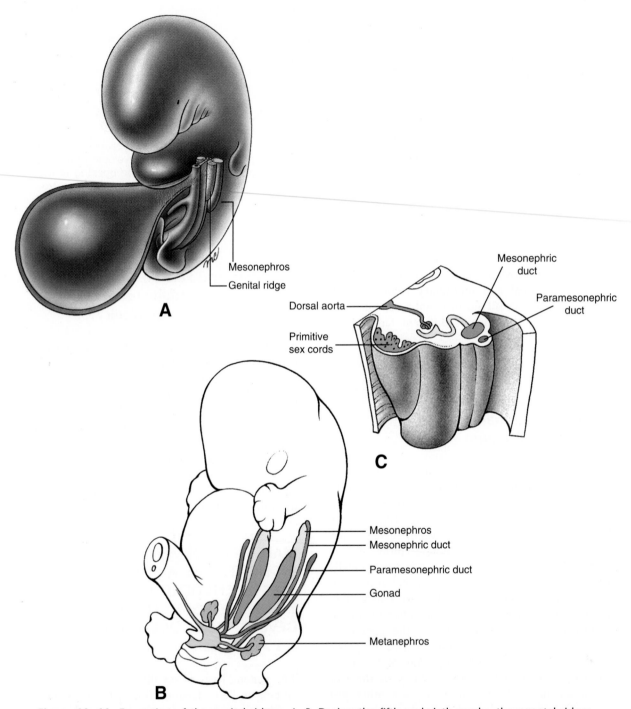

Figure 10–11. Formation of the genital ridges. *A, B,* During the fifth and sixth weeks, the genital ridges form in the posterior abdominal wall just medial to the developing mesonephroi in response to colonization by primordial germ cells migrating from the yolk sac. *C,* The primordial germ cells induce the coelomic epithelium lining the peritoneal cavity as well as cells of the mesonephros to proliferate and form the sex cords.

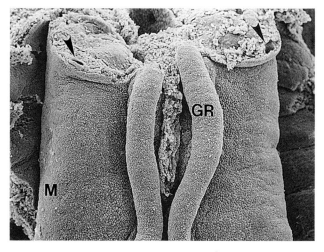

Figure 10–12. Scanning electron micrographs showing the relationship between the developing genital ridges (GR) and the mesonephroi (M). Arrowheads: Mesonephric ducts. (From Evan AP, Gattone VC II, Blomgren PM. 1984. Application of scanning electron microscopy to kidney development and nephron maturation. Scanning Electron Microsc 1:455.)

quent phases of sexual development are controlled not only by sex chromosome genes but also by hormones and other factors, most of which are encoded on the autosomes (see the Experimental Principles section of this chapter). A single sex-determining factor appears to control a cascade of events leading to male and female sexual dimorphism. This sex-determining transcription factor is encoded on the **sex-determining region of the Y chromosome (SRY).** When this factor is synthesized in the sex cord cells of the indifferent presumptive gonad, male development is triggered. If the factor is absent or defective, female development occurs. Thus, femaleness could be seen as the basic developmental path for the human embryo, which is followed unless maleness is actively induced. (The sex-determining protein is discussed further in the Experimental Principles section at the end of this chapter.)

Male Genital Development Begins With the Differentiation of Sertoli Cells in the Medullary Sex Cords

The first event in male genital development is the elaboration of SRY protein within the sex cord cells (see Fig. 10–13). Under the influence of this factor, cells in the *medullary* region of the primitive sex cords begin to differentiate into **Sertoli cells,** while the cells of the *cortical* sex cords degenerate (Fig. 10–14). Sex cord cells will differentiate into Sertoli cells only if they contain the SRY and produce SRY protein; if these are absent, the sex cords differentiate into ovarian follicles.

During the seventh week, the differentiating Sertoli cells organize to form the **testis cords** (Fig. 10–14). At puberty, the testis cords associated with the germ cells will become canalized and differentiate into a system of **seminiferous tubules.** The testis cords distal to the presumptive seminiferous tubules also develop lumina and differentiate into a set of thin-walled ducts called the **rete testis** at puberty. Just medial to the developing gonad, the tubules of the rete testis will become connected with 5 to 12 residual mesonephric tubules. Because these mesonephric tubules drain into the mesonephric duct, it is not surprising that the mesonephric ducts become the **spermatic ducts** or **vasa deferentia** (singular, vas deferens), as discussed later.

During the seventh week, the testis begins to round up, reducing its area of contact with the mesonephros (see Fig. 10–14). This physical isolation of the testis is important, because the mesonephros exerts a feminizing influence on the developing gonad. As the testes continue to develop, the degenerating cortical sex cords become separated from the coelomic epithelium by an intervening layer of connective tissue called the **tunica albuginea.**

In genetic males, the testis-determining factor gene in the sex-determining region (*SRY*) of the Y chromosome is expressed in the sex cord cells, resulting in the production of SRY protein. Genetic females lack this gene and do not produce SRY protein.

SRY Protein

In response to SRY protein, the cells of the medullary sex cords differentiate into Sertoli cells and secrete antimüllerian hormone (AMH), whereas the cells of the cortical sex cords degenerate.

AMH

Signal resulting from the expression of SRY protein causes mesenchymal cells in the gonadal ridge to differentiate into Leydig cells, which secrete testosterone.

AMH induces degeneration of the paramesonephric (müllerian) ducts.

Testosterone ⟶ **Dihydrotestosterone**

During fetal life, testosterone induces the male differentiation of many structures, including the genital duct system and the brain.

During fetal life, conversion of testosterone to dihydrotestosterone within the relevant target tissues causes the indifferent external genitalia to differentiate into a penis and scrotum and also induces the development or differentiation of some other male structures, such as the prostate.

The testosterone surge at puberty causes the seminiferous tubules to canalize, mature, and commence spermatogenesis, and induces the other pubertal changes in primary and secondary sexual characteristics.

Figure 10–13. Differentiation cascade of male genital system development.

Contact Between the Pre-Sertoli Cells and the Germ Cells Regulates the Development of the Male Gametes

Although the mechanism has not been elucidated, it is clear that direct cell-to-cell contact between pre-Sertoli cells and primordial germ cells within the medullary sex cords plays a key role in the development of the male gametes. This interaction occurs shortly after the arrival of the primordial germ cells in the region of the presumptive genital ridge. It has the immediate effect of inhibiting further mitosis and also prevents the germ cells from entering meiosis. The remaining phases of male

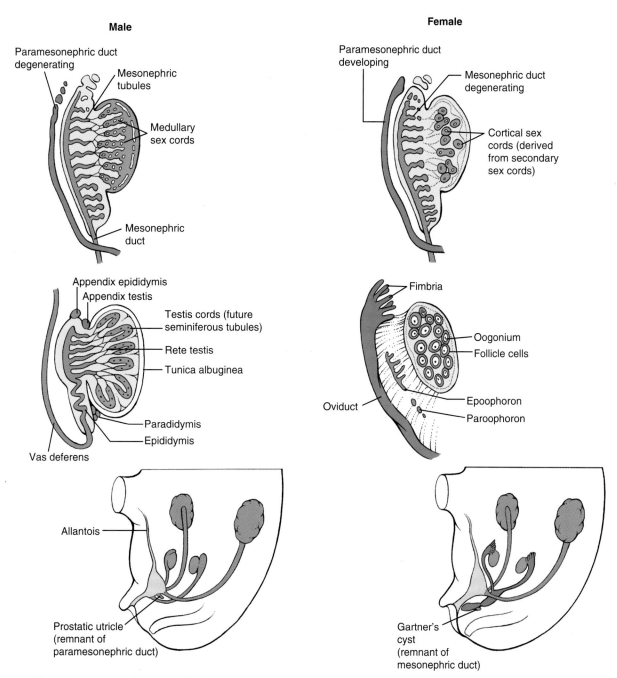

Figure 10–14. Male gonadal development compared with that of the female. The male and female genital systems are virtually identical through the seventh week. In the male, SRY protein produced by the pre-Sertoli cells causes the medullary sex cords to develop into presumptive seminiferous tubules and rete testis tubules and causes the cortical sex cords to regress. Antimüllerian hormone produced by the Sertoli cells then causes the paramesonephric ducts to regress and Leydig cells also develop, which in turn produce testosterone, the hormone that stimulates development of the male genital duct system, including the vas deferens and the presumptive efferent ductules. (See Fig. 10–16 for a description of female gonadal development.)

gametogenesis—further germ cell mitosis, differentiation into spermatogonia, meiosis, and spermatogenesis—are thus delayed until puberty (see Ch. 1).

Antimüllerian Hormone Secreted by the Pre-Sertoli Cells Controls Several Steps in Male Genital Development

As the pre-Sertoli cells begin their morphologic differentiation in response to SRY, they also begin to secrete a glycoprotein hormone called **antimüllerian hormone (AMH)** or **müllerian-inhibiting substance (MIS).** The protein portion of this hormone, which has been sequenced, turns out to closely resemble transforming growth factor-β, a molecule that has been implicated in a variety of developmental processes, including mesoderm induction (see the Experimental Principles section of Ch. 4) and angiogenesis (see the Experimental Principles section of Ch. 8).

AMH Causes the Paramesonephric Ducts to Regress in the Male. In male embryos, AMH secreted by the pre-Sertoli cells causes the paramesonephric (müllerian) ducts to regress rapidly between the eighth and tenth weeks (see Figs. 10–13 and 10–14). Small paramesonephric duct remnants can be detected in the adult male, however, including a small cap of tissue associated with the testis, called the **appendix testis,** and an expansion of the prostatic urethra called the **utriculus prostaticus** (see Fig. 10–14). In female embryos, as described later, the paramesonephric ducts do not regress.

The existence of AMH was first postulated in 1916 on the basis of the existence of **freemartin calves.** Freemartin calves are female calves that share the womb with a male twin. These calves possess ovaries, but, like their male twins, they lack the derivatives of the paramesonephric ducts and are therefore sterile. It was hypothesized that some substance (now known to be AMH) circulates from the bloodstream of the male calf to the bloodstream of the female calf and induces the paramesonephric ducts to regress.

Occasionally, genetic male humans have persistent paramesonephric ducts. In these individuals, AMH and AMH receptor gene mutations have been identified. This observation suggests that paramesonephric duct regression is an active process rather than a consequence of cessation of growth of the paramesonephric ducts.

AMH signaling appears to be indirect through interaction with the AMH receptor in the mesenchyme surrounding the paramesonephric duct. Upon receptor activation, mesenchyme-epithelial signaling induces duct regression. Epithelial to mesenchyme signaling is also important in this process to maintain AMHr expression in the mesenchyme. In the absence of normal Wnt7a expression in the duct, AMHr is not expressed in the mesenchyme, and paramesonephric structures do not regress in the male.

SRY Protein Initiates a Cascade That Induces the Differentiation of Testosterone-Secreting Leydig Cells in the Testis. In the ninth or tenth week, **Leydig cells** differentiate from mesenchymal cells within the genital ridges, probably in response to the expression of SRY protein by the pre-Sertoli cells (see Fig. 10–13). These endocrine cells produce the male sex steroid hormone **testosterone,** which promotes survival of the mesonephric duct. At this early stage of development, testosterone secretion is regulated by the peptide hormone **chorionic gonadotropin,** secreted by the placenta, but later in development, the pituitary gonadotropins of the male fetus take over control of the masculinizing sex steroids (androgens).

The Mesonephric Ducts and the Accessory Glands of the Male Urethra Differentiate in Response to Testosterone

The Mesonephric Duct and Mesonephric Tubules Give Rise to the Vas Deferens and Ductuli Efferentes. Between 8 and 12 weeks, the initial secretion of testosterone stimulates the mesonephric ducts to transform into the spermatic ducts called the **vasa deferentia** (see Fig. 10–14). The most cranial end of each mesonephric duct degenerates, leaving a small remnant called the **appendix epididymis,** and the region of the vas deferens adjacent to the presumptive testis differentiates into the convoluted **epididymis.** During the ninth week, 5 to 12 mesonephric ducts in the region of the epididymis make contact with the cords of the future rete testis. It is not until the third month, however, that these **epigenital mesonephric tubules** actually unite with the presumptive rete testis. The epigenital mesonephric tubules are thereafter called the **ductuli efferentes,** and they will provide a pathway from the seminiferous tubules and rete testis tubules to the vas deferens. Meanwhile, the mesonephric tubules at the inferior pole of the developing testis (called the **paragenital mesonephric tubules**) degenerate, leaving a small remnant called the **paradidymis.**

The Seminal Vesicle Buds From the Distal Mesonephric Duct, Whereas the Prostate and Bulbourethral Glands Bud From the Urethra. The three accessory glands of the male genital system all develop near the junction between the mesonephric ducts and the pelvic urethra (Fig. 10–15). The glandular **seminal vesicles** sprout during the 10th week from the mesonephric ducts near their attachment to the pelvic urethra. The portion of the vas deferens (mesonephric duct) distal to each seminal vesicle is thereafter called the **ejaculatory duct.**

The **prostate gland** also begins to develop in the 10th week as a cluster of endodermal evaginations that bud from the pelvic urethra. These presumptive prostatic outgrowths are probably induced by the surrounding mesenchyme, the inductive activity of which probably depends on the conversion of secreted testosterone to another androgenic hormone, **dihydrotestosterone.** The

prostatic outgrowths initially form at least five independent groups of solid prostatic cords. By 11 weeks, these cords develop a lumen and glandular acini, and by 13 to 15 weeks (just as testosterone concentrations reach a high level), the prostate begins its secretory activity. The mesenchyme surrounding the endoderm-derived glandular portion of the prostate differentiates into the smooth muscle and connective tissue of the prostate.

As the prostate is developing, the paired **bulbourethral glands** sprout from the urethra just inferior to the prostate. As in the prostate, the mesenchyme surrounding the endodermal glandular tissue gives rise to the connective tissue and smooth muscle of this gland.

Eventually, the secretions of the seminal vesicles, prostate, and bulbourethral glands all contribute to the seminal fluid that protects and nourishes the spermatozoa after ejaculation. It should be noted, however, that these secretions are not absolutely necessary for sperm function; spermatozoa removed directly from the epididymis can fertilize oocytes.

IN THE ABSENCE OF A Y CHROMOSOME, FEMALE DEVELOPMENT OCCURS

In the female embryo, the somatic sex cord cells do not contain a Y chromosome or SRY region, do not elaborate SRY protein, and therefore do not differentiate into Sertoli cells. In the absence of Sertoli cells and SRY protein, AMH, Leydig cells, and testosterone are not produced. Male development of the genital ducts and accessory sexual structures therefore is not stimulated, and female development ensues (Fig. 10–16).

In the Presumptive Ovary, the Primitive Sex Cords Degenerate and Follicle Cells Form From Secondary Cortical Sex Cords

In genetic females, the primitive sex cords degenerate and the mesothelium of the genital ridge forms secondary cortical sex cords (see Fig. 10–16). These secondary sex cords then invest the pri-

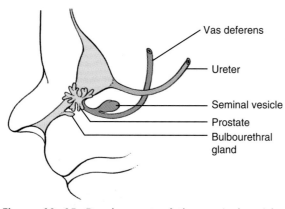

Figure 10–15. Development of the seminal vesicles, prostate, and bulbourethral glands. These glands are induced by androgens between the 10th and 12th weeks.

Vas deferens

Ureter

Seminal vesicle

Prostate

Bulbourethral gland

Female

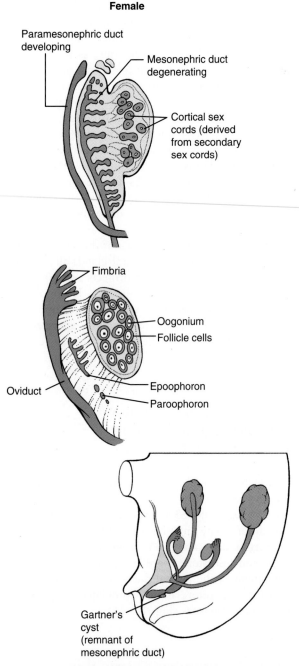

Figure 10–16. Female gonadal development. In the absence of testis-determining factor, the medullary sex cords of the female disappear and the cortical sex cords differentiate into follicle cells. The mesonephric ducts and mesonephric tubules disappear except for remnants such as the epoophoron, the paroophoron, and Gartner's cysts. The paramesonephric ducts continue to develop to form the oviducts, the uterus, and the superior part of the vagina. (See Fig. 10–14 for a description of male gonadal development.)

mordial germ cells to form the follicle cells of the ovary (see Ch. 1).

The Female Germ Cells Enter Meiosis, but Further Nuclear Development Is Inhibited by the Follicle Cells. In the male, the pre-Sertoli cells inhibit germ cell development before meiosis begins. In the female fetus, the germ cells differentiate into oogonia and enter the first meiotic division as primary oocytes before they develop close interactions with the investing follicle cells. The follicle cells then arrest germ cell development until puberty, at which point individual oocytes resume gametogenesis in response to each monthly surge of gonadotropins. The close physical contact between the genital ridge and the mesonephros in females seems to play a role in inducing the initial stages of gamete maturation.

In the Absence of Testosterone and AMH, the Mesonephric Ducts Degenerate and the Paramesonephric Ducts Give Rise to the Fallopian Tubes, Uterus, and Superior Vagina

The mesonephric ducts and mesonephric tubules require testosterone for their development. In the female, therefore, they rapidly disappear except for a few vestiges. Two remnants, the **epoophoron** and **paroophoron,** are found in the mesentery of the ovary, and a scattering of tiny remnants called **Gartner's cysts** cluster near the vagina (Fig. 10–17C; see also Fig. 10–16). The paramesonephric ducts, in contrast, develop uninhibited.

Recall that the distal tips of the growing paramesonephric ducts adhere to each other just before they contact the posterior wall of the pelvic urethra. The wall of the pelvic urethra at this point forms a slight thickening called the **sinusal tubercle** (see Fig. 10–17A). As soon as the fused tips of the paramesonephric ducts connect with the sinusal tubercle, the paramesonephric ducts begin to fuse from their caudal tips cranially, forming a tube with a single lumen (see Fig. 10–17B, C). This tube, called the **genital canal** or **uterovaginal canal,** becomes the superior portion of the vagina and the uterus. The unfused, superior portions of the paramesonephric ducts become the fal-

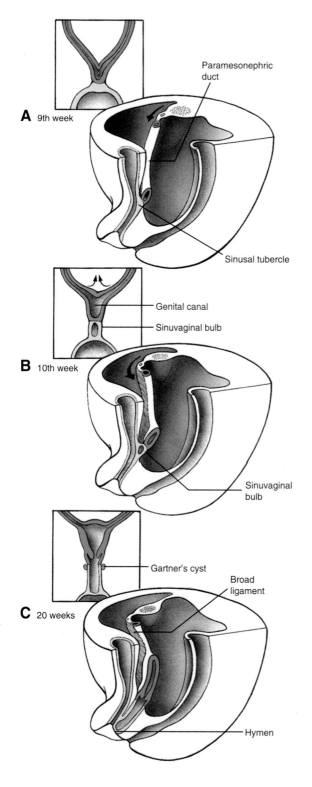

lopian tubes (oviducts), and the funnel-shaped superior openings of the paramesonephric ducts become the infundibula of the oviducts.

While the uterovaginal canal is forming during the third month, the endodermal tissue of the sinusal tubercle in the posterior urethra continues to thicken, forming a pair of swellings called the **sinuvaginal bulbs** (see Fig. 10–17). These structures give rise to the inferior 20 percent of the vagina. The most inferior region of the uterovaginal canal meanwhile becomes occluded by a block of tissue called the **vaginal plate.** The origin of the vaginal plate tissue is unclear; it may arise from the sinuvaginal bulbs, from the walls of the paramesonephric ducts, from the nearby mesonephric ducts, or from a combination of these tissues. The vaginal plate elongates from the third to the fifth month and subsequently becomes canalized by a process of **desquamation** (cell shedding) to form the inferior vaginal lumen.

As the vaginal plate forms, the lower end of the vagina lengthens, and its junction with the urogenital sinus migrates caudally until it comes to rest during the fourth month on the posterior wall of the definitive urogenital sinus (see Fig. 10–17C). This migration may be caused by the physical lengthening of the vaginal plate itself. However, an endodermal membrane temporarily separates the lumen of the vagina from the cavity of the definitive urogenital sinus, which differentiates into the **vestibule of the vagina.** This barrier degenerates partially after the fifth month, but its remnant persists as the vaginal **hymen.** The mucous membrane that lines the vagina and cervix may also be derived from the endodermal epithelium of the definitive urogenital sinus.

Figure 10–17. Formation of the uterus and vagina. *A,* The uterus and superior end of the vagina begin to form as the paramesonephric ducts fuse together near their attachment to the posterior wall of the primitive urogenital sinus. *B, C,* The ducts then zipper together in a superior direction between the third and fifth months. As the paramesonephric ducts are pulled away from the posterior body wall, they drag a fold of peritoneal membrane with them, forming the broad ligaments of the uterus. *A–C,* The inferior end of the vagina forms from the sinuvaginal bulbs on the posterior wall of the primitive urogenital sinus.

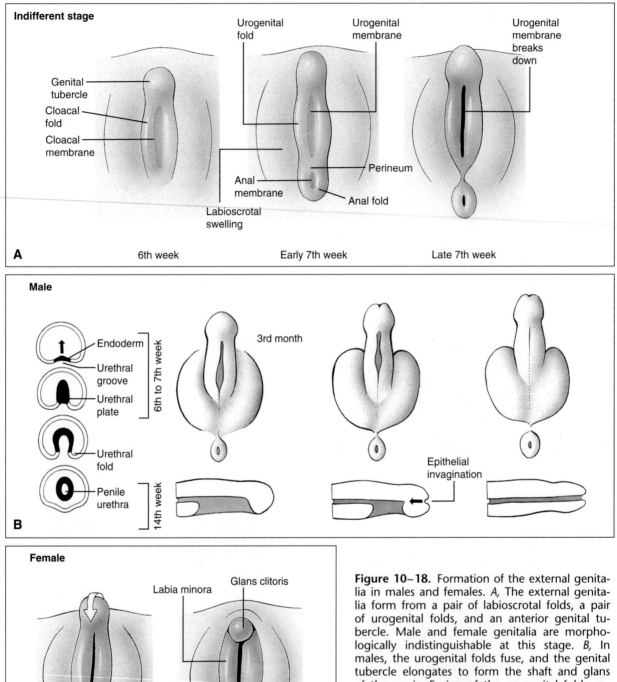

Figure 10–18. Formation of the external genitalia in males and females. *A,* The external genitalia form from a pair of labioscrotal folds, a pair of urogenital folds, and an anterior genital tubercle. Male and female genitalia are morphologically indistinguishable at this stage. *B,* In males, the urogenital folds fuse, and the genital tubercle elongates to form the shaft and glans of the penis. Fusion of the urogenital folds encloses the definitive urogenital sinus to form most of the penile urethra. A small region of the distal urethra is formed by the invagination of ectoderm covering the glans. The labioscrotal folds give rise to the scrotum. *C,* In females, the genital tubercle bends inferiorly to form the clitoris, and the urogenital folds remain separated to form the labia minora. The labioscrotal folds form the labia majora.

THE EXTERNAL GENITALIA DEVELOP FROM THE SAME PRIMORDIA IN BOTH SEXES

The early development of the external genitalia is similar in males and females. Early in the fifth week, a pair of swellings called **cloacal folds** develop on either side of the cloacal membrane (Fig. 10–18A). These folds meet just anterior to the cloacal membrane to form a midline swelling called the **genital tubercle.**

The fusion of the urorectal septum with the cloacal membrane in the seventh week creates the **perineum,** which divides the cloacal membrane into an anterior urogenital membrane and a posterior anal membrane. The portion of the cloacal fold flanking the urogenital membrane is now called the **urethral fold** (also the **genital** or **urogenital fold**), and the portion flanking the anal membrane is called the **anal fold.** A new pair of swellings, the **labioscrotal swellings,** then appear on either side of the urethral folds (see Fig. 10–18A).

The cavity of the definitive urogenital sinus extends onto the surface of the enlarging genital tubercle in the form of an endoderm-lined **urethral groove** during the sixth week (see Fig. 10–18B). This groove becomes temporarily filled by a solid endodermal **urethral plate,** but the urethral plate then recanalizes to form an even deeper groove. In males this groove is relatively long and broad, whereas in females it is shorter and more sharply tapered. In both sexes, an **epithelial tag** is now present at the tip of the genital tubercle. Table 10–1 lists the adult derivatives of the embryonic external genital structures.

The urogenital membrane ruptures in the seventh week, opening the cavity of the urogenital sinus to the amniotic fluid. The genital tubercle elongates to form the **phallus,** and a primordium of the glans clitoris and glans penis is demarcated from the phallic shaft by a **coronary sulcus.**

The appearance of the external genitalia is similar in male and female embryos through the 12th week, and embryos of this age are difficult to sex on the basis of their external appearance.

In the Male, the Urethral Groove Becomes the Penile Urethra and the Labioscrotal Swellings Form the Scrotum

Starting in the fourth month, the effects of dihydrotestosterone on the male external genitalia become readily apparent (see Fig. 10–18B). The perineal region separating the definitive urogenital sinus from the anus begins to lengthen. The labioscrotal folds fuse at the midline to form the **scrotum,** and the urethral folds also fuse to enclose the **penile urethra.** The penile urethra is completely enclosed by 14 weeks. However, because the urethral groove does not extend onto the glans of the penis, the penile urethra is initially blind ended. The terminal portion of the urethra is created by an ectodermal invagination from the tip of the glans.

It should be noted that the aforementioned generally accepted explanation for the closure of the urethral groove has been questioned. An alternative mechanism has been proposed in which the penile urethra is enclosed by an anterior growth of perineal mesoderm, with little or no involvement of the genital folds.

Table 10–1
Development of Male and Female External Genitalia

PRESUMPTIVE ANLAGE	MALE STRUCTURE	FEMALE STRUCTURE
Genital tubercle	Glans and shaft of penis	Glans and shaft of clitoris
Definitive urogenital sinus	Penile urethra	Vestibule of vagina
Urethral fold	Penis surrounding penile urethra	Labia minora
Labioscrotal fold	Scrotum	Labia majora

In the Female, the Perineum Does Not Lengthen and the Labioscrotal and Urethral Folds Do Not Fuse

In the absence of dihydrotestosterone in female embryos, the primitive perineum does not lengthen, and the labioscrotal and urethral folds do not fuse across the midline (see Fig. 10–18C). The phallus bends inferiorly, becoming the clitoris, and the definitive urogenital sinus becomes the vestibule of the vagina. The urethral folds become the labia minora, and the labioscrotal swellings become the labia majora.

THE TESTES AND OVARIES BOTH DESCEND UNDER THE CONTROL OF A GUBERNACULUM

During embryonic and fetal life, the testes and the ovaries both descend from their original position at the 10th thoracic level, although the testes ultimately descend much farther. In both sexes, the descent of the gonad depends on a ligamentous cord called the **gubernaculum**. The gubernaculum condenses during the seventh week within the subserous fascia of a longitudinal peritoneal fold on either side of the vertebral column (Fig. 10–19). The superior end of this cord attaches to the gonad, and its expanded inferior end (the **gubernacular bulb**) attaches to the fascia between the developing external and internal oblique muscles in the region of the labioscrotal swellings. At the same time, a slight evagination of the peritoneum, called the **processus vaginalis** or **vaginal process**, develops just adjacent to the inferior root of the gubernaculum.

Inguinal Canals Develop in Both Sexes

The **inguinal canal** is a caudal evagination of the abdominal wall that forms when the processus vaginalis grows inferiorly, pushing out a socklike evagination consisting of the various layers of the abdominal wall (see Fig. 10–19). In the male, the inguinal canal extends into the scrotum and transmits the descending testes. A complete inguinal canal also forms in females but plays no role in

genital development. The processus vaginalis normally degenerates. Occasionally, however, it remains patent, in which case the inguinal canal may later become the site of an **indirect inguinal hernia** (Fig. 10–20).

In the Male, the Inguinal Canal Conveys the Testes to the Scrotum and Forms the Sheath of the Spermatic Cord. Figure 10–19 illustrates the development of the inguinal canal in the male. During the eighth week, the processus vaginalis begins to elongate caudally, carrying along the bulb of the gubernaculum. The elongating processus successively encounters three layers of the differentiating abdominal wall and pushes them out to form a socklike evagination (see Fig. 10–19D). The first layer encountered by the processus is the **transversalis fascia**, lying just deep to the transversus abdominis muscle. This layer will become the **internal spermatic fascia of the spermatic cord**. The processus does not encounter the transversus abdominis muscle itself, because this muscle has a large hiatus in this region. Next, the processus picks up the fibers and fascia of the **internal oblique muscle**. These become the **cremasteric fascia of the spermatic cord**. Finally, the processus picks up a thin layer of **external oblique muscle**, which will become the **external spermatic fascia**. In males, the processus vaginalis pushes this entire inguinal "sock" out into the scrotal swelling.

The inguinal canal can be thought of as a series of weakenings in the layers of the abdominal wall, which become stretched out to allow the testes to descend into the scrotum. The superior rim of the canal—the point of weakening and eversion of the transversalis fascia—is called the **deep ring of the inguinal canal** (see Fig. 10–19D). The inferomedial rim of the canal formed by the point of eversion of the external oblique muscle is called the **superficial ring of the inguinal canal**.

The Testes Descend to the Deep Ring of the Inguinal Canal by the Third Month and Complete Their Descent in the Seventh to Ninth Months. Between the 7th and 12th weeks, the extrainguinal portions of the gubernacula shorten and pull the testes down to the vicinity of the deep inguinal ring within the plane of the subserous fascia. The gubernacula shorten mainly by getting fatter at their base; this serves the secondary purpose of enlarging the inguinal canal.

The testes remain in the vicinity of the deep

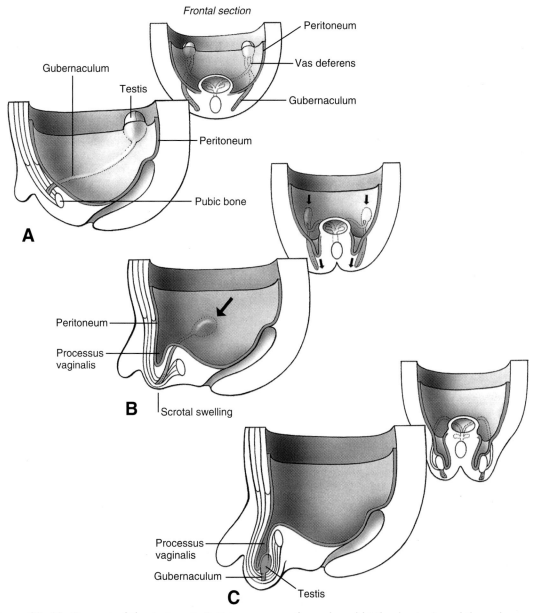

Figure 10–19. Descent of the testes. *A–C,* Between seventh week and birth, shortening of the gubernaculum testis causes the testes to descend from the 10th thoracic level into the scrotum. The testes pass through the inguinal canal in the anterior abdominal wall.

Illustration continued on following page

ring from the third to the seventh month but then enter the inguinal canal in response to renewed shortening of the gubernaculum. The testes remain within the subserous fascia of the processus vaginalis through which they descend toward the scrotum (see Fig. 10–19). This second phase of gubernacular shortening is caused by actual reduction

and regression of the gubernaculum as a result of the loss of the mucoid extracellular matrix that forms much of its substance. The movement of the testes through the canal is also aided by the increased abdominal pressure created by the growth of the abdominal viscera. By the ninth month, just before normal term delivery, the testes have com-

Figure 10–19. *Continued. D,* After the eighth week, a peritoneal evagination called the processus vaginalis forms just anterior to the gubernaculum and pushes out socklike extensions of the transversalis fascia, the internal oblique muscle, and the external oblique muscle, thus forming the inguinal canal. The inguinal canal extends from the base of the everted transversalis fascia (the deep ring) to the base of the everted external oblique muscle (the superficial ring). After the processus vaginalis has evaginated into the scrotum, the gubernaculum shortens and simply pulls the gonads through the canal. The gonads always remain within the plane of the subserous fascia associated with the posterior wall of the processus vaginalis, however.

Figure 10–20. Normal and abnormal development of the processus vaginalis. *A*, The proximal end of the processus vaginalis normally disintegrates during the first year after birth, leaving a distal remnant called the tunica vaginalis. *B*, Some proximal remnants may remain, and these and the tunica vaginalis may fill with serous fluid, forming testicular hydroceles in pathologic conditions or subsequent to injury. *C*, If the proximal end of the processus vaginalis does not disintegrate, abdominal contents may herniate through the processus and inguinal canal into the scrotum. This condition is called congenital inguinal hernia. *D*, Infant with a testicular hydrocele. (Fig. 10–20D photo courtesy of Children's Hospital Medical Center, Cincinnati, OH.)

pletely entered the scrotal sac and the gubernaculum is reduced to a small ligamentous band attaching the inferior pole of the testis to the scrotal floor. The action of testosterone and other **androgens** (male sex steroids) seems to be important for

this second phase of testicular descent. Cryptorchidism (undescended testes) is a common condition and is a risk factor for development of malignancy within the gonad. Patients with this condition will sometimes respond to treatment

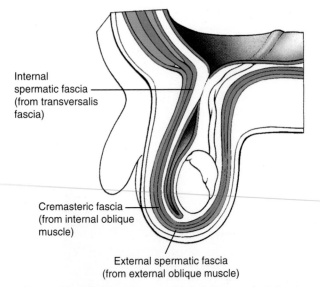

Internal
spermatic fascia
(from transversalis
fascia)

Cremasteric fascia
(from internal oblique
muscle)

External spermatic fascia
(from external oblique muscle)

Figure 10–21. The three extruded layers of abdominal wall pushed into the scrotum by the evaginating processus vaginalis from three layers of spermatic fascia. These three layers enclose the tunica vaginalis and the testis in a common compartment.

The Ovaries Descend and Become Suspended in the Broad Ligaments of the Uterus. Like the male embryo, the female embryo develops a gubernaculum extending initially from the inferior pole of the gonad to the subcutaneous fascia of the presumptive labioscrotal folds and later penetrating the abdominal wall as part of a fully formed inguinal canal (Fig. 10–22). In the female, the gubernaculum does not shorten, deform, or regress. Nevertheless, it causes the ovaries to descend during the third month and to be swept out into a peritoneal fold called the **broad ligament of the uterus** (see Fig. 10–22; see also Fig. 10–17). This translocation occurs because during the seventh week the gubernaculum becomes attached to the developing paramesonephric ducts, where these two structures cross each other on the posterior body wall. As the paramesonephric ducts zipper together from their caudal ends, they sweep out the broad ligaments and simultaneously pull the ovaries into these peritoneal folds.

In the absence of male hormones, the female gubernaculum remains intact and grows in step with the rest of the body. The inferior gubernaculum becomes the **round ligament of the uterus**

with hCG (human chorionic gonadotropin) hormonal therapy.

Within the first year after birth, the superior portion of the processus vaginalis is usually obliterated, leaving only a distal remnant sac, the **tunica vaginalis,** which lies anterior to the testis (see Figs. 10–20, 10–21). During infancy this sac wraps around most of the testis. Its lumen is normally collapsed, but under pathologic conditions it may fill with serous secretions, forming a testicular hydrocele (see Fig. 10–20B, D).

As mentioned earlier, it is not rare for the entire processus vaginalis to remain patent, forming a connection between the abdominal cavity and the scrotal sac. During childhood, loops of intestine may herniate into the processus, resulting in an **indirect inguinal hernia** (see Fig. 10–20C). Repair of these hernias is the second most common childhood operation.

The hormonal control of testicular descent is not completely understood. Androgens and pituitary hormones are important, but other unknown testicular factors or hormones apparently play a role, as does neural input via the genitofemoral nerve.

*Derivatives
of the
gubernaculum:*

Ovarian
ligament

Round
ligament
of the uterus

Labia majora

Figure 10–22. The ovaries descend to some degree during development and are swept into the broad ligaments, whereas the paramesonephric ducts zipper together to form the uterus. The gubernaculum in the female grows in pace with the body and is attached to the paramesonephric ducts at a crossover point on the posterior body wall. In consequence, the remnant of the female gubernaculum connects the labia majora with the wall of the uterus and is then reflected laterally, attaching to the ovary.

connecting the fascia of the labia majora to the uterus, and the superior gubernaculum becomes the **ligament of the ovary** connecting the uterus to the ovary.

As in males, the processus vaginalis of the inguinal canal is normally obliterated, but occasionally remains patent and may become the site of an **indirect inguinal hernia.**

Clinical Applications

Abnormalities of the Urinary and Genital Systems

URINARY TRACT ANOMALIES MAY ARISE FROM DEFECTS OF THE URETERIC BUD OR METANEPHRIC MESENCHYME

About 10 percent of all newborns have a developmental abnormality of the urinary tract. Most of these anomalies do not cause clinical problems. About 45 percent of all cases of childhood renal failure, however, result from anomalous development of the ureteric bud or metanephric mesenchyme. Because the development of each of these anlagen is dependent on inductive signals from the other, abnormalities in one often cause abnormalities in the other (see the Experimental Principles section of this chapter).

The Ureter May Be Partially or Completely Duplicated. *Premature bifurcation of the ureteric bud results in a bifid ureter.* The ureteric bud normally does not bifurcate until it enters the substance of the metanephric blastema. Occasionally, however, it bifurcates prematurely, resulting in a Y-shaped **bifid ureter** (Fig. 10–23). The undivided inferior end of the ureter attaches normally to the bladder. Typically, most of the kidney is drained by the branch attached to its lower pole. One of the branches occasionally ends blindly.

A bifid ureter is not always asymptomatic. Although the two branches of the Y arise from the same ureteric bud, the contractions of their muscular walls appear to be asynchronous. Urine may therefore reflux from one branch into the other, resulting in stagnation of urine and predisposing the individual to infections of the ureter.

Complete Duplicate Ureters Result From the Growth of Two Ureteric Buds. Occasionally, a mesonephric duct sprouts two ureteric buds, which penetrate

the metanephric blastema independently (Fig. 10–24). The more cranial bud induces formation of the cranial pole of the kidney, and the caudal bud induces the formation of the caudal pole. As the mesonephric duct undergoes exstrophy into the posterior wall of the bladder, the caudal ureteric bud is incorporated into the bladder wall in the normal manner. The cranial bud, however, is carried inferiorly along with the descending mesonephric duct (recall that the exstrophy is a craniocaudal process) and may form its final connection with any derivative of the distal mesonephric duct, pelvic urethra, or definitive urogenital sinus (see Fig. 10–24). The caudal ureteric bud thus forms a normal, or *orthotopic*, ureter connected to the bladder, whereas the cranial bud forms an inferior *ectopic* ureter. Because the normal ureter drains the *lower* pole of the kidney and the ectopic ureter drains the *upper* pole, the two ureters cross each other. This crossing of the normal and ectopic ureters, called the **Weigert-Meyer rule,** is part of the evidence from which the mechanism of mesonephric duct exstrophy was deduced.

In males, an ectopic ureter may drain into the prostatic urethra, the ejaculatory duct, the vas deferens, or the seminal vesicle. These ectopic ureters thus always open superior to the sphincter urethra muscle and do not result in incontinence, although they may cause painful urination or recurrent infections. In females, ectopic ureters often connect to the vestibule, the vagina, or, less often, the uterus. These **extrasphincteric outlets** of the ectopic ureter result in continuous dribbling of urine unless surgically corrected. Anomalous insertion of the ureter within the bladder can also be a problem because the valve mechanism preventing reflux of urine to the kidney fails to develop. Reflux predisposes individuals to urinary tract infection. Although the majority of individuals with this

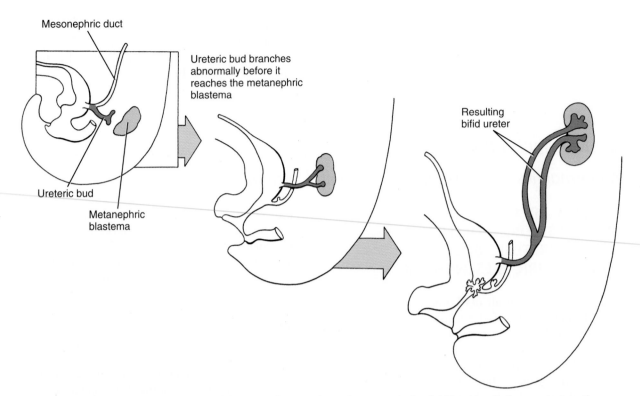

Figure 10–23. Bifid ureter. A bifid ureter forms when the ureteric bud bifurcates before entering the metanephric blastema.

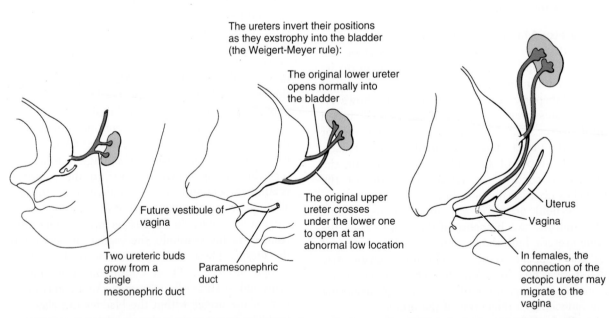

Figure 10–24. Ectopic ureter. An ectopic ureter forms from an anomalous "extra" ureteric bud. The mechanisms of formation of the trigone and placement of the vas deferens and ureters on the posterior wall of the primitive urogenital sinus were largely deduced from the Weigert-Meyer rule.

defect have no known genetic cause, some are found to have mutations in *Hoxa 13.*

Defects in the Inductive Interaction Between the Ureteric Bud and Metanephric Blastema May Cause Renal Agenesis or Dysplasia

The Kidney May Fail to Develop on One or Both Sides. In the absence of inductive signals from the ureteric bud, the metanephros fails to develop. Infants with **bilateral renal agenesis** are stillborn or die within a few days of birth. Infants with **unilateral renal agenesis,** in contrast, often live, because the remaining kidney undergoes compensatory hypertrophy. For unknown reasons, about 75 percent of infants with renal agenesis are male. Although the relative frequencies of unilateral and bilateral renal agenesis are difficult to determine because unilateral renal agenesis often goes undetected, autopsy data suggest that unilateral renal agenesis is about four to eight times more common than bilateral renal agenesis.

Renal Agenesis Is Typically Associated With Other Congenital Defects. The kidneys contribute to the production of amniotic fluid, and bilateral renal agenesis therefore results in **oligohydramnios,** or insufficient amniotic fluid. As described in the Clinical Applications section of Chapter 6, oligohydramnios allows the uterine wall to compress the growing fetus, resulting in a spectrum of abnormalities called **Potter's syndrome.** These anomalies include deformed limbs; wrinkly, dry skin; and an abnormal facies (in this context, *facies* means "facial appearance") consisting of wide-set eyes, parrot-beak nose, receding chin, and low-set ears.

   Renal agenesis is often associated with a spectrum of ipsilateral genitourinary abnormalities, including defects in structures derived from the mesonephric duct in males and paramesonephric duct in females. It is easy to understand how failure of mesonephric duct development leads to absence of both the vas deferens and kidney, because the kidney develops from an outgrowth of the duct. The association of paramesonephric duct anomalies with renal anomalies likely represents a defect in tissue interactions within the intermediate mesoderm, which are necessary for the development of both. One remaining problem is how to explain unilateral agenesis.

Abnormal Kidneys May Arise From Abnormal Inductive Interactions. In some cases, subtle defects in the interaction between ureteric bud and metanephric blastema result in **hypoplasia** or **dysplasia** of the developing kidney. The small number of nephrons in a hypoplastic kidney results either from inadequate branching of the ureteric bud or from an inadequate response by the metanephric cap tissue. In cases of **renal dysplasia,** the nephrons themselves develop abnormally and consist of primitive ducts lined by undifferentiated epithelium sheathed within thick layers of connective tissue.

   The genetic causes for some of these renal anomalies are beginning to be identified. Mutation of the transcription factor gene *Pax-2* is associated with dominant transmission of renal hypoplasia and dysplasia. Mutation in another transcription gene, *Eya1,* causes BOR (branchio-oto-renal) syndrome. In addition to renal anomalies, *Eya1* haploinsufficient individuals also develop branchial cleft cysts and have both outer and inner ear defects.

Common Forms of Congenital Polycystic Kidney Disease May Result From Mutations of Different Genes

Autosomal dominant polycystic kidney disease (ADPKD) is a common genetic disease associated with the formation of cysts in the kidneys as well as other ductal epithelia in the liver, pancreas, testis, and ovary. Mutations in the *polycystin-1* and *polycystin-2* genes account for 85 and 15 percent of ADPKD, respectively. Similarities between the clinical presentations resulting from mutations in the two genes, and evidence that the two proteins can interact, suggest their involvement in a common pathway. The precise roles of the *polycystin-1* and *polycystin-2* gene products have not yet been defined, although sequence homologies suggest receptor and ion channel functions.

Mutation of the Zinc-Finger Transcription Factor *WT1* Results in Wilms' Tumor and Malformations of the Urinary and Genital Systems

The wild-type gene **WT1,** encoded on human chromosome 11p13, is normally expressed during embryogenesis in the developing kidneys, the genital ridges of males and females, the mesothelium, and the immature hematopoietic stem cells (see the Experimental Principles section of this chapter). Mutations of *WT1* result in childhood cancers of the kidney, but these **Wilms' tumors** are relatively rare, occurring in about 8 of every one million individuals, and are apparently inherited through a dominant or dominant-negative mode of familial inheritance or acquired by sporadic mutation. Tumors are typically diagnosed in the 3- or 4-year old child and, fortunately, can be treated chemotherapeutically with a cure rate of about 90 percent.

Several distinct syndromes have been associated with mutations in the Wilms' tumor gene. For example, individuals with **Denys-Drash syndrome (DDS)** will develop renal mesangial sclerosis with progressive renal failure and streak gonads with male pseudohermaphroditism in addition to Wilms' tumors.

Cytogenetic studies have demonstrated that the mutation in DDS is restricted to the *WT1* locus, and, in a large proportion of cases, a missense mutation results in replacement of arginine for tryptophane at residue 394 in zinc-finger 3 of the WT1 protein. This is the DNA-binding region of the protein, and so it is likely that the tumor and the renal and genital anomalies can be explained by disruption of the normal function of *WT1* in respective urogenital tissues. The observation that the urogenital lesions are more profound in these individuals than in individuals with haploinsufficiency suggests a dominant-negative effect of the mutation.

Abnormalities of the eyes and brain may also occur in patients with Wilms' tumor, but these anomalies may be explained by the disruption of other genes located in close proximity to a mutated *WT1* gene on chromosome 11. For example, the WAGR syndrome is characterized by *W*ilm's tumor, *a*niridia, *g*enital abnormalities, and mental *r*etardation. Aniridia refers to the absence of irises in the eyes and is caused by deletion of the *Pax-6*

transcription factor gene. The brain-derived neurotrophic factor (*BDNF*) gene maps close by the *WT1* locus, and its disruption or deletion may contribute to the mental retardation that accompanies Wilms' tumor in WAGR.

An unusual mechanism underlies the predisposition of individuals with **Beckwith-Wiedemann syndrome** to develop renal hyperplasia and Wilms' tumor. In some cases, these individuals apparently lack the normal genomic imprinting that inactivates the insulin-like growth factor-2 (*IGF-2*) gene on the paternal chromosome (see the Clinical Applications and Experimental Principles sections of Ch. 2). Resultant overexpression of IGF-2 by the paternal gene results in an overabundance of IGF-2 and neoplastic potential. Thus, even though the *WT1* gene is normal, it does not suppress the activity of the nonimprinted paternal allele or *IGF-2*, and so these individuals express the Wilms' tumor phenotype.

WT1 Normally Functions as a Tumor Suppressor Gene

Similar to other tumor suppressor genes, the second or normal copy of the *WT1* gene is lost in Wilms' tumors. This two-hit mutational model (one abnormal-inherited allele and a second somatic mutation) explains the development of multiple primary tumors. The wild-type *WT1* zinc-finger protein transcription factor, like the products of other tumor suppressor genes, normally suppresses the activity of genes involved in cell proliferation. In addition to the regulation of insulin-like growth factors discussed above, *WT1* has also been demonstrated to suppress expression of the insulin-like growth factor receptor IGF-I-R and transforming growth factor-β. Please refer to discussions of other "developmental regulatory tumor suppressor" genes such as *DPC4* (a member of the MAD family; Ch. 3), *PTCH* (Ch. 12), and *DCC* (Ch. 13).

Defective Partitioning of the Cloaca Results in Anomalies of Urinary, Genital, and Anorectal Structures

Much of the evidence that the urorectal septum forms by fusion of a superior Tourneux fold with paired inferolateral Rathke folds (Fig. 10–25; see also Ch. 9) comes from the anatomy of the malformations that results from defective development of these structures. In as many as 1 of 5000 infants, the urorectal septum is incomplete. Depending on the location and size of the defect, a wide range of malformations involving the cloacal derivatives and their connections with the ureters and genital ducts may result. A few of the more common examples are described in the following paragraphs.

Failure of the Rathke Folds to Develop Results in Rectourethral Fistulas.

If the Rathke folds fail to grow, the inferior part of the urorectal septum does not close, resulting in abnormal **rectourethral fistulas** between the developing urogenital sinus and rectum (Fig. 10–26).

In males, these connections usually take the form of a narrow **rectoprostatic urethral fistula** connecting the rectum to the prostatic urethra (see Fig. 10–26C). In females, the situation is complicated by the presence of the paramesonephric ducts. Most often, the paramesonephric ducts attach to the pelvic urethra just superior to the rectourethral fistula. The inferior undivided region of the cloaca thus becomes a common outlet for the urethra, the vagina, and the rectum, and is called a **rectocloacal canal** (see Fig. 10–26D). Occasionally, the descending uterovaginal canal incorporates the rectourethral fistula while migrating to a more inferior position on the posterior wall of the clo-

aca. In these cases, the vagina and urethra open separately into the vestibule, but the rectum communicates with the vagina through a **rectovaginal fistula** (see Fig. 10–26E). This fistula may be located high or low in the vagina. If the rectourethral fistula is originally located at the vaginal-cloacal junction, the resulting **anovestibular fistula** will open into the vestibule of the vagina.

The Tourneux and Rathke Folds May Both Fail to Form.

This more severe defect results in the formation of an abnormal communication between the rectum and the bladder called a **rectovesical fistula** (Fig. 10–27). In females, this anomaly may interfere with the normal fusion of the inferior ends of the paramesonephric ducts, resulting in separate bilateral vaginas and uterae that empty directly into the bladder.

Malalignment of the Tourneux and Rathke Folds Results in a Urorectal Fistula.

If malalignment prevents the Tourneux fold from fusing with the Rathke folds, the distal end of the cloaca may be correctly partitioned, but a fistula will persist superiorly (Fig. 10–28). The result in males is a rectourethral fistula connecting the prostatic urethra to the rectal canal (see Fig. 10–28B). The penile urethra and the anal canal empty through their normal channels, but the penile urethra is frequently stenotic, causing urine to exit preferentially through the urorectal fistula and anorectal canal.

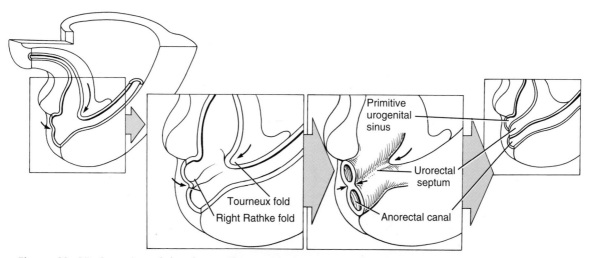

Figure 10–25. Septation of the cloaca. This process requires the coordinated behavior of three mesenchymal folds: the Tourneux fold and the left and right Rathke folds.

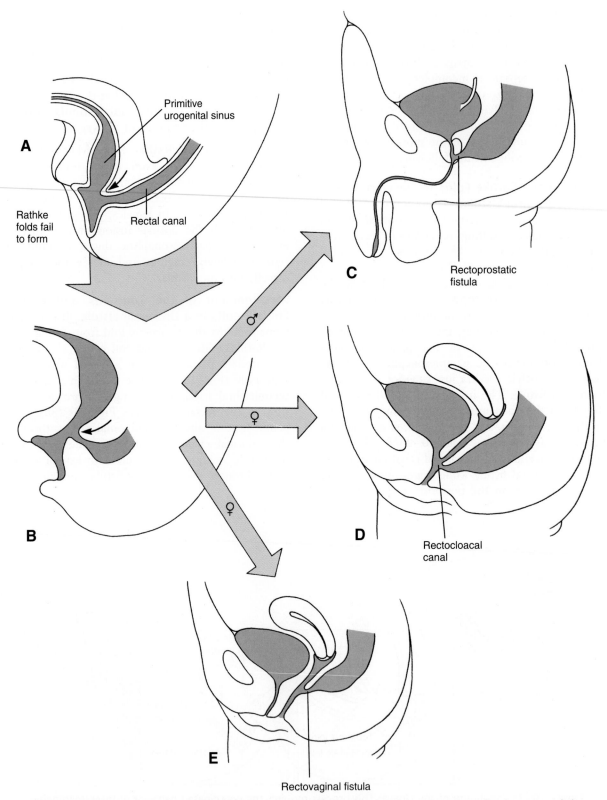

Figure 10–26. Failure of the Rathke folds to form results in characteristic anomalous development of the urogenital and lower gastrointestinal tracts in males and females.

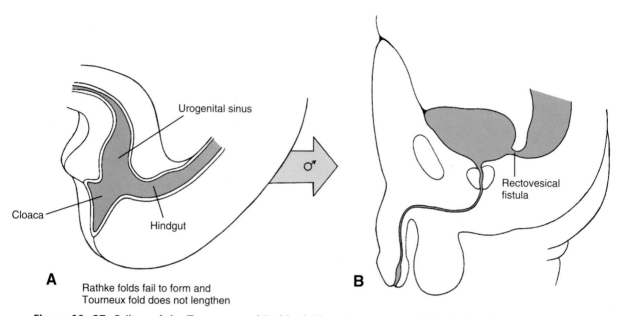

A Rathke folds fail to form and
Tourneux fold does not lengthen

B

Figure 10–27. Failure of the Tourneux and Rathke folds to form may result in the development of a fistula between the rectum and the bladder.

In females, the urogenital opening of the fistula is incorporated by the descending uterovaginal canal, resulting in a rectovaginal fistula connecting the rectum to the vagina (see Fig. 10–28D). The urethra and vagina, however, open normally to the outside.

Anal Malformations Result From Maldevelopment of the Anal Pit, the Anal Membrane, or the Genital Folds. *Failure of the anal pit to form results in a blind-ending rectum.* Because the anal pit gives rise to the distal one third of the anal canal, failure of the anal pit to form causes the rectum to end blindly in the body wall (Fig. 10–29A). This condition is called **anal agenesis.** The location of the deficient anal pit is sometimes marked by a small dimple or pigmented spot.

The Anal Membrane May Thicken and Fail to Rupture. Occasionally, the anal pit forms normally, but the anal membrane separating the ectodermal and endodermal portions of the anus is superficially thickened by tissue proliferating from the genital folds. This thickened anal membrane may fail to rupture or may rupture incompletely, resulting in

an **imperforate anal membrane** or **anal stenosis,** respectively (see Fig. 10–29B).

Excessive Posterior Fusion of the Genital Folds May Partly or Completely Cover the Anus. This condition, called **covered anus,** almost always occurs in males, because the genital folds do not normally fuse at all in females. The resulting malformation is called **anocutaneous occlusion** if the anus is completely covered. In some cases, a defect in the perineal mesoderm just anterior to the anus results in the development of a displaced anterior anal opening, a condition called **anocutaneous stenosis** or **anterior anus.**

Abnormal Development of the Genital System Can Result From Many Kinds of Errors. Many congenital defects of sexual development are caused by mutations or chromosomal anomalies affecting autosomes or sex chromosomes. Not surprisingly, mutations of the sex-determining region of the Y chromosome have drastic effects, as do deletions or duplications of the sex chromosomes. Most genital system malformations, however, arise from alterations in autosomal genes. A few examples are discussed in the following paragraphs.

A Tourneux and Rathke folds are malaligned

Tourneux fold
Rathke fold

Rectourethral fistula

♂ **B**

Development of rectovaginal fistula

♀ **C**

Rectovaginal fistula

♀ **D**

Figure 10–28. A variety of anomalies may result through failure of alignment of the Tourneux and Rathke folds.

Pseudohermaphroditism, in Which the External Genitalia of One Sex Accompany the Gonads of the Other, Is Caused by Sex Hormone Anomalies. A **pseudohermaphroditic** individual is one whose gonads and sex chromosomes indicate that one sex has genitalia exhibiting at least some traits of the other sex. Genetic males (46,XY) with feminized genitals are called **male pseudohermaphrodites,** and genetic females (46, XX) with virilized genitals are called **female pseudohermaphrodites.** Pseudohermaphroditism is always caused either by abnormal levels of sex hormones or by abnormalities in the sex hormone receptors.

In genetically male fetuses, any deficiency in androgen action will tend to allow autonomous female development to proceed, resulting in some degree of genital feminization. Which structures show feminization depends on which of the male sex steroids are affected by the block. As explained in the descriptive section of this chapter, male differentiation of the external genitalia in the fetal period depends on the hormone **dihydrotestosterone,** which is derived from testosterone. A block affecting this hormone alone will thus result in external genital feminization, whereas a block affecting testosterone (and hence all testosterone-derived androgens, including dihydrotestosterone)

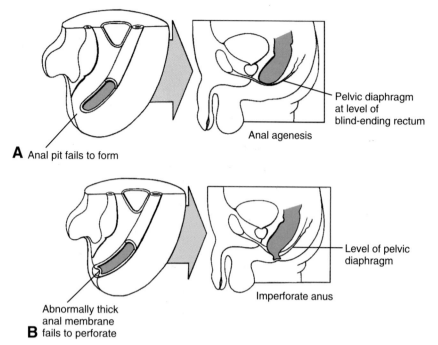

Figure 10–29. *A,* Anal agenesis resulting from failure of the anal pit to form. *B,* Imperforate anus may occur in cases where an abnormally thick anal membrane fails to rupture.

will affect many structures, including the mesonephric ducts and brain. Male pseudohermaphrodites who possess normal testes secrete AMH and do not have paramesonephric duct derivatives. However, as seen in XY individuals with *WT1* mutations, male pseudohermaphrodites with abnormal testicular development may retain paramesonephric structures.

Male Pseudohermaphroditism May Be Characterized by Incomplete Fusion of the Urethral or Labioscrotal Folds. Although not restricted to individuals with pseudohermaphroditism, one common manifestation of male pseudohermaphroditism is **hypospadias,** the condition in which the urethra opens onto the ventral surface of the penis. Hypospadias occurs in about 0.5 percent of all live births. In simple cases, a single anomalous opening is found on the underside of the glans or shaft (Fig. 10–30*A, B*). In more severe cases, the penile urethra has multiple openings or is not enclosed at all. Hypospadias of the glans is probably caused by defective development of the distal ectodermal urethral meatus, whereas openings on the penile shaft represent failures of the urethral folds to fuse completely.

A more complex condition, **penoscrotal hy-** **pospadias,** results when the labioscrotal swellings as well as the urethral folds fail to fuse (see Fig. 10–30*C, D*). If the labioscrotal folds fuse partially, the urethra will open through a hole between the base of the penis and the root of the scrotum. In the most severe form of the defect, the labioscrotal folds do not fuse at all and the urethra opens into the bottom of a depression in the perineum. This condition is usually accompanied by retarded growth of the phallus, so that the genitals appear female at birth.

Male pseudohermaphroditism affecting the external genitals may be caused by 5α-reductase deficiency. The enzyme 5α-reductase converts testosterone to the derivative androgen dihydrotestosterone. Mutations that reduce or disable this enzyme have no consequences in females, but in males the resulting absence of dihydrotestosterone results in severe penoscrotal hypospadias and genitalia that appear to be female at birth. These individuals have normal testes located either within the inguinal canals or in the labioscrotal swellings. The testes produce AMH and testosterone at the appropriate times, so paramesonephric duct derivatives are absent and the mesonephric ducts differentiate into vasa deferentia.

In male pseudohermaphrodites of this type,

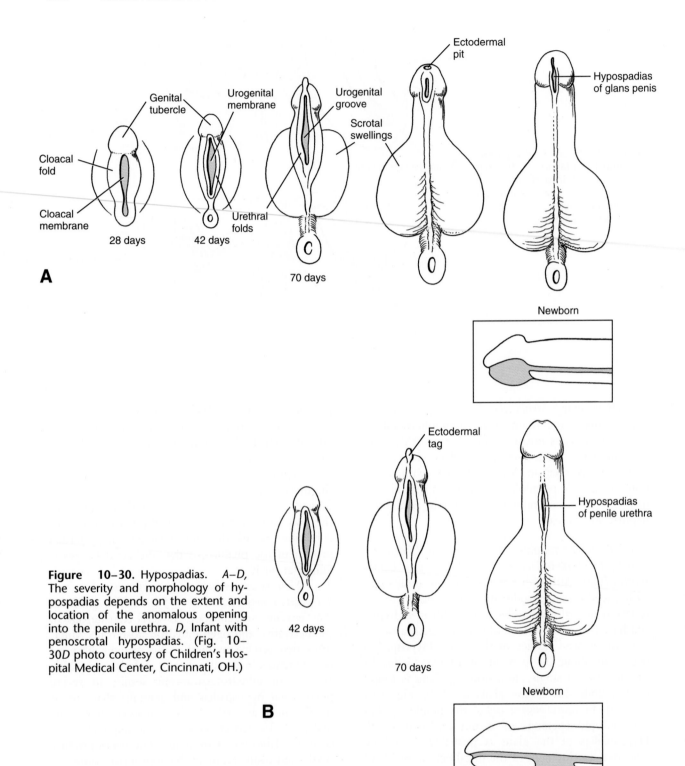

Figure 10–30. Hypospadias. *A–D,* The severity and morphology of hypospadias depends on the extent and location of the anomalous opening into the penile urethra. *D,* Infant with penoscrotal hypospadias. (Fig. 10–30*D* photo courtesy of Children's Hospital Medical Center, Cincinnati, OH.)

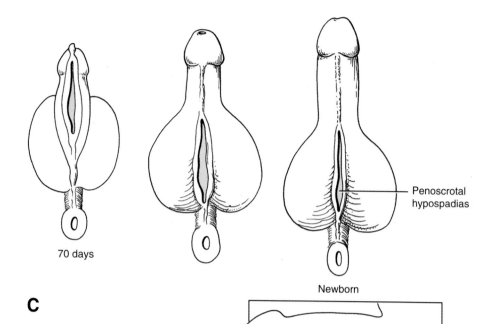

70 days

Newborn

Penoscrotal
hypospadias

C

D

Figure 10–30. *Continued.*

the sudden rise of testosterone at puberty may cause a dramatic differentiation of the external genitalia and accessory glands into typically male structures. The urethral folds and labioscrotal swellings may fuse completely, and the genital tubercle may differentiate into a penis. These former pseudohermaphrodites may be fertile and produce offspring. The normal testosterone levels during fetal life and after puberty are thought to result in normal male differentiation of the brain and, hence, a sense of male gender identity.

Male pseudohermaphroditism may be caused by testosterone deficiency. Mutations that affect enzymes required for the synthesis of testosterone, such as 20,22-desmolase, 17-hydroxylase, steroid 17,20-desmolase, and 17β-hydroxysteroid dehydrogenase, cause a deficiency or absence of testosterone. The resulting pseudohermaphroditism affects all structures that are dependent on androgens for their differentiation. The mesonephric ducts do not differentiate, the testes do not descend, and both the external genitalia and gender identity are female. Because testosterone levels do not rise at puberty, feminization is not reversed and the individual may continue to resemble a normal female. However, because testes develop and produce AMH, the paramesonephric ducts degenerate.

In Testicular Feminization Syndrome, the Androgen Receptors Are Abnormal. If the androgen receptors are disabled or absent, the male fetus may have normal or high levels of male steroid hormones, but the target issues do not respond and development proceeds as though androgens were absent. This condition is called **testicular feminization syndrome.** As in cases of primary testosterone deficiency, testes are present and AMH is produced, so the paramesonephric ducts regress, although a blind-ending vagina may form. Development is otherwise female.

Female Pseudohermaphroditism Is Rare. Female pseudohermaphrodites are genetic females who possess ovaries but whose genitalia are virilized by exposure to abnormal levels of virilizing sex steroids during fetal development. In most cases, the virilizing androgens are produced by hyperplastic fetal suprarenal glands. Some cases have apparently been caused by the administration of virilizing progestin compounds to prevent spontaneous abortion. Whatever the cause, the external genitals of female pseudohermaphrodites exhibit clitoral hypertrophy and fusion of the urethral and labioscrotal folds. Because testes and AMH are absent, however, the vagina, uterus, and fallopian tubes develop normally.

True Hermaphrodites Have Both Ovarian and Testicular Tissue. True hermaphrodites may be chromosomal males (46,XY), chromosomal females (46,XX), or mosaics (e.g. 45,X/46,XY, 46,XX/47,XXY, or 46,XX/46,XY). The mosaic cases are easiest to explain: In these individuals, ovarian tissue develops from cells without a Y chromosome, whereas testicular tissue develops from cells with a Y chromosome. There is evidence that hermaphrodites with a 46,XX karyotype may also be mosaics, with some cells that are effectively male. Apparently, the X chromosome in some cells of these individuals carries a fragment of the short arm of the Y chromosome, including the sex-determining region. This fragment was acquired by abnormal crossing over early in cleavage.

46,XY hermaphrodites are more difficult to explain. The cause may be effective mosaicism involving cells with a mutation of the Y chromosome or ovary-determining regions of the X chromosome.

The gonads of true hermaphrodites are usually streaklike, composite **ovotestes** containing both seminiferous tubules and follicles. Occasionally, however, an individual has an ovary or ovotestis on one side and a testis on the other. A fallopian tube and single uterine horn may develop on the side with the ovary. A few true hermaphrodites have ovulated and conceived, although none has carried a fetus to term. A vas deferens always develops in conjunction with a testis. The testis is usually immature, but spermatogenesis is occasionally detectable. Most true hermaphrodites are reared as males because a phallus is usually present at birth.

Failure to Enter Puberty May Be Caused by Primary or Secondary Hypogonadism. When a boy or girl fails to undergo the developmental changes associated with puberty, the cause is usually a deficiency of the appropriate sex steroids normally secreted by the gonads—testosterone in males and estrogen in females. The pubertal surge in sex steroid production is stimulated by increased levels of pituitary gonadotrophic hormones. Hypogonadism may thus be caused by a defect either in the gonads themselves or in the hypothalamus and pituitary.

Primary Hypogonadism Is Caused by a Gonadal Defect. In **primary hypogonadism,** the hypothalamus and pituitary are normal and produce high levels of circulating gonadotropins, but the gonad does not respond with an increased production of sex steroids. Most cases of primary hypogonadism are associated with one of two major chromosomal anomalies, although a few cases are of unknown (idiopathic) origin.

In males, primary hypogonadism is usually a component of **Klinefelter syndrome,** which occurs in about 1 of 500 live male births. Klinefelter syndrome is caused by a variety of sex chromosome anomalies involving the presence of an extra X chromosome. (The extra X chromosome is acquired by nondisjunction during gametogenesis or early cleavage.) The most common karyotype is 47,XXY. Other individuals with Klinefelter syndrome are mosaics: either mosaics of cells with normal male karyotype (46,XY) and cells with an abnormal karyotype (e.g., 47,XXY; 48,XXYY; 45,X; and 47,XXY) or mosaics of cells with a female 46,XX karyotype and cells with an abnormal 47,XXY karyotype. In all cases, the primary defect is a failure of the Leydig cells to produce sufficient amounts of male steroids, which results in small testes and **azoospermia** (lack of spermatogenesis) or **oligospermia** (low sperm count). Many of these individuals also exhibit **gynecomastia** (development of breasts in males) and **eunuchoidism** (elongated extremities).

Primary hypogonadism in females is usually associated with **Turner syndrome.** This condition is much less common than Klinefelter syndrome, occurring in 1 of 5000 live female births. The cause is a 45,X karyotype or 45,X/46,XX mosaicism. In addition to the failure of normal sexual maturation at puberty, Turner syndrome is characterized by a range of malformations, including short stature and webbed neck, coarctation of the aorta, and cervical lymphatic cysts (see the Clinical Applications section of Ch. 8).

Secondary Hypogonadism Is Caused by Defects of the Hypothalamus or Anterior Pituitary. Individuals with **secondary hypogonadism** have depressed levels of gonadotropins as well as sex steroids. Most often, the cause is an insufficient secretion of gonadotropin-releasing hormone (GnRH) by the hypothalamus, as in **Kallmann syndrome** and the **fertile eunuch syndrome** in males. One rare case of secondary hypogonadism in a male was shown to be due to the secretion of biologically inactive defective luteinizing hormone by the anterior pituitary. A variety of secondary hypogonadotropic disorders in males and females show autosomal recessive inheritance.

Experimental Principles

Molecular Regulation of Urogenital Development

MOLECULAR REGULATION OF KIDNEY DEVELOPMENT

Kidney Development Is a Classical Model of Reciprocal Induction. As discussed in the Descriptive Embryology section of this chapter, the ureteric bud induces the **mesenchymal to epithelial transformations** that result in formation of the nephric units within the metanephric blastema, and the metanephric blastema induces appropriate **branching of the ureteric bud.** Classic studies have postulated roles for the **extracellular matrix** and **diffusible factors** in this interactive developmental process. For example, it is well known that several components of the extracellular matrix facilitate epithelial organization of metanephric mesenchyme. Essential diffusible factors and their receptors have also been identified.

Candidate Inductive Factors and Regulatory Elements in Kidney Development Have Been Identified With Molecular Techniques. As in studies of embryogenesis and organogenesis of other systems discussed in earlier chapters, the techniques of in situ hybridization, perturbation studies with antisense oligonucleotides and transgenic technologies have also been valuable in studies of kidney development. Researchers are only in the beginning stages of understanding kidney development, but a fascinating picture is beginning to emerge.

The *initial specification of the metanephric blastema* in mice is indicated very early in development by expression of a **zinc-finger transcription factor** gene called *Wt1*. (Recall from the Clinical Applications section earlier that mutated forms of the human gene lead to genitourinary anomalies and development of the nephroblastoma Wilms' tumor). *Wt1* is expressed in the metanephric mesoderm before formation of the ureteric bud and so its expression does not require inductive signals from the ureteric bud. On the other hand, *expression of Wt1 within the metanephric blastema is required for sprouting of the ureteric bud*, because differentiation of the metanephros is disrupted and the ureteric bud fails to sprout from the mesonephric duct in transgenic knockout mice homozygous for a disrupted *Wt1* allele.

The *growth and branching of the ureteric bud* depends on signals from the metanephric mesenchyme. Glial derived neurotrophic factor (*GDNF*), made by the metanephric mesenchyme, interacts with the *c-ret* receptor tyrosine kinase on the ureteric bud to form one important component of this signaling process. Mice homozygous mutant for either the *GDNF* ligand or its *c-ret* receptor suffer **renal agenesis** or severe **renal dysgenesis** resulting from failure of ureteric bud branching morphogenesis. This process also appears to be under the inhibitory influence of BMP4, a member of the transforming growth factor beta family. Heterozygous *BMP4* mutant mice display a variety of defects, including bifid ureters, indicating that BMP4 normally functions to limit ureteric bud branching.

Induction of the metanephric mesenchyme by the ureteric bud results in its recruitment and the formation of renal excretory units. Induction and morphogenesis are parts of a multistep process that also requires rescue from apoptosis. Recently, fibroblast growth factor 2 (Fgf-2) has been shown to prevent mesenchyme apoptosis. The initial inducing event is still disputed but appears to require cell contact. Once the induced mesenchyme condenses around the ureteric bud tips, *Wnt4* is required to complete the mesenchyme to epithelial transition. In *Wnt4* mutant mice the epithelial tubules fail to form in the developing kidney. Growth and branching of the ureteric bud continues, without nephron formation. A member of the IL-6 family of cytokines, leukemia inhibitory factor (LIF), is also part of the inductive process and induces meschyme transformation. When added to isolated, dormant mesenchyme that already expresses *Wnt4*, LIF causes epithelial structures to form.

Little is known about later stages of nephron differentiation, but there are interesting changes in expression of many regulatory genes such as *Mox-1*, N-*myc*, *Mfh-1*, *Lfb-1*, *Lfb-3*, *Pax-2*, *Hoxc-9*, c-*myc* and *Wt1*. It is also interesting to note that cadherin genes are segmentally expressed in the early epithelium during nephron formation. These genes encode calcium-dependent adhesion molecules that control adhesion between cells of similar character and may play a part in segmentation of the nephron.

A single gene can function in the development of multiple organs, and at multiple genetic levels in the formation of a single organ. The *Hoxa 11* gene, for example, functions in the development of both the limb and kidney. Targeted inactivation of the *Hoxa 11* gene in mice, along with the functionally redundant *Hoxd 11* gene, results in limb malformations as well as severely hypoplastic kidneys, with dramatically reduced numbers of nephrons.

The *Pax-2* transcription factor gene provides an example of a gene that functions at more than one level in kidney development. This gene is normally expressed first in the mesonephric (also called Wolffian) duct and then in the ureteric bud. Mice with no functional *Pax-2* lack kidneys and genital tracts. In the mutants, the Wolffian ducts lose *c-ret* expression, do not extend normally to the cloaca, and degenerate without forming ureteric buds. In addition, however, the *Pax-2* gene is normally expressed in the metanephric mesenchyme after induction by the ureteric bud. There, it presumably plays a yet to be defined role in the condensation and epithelial conversion of the metanephric mesenchyme during the formation of nephrons.

Insulin-Like Growth Factor-2 Is Probably Not a Morphogen but Is Required for Growth of the Kidney. The insulin-like growth factor (IGF) family plays a role in the growth of the kidneys as well as other organs, because kidney size is reduced in mouse proportional dwarfs that lack either the *IGF-2* or *IGF-1* gene products. Moreover, knocking out the *IGF-1* gene and the gene that encodes its receptor also results in development of small kidneys that are histologically normal.

Sex Determination and Sexual Differentiation

Living organisms have evolved a variety of primary mechanisms for sex determination. In crocodiles, for example, the sex of the offspring is determined by the temperature of the incubated egg, whereas in fruit flies it is determined by the ratio of X chromosomes to autosomes.

In Humans, the Y Chromosome Instigates Development of the Testis

Although it has been known since 1921, that human males have an X and a Y sex chromosome, whereas females have two X chromosomes, the roles of these chromosomes in human sex determination were not elucidated until 1959 (Fig. 10–31). It was not clear whether femaleness was determined by the *presence* of two X chromosomes or by the *absence* of the tiny Y chromosome and, conversely, whether maleness was determined by the presence of a Y chromosome or by the presence of a *single* X chromosome.

In 1959, this question was answered by the examination of two individuals with chromosome anomalies: one female with Turner syndrome who had a 45,X karyotype and one male with Klinefelter syndrome who had a 47,XXY karyotype (see the Clinical Applications section of this chapter for a discussion of Turner and Klinefelter syndromes). Apparently, the *presence* of a Y chromosome determines maleness and its *absence* determines femaleness. By 1966, analysis of many structurally aberrant Y chromosomes in humans led to the conclusion that the information necessary to initiate development of a testis (and thus to determine male sex) was carried on the short arm of the Y chromosome.

Identification of the Testis-Determining Factor Took Almost 25 Years. The identity of the protein encoded by the testis-determining region of

Figure 10–31. A 31-year history of the search for the sex-determining region of the Y chromosome. (Modified from McLaren A. 1990. What makes a man a man? Nature 346:216.)

the Y chromosome proved elusive. Two promising candidates for this substance were investigated and rejected. One candidate that seemed to conform to all required criteria was the male-specific histocompatibility antigen H-Y. By 1984, however, mice were found that lacked this antigen but nevertheless had testes.

Exciting Advances Accompanied the Discovery of XX Males and XY Females. In the mid-1980s, a return to the strategy that originally identified the role of the Y chromosome in sex determination led to exciting new findings. First, the DNA of men with a 46,XX karyotype was examined. The genome in these individuals was found to contain very small amounts of Y chromosome DNA that had been translocated onto the X chromosome. Analysis of this DNA by using male- and female-specific cDNA probes narrowed the location of the sex-determining region of the Y chromosome to region 1, a relatively small region on the short arm. Within this region the *SRY* gene (sex-determining region of chromosome Y) was found. *SRY* encodes a transcription factor protein with an HMG box DNA binding domain.

The Role of *SRY* in Human Sex Determination Is Supported by Studies in Mice. Consistent with the idea that *SRY* initiates the genetic cascade of male sexual development is the finding that the comparable genetic locus in mice (*Sry*) is activated and expressed in the genital ridge 11.5 days after coitus, just before the initiation of testis development. Moreover, when the DNA of a female XY mouse was analyzed with DNA probes for *Sry*, part of this locus was found to be deleted.

Most importantly, it has been demonstrated that insertion of *Sry* into one of the X chromosomes of a genetically female mouse converts the mouse to a phenotypic male (see the Experimental Principles section of Ch. 1). Such transgenic mice produced by using a 14-kilobase fragment containing the *Sry* locus exhibited testes, vasa deferentia, and absence of the female reproductive tract. Although this mouse was sterile and its testes were considerably smaller than those of a normal XY mouse, these observations indicate that *Sry* alone can initiate the typical male developmental cascade that results in the synthesis of antimüllerian hormone by the developing Sertoli cells followed by the production of testosterone by the Leydig cells.

There is still much to be learned of the genetic program of gonad development, but interesting pieces of the puzzle are beginning to fall into place. In addition to *SRY*, several other genes essential for normal gonad development have now been identified. Mice with a mutation in the *Lim1* gene, for example, have no heads, kidneys, or gonads. This transcription factor gene, which encodes a protein with a Lim domain and a homeodomain, clearly occupies a high-level position in the genetic hierarchies of the development of these structures, although its downstream targets remain to be identified. For some other genes important in gonadogenesis, however, a genetic cascade is beginning to emerge, as shown in Figure 10–32.

WT1 Is Expressed Upstream From SRY and Is Required for Both Male and Female Sexual Development

As discussed above, humans heterozygous for mutations of **WT1** exhibit abnormalities of the genital system in addition to anomalies of the kidney and Wilms' tumor. In genetic males, these include hypospadias and cryptorchidism; in females, the gonads may consist of undifferentiated streaks of mesenchyme. In null alleles (homozygous knockouts) of *Wt1* in mice, normal thickening of the genital ridge does not occur, although primordial germ cells are not prevented from entering the presumptive gonadal tissue. *WT1* is expressed within the genital ridges during the early ambisexual stage of gonad development in mouse and human embryos, before expression of *SRY*. It has therefore been suggested that its gene product, a zinc-finger transcription factor, directly or indirectly induces expression of *SRY*.

Steroidogenic Factor-1 Expression Is Also Required for Development of the Bipotential Gonad

Steroidogenic factor-1 (SF-1) is an orphan nuclear receptor whose best-known functions involve binding to promoter elements that regulate expression of the **steroid hydroxylase enzymes**; these enzymes catalyze the multiple steps involved in conversion of cholesterol to testosterone. However, this factor has also been implicated in early devel-

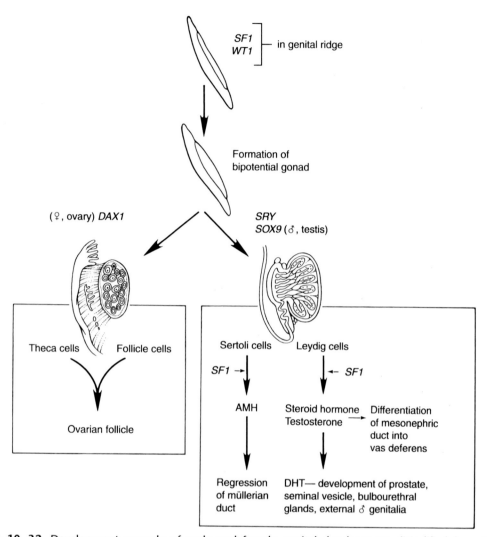

Figure 10–32. Development cascade of male and female genital development. (Modified from Marx J. 1995. Sharing the genes that divide the sexes for mammals [news]. Science 270:901.)

opment of the bipotential gonad. For example, it is expressed within the mouse gonadal ridge before differentiation of the male and female gonads. In addition, targeted disruption of **SF-1** results in the absence of gonads in male and female transgenic mice. Abnormal development of the genital ridge, however, as in the case of the *Wt1* null mutation described above, does not prevent primordial germ cell migration and infiltration.

SF-1 may also play a role in early development of the testes. As the bipotential gonad begins to differentiate, SF-1 expression is maintained in the testes, although it ceases in the ovaries. Moreover, SF-1 specifically binds to promoter sequences of the gene encoding AMH, but the nature of the functional interaction between SF-1 and *SRY* in the regulation of AMH and testes development is not known. It is unlikely, for example, that *SRY* activates the expression of SF-1, because SF-1 expression in testes both precedes and follows the expression of *SRY*. Moreover, it also seems unlikely that AMH plays a direct role in testis development per se based on the phenotype produced by targeted disruption of AMH in mice. AMH-deficient mice possess fully descended testes that produce functional spermatozoa. These animals, however, possess both male and female genital ducts, again demonstrating AMH's pivotal role in normal regression of the paramesonephric ducts in males.

Sex Reversal Without *SRY* Mutation

It is now clear that only 25 percent of sex reversals in XY females can be explained by disabling mutations of *SRY*. Indeed, autosomal chromosomal deletions of 9p and 10q and duplications of Xp can lead to a female phenotype in XY individuals with an intact *SRY*. Not only may these individuals possess normal female genital ducts, but they may also possess ovaries with normal oocytes.

Individuals suffering from a congenital skeletal disease called **camptomelic dysplasia,** for example, exhibit mutations of a gene called *SOX9,* which has been mapped to 17q24.3-q25.1. These XY individuals possess a normal *SRY* but in extreme cases may exhibit completely feminized sex organs. *SOX9* is related to *SRY* and contains a similar DNA binding HMG box. The relationship between skeletal anomalies and the mechanism by which sex reversal occurs in these individuals, however, is unknown.

The *SOX9* gene appears particularly important in sex determination. Although the *SRY* gene is restricted to mammals, the *SOX9* gene is found throughout vertebrates. As mentioned earlier, when there is only one functional copy of this autosomal gene XY individuals often develop as females, despite the presence of *SRY*. Further, XX individuals with an extra copy of *SOX9* develop as males, even though they have no Y chromosome. *SOX9* is expressed at low levels in the early genital ridges of both males and females but is soon turned off in the developing ovary. *SOX9* is upregulated in the developing testes immediately after

SRY expression and is expressed in Sertoli cells into adulthood. One candidate downstream target of *SOX9* is the *AMH* gene. Both the SF-1 and SOX9 proteins can bind the AMH promoter and cooperate to activate AMH transcription.

Duplications of part of the short arm of the X chromosome also result in sex reversal in XY males with an intact *SRY*. This duplication also results in hypoplastic development of the adrenal glands. The locus for the gene responsible for this sex reversal is a 160-kb region of Xp. The gene is called **DAX1** (or DSS-AHC critical region of the X chromosome: dosage-dependent sex reversal; adrenal hypoplasia congenita; X chromosome). Because of the feminization of the genitalia by two copies of *DAX1* in XY individuals, it is possible that *DAX1* also plays a critical role in female sexual determination and normal development of the ovary (see Fig. 10–32). It is also possible that mutations of *DAX1* may explain sex reversal in some XX males.

Estrogen Is Required for Normal Female and Male Genital Development

Null mutation of the estrogen receptor in mice does not result in lethality, as might have been predicted. Female estrogen receptor knockouts (**ERKO**), however, display anomalies of ovarian development, primarily hemorrhagic cystic ovaries that appear to result from excessive stimulation by pituitary gonadotropins (as a consequence of lack of functional negative feedback mechanism). Another somewhat surprising finding was that male ERKO mice also exhibited defects of gonadal development. The testes were reduced in size with few intact seminiferous tubules and reduction in the number of germ cells. In contrast, however, was a unique 28-year-old human male who lacked estrogen receptors but appeared to be fully masculinized. His lack of estrogen receptors, however, resulted in failure of the epiphyseal plates to close; he was 6 feet 8 inches tall and continuing to grow and wore size 19 shoes.

SUGGESTED READING

Descriptive Embryology

Buehr M, Gu S, McLaren A. 1993. Mesonephric contribution to testis differentiation in the fetal mouse. Development 117:273

Byskov AG. 1986. Differentiation of mammalian embryonic gonad. Physiol Rev 66:71

Cate RL, Mattaliano RJ, Hession C, et al. 1986. Isolation of the bovine and human genes for Müllerian inhibiting substance and expression of the human gene in animal cells. Cell 45:685

Cunha GR. 1985. Mesenchymal-epithelial interactions during androgen-induced development of the prostate, p. 15. In: Lash JW, Saxén L (eds): Developmental Mechanisms: Normal and Abnormal. Alan R Liss, New York

Ekblom P, Sariola H, Karkinen-Jaaskelainen M, Saxen L. 1982. The origin of the glomerular endothelium. Cell Differ 11:35

Fine H. 1982. The development of the lobes of the metanephros and fetal kidney. Acta Anat 113:93

Grobstein C. 1955. Inductive interaction in the development of the mouse metanephros. J Exp Zool 130:319

Huston JM, Beasely SW. 1988. Embryological controversies in testicular descent. Semin Urol 6:68

Jost A, Magre S. 1988. Control mechanisms of testicular differentiation. Philos Trans R Soc Lond B Biol Sci 322:55

Kluth D, Lambrecht W, Reich P. 1988. Pathogenesis of hypospadias—more questions than answers. J Pediatr Surg 23:1095

Marshall FF. 1978. Embryology of the lower genitourinary tract. Urol Clin North Am 5:3

McLaren A. 1988. Somatic and germ-cell sex in mammals. Philos Trans R Soc Lond B Biol Sci 322:3

McLaren A. 1990. What makes a man a man? Nature (London) 346:216

Merchant-Larios H, Moreno-Mendoza N, Buehr M. 1993. The role of the mesonephros in cell differentiation and morphogenesis of the mouse fetal testis. Int J Dev Biol 37:407

O'Rahilly R. 1977. The development of the vagina in the human. Birth Defects Orig Artic Ser 13:123

O'Rahilly R. 1977. Prenatal human development, p. 35. In Wynn RM (ed): Biology of the Uterus. Plenum Press, New York

O'Rahilly R. 1983. The timing and sequence of events in the development of the human reproductive system during the embryonic period proper. Acta Embryol 166:247

Potter EL. 1972. Normal and Abnormal Development of the Kidney. Year Book Medical Publishers, Chicago

Sariola H, Holm K, Henke-Fahle S. 1988. Early innervation of the metanephric kidney. Development 104:589

Satoh M. 1991. Histogenesis and organogenesis of the gonad in human embryos. J Anat 177:85

Saxen L, Sariola H, Lehtonen E. 1986. Sequential cell and tissue interactions governing organogenesis of the kidney. Anat Embryol 175:1

Spaulding MH. 1921. The development of the external genitalia in the human embryo. Contrib Embryol Carnegie Inst 13:67

Stephens FD. 1988. Embryology of the cloaca and embryogenesis of anorectal malformations. Birth Defects Orig Artic Ser 24:177

Wensing CGJ. 1988. The embryology of testicular descent. Horm Res 30:144

Williams HG. 1983. Regulatory features of seminal vesicle development and function. Curr Top Cell Regul 22:201

Clinical Applications

Bain J. 1986. Hypogonadal states in the male. Compr Ther 12:39

Berry AC, Chantler C. 1986. Urogenital malformations and disease. Br Med Bull 42:181

Burgoyne PS, Buehr M, Koopman P, Rossant J. 1988. Cell autonomous action of the testis-determining gene: Sertoli cells are exclusively XY in XX-XY chimeric mouse testes. Development 102:443

Churchill BM, Abara EO, McLorie GA. 1987. Ureteral duplication, ectopy, and ureteroceles. Manag Princ Pediatr Urol 34:1273

de la Chapelle A. 1986. Genetic molecular studies on 46,XX and 45,X males. Cold Spring Harbor Symp Quant Biol 51:249

deVries PA. 1984. The surgery of anorectal anomalies: its evolution, with evaluations of procedures. p. 1. In Ravitch MM (ed): Current Problems in Surgery. Year Book Medical Publishers, Chicago

Dey BR, Sukhatme VP, Roberts AB, et al. 1994. Repression of the transforming growth factor-β 1 gene by the Wilms' tumor suppressor gene product. Mol Endocrinol 8:595

DiGeorge AM. 1983. Disorders of the gonads. p. 1494. In Nelson W, Behrman RE, Vaughan VC III (eds): Nelson Textbook of Pediatrics. WB Saunders, Philadelphia

Drechsler M, Meijers-Heijboer EJ, Schneider S, et al. 1994. Molecular analysis of aniridia patients for deletions involving the Wilms' tumor gene. Human Genet 94:331

Drummond IA, Madden SL, Rohwer-Nutter P, et al. 1992. Repression of the insulinlike growth factor II gene by the Wilms tumor suppressor WT1. Science 257:674

Haber DA, Sohn RL, Buckler AJ, et al. 1991. Alternative splicing and genomic structure of the Wilms' tumor gene WT1. Proc Natl Acad Sci U S A 88:9618

Hastie ND. 1992. Dominant negative mutations in Wilms' tumor (*WT1*) gene cause Denys-Drash syndrome—proof that a tumor-suppressor gene plays a crucial role in normal genitourinary development. Hum Mol Genet 1:293

Knudson AG, Strong LC. 1972. Mutation and cancer: a model for Wilms' tumor of the kidney. J Natl Cancer Inst 48:313

Kubota T, Saitoh S, Matsumoto T, et al. 1994. Excess functional copy of allele at chromosomal region 11p15 may cause Wiedemann-Beckwith (EMG) syndrome. Am J Med Genet 49:378

Little MH, Prosser J, Condie A, et al. 1992. Zinc finger point mutations within the *WT1* gene in Wilms' tumor patients. Proc Natl Acad Sci U S A 89:4791

Luo XN, Reddy JC, Yeyati PL, et al. 1995. The tumor suppressor gene *WT1* inhibits *ras*-mediated transformation. Oncogene 11:743

Moffat DB. 1982. Developmental abnormalities of the urogenital system, p. 357. In Chisholm GD, and Williams DI (eds): Scientific Foundations of Urology. Year Book Medical Publishers, Chicago

Moyer JH, Lee-Tischler MJ, Kwon H-Y, et al. 1994. Candidate gene associated with a mutation causing recessive polycystic kidney disease in mice. Science 264:1329

Potter EL. 1946. Bilateral renal agenesis. J Pediatr 29:68

Potter EL. 1972. Extrinsic abnormalities of the kidneys. p. 83. In Potter EL: Normal and Abnormal Development of the Kidney. Year Book Medical Publishers, Chicago

Pritchard-Jones K, Fleming S, Davidson D, et al. 1990. The candidate Wilms' tumor gene is involved in genitourinary development. Nature 346:194

Rosier MF, Goguel AF, Martin A, et al. 1994. A 1.7-Mb YAC contig around the human BDNF gene (11p13): integration of the physical, genetic and cytogenetic maps in relation to WAGR syndrome. Genomics 24:69

Smith ED. 1988. Incidence, frequency of types, and etiology of anorectal malformations. Birth Defects Orig Artic Ser 24:231

Stephens FD. 1988. Embryology of the cloaca and embryogenesis of anorectal malformations. Birth Defects Orig Artic Ser 24:177

Telerman A, Dodemont H, Degraef C, et al. 1992. Identification of the cellular protein encoded by the Wilms' tumor (*WT1*) gene. Oncogene 7:2545

Thomas DFM. 1989. Cloacal malformations: embryology, anatomy and principles of management. Prog Pediatr Surg 23:135

van Niekerk WA, Retief AE. 1981. The gonads of human true hermaphrodites. Hum Genet 58:117

Wada M, Seeger RC, Mizoguchi H, Koeffler HP. 1995. Maintenance of normal imprinting of H19 and IGF2 genes in neuroblastoma. Cancer Res 55:3386

Werner H, Shen-Orr Z, Rauscher FJ 3rd, et al. 1995. Inhibition of cellular proliferation by the Wilms' tumor suppressor WT1 is associated with suppression of insulin-like growth factor I receptor gene expression. Mol Cell Biol 15:3516

Experimental Principles

Bard JBL, McConnell JE, Davies JA. 1994. Towards a genetic basis for kidney development. Mech Dev 48:3

Behringer RR. 1994. The in vivo roles of Müllerian-inhibiting substance. Curr Top Devel Biol 29:171

Behringer RR, Finegold MJ, Cate RL. 1994. Müllerian inhibiting substance function during mammalian sexual development. Cell 79:415

Bogan JS, Page D. 1994. Ovary? Testis?—a mammalian dilemma. Cell 76:603

Buhler EM. 1980. Synopsis of the human Y chromosome. Hum Genet 55:145

Burgoyne PS. 1988. Role of mammalian Y chromosome in sex determination. Philos Trans R Soc Lond Biol Sci 322:63

Burgoyne PS. 1988. Cell autonomous action of the testis-determining gene: Sertoli cells are exclusively XY in XX-XY chimeric mouse testes. Development 102:443

Burris TP, Guo W, Le T, McCabe ER. 1995. Identification of a putative steroidogenic factor-1 response element in the DAX-1 promoter. Biochem Biophys Res Commun 214:576

Chahnazarian A. 1988. Determinants of the sex ratio at birth: review of recent literature. Soc Biol 35:214

Cherfas J. 1991. Sex and the single gene. Science 252:782

Cooke H. 1990. The continuing search for the mammalian sex-determining gene. Trends Genet 60:273

de la Chapelle A. 1986. Genetic and molecular studies on 46,XX and 45,X males. Cold Spring Harbor Symp Quant Biol 51:249

Dressler GR. 1995. The genetic control of renal development. Curr Opin Nephrol Hypertens 4:253

Eccles MR, Yun K, Reeve AE, Fidler AE. 1995. Comparative in situ hybridization analysis of *PAX2*, *PAX8* and *WT1* gene transcription in human fetal kidney and Wilms' tumors. Am J Pathol 146:40

Ford CE. 1970. Cytogenetics and sex determination in man and mammals. J Biosoc Sci Suppl 2:7

Ford CE, Hammerton JL. 1956. The chromosomes of man. Nature (London) 178:1020

Ford CE, Jones KW, Polani P, et al. 1959. A sex chromosome anomaly in a case of gonadal dysgenesis (Turner's syndrome). Lancet i:711

Graves JA. 1995. The evolution of mammalian sex chromosomes and the origin of sex determining genes. Philos Trans R Soc B Biol Sci 350:305

Grobstein C. 1956. Inductive tissue interactions in development. Adv Can Res 4:187

Grubb GR, Yun K, Williams BR, et al. 1994. Expression of WT1 protein in fetal kidneys and Wilms' tumors. Lab Invest 71:472

Gubbay J, Collignon J, Koopman P, et al. 1990. A gene mapping to the sex-determining region of the mouse Y chromosome is a member of a novel family of embryologically expressed genes. Nature (London) 346:245

Hacker A, Capel B, Goodfellow P, Lovell-Badge R. 1995. Expression of *Sry*, the mouse sex-determining gene. Development 121:1603

Haqq CM, King CY, Donahoe PK, Weiss MA. 1993. SRY recognizes conserved DNA sites in sex-specific promoters. Proc Natl Acad Sci U S A 90: 1097

Haqq CM, King CY, Ukiyama E, et al. 1994. Molecular basis of mammalian sexual determination: activation of Müllerian inhibiting substance gene expression by SRY. Science 266:1994

Ingraham HA, Lala DS, Ikeda Y, et al. 1994. The nuclear receptor steroidogenic factor 1 acts at multiple levels of the reproductive axis. Genes Dev 8: 2302

Jacobs PA, Ross A. 1966. Structural analyses of the Y chromosome in man. Nature (London) 210:352

Jacobs PA, Strong JA. 1959. A case of human intersexuality having a possible XXY sex determining mechanism. Nature (London) 183:302

Koopman P, Gubbay J, Vivian N, et al. 1991. Male development of chromosomally female mice transgenic for Sry. Nature (London) 351:117

Korach K. 1994. Insights from the study of animals lacking functional estrogen receptor. Science 266: 1524

Kreidberg JA, Sariola H, Loring JM, et al. 1993. WT-1 is required for early kidney development. Cell 74: 679

Lala DS, Ikeda Y, Luo X, et al. 1995. A cell-specific nuclear receptor regulates the steroid hydroxylases. Steroids 60:10

Lovell-Badge R, Hacker A. 1995. The molecular genetics of Sry and its role in mammalian sex determination. Philos Trans R Soc B Biol Sci 350:205

McElreavey K, Barbaux S, Ion A, Fellous M. 1995. The genetic basis of murine and human sex determination: a review. Heredity 75:599

McElreavey K, Vilain E, Abbas N, et al. 1993. A regulatory cascade hypothesis for mammalian sex determination: SRY represses a negative regulator of male development. Proc Natl Acad Sci U S A 90: 3368

McLaren A. 1990. What makes a man a man? Nature (London) 346:216

McLaren A. 1991. The making of male mice. Nature (London) 351:96

McLaren A, Simpson E, Tomonari K, et al. 1984. Male sexual differentiation in mice lacking H-Y antigen. Nature (London) 312:552

Mittwoch U. 1992. Sex determination and sex reversal: genotype, phenotype, dogma and semantics. Hum Genet 89:467

Müller U. 1987. Mapping of testis-determining locus on Yp by the molecular analysis of XX males and XY females. Development 101:52

Mundlos S, Pelletier J, Darveau A, et al. 1993. Nuclear localization of the protein encoded by the Wilms' tumor gene *WT1* in embryonic and adult tissues. Development 119:1329

Nomura M, Bartsch S, Nawata H, et al. 1995. An E box element is required for the expression of the *ad4bp* gene, a mammalian homolog of *fiz-fl* gene, which is essential for adrenal and gonadal development. J Biol Chem 270:7453

Page DC, Fisher EMC, McGillivray B, Brown LG. 1990. Additional deletion in sex-determining region of human Y chromosome resolves paradox of X,t(Y,22) female. Nature (London) 346:279

Page DC, Mosher R, Simpson EM, et al. 1987. The sex-determining region of the Y chromosome encodes a finger protein. Cell 51:1091

Patterson LT, Dressler GR. 1994. The regulation of kidney development: new insights from an old model. Curr Opin Genet Dev 4:696

Perantoni AO, Dove LF, Karanova I. 1995. Basic fibroblast growth factor can mediate the early inductive events in renal development. Proc Natl Acad Sci U S A 92:4696

Pontiggia A, Whitfield S, Goodfellow PN, et al. 1995. Evolutionary conservation in the DNA-binding and e-binding properties of HMG-boxes from SRY proteins of primates. Gene 154:277

Pritchard-Jones K, Fleming S, Davidson D, et al. 1990. The candidate Wilms' tumor gene is involved in genitourinary development. Nature 346:194

Richards JS, Fitzpatrick SL, Clemens JW, et al. 1995. Ovarian cell differentiation: a cascade of multiple hormones, cellular signals, and regulated genes. Recent Prog Horm Res 50:223

Rimini R, Pontiggia A, Spada F, et al. 1995. Interaction of normal and mutant Sry proteins with DNA. Philos Trans R Soc B Biol Sci 350:215

Roberts L. 1988. Zeroing in on the sex switch. Science 239:21

Ryner LC, Swain A. 1995. Sex in the '90s. Cell 81:483

Saxen L, Karkinen-Jaaskelainen M, Lehtonen E, et al. 1976. Inductive tissue interactions. p. 331. In Poste G, Nicholson GL (eds): The Cell Surface in Animal Embryogenesis and Development. Elsevier/North Holland, Amsterdam.

Saxen L, Lehtonen E. 1987. Embryonic kidney in organ culture. Differentiation 36:2

Schuchardt A, D'Agati V, Larsson-Blomberg L, et al. 1994. Defects in the kidney and enteric nervous system of mice lacking the tyrosine kinase receptor Ret. Nature 367:380

Shen W-H, Moore CCD, Ikeda Y, et al. 1994. Nuclear receptor steroidogenic factor 1 regulates the Müllerian inhibiting substance gene: a link to the sex determination cascade. Cell 77:651

Sinclaire AH, Berta P, Palmer MS, et al. 1990. A gene from the human sex-determining region encodes a protein with homology to a conserved DNA-binding motif. Nature (London) 346:240

Tommerup N, Schempp W, Meinecke P, et al. 1993. Assignment of an autosomal sex reversal locus (*SRA1*) and campomelic dysplasia (*CMPD1*) to 17q24. 3-q25.1. Nature Genet 4:170

11

Development of the Limbs

Summary

The upper **limb buds** appear on day 24 as small bulges on the lateral body wall at about the level of C5 to C8. By the end of the fourth week, they have grown to form noticeable, coronally oriented ridges, and the lower limb buds appear at the level of L3 to L5. Limb morphogenesis takes place from the fourth to the eighth weeks, with the development of the lower limbs lagging slightly behind the development of the upper limbs. Each limb bud consists of a **mesenchymal core** of mesoderm covered by an **ectodermal cap.** Along the distal margin of the limb bud, the ectoderm thickens to form an **apical ectodermal ridge.** This structure stimulates the outgrowth of the limb bud along the proximodistal axis.

By 33 days, the **hand plates** are visible at the end of the lengthening upper limb buds, and the lower limb buds have begun to elongate. By the end of the sixth week, the segments of the upper and lower limbs can be distinguished. **Digital rays** appear on the hand and foot plates during the sixth week (upper limbs) and the seventh week (lower limbs). A process of programmed cell death sculpts out these rays to free the fingers and toes. By the end of the eighth week, all the components of the upper and lower limbs are distinct.

The **skeletal elements** of the limbs develop from column-like mesodermal condensations that appear along the long axis of the limb bud during the fifth week. The cartilaginous precursors of the limb bones develop by chondrification within this mesenchymal condensation, starting in the sixth week. Ossification of these cartilaginous precursors begins in the 8th to 12th weeks.

The bones and blood vessels of the limbs arise from the lateral plate mesoderm of the limb buds, but the limb muscles are formed by somitic mesoderm that invades the limb buds. In general, the muscles that form on the ventral side of the developing long bones become the flexors and pronators of the upper limbs and the flexors and adductors of the lower limbs. These muscles are innervated by ventral branches of the ventral primary rami of the spinal nerves. The muscles that form on the dorsal side of the long bones generally become the extensor and supinator muscles of the upper limbs and the extensor and abductor muscles of the lower limbs. These muscles are innervated by dorsal branches of the ventral primary rami. However, muscles of the limbs may shift their position dramatically during development either by migration or by slight lateral rotation of the upper limb and medial rotation of the lower limb.

Development of the Limb Buds

Functions of the Apical Ectodermal Ridges and Mesodermal Core

Formation of the Hand and Foot Plates

Development of the Appendicular Skeleton and Musculature

Timeline. Development of the limbs.

THE LIMBS DEVELOP THROUGH A SERIES OF RECIPROCAL INDUCTIVE INTERACTIONS BETWEEN ECTODERM AND MESODERM

The Formation of Limb Buds in the Lateral Plate Mesoderm Is Reduced by the Adjacent Somites

The upper and lower **limb buds** are formed by proliferation of the somatopleuric lateral plate mesoderm in the limb regions of the flank (Fig. 11-1*A*, *B*). The upper limb bud appears in the lower cervical region at 24 days, and the lower limb bud appears in the lower lumbar region at 28 days. Each limb bud consists of an outer ectodermal cap and an inner mesodermal core.

The Apical Ectodermal Ridge Induces Proximodistal Elongation of the Limb Buds

As each limb bud forms, the ectoderm along the apex of the bud, induced by the underlying somatopleuric mesoderm, differentiates into a ridgelike thickening called the **apical ectodermal ridge** (AER) (see Fig. 11-1*C*, *D*). This structure plays an essential role in the outgrowth of the limb. Surgical removal of the AER arrests further outgrowth of distal limb elements at the stage corresponding to its removal. Limbs do not develop in a chick mutant that forms normal limb buds but fails to develop an AER. Transplantation experiments show that the absence of limbs in these chicks is not due to a defect in the mesodermal core: Limb bud mesoderm from this "limbless" mutant is capable of inducing the development of an apical ectodermal ridge and a normal limb if transplanted to the flank of a normal host.

The Identity of the Proximodistal Limb Segments Is Determined by the Age of the Corresponding Portions of Core Mesoderm

Transplantation experiments in chicks demonstrate that the AER induces growth in the distal subridge mesoderm termed the *progress zone* but does not specify which part of the bud will form which segment of the limb. That "decision" is made by the mesodermal core, apparently on the basis of its age: The late-formed mesenchyme at the tip of the elongating limb bud differentiates into the distal segments of the limb, whereas the early-formed mesenchyme at the base of the bud differentiates into the proximal segments of the limb after leaving the influence of the AER.

This conclusion is based partly on a series of transplantation experiments carried out on chick wing buds (Fig. 11-2). For example, if a composite artificial wing bud is made by combining the late-formed mesenchyme from the tip of an older bud with the ectodermal cap of a bud of any age, only the distal parts of the wing will form. Conversely, a composite wing bud made by combining an ectodermal cap of any age with the early-formed mesodermal core of a young bud will form an entire limb. On the basis of these and other experiments, it has been suggested that the factor that specifies which limb segment will be formed by a given zone of mesenchyme is the amount of time the mesenchyme has spent under the influence of the apical ridge and that the mesenchymal cells may measure this time by the number of cell divisions they have undergone under the influence of the apical ridge.

Development of the Limb Buds Occurs Between the Fourth and Eighth Weeks

Limb development takes place over a 5-week period from the fourth to the eighth weeks. The upper limbs develop slightly in advance of the lower limbs, although by the end of the period of limb development, the two limbs are nearly synchronized. Development takes place as follows (Fig. 11-3):

Day 33. In the upper limb, the **hand plate, forearm, arm,** and **shoulder** regions can be distinguished. In the lower limb, a somewhat rounded cranial part can be distinguished from a more tapering caudal part. The distal tip of the tapering caudal part will form the foot.

Day 37. In the hand plate of the upper limb, a

Figure 11–1. Scanning electron micrographs showing limb buds. The limb buds are formed when somitic mesoderm induces the proliferation of overlying lateral plate mesoderm. *A,* Embryo with newly formed upper limb bud (arrow). *B,* By day 29, the upper limb bud (arrow) is flattened. *C,* By day 32, the apical ectodermal ridge (arrow) is visible as a thickened crest of ectoderm at the distal edge of the growing upper limb bud. Rectangle indicates plane of sectioning of part *D. D,* Limb bud sectioned to show the inner mesenchymal core (M) and the outer ectodermal cap *E.* Arrow: apical ectodermal ridge. (From Kelley RO. 1985. Early development of the vertebrate limb: an introduction to morphogenetic tissue interactions using scanning electron microscopy. Scanning Microsc II:827.)

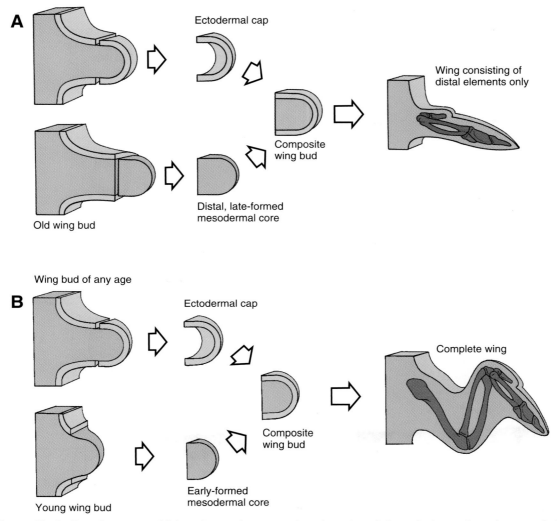

Figure 11–2. Experiment on chick embryos demonstrating the roles of the apical ectodermal cap and the mesodermal core in limb bud development. *A,* If an ectodermal cap of any age (even very young) is recombined with the distal end of an old mesenchymal core, the hybrid bud will form only distal elements of the limb. *B,* If an ectodermal cap from a bud of any age (even very old) is recombined with a complete mesodermal core from a young limb bud, the hybrid bud will form an entire limb. (Modified from Rubin L, Saunders TW. 1972. Ectodermal-mesodermal interactions in the growth of limb buds in the chick embryo: constancy and temporal limits of the ectodermal induction. Dev Biol 28:94.)

central **carpal region** is surrounded by a thickened crescentic flange, the **digital plate,** which will form the fingers. In the lower limb, the **thigh, leg,** and **foot** have become distinct.

Day 38. Finger rays (more generally, **digital rays**) are visible as radial thickenings in the digital plate of the upper limb. The tips of the finger rays project slightly, producing a crenulated rim on the digital plate. A process of programmed cell death will gradually sculpt the digital rays out of the digital plate to form the fingers and toes. Programmed cell death takes place in radial **necrotic zones** between the digital rays. The lower limb

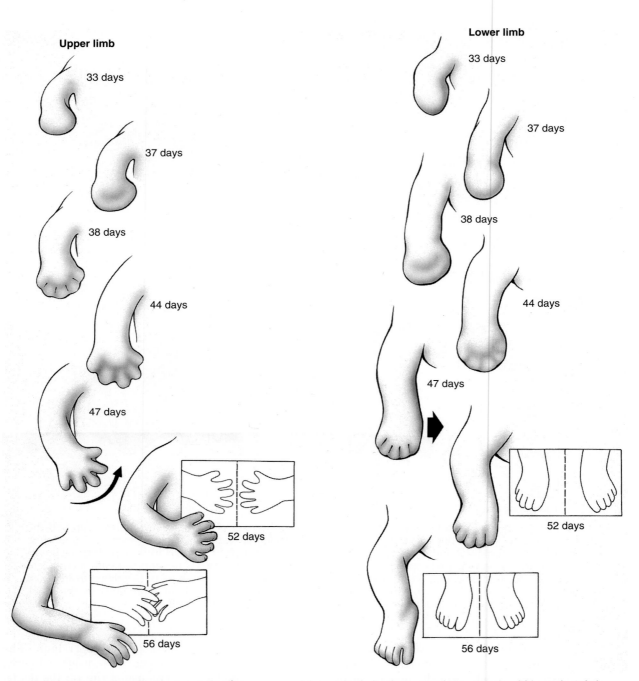

Figure 11–3. The development of the upper and lower limb buds occurs between the fifth and eighth weeks. Nearly every stage in the development of the lower limb bud takes place several days later than in the upper limb bud.

bud has increased in length and become demarcated from the trunk, and a clearly defined **foot plate** is apparent on the caudal side of the distal end of the bud.

Day 44. In the upper limb, the margin of the digital plate is deeply notched and the grooves between the finger rays are deeper. The elbow is obvious. **Toe rays** are visible in the digital plate of the foot, but the rim of the plate is not yet crenulated.

Day 47. The entire upper limb has undergone **horizontal flexion** so that it lies in a parasagittal rather than a coronal plane (Fig. 11–4A). The lower limb has also begun to flex toward a parasagittal plane. The toe rays are more prominent, although the margin of the digital plate is still smooth.

Day 52. The upper limbs are slightly bent at the elbows, and the fingers have developed distal swellings called **tactile pads** (see Fig. 11–4B). The hands are slightly flexed at the wrists and meet at the midline in front of the cardiac eminence.

The legs are longer, and the feet have begun to approach each other at the midline. The rim of the digital plate is notched.

Day 56. All regions of the arms and legs are well defined, including the toes. The fingers of the two hands overlap at the midline.

The Somites, Lateral Plate Mesoderm, and Neural Crest Contribute to Different Components Within the Limb

The quail–chick chimera system has been used to study the cell populations that give rise to the various elements of the limbs. One discovery was that although the lateral plate mesoderm gives rise to the bones, ligaments, and vasculature of the limbs, the limb *musculature* is derived from somitic mesoderm that migrates into the developing limb bud. A quail–chick chimera experiment demonstrating this point is illustrated in Fig. 11–5. If the chick somites at the level of the wing bud are replaced with the corresponding somites from a

A 7 weeks

B 8 weeks

Figure 11–4. *A,* By 7 weeks, the digits are clearly visible in both upper and lower extremities. *B,* At 8 weeks, tactile pads are apparent on the distal tips of the fingers. (*A,* Photo courtesy of Dr. Arnold Tamarin.)

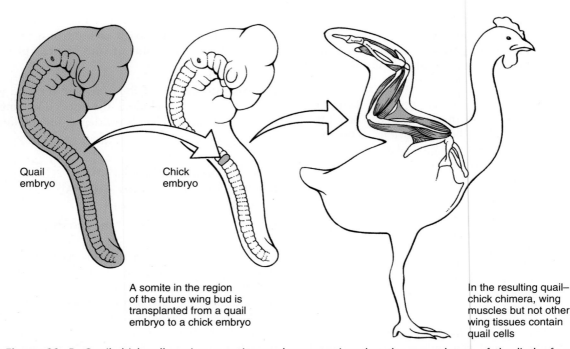

Quail embryo

Chick embryo

A somite in the region of the future wing bud is transplanted from a quail embryo to a chick embryo

In the resulting quail–chick chimera, wing muscles but not other wing tissues contain quail cells

Figure 11–5. Quail-chick cell tracing experiment demonstrating that the musculature of the limbs forms from somitic mesoderm, whereas the bones form from lateral plate mesoderm. Transplanted somites in the region of limb bud development give rise to limb myocytes. (Modified from Chevallier A, Kieny M, Mauger A. 1977. Limb–somite relationship: origin of the limb musculature. J Embryol Exp Morphol 41: 245.)

quail, the wing muscles will be made of quail cells, although the other wing tissues will be made of chick cells.

Other quail–chick experiments involving transplantation of parts of the neural tube have shown that the **melanocytes** and **Schwann cells** of the limb are derived from migrating ectomesenchymal cells of the neural crest.

The Limb Bones Form as Mesenchymal Condensations That First Chondrify and Then Ossify

With the exception of the clavicle, the bones of the limbs and girdles (constituting the **appendicular skeleton**) form by ossification of a cartilaginous precursor, a process known as **endochondral ossification.** The clavicle, in contrast, is a **membrane bone:** It forms by direct ossification from

mesenchyme in the dermis and lacks a cartilaginous precursor.

The endochondral bones of the limb and their intervening joints form from a rodlike condensation of lateral plate mesenchyme that develops along the long axis of the limb bud (Fig. 11–6). In response to growth factors, **chondrocytes** (cartilage cells) differentiate within this mesenchyme and begin to secrete molecules characteristic of the extracellular matrix of cartilage, such as collagen type II and proteoglycans.

The initial phase of chondrification in the developing limbs results in the deposition of cartilage around the entire axial mesenchymal condensation. This cartilaginous envelope is called the **perichondrium.** Further chondrification is limited to the sites of the future bones, where it creates a cartilaginous model (anlage) of each bone. The mesenchyme in the **interzones**—the sites of the future joints—differentiates into fibrous connective tissue.

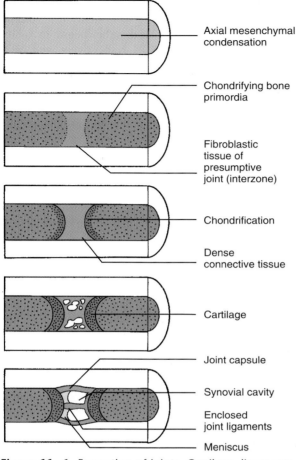

Axial mesenchymal condensation

Chondrifying bone primordia

Fibroblastic tissue of presumptive joint (interzone)

Chondrification

Dense connective tissue

Cartilage

Joint capsule

Synovial cavity

Enclosed joint ligaments

Meniscus

Figure 11–6. Formation of joints. Cartilage, ligaments, and capsular elements of the joints develop from the interzone regions of the axial mesenchymal condensations that form the long bones of the limbs.

After the anlage of each endochondral limb bone has chondrified, the process of **ossification** commences in a region of the bone called the **primary ossification center.** First, mesenchymal cells in the perichondrium differentiate into **osteoblasts** or bone cells, apparently in response to transforming growth factor-β–like molecules. These cells secrete the calcium salt matrix of mineralized bone and form a **primary bone collar** around the circumference of the bone. This primary bone collar thickens as osteoblasts differentiate in progressively more peripheral layers of the perichondrium. Cells called **osteoclasts,** which break down previously formed bone, also appear and begin to remodel the

growing bone. Bone is continually remodeled throughout development and adult life. Ossification also spreads from the primary ossification center toward the ends of the anlage, and the cartilaginous core enclosed by the primary bone collar also begins to ossify to form a loose **trabecular network** of bone.

Shortly after ossification begins, the developing bone is invaded by multiple blood vessels that branch from the limb vasculature (see Ch. 8). One of these vessels eventually becomes dominant and gives rise to the **nutrient artery** that nourishes the bone.

At birth, the **diaphyses** or shafts of the limb bones (consisting of a bone collar and trabecular core) are completely ossified, whereas the ends of the bones, called the **epiphyses,** are still cartilaginous. After birth, **secondary ossification centers** develop in the epiphyses, which gradually ossify. However, a layer of cartilage called the **epiphyseal cartilage plate (growth plate** or **physis)** persists between the epiphysis and the growing end of the diaphysis **(metaphysis).** Continued proliferation of the chondrocytes in this growth plate allows the diaphysis to lengthen. Finally, when the growth of the body is complete at about 20 years of age, the epiphyses and diaphyses fuse.

Most of the Limb Bones Form Between the Fifth and Twelfth Weeks

The axial mesenchyme of the limb buds first begins to condense in the fifth week. In general, the bones of the upper limb form slightly earlier than their counterparts in the lower limb.

By the end of the fifth week, the portion of the axial mesenchymal condensation that will give rise to the proximal limb skeleton (the scapula and humerus in the upper limb; the pelvic bones and femur in the lower limb) is distinct. By the early sixth week, the mesenchymal precursor of the distal limb skeleton is distinct in the upper and lower limbs, and chondrification commences in the humerus, ulna, and radius. By the end of the sixth week, the carpal and metacarpal bones also begin to chondrify. In the lower limb, the femur, the tibia, and, to a lesser extent, the fibula begin to

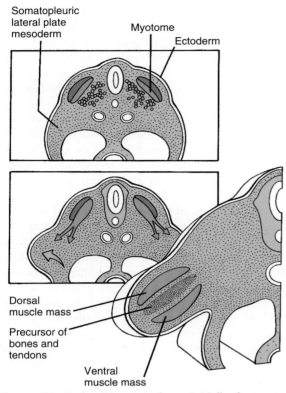

Somatopleuric
lateral plate
mesoderm
Myotome
Ectoderm

Dorsal
muscle mass

Precursor of
bones and
tendons

Ventral
muscle mass

Figure 11–7. Somitic mesoderm initially forms two major muscle masses in each limb bud. The ventral mass gives rise mainly to flexors, pronators, and adductors, whereas the dorsal muscle mass gives rise mainly to extensors, supinators, and abductors.

chondrify by the middle of the sixth week, and the tarsals and metatarsals begin to chondrify near the end of the sixth week. By the early seventh week, all the bones of the upper limb except the distal phalanges of the second to fifth digits are undergoing chondrification. By the end of the seventh week, the distal phalanges of the hand have begun to chondrify, and chondrification is also under way in all the bones of the lower limb except the distal row of phalanges. The distal phalanges of the toes do not chondrify until the eighth week.

The primary ossification centers of most of the limb bones appear in the seventh to twelfth weeks. By the early seventh week, ossification has commenced in the clavicle, followed by the humerus, radius, and ulna at the end of the seventh week. Ossification begins in the femur and tibia in the eighth week. During the ninth week, the scapula and ilium begin to ossify, followed in the next

3 weeks by the metacarpals, metatarsals, distal phalanges, proximal phalanges, and, finally, the middle phalanges. The ischium and pubis begin to ossify in the 15th and 20th weeks, respectively, and ossification of the calcaneus finally begins at about 16 weeks. Some of the smaller carpal and tarsal bones do not ossify until early childhood.

The Joints of the Limbs Develop From the Mesenchymal Interzones

Figure 11–6 illustrates the process by which the **diarthrodial (synovial) joints** connecting the limb bones develop. First, the mesenchyme of the interzones between the chondrifying bone primordia differentiates into **fibroblastic tissue** (undifferentiated connective tissue). This tissue then further differentiates into three layers: a cartilage layer at either end of the future joint, in contact with the adjacent bone primordia, and a central layer of dense connective tissue. The connective tissue of this central layer gives rise to the internal elements of the joint. Proximally and distally, it condenses to form the **synovial tissue** that will line the future joint cavity. Its central zone gives rise to the **menisci** and to **enclosed joint ligaments** such as the cruciate ligaments of the knee. Vacuoles appear within this tissue and coalesce to form the **synovial cavity.** The **joint capsule** arises from the mesenchymal sheath surrounding the entire interzone.

Synchondroidal joints, such as those connecting the bones of the pelvis, also develop from interzones, but the interzone mesenchyme simply differentiates into a single layer of fibrocartilage.

The Limb Musculature Develops From Ventral and Dorsal Condensations of Somitic Mesoderm

During the fifth week, somitic mesoderm invades the limb bud and forms two large condensations, one dorsal to the axial mesenchymal column and one ventral to it (Fig. 11–7). The cells of the condensations form the anlagen of the limb muscles and differentiate into **myoblasts** (muscle cell precursors). Myoblasts proliferate and begin to make myofibrils. These cells fuse to form single cells (myocytes) with multiple nuclei (called a syncytium). The nuclei can no longer synthesize DNA in the syncytium. Myocytes grow by increasing myofibrils. The number of nuclei in a syncytial cell is a limiting factor in its growth; when the limit is reached, addition of myoblast nuclei by fusion is required. In adults, there is a reserve of myoblast-like cells called satellite cells that can proliferate and fuse with the syncytium to permit further growth (e.g., in response to exercise).

The dorsal muscle mass gives rise in general to the **extensors** and **supinators** of the upper limb and to the **extensors** and **abductors** of the lower limb, whereas the ventral muscle mass gives rise to the **flexors** and **pronators** of the upper limb and to the **flexors** and **adductors** of the lower limb (Table 11–1). However, this rule is not absolute. Some muscles migrate from their site of origin and acquire different functions.

SPINAL NERVE AXONS INNERVATE SPECIFIC LIMB STRUCTURES BY A MULTISTEP PATHFINDING PROCESS

As described in Chapter 5, each spinal nerve splits into main branches, the dorsal and ventral primary rami, shortly after it exits the spinal cord. The limb muscles are innervated by branches of the ventral primary rami of spinal nerves C5 through T1 (for the upper limb) and L4 through S3 (for the lower limb). Muscles originating in the dorsal muscle mass are served by *dorsal* branches of these ventral primary rami, whereas muscles originating in the ventral muscle mass are served by *ventral* branches of the ventral primary rami. Thus, the innervation of a muscle shows whether it originated in the dorsal or the ventral muscle mass.

As illustrated in Figure 11–8, the motor ax-

Table 11–1

Muscles Derived from the Ventral and Dorsal Muscle Masses of the Limb Buds

VENTRAL MUSCLE MASS		DORSAL MUSCLE MASS
Upper Limb	*Upper Limb*	*Lower Limb*
Anterior compartment of the arm and forearm	Posterior compartment muscles of the arm and forearm	Anterior compartment muscles of the thigh and leg
All muscles on the palmar surface of hand	Deltoid	Tensor fasciae latae
Lower Limb	Lateral compartment muscles of the forearm and hand	Short head of the biceps femoris
Medial compartment muscles of the thigh	Latissimus dorsi	Lateral compartment muscles of the leg
Posterior compartment muscles of the thigh except for the short head of the biceps femoris	Rhomboids	Muscles of the dorsum of the foot
	Levator scapulae	Gluteus maximus, medius, and minimus
	Serratus anterior	Piriformis
Posterior compartment muscles of the leg	Teres major and minor	Iliacus
	Subscapularis	Psoas
All muscles on the plantar surface of the foot	Supraspinatus (?)	
	Infraspinatus (?)	
Obturator internus		
Gemellus superior and inferior		
Quadratus femoris		

Data from Crafts RC. 1985. A Textbook of Human Anatomy. 3rd Ed. Churchill Livingstone, New York.

Figure 11–8. Scanning electron micrograph of a sectioned embryo showing axons entering the limb bud (dotted area). (From Tosney KW, Landmesser LT. 1985. Development of the major pathways for neurite outgrowth in the chick hindlimb. Dev Biol 109:193.)

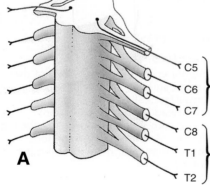

A

Grow to the craniodorsal parts of the upper limb bud

C5
C6
C7

Grow to the ventrocaudal parts of the upper limb bud

C8
T1
T2

B

Nerves diverge after leaving the plexus to enter the craniodorsal or ventrocaudal part of the limb bud

Axons diverge to specific muscles in the limb bud

C

Figure 11–9. Growth of spinal nerve axons into the limb buds. *A, B,* Axons grow into the limb buds along permissive pathways. As the axons of the various spinal nerves mingle at the base of the limb buds to form the brachial and lumbosacral plexuses, each axon must "decide" whether to grow into the dorsal or ventral muscle mass. Factors that may play a role in directing axon growth include areas of dense mesenchyme or glycosaminoglycan-containing mesenchyme, which are avoided by outgrowing axons. *C,* Once the axons grow into the bud, decision points (arrows) under the control of "local factors" may regulate the invasion of specific muscle anlagen by specific axons. (Modified from Tosney K, Landmesser LT. 1984. Pattern and specificity of axonal outgrowth following varying degrees of chick limb bud ablation. J Neurosci 4:2518.)

ons that innervate the limbs perform an intricate feat of pathfinding to reach their target muscles. The ventral ramus axons destined for the limbs apparently travel to the base of the limb bud by growing along **permissive pathways** (Fig. 11–9*A*). The growth cones of these axons avoid or are unable to penetrate regions of dense mesenchyme or mesenchyme containing glycosaminoglycans. The axons heading for the lower limb are thus deflected around the developing pelvic anlagen. In both the upper and lower limb buds, the axons from the nerves cranial to the limb bud grow toward the craniodorsal side of the limb bud, whereas the axons from the nerves caudal to the limb bud grow toward the ventrocaudal side of the limb bud (see Fig. 11–9*B*).

Once the motor axons arrive at the base of the limb bud, they mix in a specific pattern to form the **brachial plexus** of the upper limb and the **lumbosacral plexus** of the lower limb. This zone thus constitutes a **decision-making region** for the axons (see the Experimental Principles section of Ch. 13 for a further discussion of axonal decision-making). The identities of the factors that

control the formation of the brachial and lumbosacral plexuses are not well known, but hepatocyte growth factor has been implicated as a tropic substance. However, some sorting along the dorsoventral axis occurs correctly in the absence of the limb bud.

Once the axons have sorted out in the plexus, the growth cones continue into the limb bud, presumably traveling along permissive pathways that lead in the general direction of the appropriate muscle compartment. Axons from the dorsal divisions of the plexuses tend to grow into the dorsal side of the limb bud and thus innervate mainly extensors, supinators, and abductors; axons from the ventral divisions of the plexus grow into the ventral side of the limb bud and thus innervate mainly flexors, pronators, and adductors. Over the last part of an axon's path, from the point where it leaves its major nerve trunk to the point where it innervates a specific muscle, axonal pathfinding is probably regulated by cues produced by the muscle itself (see Fig. 11–9*C*).

Once the motor axons have found their targets, sensory fibers innervate the sensory end or-

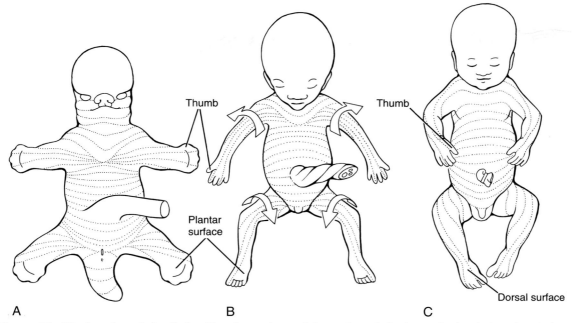

Figure 11–10. Rotation of the limbs. The dramatic medial rotation of the lower limbs during the sixth to eighth weeks causes the mature dermatomes to spiral down the limb. The configuration of the upper limb dermatomes is partially modified by more limited lateral rotation of the upper limb during the same period.

gans in the limbs. The sensory axons apparently grow along the motor axons to the vicinity of the appropriate sensory end organs. Local cues then direct their final branching and innervation of the end organs.

The Segmental Pattern of Limb Innervation Is Complicated by Limb Bud Rotation

As described earlier, the upper and lower limb buds rotate from their original coronal orientation into a roughly parasagittal orientation. Subsequently (between the sixth and eighth weeks), they also rotate around their long axis. The upper limb rotates laterally so that the elbow points caudally and the original ventral surface of the limb bud becomes the cranial surface of the limb. The lower limb rotates medially so that the knee points cranially and the original ventral surface of the limb bud becomes the caudal surface of the limb. As shown in Figure 11–10, this rotation causes the originally straight segmental pattern of lower limb innervation to twist into a spiral. The rotation of the upper limb is less extreme than that of the lower limb and is accomplished partly through the caudal migration of the shoulder girdle. Moreover, some of the dermatomes in the upper limb bud exhibit overgrowth and come to dominate the limb surface.

Clinical Applications

Congenital Anomalies of the Limbs

Humans exhibit a wide variety of limb defects. In general, these defects fall into three categories: (1) **reduction defects,** in which part of a limb (**meromelia;** Fig. 11–11*A*) or an entire limb (**amelia;** see Fig. 11–11*B*) is missing; (2) **duplication defects,** in which *super-numerary* limb elements are present (**polydactyly,** or the presence of extra digits, is the most common example; see Fig. 11–11*C*); and (3) **dysplasia** (malformation) of the limb. Limb dysplasias include **syndactyly,** or fusion of digits (Fig. 11–12), and **gigantism,** or excessive growth of parts of the limb. Limb malformations may involve virtually any part of the limb and may be local or involve the whole limb.

Historically, the nomenclature of limb defects has been somewhat imprecise. Table 11–2 lists a number of terms in common use. Despite the variations in pathogenesis, location, and complexity that confuse the classification of limb abnormalities, several schemes of rational classification have been proposed. First, it is generally agreed that limb defects can be attributed to the following general causes: (1) *arrest of development* (failure of components to form); (2) *failure of differentiation* of component primordia; (3) *duplication* of components; (4) *overgrowth*; (5) *hypoplasia* (undergrowth); (6) *focal defects*, such as amniotic band syndrome; and (7) *general skeletal abnormalities* that incidentally affect the limbs, such as osteogenesis imperfecta. Limb abnormalities can also be further characterized with respect to the part of the limb affected (e.g., the limb **segment** [such as forearm or thigh] or **compartment** [extensor versus flexor or radial versus ulnar]).

The Etiology of Most Limb Defects Is Unknown

Ideally, a limb malformation could be assigned a specific **genetic** or **teratogenic** cause. However, most human limb defects appear to have a multifactorial etiology, arising from an ill-defined interaction between environmental influences and the individual's genetic makeup (see the Clinical Applications section of Ch. 7). In a few cases, a familial association or a history of exposure to a known teratogen makes it possible to ascribe a specific genetic or teratogenic cause to a given limb abnormality.

Familial Associations Indicate a Genetic Basis for Some Limb Anomalies. Both polydactyly and ectrodactyly often run in families, and these defects may show an autosomal dominant, autosomal recessive, or X-linked pattern of inheritance. Other limb defects known to be transmitted as autosomal dominant traits include partial tibia defect, general micromelia, triphalangeal thumbs, lobster claw hand and foot (Fig. 11–13), and the Adams-Oliver syndrome (characterized by limb anomalies and defects of the scalp and skull). An autosomal recessive disease characterized by the fusion of digits and the transformation of metacarpal and metatarsal segments to carpals and tarsals, respectively, results from mutation of the *HOX* gene *HOXD13* (Fig. 11–14; see the Experimental Principles section of this chapter). Some chromosomal anomalies, such as trisomy 18, cause limb defects. In addition, a variety of specific gene mutations causing limb anomalies have been characterized in humans. (Table 11–3)

Some Environmental Teratogens Cause Limb Defects. A variety of drugs, metabolic poisons, and other environmental teratogens have been shown to cause limb defects in experimental animals. Some of these agents are also associated with limb defects in humans. Not surprisingly, agents that influence general cell metabolism or cell proliferation are likely to cause limb defects if administered during the period of limb morphogenesis. Such agents include **5′-fluoro-2-deoxyuridine,** an inhibitor of thymidylate synthetase; **acetazolamide,** a carbonic anhydrase inhibitor; and alkylating agents such as **triethylene melamine. Cadmium,** which inhibits a wide range of zinc metalloenzymes including carbonic anhydrase, is also known to induce limb deformities in mice and rats.

Hyperthermia may also be a significant cause of limb defects. Increases in body temperature of only 1 to 2.5°C can induce limb malforma-

Figure 11–11. *A,* Meromelia. In this example, the distal end of a lower limb has not completely formed. (Photo courtesy of Children's Hospital Medical Center, Cincinnati, OH.) *B,* Amelia. In this example, an entire upper limb failed to form. (Photo courtesy of Children's Hospital Medical Center, Cincinnati, OH.) *C,* Polydactyly. One of the hands has six digits. (Photo courtesy of Children's Hospital Medical Center, Cincinnati, OH.)

Figure 11–12. Syndactyly. In this severe case, even the bony elements of digits 2 and 3 are fused. Less severe cases may exhibit only a web of skin between the digits. (Photo courtesy of Children's Hospital Medical Center, Cincinnati, OH.)

Table 11–2
Some Common Terms for Limb Malformations

TERM	DEFINITION
Meromelia	Absence of part of a limb
Amelia, ectromelia	Absence of one or more limbs
Phocomelia	Absence of proximal limb structures—named for their resemblance to the flippers of a seal
Hemimelia	Absence of distal limb segments in the cranial or caudal half of the limb e.g., radial hemimelia
Acrodolichomelia	Disproportionately large hands or feet
Ectrodactyly	Absence of any number of fingers or toes
Polydactyly	Presence of extra digits or parts of digits
Syndactyly	Fusion of digits
Adactyly	Absence of all the digits on a limb

tions in several species, including some nonhuman primates. These findings suggest that febrific (fever-causing) diseases may be teratogenic agents causing limb defects in humans.

Of particular importance to clinicians are the teratogenic effects of therapeutic drugs. The possible teratogenicity of a drug is usually investigated in animal studies, and the actual effects of the drug on human embryos are rarely known. Two drugs that induce limb malformations in laboratory animals and humans are the anticonvulsant *valproic acid* and the antileprosy drug *thalidomide*.

The thalidomide incident is a tragic example of drug teratogenicity. In 1957, the drug thalidomide was first marketed as a nonbarbiturate sedative under the trade name Contergan. The drug was recommended for a variety of indications and for several years was thought to be virtually free of side effects.

On December 25, 1956, a girl with no ears (anotia) was born in Stolberg, West Germany, the town in which Contergan was manufactured. The girl's father worked for the manufacturer of Contergan and had been given free samples of the new drug for his pregnant wife. Approximately 1 year later, an epidemic of congenital limb malforma-

tions commenced throughout West Germany. Hindsight shows that the incidence of these malformations exactly paralleled the West German sales figures for thalidomide, with a lag of about 7 to 8 months (Fig. 11–15). Indeed, the incidence of limb embryopathy in the late 1950s and early 1960s closely matched the sales of thalidomide-

Figure 11–13. Some limb anomalies, such as lobster claw hand or foot, are sometimes inherited as autosomal dominant traits. (Photo courtesy of Children's Hospital Medical Center, Cincinnati, OH.)

Figure 11–14. *A,* Hand and *B,* radiograph of homozygous individual. Note syndactyly of digits III, IV, and V, their single knuckle, the transformation of metacarpals I, II, III, and V to short carpal-like bones (stars), two additional carpal bones (asterisks), and short second phalanges. The radius, ulna, and proximal carpal bones appear normal. (From Muragaki Y, Mundlos S, Upton J, et al. 1996. Altered growth and branching patterns in synpolydactyly caused by mutations in *HOXD13.* Science 272:548.)

based products in 20 countries. These malformations included major defects such as amelia and phocomelia (Fig. 11–16), as well as minor deformities such as hypoplasia of the thumb and syndactyly between the thumb and index finger. The limb malformations were sometimes accompanied by other defects such as anotia, duodenal stenosis, and cardiac defects. It is estimated that approximately 5850 individuals were affected. About 40 percent of these "thalidomide babies" died soon after birth, leaving 3900 survivors.

Thalidomide apparently exerts its effects only when taken during the **sensitive period** of limb morphogenesis, between about 3 and 5 weeks of gestation. Presumably, the type of defect depends on the amount of thalidomide ingested, the general susceptibility of the individual embryo to the drug, and the precise period during which the teratogen was present.

Although realization of thalidomide's teratogenicity in the early 1960s led to universal prohibitions of its use, a limited amount of subsequent research has provided insights into its mechanism of action. There is some limited evidence to suggest that thalidomide's teratogenicity in humans may be mediated by its ability to disrupt cell adhesion in the limb by downregulating cell surface adhesion receptors (integrins and selectin) or by inhibiting angiogenesis. Understanding these fundamental mechanisms, however, is no longer of purely academic value, because studies have demonstrated that thalidomide may have many beneficial uses, and the drug has been sanctioned for use by the Food and Drug Administration for treatment of leprosy. It has also been used in the treatment of several autoimmune and inflammatory conditions, including symptoms of **AIDS, lupus erythematosus, Jessner-Kanof lymphocytic infil-**

Table 11–3
Human Mutations Affecting Limb Development

GENE	HUMAN ABNORMALITY	EFFECT ON LIMBS	REFERENCE
HOXD13	Type II syndactyly	Syndactyly (synostotic), polydactyly, meromelia, hemimelia	Goodman et al. 1997 Muragaki et al. 1996
HOXA13	Hand-foot-genital syndrome	Hemimelia/hypoplasia, syndactyly (synostotic), carpal fusion, delayed ossification	Mortlock and Innis 1996
GL13	Greig cephalopolysyndactyly	Polydactyly, syndactyly	Kang et al. 1997
	Pallister-Hall syndrome	Polydactyly	Vortkamp et al. 1991 Wild et al. 1997
LMX1B	Nail-patella syndrome	Meromelia, nail hypoplasia or dysplasia	Dreyer et al. 1998 Vollrath et al. 1998
CDMP1	Chondrodysplasia Grebe type	Brachydactyly, polydactyly, hemimelia, hypoptasia, aplasia	Thomas et al. 1997
MSX2	Autosomal dominant craniosynostosis	Brachydactyly, finger-like thumb	Jabs et al. 1993
SHOX	Léri-Weill dyschondrosteosis	Meromelia, brachydactyly	Belin et al. 1998 Shears et al. 1998
SALL1	Townes-Brocks syndrome	Polydactyly, finger-like thumb	Kohlhase et al. 1998
TWIST	Saethre-Chotzen syndrome	Brachydactyly, syndactyly (soft tissue)	el Ghouzzi et al. 1997 Howard et al. 1997
TBX3	Ulnar-mammary syndrome	Meromelia, nail duplicated ventrally, hypoplasia, carpal fusion	Bamshad et al. 1997
TBX5	Holt-Oram syndrome	Ectrodactyly, finger-like thumb, meromelia	Basson et al. 1997 Li et al. 1997
FGFR1	Pfeiffer syndrome	Syndactyly (soft tissue), broad digit 1, brachydactyly	Muenke et al. 1994
FGFR2	Pfeiffer syndrome	As above	Meyers et al. 1996
	Apert syndrome	Syndactyly (synostotic)	Muenke et al. 1994
	Jackson-Weiss	Syndactyly (synostotic)	Wilkie et al. 1995
FGFR3	Achondroplasia	Brachydactyly, hemimelia	Bellus et al. 1995
	Hypochondroplasia	Milder form of the above	Rousseau et al. 1994 Shiang et al. 1994
SOX9	Campomelic dysplasia	Bowed long bones	Foster et al. 1994
ATPSK2	Spondyloepimetaphyseal dysplasia	Bowed long bones, hemimelia, brachydactyly, enlarged knee joints, joint degeneration (early onset)	Haque et al. 1998

From Cohn MJ, Bright, PE. 1999. Molecular control of vetebrate limb development, evolution, and congenital malformations. Cell Tissue Res 296:3.

tration of the skin, cutaneous and **pulmonary sarcoidoses, chronic graft-versus-host disease,** and **oral** and **genital ulceration** (in **Behçet's disease**) and has shown therapeutic utility in the treatment of cancer, specifically in multiple myeloma. In Brazil, where leprosy is more common, thalidomide has been used for several years. As a consequence, at least 46 new cases of thalidomide embryopathy have occurred. For these reasons, it is more important than ever that physicians be aware

of thalidomide's teratogenic potency when treating women of reproductive age.

Limb Deformities Can Be Caused by Amniotic Bands, Oligohydramnios, and Local Vascular Disruption.

Occasionally, a band of tissue detaches from the amnion and wraps around part of the embryo, constricting its growth and causing malformations. Congenital deformities of this type are referred to as **amniotic band syndrome**. Am-

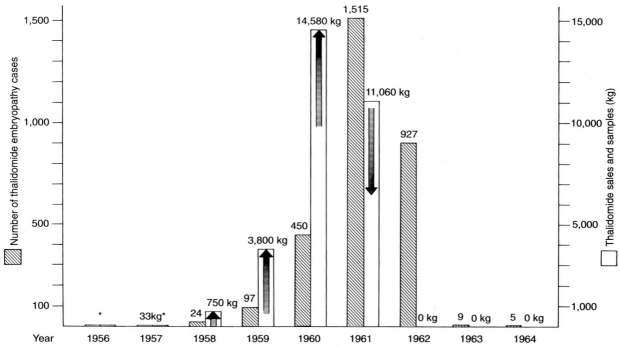

Figure 11–15. The frequency of limb embryopathy in Germany between 1956 and 1967 compared with the sales of thalidomide. The correlation of thalidomide sales with limb embryopathies strongly indicated the teratogenic role of the drug. *Premarketing samples (low volume of samples in 1956).

niotic bands may amputate or constrict a developing limb or may induce facial dysplasia by entangling the head and face (Fig. 11–17). A malformation involving the limbs and body wall, called **limb body wall malformation complex,** has been attributed to the effects of amniotic bands. It has been argued, however, that some cases may be due to local disruption of vasculature. Conditions that result in a constricted uterine environment can cause limb reduction anomalies, both as a direct consequence of compression of the fetus by the uterine wall and, apparently, as an indirect effect of compression-induced vascular disruption. The Clinical Applications section of Chapter 6 describes fetal compression due to oligohydramnios (insufficient amniotic fluid). Limb defects have also been associated with constricted uterine environments caused by **bicornuate uterus** (a Y-shaped uterus resulting from incomplete fusion of the paramesonephric ducts during forma-

tion of the uterovaginal canal; see Ch. 10) and by large benign tumors of the uterine myometrium.

Studies on Mice and Chicks Have Elucidated Some Mechanisms Underlying Limb Malformations

Studies on several mouse mutants indicate that many limb abnormalities arise through generalized defects in skeletal morphogenesis. A variety of mouse mutants with limb deformities that mimic human conditions exhibit generalized disturbances either in the development of the mesenchymal anlagen of the limb bones or in their chondrification or ossification. For example, the autosomal mutation brachypod (*pb tH/bp H*) disrupts the development of the mesenchymal precartilage anlagen in

Figure 11–16. Phocomelia. Although phocomelia may be inherited, it was also a common limb defect in offspring of pregnant women who ingested thalidomide. (Photo courtesy of Children's Hospital Medical Center, Cincinnati, OH.)

Figure 11–17. Amniotic band syndrome. Generalized limb defects as well as craniofacial and trunk anomalies may arise when bands of amniotic membrane detach from the chorion and wrap around growing body structures. (Photo courtesy of Children's Hospital Medical Center, Cincinnati, OH.)

the limb (presumably by affecting the plasma membrane-associated enzyme galactosyltransferase), leading to brachydactyly and postaxial hemimelia. Mice homozygous for the mutation *cmd* (cartilage-matrix deficiency) have short limbs and are characterized by deficient cartilage development throughout the body. The limb dysplasia of *Dmm* (disproportional micromelia) mice appears to result from incomplete incorporation of collagen into the cartilage matrix.

Errors in the pattern of programmed cell death can also cause limb defects. For example, a dominant mutation of the mouse that alters the pattern of cell death in the distal foot results in hemimelia and the presence of an extra toe. The polydactyly typical of mouse embryos treated with retinoic acid may arise by a similar mechanism. Other mechanisms implicated in the pathogenesis of various limb malformations include perturbations of limb bud cell proliferation, mesenchymal

cell adhesiveness, and the migratory capacity of myoblasts.

Investigations of the mechanisms responsible for retinoic acid-induced limb deformities support the idea that retinoic acid can induce the synthesis of morphogenetic molecules regulating pattern formation in the limb. The administration of retinoic acid to pregnant mice during the critical period for limb morphogenesis results in a dose-dependent induction of limb abnormalities. Low doses produce relatively minor abnormalities, whereas high doses result in a 100 percent incidence of limb reduction defects. Moreover, the dose-dependent effects of retinoic acid are paralleled by the measured concentrations of the agent in the limb bud: at mildly teratogenic doses the limb bud retinoic acid content is increased 50-fold, whereas at highly teratogenic doses it is raised as much as 300-fold.

Retinoic acid has been shown to inhibit chondrogenesis in cultured limb buds, but its effects in living embryos seem to be much more complex.

Experimental Principles

A Molecular Basis for Pattern Formation in the Limbs

How do the cells of the embryo sort themselves out and differentiate into the morphologically complex structures and tissues of the organism? The mechanisms by which cells "know" where to migrate, when to divide, and what to become are fundamental problems of developmental research. The spatial organization of differentiating cells and tissues, which accounts for the morphogenesis of the organs and, ultimately, of the body as a whole, is called **pattern formation.** Some of the mechanisms and processes that underlie pattern formation have been discussed previously: gastrulation (Ch. 3), the differentiation of the trunk (Ch. 4), the migration and differentiation of the neural crest (Ch. 5), and the development of the handed asymmetry of the viscera (Ch. 9). The patterns that arise as a result of the segmentation of the pharyngeal arches are discussed in Chapter 12.

Pattern Formation Plays a Fundamental Role in Limb Development

Not only must a cell in the limb bud differentiate into the correct tissue (such as cartilage or muscle),

but also it must adopt the correct position relative to other cells in an exceptionally complex and irregular structure. How does one part of the limb bud form the upper arm and another the wrist? How does one digital ray in the hand plate form an index finger and another give rise to the thumb? How do dorsal and ventral sides of the limb become differentiated from each other?

A Cell in the Limb Bud Must "Know" Its Position With Respect to Three Axes

The limb bud differentiates with respect to three axes: its own proximal distal long axis and the craniocaudal and dorsoventral axes of the organism as a whole (Fig. 11–18). The long axis of the limb bud defines the sequence of the limb segments (girdle-arm/thigh-forearm/leg-wrist/ankle-hand/foot); the craniocaudal axis defines the differentiation from the first-digit side of the limb to the fifth-digit side; and the dorsoventral axis defines the differentiation of extensor from flexor compartments. A cell in the limb bud must respond appropriately to

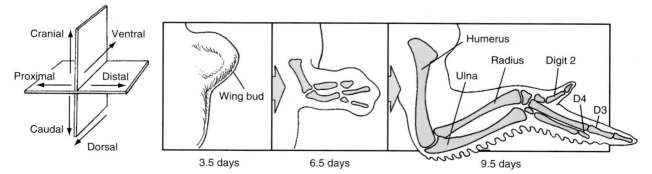

Figure 11–18. The limb buds of birds and other vertebrates grow with respect to three axes of symmetry: craniocaudal, dorsoventral, and proximodistal. (Modified from Alberts B, Bray D, Lewis J, et al. 1983. Molecular Biology of the Cell. Garland, New York.)

its position relative to all three axes. The experimental work discussed in this section provides some insight into the mechanisms of **positional signaling** responsible for differentiation with respect to the proximal distal, craniocaudal, and dorsoventral axes.

Limb Bud Outgrowth Requires Reciprocal Interactions Between the Apical Ectodermal Ridge and the Underlying Mesenchyme

Classic transplantation barrier studies suggest that a signal for the lateral plate mesoderm to initiate limb bud formation may arise from an axial source near the midline, perhaps the paraxial mesoderm or Hensen's node. Molecular studies indicate a crucial role of the fibroblast growth factor (FGF) family in limb initiation. This concept originated from the extraordinary demonstration that beads soaked in FGF and applied to the flank of chick embryos could induce formation of a supernumerary limb in the region between the fore- and hind limbs (Fig 11–19). This demonstration was supported by expression studies indicating that

FGF family members are present in the lateral plate mesoderm and intermediate mesoderm before limb bud initiation. Also, the concept draws support from the demonstration that loss of a gene for an FGF receptor (by targeted gene knockout) leads to an inhibition of limb initiation.

FGFs are also involved in the interaction whereby the AER induces outgrowth of the limb mesenchyme along the proximodistal axis. Many members of the FGF family are expressed in the AER (Fig. 11–20), and FGFs applied by beads can rescue a limb in which the AER has been surgically removed. Otherwise AER removal leads to truncated limbs whose proximodistal extent is directly correlated to the stage of limb bud development when the AER is removed.

A third interaction between the two tissues composing the early limb bud is maintenance of the AER structure and its function by the underlying mesenchyme. There is evidence that this function may also arise from FGF family members that are different from those FGFs in the AER. The maintenance of the AER also depends on another growth factor family, the transforming growth factor βs (TGFβs), through members in the bone morphogenetic protein, (BMP) subgroup. Whether the FGFs and BMPs act independently or through

Figure 11–19. FGF-soaked bead produces supernumerary limb. FGF = fibroblast growth factor.

Figure 11-20. In situ hybridization showing mRNA transcripts for fibroblast growth factor-8 (FGF-8) is expressed in the ectoderm prior to limb bud outgrowth (note lower limb) and then becomes discretely contained within the apical ectodermal ridge (AER) during later development (note upper limb bud). (Photo courtesy of Sheila Bell and W. Scott.)

some sequential pathway to maintain the AER is not yet clear.

Identity of Skeletal Elements Along the Proximodistal Axis Arises During the Residence of a Cell in the Progress Zone

A specific role for the AER, and thereby presumably for FGFs as well, is the maintenance of an active zone of mesenchymal proliferation at the distal end of the limb, a region called the **progress zone.** This is a narrow zone of mesenchyme about 300 μm in width, where cells are thought to acquire **positional information** that will inform

them of their final address along the proximodistal axis. Cells that exit the progress zone after a short residence are destined to form proximal structures such as the humerus. Cells with the longest residence in the progress zone become distal structures, the phalanges. The mechanism of acquiring this positional information during residence in the progress zone is unknown. A timing mechanism whereby a cell counts the number of mitotic divisions was proposed in the late 1970s and has neither been confirmed or denied by subsequent experimentation.

Hox Genes Are Regionally Expressed in the Limb Bud

As described in Chapters 3 and 4, four clusters of *Hox* genes are expressed in vertebrates (including humans) in a 3' to 5' sequence along the DNA of four respective chromosomes. Moreover, members of the most 5' members of the *Hoxd* and *Hoxa* clusters (9 to 13) are expressed in a distal to proximal transcriptional cascade within the growing limb bud (Fig. 11–21). Ultimately, the expression of each of the 5 *Hoxd* genes (along with those of the *Hoxa* group) can be correlated with development of specific skeletal elements of upper and lower limb segments. For example, in the upper extremity, *Hoxd-9* is expressed within the segment forming the scapula; *Hoxd-9* and *Hoxd-10* within the arm (containing the humerus); *Hoxd-9*, *Hoxd-10*, and *Hoxd-11* within the forearm and proximal wrist (containing ulna, radius, and proximal carpals); *Hoxd-9*, *Hoxd-10*, *Hoxd-11*, *Hoxd-12* within the distal wrist (containing distal carpals); and *Hoxd-9*, *Hoxd-10*, *Hoxd-11*, *Hoxd-12*, and *Hoxd-13* within the hand and fingers (containing metacarpals and phalanges; Fig. 11–22).

A direct test of the developmental role of *Hox* gene expression in proximodistal differentiation of the limb is a double knockout of *Hoxa-11* and *Hoxd-11* genes. While the disruption of one or the other of these genes has subtle effects on skeletal morphology, the double null mutation of *Hoxa-11* and *Hoxd-11* results in complete absence of the ulna and radius. Another direct test of *Hox* gene regulation of proximodistal differentiation of limb segments is the spontaneous human mutation of *Hoxd-13* described in the Clinical Applications section above. In these individuals, disruption of normal *Hoxd-13* expression transforms the metacarpals to carpals and metatarsals to tarsals (see Fig. 11–14).

Of course, the sequence of regulatory gene activation is not as simple as described. It has been demonstrated, for example, that each of the *Hoxa* and *Hoxd* genes is regulated in as many as three independent phases and that each of these phases coincides with specification of each limb segment of the upper limb (arm, forearm, and hand).

Transplantation Experiments Suggest That Craniocaudal Limb Differentiation Is Regulated by a Morphogen Gradient

The classic series of experiments on craniocaudal limb differentiation was performed in the 1960s by using chick wing buds. When a small piece of tissue was transplanted from the caudal edge of a donor wing bud to the leading edge of a host wing bud, the cranial half of the wing bud formed extra digits that were a mirror image of the normal digits on the caudal half of the wing bud (Fig. 11–23). Investigators proposed that the transplanted tissue fragment produced a morphogenetic substance, or **morphogen,** that diffused to form a gradient across the wing bud and determined which digit would be induced in each position: a high morphogen concentration would induce digit 4, and progressively lower concentrations would induce digits 3 and 2. (Digits 1 and 5 do not form in chick wings.) The caudal tissue region responsible for this digit-determining activity was called the **zone of polarizing activity** (ZPA) (see Fig. 11–23).

Sonic Hedgehog Plays a Pivotal Role in Craniocaudal Patterning of the Limb Bud

A definitive candidate for the polarizing function of the ZPA, is the protein **sonic hedgehog (SHH),** a factor identified in avian and mammalian embryos and the gene mapped to human chromosome 7q (see Chs. 3, 4, 9, and 12).

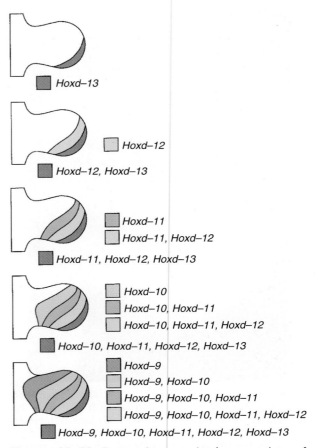

Figure 11–21. Progressive proximal expression of *Hoxd* paralogs. (Modified from Izpisua-Belmonte JC, Duboule D. 1992. Homeobox genes and pattern formation in the vertebrate limb. Dev Biol 152:26.)

In chicks and mice, limb bud *Shh* is normally expressed endogenously only within the caudal region of the limb bud mesenchyme, in the region of the ZPA. Moreover, *Shh* is expressed at the cranial edge of the inverted limb buds ectopically induced with an FGF-4-soaked bead (Fig. 11–24*A*). Shh is also expressed at both caudal and cranial edges of limb buds in Luxoid mouse mutants; such mice are characterized by mirror-image polydactyly (see Fig. 11–24*B*). Indeed, several other mouse mutants exhibiting mirror-image polydactyly also exhibit duplication of *Shh* expression in an ectopic ZPA at the cranial edge of the limb buds. Perhaps the strongest evidence that SHH protein supports craniocaudal patterning is derived from ectopic expression studies. Grafting of an SHH loaded bead

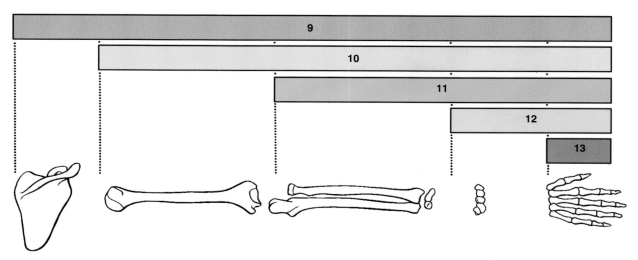

Figure 11–22. *Hoxd* gene expression patterns in relation to definitive segments of the upper extremity. (Modified from Davis AP, Witte DP, Hsieh-Li HM, et al. 1995. Absence of radius and ulna in mice lacking *Hoxa-11* and *Hoxd-11*. Nature. 375:791.)

Figure 11–23. Transplantation of the zone of polarizing activity (ZPA) of one limb bud to the cranial edge of another will induce mirror polydactyly. (Modified from Alberts B, Bray D, Lewis J, et al. 1983. Molecular Biology of the Cell. Garland, New York.)

Figure 11–24. *A,* Whole mount in situ hybridization (sonic hedgehog [Shh] mRNA) shows Shh expression in a chick embryo 48 hours after application of an FGF-2 bead similar to that in Figure 2 in Cohn et al (1995). Cell 80:739. (With permission from Martin J. Cohn.) *B,* In situ hybridization showing both Shh and Fgf-4 mRNA in normal caudal ZPA and at ectopic cranial location (arrowheads). (From Chan DC, Laufer E, Tabin C, Leder P. 1995. Polydactylous limbs in Strong's Luxoid mice result from ectopic polarizing activity. Development 121:1971.)

in the anterior mesenchyme of a chick wing bud, infection of a chick wing bud with a retrovirus expressing *Shh,* or placement of a pellet of *Shh* expressing cells in the anterior mesenchyme can all induce polarized digit formation much like a graft of ZPA tissue.

Taken together all this evidence points toward SHH protein as the factor responsible for craniocaudal patterning. How does it accomplish this task? Apparently not by forming a gradient as was predicted by the earlier transplantation studies. Expression of the SHH protein appears restricted to the posterior mesoderm where it is produced. The non-gradient concept is further strengthened by experimental modification of SHH to create a membrane-tethered form of the protein unable to leave the cell for diffusion to faraway sites. This membrane-tethered form of SHH had similar polarizing activity to endogenous SHH indicating that the initiation of craniocaudal patterning begins locally. A direct downstream target of SHH signal-

ing, Gli-3, a transcription factor that is mutated in clinical preaxial (cranial) polydactyly (Greig cephalopolysyndactyly, see Table 11–3) has been found in a gradient across the craniocaudal extent of the chick wing, but how the gradient is set up remains unknown.

Dorsoventral Patterning of the Limb Bud Is Regulated by Wnt-7a and Engrailed-1

Function of the cell surface-associated and extracellular matrix-associated wnt family member *Wnt-7a* in dorsoventral differentiation of the limbs is implied by its restricted expression within the dorsal limb bud ectoderm. Moreover, if the ectodermal covering of the limb bud is surgically reversed, dorsoventral polarity of the skeletal elements determined after the ectoderm reversal is also reversed. Consistent with this observation, striking dorsal-to-ventral transformations of the paw are exhibited in null mutants of mice in which the gene expressing *Wnt-7a* is disrupted. Although ventral structures remain relatively normal, the dorsal side of the paw assumes ventral characteristics. For example, both dorsal skin and ventral skin now develop foot pads, and the large ventral central tendon of each digit is duplicated on the dorsal side. Although sesamoid bones are formed in their normal ventral positions, they are also duplicated dorsally. Apparently, the dorsoventral signaling mechanism must involve factors other than *Wnt-7a*, however, because only the paw is affected in this knockout. Indeed, *Wnt-7a* has been shown to induce the expression of *Lmx-1*, a *Lim* homeobox gene and thus to dorsalize the limb bud in a manner similar to dorsalization of the embryo as a whole (see Experimental Principles section of Ch. 3). Moreover, ectopic expression of *Lmx-1* is able to dorsalize the limb, showing that this homeobox gene mediates the dorsalizing signal expressed by *Wnt-7a* within the dorsal ectoderm. Mutation of *Lmx-1* leads to Nail-Patella syndrome (see Table 11–3) indicating that dorsal structures in the limb are primarily affected when this gene is not functional.

Ventral properties of the limb are attributable to Engrailed, a homeodomain protein expressed only in the ventral ectoderm of the limb bud. In contrast to the *Wnt-7a* knockout, the loss of *En-1* function leads to double dorsal limbs. How the information from these genes is translated into dorsalization or ventralization is unknown.

Mechanisms Underlying Differentiation of the Proximodistal, Craniocaudal, and Dorsoventral Axes Are Integrated

Although *Wnt-7a* plays a critical role in dorsoventral signaling, it also interacts with factors that regulate organization of the proximodistal and craniocaudal axes. For example, *Wnt-7a* may play a role in maintenance of *Shh* expression within the ZPA. First, the surgical removal of the dorsal ectoderm leads to absence of caudal skeletal elements. Second, the loss of these caudal skeletal elements can be rescued by the application of *Shh* to the limb bud. Moreover, in experiments in which the dorsal ectoderm and the apical ectodermal ridge are both removed from the limb bud, recovery of *Shh* expression requires the application of both WNT-7A and FGF-4, indicating that WNT-7A and FGF-4 may act together to maintain *Shh* expression in the ZPA. The requirement for these interactions should be viewed with caution because a recent conditional knockout of Fgf-4 did not cause any abnormality of limb development.

In summary, it has been suggested that *Shh* expression within the ZPA and its long-term influence on proximodistal, craniocaudal, and dorsoventral patterning of the limb bud may involve the activity of a **positive feedback loop** between the AER and the ZPA.

Tbx Genes Contribute to the Development of a Limb Bud as a Forelimb or Hindlimb

Although forelimbs and hindlimbs utilize the same developmental signaling centers, the AER and ZPA, the final outcome is somewhat different, especially if one compares the chick wing to the chick leg. At least part of this difference can be attributed to the differential expression of T-box genes. T-box genes are a family of transcription factors, two of which have restricted expression in forelimb or hindlimb. *Tbx-5* is expressed only in the forelimb, whereas *Tbx-4* is restricted to the hindlimb. The ability of the protein products of these genes to direct the identity of the limb is evident from misexpression studies. When *Tbx-5* is misexpressed in the chick embryonic hindlimb, the leg takes on characteristics of the wing, including three rather than four digits, and feathers instead of scales. Conversely, if *Tbx-4* is misexpressed in the wing, the limb develops features consistent with a leg. In neither case is the transformation complete, suggesting that other factors, not completely understood, also contribute to forelimb and hindlimb identity.

Clinically, these findings are supported as a mutation of *Tbx-5* (Holt-Oram syndrome) which leads to malformations only in the forelimbs. No mutation of *Tbx-4* has yet been identified.

Loss of Cells Through Programmed Cell death Is Required for Normal Development of the Vertebrate Limb

Loss of cells from most organs and tissue is a common feature of vertebrate embryos. These episodes have been termed **programmed cell death** because they consistently occur at the same time and place during the development of an organ system. Many episodes of programmed cell death occur during limb development. The best known of these episodes is the loss of tissue in the developing hand and footplate where its obvious function is to remove the interdigital tissue so that the digits are freed for the mobility to carry out their specialized tasks. The lack of this episode can be seen in the duck foot, specialized for swimming, and in the occurrence of soft tissue syndactyly as a frequent clinical observation. Considerable experimental evidence indicates that the signaling molecule responsible for the cascade of events leading to cell death belongs to the BMPs subfamily of the TGFβ family. Manipulation that increases BMP activity leads to increased cell death in the interdigital necrotic zone (INZ) whereas lowering BMP activity by expressing dominant negative BMP receptors prevents INZ cell death and leads to digital webbing.

Other episodes of cell death during limb morphogenesis are seen in the AER and the anterior and posterior mesenchyme. Here again BMPs have been indicated as the important signaling pathway leading these cells to die. The developmental function of these cell death episodes is less clear. AER cell death is thought to modulate its inductive activity on the underlying mesenchyme. Cell death in the anterior mesenchyme has been related to digital morphogenesis, the absence of this episode leading to anterior (preaxial) polydactyly. Teratogens, especially retinoic acid, have been postulated to act by changing the size of this episode of programmed cell death.

The Immense Vitality of the Field of Limb Research Promises New and Significant Discoveries

In spite of the astounding progress in this area of developmental biology, numerous intriguing questions remain. For example, what role does vitamin A or RA play in normal limb development, and how does it interact with other regulatory factors? What other signal molecules act in concert with the dorsalizing signal WNT-7A, and what are the downstream targets of WNT-7A and LMX-1? In other words, how is the dorsoventral patterning of proximal limb segments regulated? An interesting area of study, not fully explored, is the mechanism of limb regeneration in amphibians and its possible relationship to limb development in higher organisms.

SUGGESTED READING

Descriptive Embryology

Bardeen CR, Lewis WH. 1901. Development of the limbs, body wall, and back in man. Am J Anat 1:1

Bowen R, Hinchliffe JR, Horder TJ, Reeve AMF. 1989. The fate map of the chick forelimb-bud and its bearing on hypothesized development control mechanisms. Anat Embryol 179:269

Brookes M. 1955. The vascularization of long bones in the human fetus. J Anat 92:261

Carrington JL, Fallon JF. 1988. Initial budding is independent of apical ectodermal ridge activity: evidence from a limbless mutant. Development 104: 361

Chevallier A, Kieny M, Mauger A. 1977. Limb-somite relationship: origin of the limb musculature. J Embryol Exp Morphol 41:245

Christ B, Jacob HJ. 1980. Origin, distribution, and determination of chick limb bud mesenchymal cells. p. 67. In Merker H-J, Nau H, Neubert D (eds): Teratology of the Limbs. Walter D. Gruyter, Berlin

Christ B, Jacob HJ, Jacob M. 1977. Experimental analysis of origin of the wing musculature in avian embryos. Anat Embryol 150:171

Christ B, Jacob HJ, Jacob M, Brand B. 1986. Principles of hand ontogenesis in man. Acta Morphol Neerl-Scand 24:249

Cohn MJ, Bright PE. 1999. Molecular control of vertebrate limb development, evolution and congenital malformations

Gardner E. 1968. The embryology of the clavicle. Clin Orthop 58:9

Heine UI, Munoz EF, Flanders KC, et al. 1987. Role of transforming growth factor-β in the development of the mouse embryo. J Cell Biol 105:2861

Hinrichsen KV, Jacob HJ, Jacob M, et al. 1994. Principles of ontogenesis of leg and foot in man. Ann Anat 176:121

Honig MG, Lance-Jones C, Landmesser L. 1986. The development of sensory projection patterns in embryonic chick hind-limb under experimental conditions. Dev Biol 118:532

Jacob M, Christ B, Jacob HJ. 1980. On the migration of myogenic stem cells into the prospective wing region of chick embryos. Anat Embryol (Berl) 153:179

Kelley RO. 1985. Early development of the vertebrate limb: an introduction to morphogenetic tissue interactions using scanning electron microscopy. Scanning Microsc II:827

Kelly RO, Fallon JF. 1981. The developing limb: an analysis of interacting cells and tissues in a model morphogenetic system. p. 49. In Connelly TG, Brinkley LL, and Carlson BM (eds): Morphogenesis and Pattern Formation. Raven Press, New York

Kieny M, Chevallier A. 1979. Anatomy of tendon development in the embryonic chick wing. J Embryol Exp Morphol 49:153

Landmesser L. 1988. Peripheral guidance cues and the formation of specific motor projections in the chick. p. 121. In Easter SS Jr., Berald KF, Carlson BM (eds): From Message to Mind. Sinauer Associates, Inc, Sunderland, MA

Landmesser L, Honig MG. 1986. Altered sensory projections in the chick hind limb following the early removal of motoneurons. Dev Biol 118:511

Lehnert SA, Akhurst RJ. 1988. Embryonic expression pattern of TGF-beta type 1 RNA suggests both paracrine and autocrine mechanisms of action. Development 104:263

Muneoka K, Wanek N, Bryant SV. 1989. Mammalian limb bud development: in situ fate maps of early hind-limb buds. J Exp Zool 249:50

Noback CR, Robertson GG. 1951. Sequences of appearance of ossification centers in the human skeleton during the first five prenatal months. Am J Anat 89:1

O'Rahilly R, Gray DJ, Gardner E. 1957. Chondrification in the hands and feet of staged human embryos. Contrib Embryol Carnegie Inst 36:183

O'Rahilly R, Meyer DB. 1956. Roentgenographic investigation of the human skeleton during early fetal life. Am J Roentgenol 76:455

O'Rahilly R, Muller F. 1987. Development stages in human embryos. Carnegie Inst Wash Publ 637:1

Rubin L, Saunders JW Jr. 1972. Ectodermal-mesodermal interactions in the growth of limb buds in the chick embryo: constancy and temporal limits of the ectodermal induction. Dev Biol 28:94

Rutz R, Haney C, Hauschka S. 1982. Spatial analysis of limb bud myogenesis: a proximodistal gradient of muscle colony-forming cells in chick embryo leg buds. Dev Biol 90:399

Saunders JW. 1948. The proximo-distal sequence of origin of the parts of the chick wing and the role of the ectoderm. J Exp Zool 108:363

Saunders JW, Gasseling MT. 1983. New insights into the problem of pattern regulation in the limb bud of the chick embryo. p. 67. In Fallon JF, Caplan AI (eds): Limb Development and Regeneration. Part A. Alan R Liss, New York

Solursh M, Drake C, Meier S. 1987. The migration of myogenic cells from the somites at the wing level in avian embryos. Dev Biol 121:389

Sporn MB, Roberts AB. 1989. Transforming growth factor-β: multiple actions and potential clinical applications. JAMA 262:938

Stephens TD, Beier RLW, Bringhurst DC et al. 1989. Limbness in the early chick embryo lateral plate. Dev Biol 133:1

Summerbell D, Honig LS. 1982. The control of pattern across the antero-posterior axis of the chick limb bud by a unique signaling region. Am Zool 22:105

Summerbell D, Lewis JH, Wolpert L. 1973. Positional information in chick limb morphogenesis. Nature (London) 244:492

Tosney K, Landmesser LT. 1984. Pattern and specificity of axonal outgrowth following varying degrees of chick limb bud ablation. J Neurosci 4:2518

Tosney K, Watanabe M, Landmesser L, Rutishauser U. 1986. The distribution of NCAM in the chick hindlimb during axon outgrowth and synaptogenesis. Dev Biol 114:437

Wachtler F, Christ B, Jacob HJ. 1982. Grafting experiments on determination and migratory behavior of presomitic, somitic, and somatopleural cells in avian embryos. Anat Embryol (Bed) 164:369

Wolpert L. 1978. Pattern formation in biological development. Sci Am 239:154

Wolpert L. 1981. Cellular basis of skeletal growth during development. Br Med Bull 37:215

Clinical Applications

Bhat BV, Ashok BA, Puri RK. 1987. Lobster claw hand and foot deformity in a family. Indian Pediatr 24:675

Brown KS, Cranley RE, Greene R, et al. 1981. Disproportionate micromelia (*Dmm*): an incomplete dominant mouse dwarfism with abnormal cartilage matrix. J Embryol Exp Morphol 62:165

Collins MD, Fradkin R, Scott WJ. 1990. Induction of postaxial forelimb ectrodactyly with anticonvulsive agents in A/J mice. Teratology 41:61

Cusic AM, Dagg CP. 1985. Spontaneous and retinoic acid-induced postaxial polydactyly in mice. Teratology 31:49

D'Amato RJ, Loughnan MS, Flynn E, Folkman J. 1994.

Thalidomide is an inhibitor of angiogenesis. Proc Natl Acad Sci U S A 91:4082

Ehninger G, Eger K, Stuhler A, Schuler U. 1993. Thalidomide—the need for a new clinical evaluation of an old drug. Bone Marrow Transplant 12(suppl 3):S26

Elmer WA, Pennybacker MF, Knudsen TB, Kwasigroch TE. 1988. Alterations in cell surface galactosyltransferase activity during limb chondrogenesis in *Brachypod* mutant mouse embryos. Teratology 38:475

Graham JM. 1985. The association between limb anomalies and spatially-restricting uterine environments. Prog Clin Biol Res 163c:99

Hartwig NG, Vermeij-Keers C, De Vies HE, et al. 1989. Limb body wall malformation complex: an embryologic etiology? Hum Pathol 20:1071

Higginbottom MC, Jones KL, Hall BD, Smith DW. 1979. The amniotic band disruption complex: timing of amniotic rupture and variable spectra of consequent defects. J Pediatr 95:544

Jaeggi E, Kind C, Morger R. 1990. Congenital scalp and skull defects with terminal transverse limb anomalies (Adams-Oliver syndrome): report of three additional cases. Eur J Pediatr 149:565

Klein KL, Scott WJ, Wilson JG. 1981. Aspirin-induced teratogenesis: a unique pattern of cell death and subsequent polydactyly in the rat. J Exp Zool 216:107

Knudsen TB, Kochhar DM. 1981. The role of morphogenetic cell death during abnormal limb-bud outgrowth in mice heterozygous for the dominant mutation *He-mimelia-extra toe (Hmx)*. J Embryol Exp Morphol 65:289

Kocher W, Kocher-Becker U. 1980. Bilaterally symmetric and asymmetric realization of limb malformations. p. 259. In Merker HJ, Nau H, Neubert D (eds): Teratology of the Limbs. Walter de Gruyter, Berlin

Kochhar DM. 1985. Cellular expression of a mutant gene (*cmd/cmd*) causing limb and other defects in mouse embryos. Prog Clin Biol Res 163c:131

Lenz W. 1988. A short history of thalidomide embryopathy. Teratology 38:203

Lenz W, Knapp K. 1962. Foetal malformation due to thalidomide. German Med Monthly 7:253

Merker H-J. 1977. Considerations of the problem of critical period during development of the limb skeleton. Birth Defects Orig Artic Ser 13:179

Mundlos S, Mulliken JB, Abramson DL, et al. 1996. Genetic mapping of cliedocranial dysplasia and evidence of a microdeletion in one family. Hum Mol Genet 4:71

Muragaki Y, Mudlos S, Upton J, Olsen B. 1996. Altered growth and branching patterns in synpolydactyly caused by mutations in *HOXD13*. Science 272:548

Neubert R, Helge H, Neubert D. 1995. Thalidomide and the immune system. 4. Down-regulation of the CD26 receptor, probably involved in the binding of HIV components to T cells in primates. Life Sci 56:407

Neubert R, Hinz N, Thiel R, Neubert D. 1995. Down-regulation of adhesion receptors on cells of primate embryos as a probable mechanism of the teratogenic action of thalidomide. Life Sci 58:295

Olsen B. 1995. Mutations in collagen genes resulting in metaphyseal and epiphyseal dysplasias. Bone 17:45S

O'Rahilly R. 1985. The development and classification of anomalies of the limbs in the human. Prog Clin Biol Res 163c:85

Regemorter NV, Milare J, Ramet J, et al. 1982. Familial ectrodactyly and polydactyly: variable expressivity of one single gene—embryological considerations. Clin Genet 22:206

Rooze MA. 1977. The effects of the *Dh* gene on limb morphogenesis in the mouse. Birth Defects Orig Artic Ser 13:69

Ruffing L. 1977. Evaluation of thalidomide children. Birth Defects Orig Artic Ser 13:287

Satre MA, Kochhar DM. 1989. Elevations in the endogenous levels of the putative morphogen retinoic acid in embryonic mouse limb-buds associated with limb dysmorphogenesis. Dev Biol 133:529

Scott WJ. 1985. Asymmetric limb malformations induced by drugs or mutant genes. Prog Clin Biol Res 163c:111

Silengo MC, Biagli M, Bell GL, et al. 1987. Triphalangeal thumb and brachyectrodactyly syndrome. Clin Genet 31:13

Sulik K, Dehart DB. 1988. Retinoic-acid-induced limb malformations resulting from apical ectodermal ridge death. Teratology 37:527

Torpin R. 1968. Amniochorionic mesoblastic fibrous strings and amniotic bands. Am J Obstet Gynecol 91:65

Van Allen MI, Curry C, Gallagher L. 1987. Limb body wall complex. I. Pathogenesis. Am J Med Genet 28:529

Viljoen DL, Kidson SH. 1990. Mirror polydactyly: morphogenesis based on a morphogen gradient theory. Am J Med Genet 35:229

Weaver T, Scott WJ 1984. Acetazolamide teratogenesis: interaction of maternal metabolic and respiratory acidosis in the induction of ectrodactyly in C57BL/6J mice. Teratology 30:195

Wulfsberg EA, Mirkinson LJ, Meister SJ. 1993. Autosomal dominant tetramelic postaxial oligodactyly. Am J Med Genet 46:579

Experimental Principles

Bitgood MJ, McMahon AP. 1995. Hedgehog and BMP genes are coexpressed at many diverse sites of cell-cell interaction in the mouse embryo. Dev Biol 172:126

Bryant SV. 1996. Digit induction by Henson's node and notochord involves the expression of shh but not RAR-β 2. Dev Biol 173:318

Bryant SV, Muneoka K. 1986. Views of limb development and regeneration. Trends Genet 2:153

Chan DC, Laufer E, Tabin C, Leder P. 1995. Polydactylous limbs in Strong's Luxoid mice result from ectopic polarizing activity. Development 121:1971

Chan DC, Wynshaw-Boris A, Leder P. 1995. Formin isoforms are differentially expressed in the mouse embryo and are required for normal expression of fgf-4 and shh in the limb bud. Development 121:3151

Charite J, de Graaff W, Shen S, Deschamps J. 1994. Ectopic expression of *Hoxb-8* causes duplication of the ZPA in the forelimb and homeotic transformation of axial structures. Cell 78:589

Chen Y, Dong D, Kostetskii I, Zile MH. 1996. Henson's node from viamin A-deficient quail embryo induces chick limb bud duplication and retains its normal symmetric expression of sonic hedgehog (Shh). Dev Biol 173:256

Cohn MJ, Bright PE. 1999. Molecular control of vertebrate limb development, evolution, and congenital malformations. Cell Tissue Res 296:3

Cohn MJ, Izpisua-Belmonte JC, Abud H, et al. 1995. Fibroblast growth factors induce additional limb development from the flank of chick embryos. Cell 80:739

Crossley PH, Martin GR. 1995. The mouse *Fgf8* gene encodes a family of polypeptides and is expressed in regions that direct outgrowth and patterning in the developing embryo. Development 121:439

Davis AP, Capecchi MR. 1994. Axial homeosis and appendicular skeleton defects in mice with a targeted disruption of *hoxd-11*. Development 120:2187

Davis AP, Witte DP, Hsieh-Li Hm, et al. 1995. Absence of radius and ulna in mice lacking *hoxa-11* and *hoxd-11*. Nature 375:791

Dealy CN, Kosher RA. 1996. IGF-I and insulin in the acquisition of limb-forming ability by the embryonic lateral plate. Develop Biol 177:291

Dealy CN, Kosher RA. 1996. IGF-I, insulin and FGFs induce outgrowth of the limb buds of amelic chick embryos. Development 122:1323

Dolle P, Izpisua-Belmonte J-C, Falkenstein H, et al. 1989. Coordinate expression of the murine *Hox-5* complex homeobox-containing genes during limb pattern formation. Nature (London) 342:767

Duboule D. 1993. The function of *Hox* genes in the morphogenesis of the vertebrate limb. Ann Genet 36:24

Fawcett D, Pasceri P, Fraser R, et al. 1995. Postaxial polydactyly in forelimbs of CRABP-II mutant mice. Development 121:671

Francis PH, Richardson MK, Brikell PM, Tickle C. 1994. Bone morphogenetic proteins and a signalling pathway that controls patterning in the developing chick limb. Development 120:209

Francis-West PH, Robertson KE, Ede DA, et al. 1995. Expression of genes encoding bone morphogenetic proteins and sonic hedgehog in talpid (ta3) limb buds: their relationships in the signalling cascade involved in limb patterning. Dev Dyn 203:187

Gould SE, Upholt WB, Kosher RA. 1995. Characterization of chicken syndecan-3 as a heparan sulfate proteoglycan and its expression during embryogenesis. Dev Biol 168:438

Haramis AG, Brown JM, Zeller R. 1995. The limb deformity mutation disrupts the SHH/FGF-4 feedback loop and regulation of 5' *HoxD* genes during limb pattern formation. Development 121:4237

Hardy A, Richardson MK, Francis-West PH, et al. 1995. Gene expression, polarising activity skeletal patterning in reaggregated hind limb mesenchyme. Development 121:4329

Hayamizu TF, Bryant SV. 1994. Reciprocal changes in *Hox D13* and RAR-beta 2 expression in response to retinoic acid in chick limbs. Dev Biol 166:123

Helms J, Thaller C, Eichele G. 1994. Relationship between retinoic acid and sonic hedgehog, two polarizing signals in the chick wing bud. Development 120:3267

Hornbruch A, Wolpert L. 1986. Positional signalling by Henson's node when grafted to the chick limb bud. J Embryol Exp Morphol 94:257

Itoh N, Mima T, Mikawa T. 1996. Loss of fibroblast growth factor receptors is necessary for terminal differentiation of embryonic limb muscle. Development 122:291

Izpisua-Belmonte JC, Duboule D. 1992. Homeobox genes and pattern formation in the vertebrate limb. Dev Biol 152:26

Kochar DM. 1973. Limb development in mouse embryos. I. Analysis of teratogenic effects of retinoic acid. Teratology 7:289

Laufer E, Nelson CE, Johnson RL, et al. 1994. Sonic hedgehog and FGF-4 act through a signaling cascade and feedback loop to integrate growth and patterning of the developing limb bud. Cell 79:993

Lopez-Martinez A, Chang DT, Chiang C, et al. 1995. Limb-patterning activity and restricted posterior localization of the amino-terminal product of the Sonic hedgehog cleavage. Curr Biol 5:791

Lyons KM, Hogan BL, Robertson EJ. 1995. Colocalization of BMP 7 and BMP 2 RNAs suggests that these factors cooperatively mediate tissue interactions during murine development. Mech Dev 50:71

Maas RL, Zeller R, Woychik RP, et al. 1990. Disruption of formin-encoding transcripts in two mutant limb deformity alleles. Nature (London) 346:853

MacArthur CA, Lawshe A, Xu J, et al. 1995. FGF-8 isoforms activate receptor splice forms that are expressed in mesenchymal regions of mouse development. Development 121:3603

MacCabe JA, Errick J, Sauders JW. 1974. Ectodermal control of the dorsoventral axis of the leg bud of the chick embryo. Dev Biol 39:69

Mahmud R, Bresnick J, Hornbruch A, et al. 1995. A role for FGF-8 in the initiation and maintenance of vertebrate limb bud outgrowth. Curr Biol 5:797

Marigo V, Roberts DJ, Lee SM, et al. 1995. Cloning, expression, and chromosomal location of SHH and IHH: two human homologues of the *Drosophila* segment polarity gene hedgehog. Genomics 28:44

Masuya H, Sagai T, Wakana S, et al. 1995. A duplicated

zone of polarizing activity in polydactylous mouse mutants. Genes Dev 9:1645

McGinnis W, Garber RL, Wirz J, et al. 1984. A homologous protein coding sequence in *Drosophila* homeotic genes and its conservation in other metazoans. Cell 37:403

McNeisch JD, Scott WJ, Potter SS. 1988. Legless, a novel mutation found in PHT1-1 transgenic mice. Science 241:837

Mima T, Ohuchi H, Noji S, Mikawa T. 1995. FGF can induce outgrowth of somatic mesoderm both inside and outside of limb-forming regions. Dev Biol 167:617

Morgan BA, Tabin C, 1994. *Hox* genes and growth: early and late roles in limb bud morphogenesis. Development (suppl): 181

Nelson CE, Morgan BA, Burke AC, et al. 1996. Analysis of HOX gene expression in the chick limb bud. Development 122:1449

Niswander L, Jeffery S, Martin GR, Tickle C. 1994. A positive feedback loop coordinates growth and patterning in the vertebrate limb. Nature 371:609

Niswander L, Martin G. 1993. FGF-4 regulates expression of *Evx-1* in the developing mouse limb. Development 119:287

Niswander L, Martin GR. 1993. Mixed signals from the AER: FGF-4 and BMP-2 have opposite effects on limb growth. Prog Clin Biol Res 383B:625

Niswander L, Tickle C, Vogel A, et al. 1993. FGF-4 replaces the apical ectodermal ridge and directs outgrowth and patterning of the limb. Cell 75:579

Noji S, Nohno T, Koyama E, et al. 1991. Retinoic acid induces polarizing activity but is unlikely to be a morphogen in the chick limb bud. Nature (London) 350:83

Ochiya T, Sakamoto H, Tsukamoto M, et al. 1995. Hst-1 (FGF-4) antisense oligonucleotides block murine limb development. J Cell Biol 130:997

Ohuchi H, Yoshioka H, Tanaka A, et al. 1994. Involvement of androgen-induced growth factor (FGF-8) gene in mouse embryogenesis and morphogenesis. Biochem Biophys Res Commun 204:882

Oster GF, Murray JD, Maini PK. 1985. A model for chondrogenic condensations in the developing limb: the role of extracellular matrix and cell interactions. J Embryol Exp Morphol 89:93

Parr BA, McMahon AP. 1995. Dorsalizing signal Wnt-7a required for normal polarity of D-V and A-P axes of mouse limb. Nature 374:350

Patou M-P. 1977. Dorsoventral axis determination of chick limb bud development. p. 257. In (Ede DA, Hinchiliffe JR, Balls M (eds): Vertebrate Limb and Somite Morphogenesis. Cambridge University Press, Cambridge, England

Perrimon N. 1995. Hedgehog and beyond. Cell 80:517

Reid L. 1990. From gradients to axes, from morphogenesis to differentiation. Cell 63:875

Riddle RD, Ensini M, Nelson C, et al. 1995. Induction of the *LIM* homeobox gene *Lmx1* by Wnt7a establishes dorsoventral pattern in the vertebrate limb. Cell 83:631

Riddle RD, Johnson RL, Laufer E, Tabin C. 1993. Sonic hedgehog mediates the polarizing activity of the ZPA. Cell 75:1401

Robert B, Sassoon D, Jacq B, et al. 1989. *Hox-7*, a mouse homeobox gene with a novel pattern of expression during embryo-genesis. EMBO J 8:91

Saunders JW, Gasseling MT. 1968. Ectodermal-mesenchymal interactions in the origin of wing symmetry. p. 78. In Fleischmajer R, Billingham E (eds): Epithelial-Mesenchymal Interactions. Williams & Wilkins, Baltimore

Savage MP, Fallon JF. 1995. FGF-2 mRNA and its antisense message are expressed in a developmentally specific manner in the chick limb bud and mesonephros. Dev Dyn 202:343

Slack JMW. 1987. Morphogenetic gradients—past and present. Trends Biochem Sci 12:200

Small KM, Potter SS. 1993. Homeotic transformations and limb defects in *Hox All* mutant mice. Genes Dev 7:2318

Smith SM, Pang K, Sundin O, et al. 1989. Molecular approaches to vertebrate limb morphogenesis. Development (suppl):107:121

Storm EE, Huynh TV, Copeland NG, et al. 1994. Limb alterations in brachipodism mice due to mutations in a new member of the TGF-beta-superfamily. Nature 368:639

Tabin C. 1995. The initiation of the limb bud: growth factors, *Hox* genes, and retinoids. Cell 80:671

Tanaka EM, Gann AF. 1995. Limb development. The budding role of FGF. Curr Biol 5:594

Taylor GP, Anderson R, Reginelli AD, Muneoka K. 1994. FGF-2 induces regeneration of the chick limb bud. Dev Biol 163:282

Thaller C, Eichele G. 1987. Identification and spatial distribution of retinoids in the developing chick limb bud. Nature (London) 327:625

Tickle C. 1995. Vertebrate limb development. Curr Opin Genet Dev 5:478

Tickle C, Alberts B, Wolpert L, Lee J. 1982. Local application of retinoic acid to the limb bud mimics the action of the polarizing region. Nature (London) 296:564

Tickle C, Summerbell D, Wolpert L. 1975. Positional signalling and specification of digits in chick limb morphogenesis. Nature (London) 254:199

Vogel A, Roberts-Clarke D, Niswander L. 1995. Effect of FGF on gene expression in chick limb bud cells in vivo and in vitro. Dev Biol 171:507

Vogel A, Rodriguez, Warnken W, Belmonte JCI. 199. Dorsal cell fate specified by chick *Lmx1* during vertebrate limb development. Nature 378:716

Vogel A, Tickle C. 1993. FGF-4 maintains polarizing activity of posterior limb bud cells in vivo and in vitro. Development 119:199

Vogt TF, Jackson-Grusby L, Rush J, Leader P. 1993. Formins: phosphoprotein isoforms encoded by the mouse limb deformity locus. Proc Natl Acad Sci U S A 90:5554

Wanek N, Gardiner DM, Muneoka K, Bryant SV. 1991. Conversion by retinoic acid of anterior cells into

ZPA cells in the chick wing bud. Nature (London) 350:81

Wang Y, Sassoon D. 1995. Ectoderm-mesenchyme and mesenchyme-mesenchyme interactions regulate *Msx-1* expression and cellular differentiation in the murine limb. Dev Biol 168:374

Warkany PJ, Nelson R. 1940. Appearance of skeletal abnormalities in the offspring of rats reared on a deficient diet. Science 92:383

Wolpert L. 1989. Positional information revisited. Development (suppl) 107:3

Yamaguchi TP, Rossant J. 1995. Fibroblast growth factors in mammalian development. Curr Opin Genet Dev 5:485

Yang Y, Niswender L. 1995. Interaction between the signaling molecules WNT7a and SHH during vertebrate limb development: dorsal signals regulate anteroposterior patterning. Cell 80:939

Yokouchi Y, Nakzato S, Yamamoto M, et al. 1995. Misexpression of *Hoxa-13* induces cartilage homeotic transformation and changes cell adhesiveness in chick limbs. Genes Dev 9:2509

Yuan H, Corbi N, Basilico C, Dailey L. 1995. Developmental-specificity activity of the FGF-4 enhancer requires the synergistic action of *Sox2* and *Oct-3*. Genes Dev 9:2635

Zeller R, Jackson-Grusby L, Leder P. 1989. The limb deformity gene is required for apical ectodermal ridge differentiation and anteroposterior limb pattern formation. Genes Dev 3:1481

Zou H, Niswander L. 1996. Requirement for BMP signaling in interdigital apoptosis and scale formation. Science 272:738

Development of the Head, the Neck, the Eyes, and the Ears

Part One

Development of the Head and Neck

Summary

In all vertebrates, the skeleton of the head and pharynx is made up of the **chondrocranium (neurocranium),** which supports the brain; the **sensory capsules,** which support the olfactory organs, eyes, and inner ears; the **membrane bones,** which roof the skull; and the **viscerocranium,** which supports the pharyngeal arches and their derivatives. The chondrocranium of primitive fishes protects the brain and carries the three pairs of sensory capsules. In humans, the chondrocranium ossifies to form the bones of the skull base, and the sensory capsules give rise to some bones of the nasal cavities and orbits and to portions of the temporal bone. Membrane bones form an additional secondary armor that completely roofs the skull in an evolutionary line of fishes that led to humans. In humans, these bones become the skull vault. The membrane bones ossify directly from ectomesenchyme rather than from a cartilaginous precursor.

In humans, five pairs of **pharyngeal arches** form on either side of the pharyngeal foregut, starting on day 22. These arches correspond to numbers 1, 2, 3, 4, and 6 of the primitive vertebrate gill bars, or branchial arches. Each arch has an outer covering of ectoderm, an inner covering of endoderm, and a core of mesenchyme that is derived from the lateral plate mesoderm and also includes contributions from the adjacent somitomeres or somites and from the neural crest. Each arch contains a cartilaginous supporting element, an aortic arch artery (described in Ch. 8), and an arch-associated cranial nerve (comprising cranial nerves V, VII, IX, and X). The arches are separated externally by ectoderm-lined **pharyngeal clefts** and internally by endoderm-lined **pharyngeal pouches.**

The elements of the viscerocranium arise evolutionarily from the pharyngeal arch cartilages, which develop from a mesenchymal condensation within each arch. This mesenchymal condensation of the first arch consists of neural crest-derived ectomesenchyme. In primitive vertebrates, the first-arch cartilage gives rise to the bones of the upper and lower jaws. The jaws of higher vertebrates, including humans, are formed almost entirely of membrane bone, and in humans the cartilage of the first arch gives rise principally to the incus and malleus of the middle ear. The cartilage of the second arch is also derived from ectomesenchyme and gives rise to the stapes, the stylohyoid, and the upper rim of the hyoid. (The lower rim of the hyoid is derived from neural crest cells in the third pharyngeal arch.) The supporting elements of the remaining two arches are derived from lateral plate mesoderm and give rise to the cartilages of the larynx.

The muscles associated with each arch skeletal element are derived

Formation of the Skull

Differentiation of the Pharyngeal Arch Cartilages, Muscles, and Nerves

Development of the Tongue and Pharyngeal Pouch Derivatives

Morphogenesis of the Face

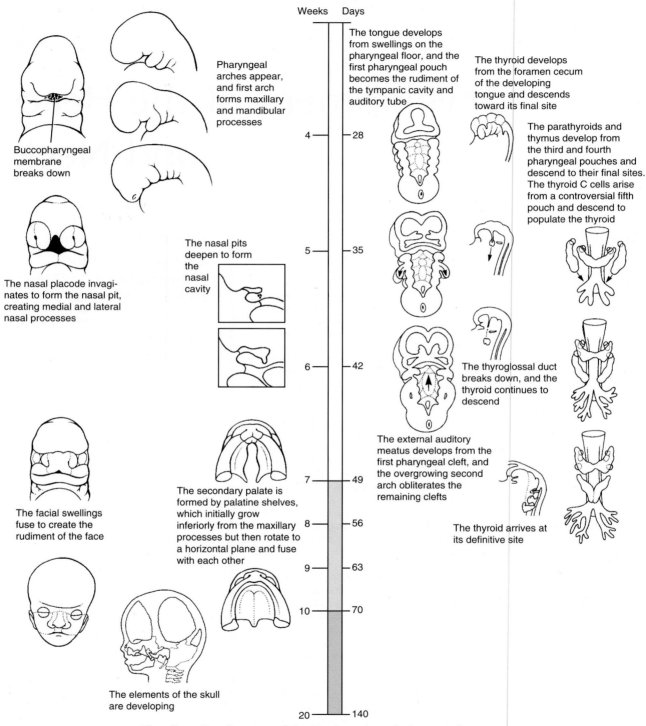

Weeks   Days

Pharyngeal arches appear, and first arch forms maxillary and mandibular processes

Buccopharyngeal membrane breaks down

The nasal placode invaginates to form the nasal pit, creating medial and lateral nasal processes

The nasal pits deepen to form the nasal cavity

The facial swellings fuse to create the rudiment of the face

The secondary palate is formed by palatine shelves, which initially grow inferiorly from the maxillary processes but then rotate to a horizontal plane and fuse with each other

The elements of the skull are developing

The tongue develops from swellings on the pharyngeal floor, and the first pharyngeal pouch becomes the rudiment of the tympanic cavity and auditory tube

The thyroid develops from the foramen cecum of the developing tongue and descends toward its final site

The parathyroids and thymus develop from the third and fourth pharyngeal pouches and descend to their final sites. The thyroid C cells arise from a controversial fifth pouch and descend to populate the thyroid

The thyroglossal duct breaks down, and the thyroid continues to descend

The external auditory meatus develops from the first pharyngeal cleft, and the overgrowing second arch obliterates the remaining clefts

The thyroid arrives at its definitive site

4 — 28
5 — 35
6 — 42
7 — 49
8 — 56
9 — 63
10 — 70
20 — 140

Timeline. Development of the head, neck, and pharyngeal structure.

from the somitic or somitomeric mesoderm that migrates into the arch. The principal arch-derived muscles are the muscles of mastication and facial expression, the pharyngeal muscles, and the intrinsic muscles of the larynx. The muscles derived from each arch are innervated by a corresponding cranial nerve.

The human face is formed between the 4th and 10th weeks by the fusion of five **facial swellings:** an unpaired **frontonasal process,** a pair of **maxillary swellings,** and a pair of **mandibular swellings.** The maxillary and mandibular swellings constitute dorsal and ventral regions, respectively, of the first pharyngeal arch and give rise to the upper and lower jaws. The frontonasal process forms the forehead and temples. In addition, a pair of thickened ectodermal **nasal placodes** develop on the frontonasal process. The center of each placode invaginates to form the epithelium of the nasal passages, whereas the raised margin of the placode gives rise to the nose, the philtrum of the upper lip, and the primary palate. The secondary palate is formed by shelves that grow from the maxillary swellings. Some of the paranasal air sinuses begin to grow during fetal life, whereas others do not appear until after birth. The **auricle (pinna)** of the outer ear develops from six **auricular hillocks** that develop on the facing edges of the first and second arches.

The **external auditory meatus** develops from the first pharyngeal cleft (the cleft separating the first and second pharyngeal arches), and the corresponding first pharyngeal pouch gives rise to the **tympanic cavity** of the middle ear and to the **auditory (eustachian) tube.** The other pharyngeal clefts are normally obliterated by overgrowth of the second pharyngeal arch, although they occasionally persist as abnormal cervical cysts or fistulae.

The tongue develops from endoderm-covered swellings on the floor of the pharynx. The anterior two thirds of the tongue mucosa is derived from first-arch swellings, whereas the posterior one third is contributed by the third and fourth arches. The tongue muscles, in contrast, are formed by myocytes arising from the occipital somites. For this reason, the motor and sensory nerve fibers of the tongue are carried by separate sets of cranial nerves.

The thyroid gland forms as an endodermal invagination of the **foramen cecum** of the tongue. This primordium elongates, detaches from the pharyngeal endoderm, and finally migrates to its definitive location just inferior and ventral to the larynx.

Each of the pharyngeal pouches gives rise to an adult structure. The first pouch becomes the tympanic cavity and auditory tube, as mentioned earlier. The second pouch gives rise to the palatine tonsils; the third to the thymus gland; and the third and fourth to the inferior and superior parathyroid glands, respectively. A controversial fifth pouch may give rise to the parafollicular cells of the thyroid (ultimobranchial body).

A HEAD AND NECK SPECIALIZED FOR ACTIVE PREDATION AROSE DURING EARLY VERTEBRATE EVOLUTION: OUR PROGENITORS HAD SMALL AND SIMPLE HEADS

The vertebrates arose from a group of simple, filter-feeding aquatic organisms called **protochordates.** A prominent structure of living protochordates is the expanded **pharyngeal chamber** used in filter feeding. This chamber is supported by a cartilaginous **branchial basket.** Water and suspended food particles are drawn into the pharynx through the mouth; the water is expelled through **gill pores** or **gill slits** located on either side of the pharynx; and the edible particles proceed down the gut tube.

Some other characteristic vertebrate features—particularly the presence of a notochord, segmented axial musculature, and a head—probably developed in response to the active life of larval protochordates. Many living protochordates are sessile (remain attached to one spot) as adults, but the larvae appear always to have been free-living. A notochord flanked by muscles makes possible the vertebrate mode of swimming, and the concentration of sense organs and central nervous system centers at the leading end of the animal creates a head.

The most primitive vertebrates, the **jawless fishes (agnathans),** do not have a movable jaw. Most extinct forms appear to have been filter feeders or detritus feeders (Fig. 12–1A), although the living forms, the lamprey and hagfishes, pursue specialized bloodsucking and scavenging modes of life. The brain of agnathans (which is large compared with that of protochordates) is cradled in a bony or cartilaginous **chondrocranium,** which is connected to the persistent notochord as well as to the newly developed spinal column (see Fig. 12–1A). The branchial skeleton supports the **branchial bars (gill bars)** between the gill slits or gill pores and is also anchored to the chondrocranium. The gill bars bear gills in which the blood is oxygenated, and each is therefore served by a **branchial arch artery** (see later in this chapter and Ch. 8).

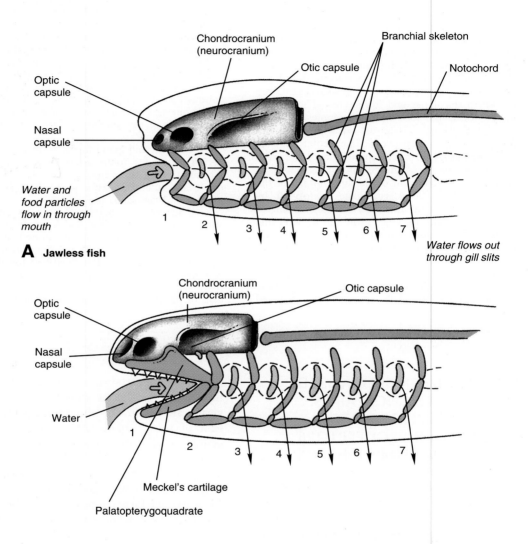

Figure 12–1. The evolutionary origin of the human skull from the pharyngeal arch skeleton, braincase, and dermal bones of primitive vertebrates. *A, B,* The pharyngeal arches of humans are modified from the gill apparatus (branchial arches) of primitive vertebrates. The skeletal elements of the gill bars formed the foundation for the development of the human jaw and neck skeleton. *C, D,* The expanding brain in the line of fishes leading to humans was housed in a cranium formed partly by the chondrocranium and partly by membrane bones derived from the dermis. Membrane bones also form a large part of the highly modified facial skeleton of humans.

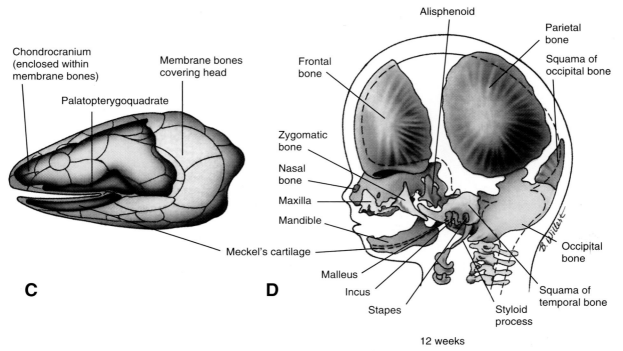

Figure 12–1. *Continued*

In an extinct line of fishes, the first gill bar became hinged and eventually was transformed into a pair of upper and lower jaws (see Fig. 12–1B). This innovation made possible the pursuit and capture of living prey. The improvements to the sensory and propulsive apparatus necessitated by this new mode of life made additional demands on the brain, which progressively enlarged. All these developments together laid the foundations for the evolution of the familiar human head and neck.

THE HUMAN SKULL IS COMPOSED OF DISTINCT GROUPS OF BONES DERIVED FROM DISCRETE EVOLUTIONARY PRECURSORS

The cranial skeleton of fishes is composed of (1) the **chondrocranium,** which encloses the brain and helps to form the **sensory capsules** that support the olfactory organs, eyes, and inner ears; (2) an external armor of **membrane (dermal) bones;** and (3) the **visceral skeleton** or **viscerocranium** that supports the gill bars and jaws. These compo-

nents can still be distinguished in the genesis of the human skull (see Fig. 12–1C, D).

The Brain Is Cradled in the Chondrocranium and Roofed by the Membrane Bones of the Skull Vault

The chondrocranium of primitive fishes is the forerunner of the human **skull base.** In humans, as in fishes, the chondrocranium develops from three pairs of cartilaginous precursors—the **prechordal cartilages (trabeculae cranii),** the **hypophyseal cartilages,** and the **parachordal cartilages**—which are arranged in series and underlie the brain from the interorbitonasal region to the cranial end of the vertebral column (Fig. 12–2A). The caudal-most pair of elements, the parachordal cartilages, are derived from the occipital sclerotomes plus the first cervical sclerotome and thus represent modified vertebral elements (see Ch. 4). The cranial two pairs of elements appear to be derived mostly from neural crest. The bones of the chondrocra-

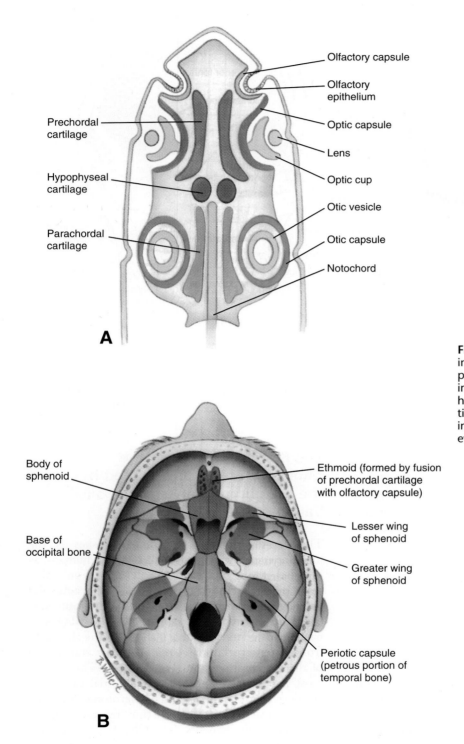

Olfactory capsule

Olfactory epithelium

Optic capsule

Lens

Optic cup

Otic vesicle

Otic capsule

Notochord

Prechordal cartilage

Hypophyseal cartilage

Parachordal cartilage

A

Body of sphenoid

Base of occipital bone

Ethmoid (formed by fusion of prechordal cartilage with olfactory capsule)

Lesser wing of sphenoid

Greater wing of sphenoid

Periotic capsule (petrous portion of temporal bone)

B

Figure 12–2. The base of the skull in humans is derived from three pairs of cartilaginous plates formed in early ancestors: the prechordal, hypophyseal, and parachordal cartilages. Sensory capsules became increasingly complex throughout evolutionary history.

nium (as the name indicates) are preformed in cartilage and ossify by the process of **endochondral ossification** (see Ch. 11).

The membrane-bone armor that covers the skull of our piscene ancestors (bony fishes) is represented in humans by the membrane bones of the skull, comprising the flat bones of the **cranial vault,** or **calvaria,** as well as many bones of the face (see Fig. 12–1*C, D*). These bones grow by the direct ossification of mesenchyme in the presumptive dermis and therefore are not preformed in cartilage. The mesenchyme from which they develop is derived from the neural crest.

The bones of the cranial vault do not complete their growth during fetal life. The soft, fibrous sutures that join them at birth permit the skull vault to deform as it passes through the birth canal and also allow it to continue growing throughout infancy and childhood. Six large, membrane-covered **fontanelles** occupy the areas between the corners of cranial vault bones at birth (Fig. 12–3). The posterior fontanelle closes by 3 months after birth, but the anterior fontanelle normally remains open until 1.5 years of age. Palpa-

tion of this fontanelle can be used to detect elevated intracranial pressure or premature closure of the skull sutures (see the Clinical Applications section of this chapter).

The Special Sense Organs Are Protected by Sensory Capsules

As the simple sense organs of the protochordates gave way to the more sophisticated olfactory, ocular, and auditory/vestibular systems of the vertebrates, three pairs of skeletal capsules evolved to house and protect these organs. In humans, these capsules are formed from portions of the prechordal and hypophyseal cartilages and from bones derived from elements of the primitive capsules of evolutionary ancestors (see Fig. 12–2). The nasal capsules of humans include the **ethmoid** bone, derived from the prechordal cartilages, and the **nasal** and **turbinate** bones. The human orbit includes the body of the sphenoid bone, which is derived from the hypophyseal cartilages, and the greater

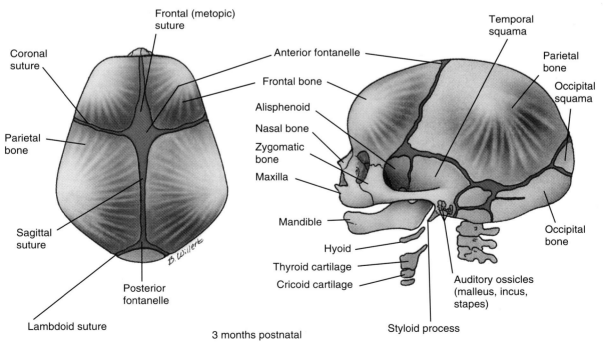

3 months postnatal

Figure 12–3. The brain in humans is mostly enclosed by the dermal bones of the cranial vault. These bones do not fuse together until early childhood. The unfused sutures allow the cranium to deform during birth and to expand during childhood as the brain grows.

and lesser wings of the sphenoids. The otic capsules of humans are descendents of primitive otic capsule ossification centers, which fuse together into a single mass called the **periotic** or **petromastoid bone.**

The sensory capsules arise from cranial somitomeres, occipital somites, and neural crest.

Much of the Human Face and Neck Is Derived From the Ancient Gill Apparatus

The jawless fishes improved the respiratory and filter-feeding systems of the protochordates by transforming the rigid branchial basket into a series of movable gill bars on either side of the pharynx. These arches still develop embryonically in all vertebrates. In jawed vertebrates, the first arch gives rise to the upper and lower jaws. The remaining arches form the gills in fishes and many structures of the face and neck in humans.

Each embryonic arch (branchial or pharyngeal) consists of a mesodermal core lined on the outside with ectoderm and on the inside with endoderm (Fig. 12–4D). Each contains a central cartilaginous skeletal element, striated muscle anlagen innervated by an arch-specific cranial nerve, and an aortic arch artery. The embryonic aortic arch artery system of humans was discussed in Chapter 8. In fishes, the blood pumped out of the single ventricle is distributed to the arch arteries and thence to the capillary beds of the gills. The blood is oxygenated in the gills by the water flowing through the gill slits and then reenters the dorsal portion of the arch artery for distribution to the body via the dorsal aortae (see Fig. 8–2).

In jawed fishes, forcible expansion of the pharyngeal cavity is often used to suck prey into the mouth. Thus, the branchial arches of jawed fishes, like those of filter-feeding jawless fishes, may function in feeding as well as respiration. The pharyngeal arches of humans also participate in both these functions: they give rise, for example, to the jaws and the muscles of chewing and swallowing. Other human pharyngeal arch derivatives have been adapted to the new function of communication: the second arch contributes to the muscles of facial expression, and the fourth and sixth arches contribute to the tongue and larynx, which are used in vocalization.

The Five Human Pharyngeal Arches Form in Craniocaudal Sequence. The pharyngeal arches of human embryos initially resemble the gill arches of fish except that the gill slits never become perforated. Instead, the external **pharyngeal clefts** between the arches remain separated from the apposed, internal **pharyngeal pouches** by thin **pharyngeal membranes.** These membranes are three layered, consisting of ectoderm, mesoderm, and endoderm.

Although the number of pharyngeal arches is somewhat variable among the fishes, the five that develop in human embryos correspond to numbers 1, 2, 3, 4, and 6 of the primitive complement in the evolutionary line leading to land vertebrates. Arch 5 either never forms in humans or forms as a short-lived rudiment and promptly regresses. Like so many other structures in the body, the pharyngeal arches form in craniocaudal succession (see Fig. 12–4A–C): the first arch appears on day 22; the second and third arches appear sequentially on day 24; and the fourth and sixth arches appear sequentially on day 29. Table 12–1 summarizes the origin and fate of the skeletal element, artery, muscles, and cranial nerve of each of the pharyngeal arches.

The Skeletal Elements of the Pharyngeal Arches Are Derived From Midbrain and Hindbrain Neural Crest and From Lateral Plate Mesoderm. Most of the cartilages that form within the pharyngeal arches develop from the neural crest of the midbrain and hindbrain regions, although the cartilages of arches 4 and 6 apparently develop from lateral plate mesoderm. As discussed in Chapter 5, the neural crest in the trunk region migrates mainly by the active movement of the neural crest cells. The neural crest of the cranial region also tends to migrate passively along with the displacement of the surrounding tissue.

Figure 12–5 shows the skeletal elements derived from each arch. All the bones that develop from the pharyngeal arch cartilages themselves are endochondral. Some of these cartilages in humans, however, become completely encased within membrane bones that form by the direct ossification of dermal mesenchyme (also of neural crest origin).

In Mammals, the First Arch Gives Rise to the Incus and Malleus of the Middle Ear and to the Endochondral and Dermal Bones of the Upper and Lower Jaw. As the first pharyngeal arch develops, it is remodeled to form a cranial

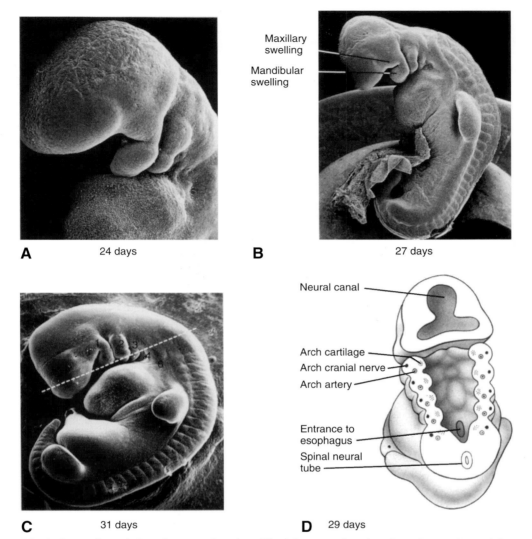

Figure 12–4. Formation of the pharyngeal arches. The pharyngeal arches form in craniocaudal sequence during the fourth and fifth weeks. *A,* By day 24, the first two arches have formed. *B,* By day 27, the first three arches have formed, and the left first arch is visibly divided into maxillary and mandibular swellings. *C,* By the early fifth week, all five arches have formed. The dashed line indicates the plane of the section shown (at a slightly earlier stage) in part *D. D,* Schematic cross section through the pharyngeal arches, showing the cartilage, artery, and cranial nerve in each arch. (*A, B,* Photos courtesy of Dr. Arnold Tamarin.)

maxillary swelling and a caudal **mandibular swelling** (see Fig. 12–4*A–C*). These processes give rise to the upper and lower jaws, respectively. Each process contains a central cartilaginous element. The central cartilages are produced by neural crest cells arising in the region of the embryonic midbrain (mesencephalon) and cranial portion of the hindbrain (metencephalon). The central cartilages of the maxillary swellings are called **pala-**

topterygoquadrate bars, and the central cartilages of the mandibular swellings are called **Meckel's cartilages.**

In humans and other mammals, the jaws consist almost entirely of membrane bones that ensheathe some of the cartilages of the first arch and therefore receive little contribution from the viscerocranium (see Fig. 12–1*D*). Instead, the first-arch cartilages of mammals give rise mainly to two

Table 12–1
The Derivatives of the Pharyngeal Arches and Their Tissues of Origin

PHARYNGEAL ARCH	ARCH ARTERY*	SKELETAL ELEMENTS	MUSCLES	CRANIAL NERVE†

1	Terminal branch of maxillary artery	Derived from arch cartilages (originating from neural crest):
		  From maxillary cartilage: alisphenoid, incus
		  From mandibular (Meckel's) cartilage: malleus
		Derived by direct ossification from arch dermal mesenchyme: maxilla, zygomatic, squamous portion of temporal bone, mandible
			Muscles of mastication (temporalis, masseter, and pterygoids), myelohyoid, anterior belly of the digastric, tensor tympani, tensor veli palatini (originate from cranial somitomere 4)	Maxillary and mandibular division of trigeminal nerve (V)

2	Stapedial artery (embryonic), corticotympanic artery (adult)	Stapes, styloid process, stylohyoid ligament, lesser horns and upper rim of hyoid (derived from the second-arch [Reichert's] cartilage; originate from neural crest)	Muscles of facial expression (orbicularis oculi, orbicularis oris, risorius, platysma, auricularis, fronto-occipitalis, and buccinator), posterior belly of the digastric, stylohyoid, stapedius (originate from cranial somitomere 6)	Facial nerve (VII)
3	Common carotid artery, root of internal carotid	Lower rim and greater horns of hyoid (derived from the third-arch cartilage; originate from neural crest)	Stylopharyngeus (originate from cranial somitomere 7)	Glossopharyngeal nerve (IX)
4	Arch of aorta, right subclavian artery; original sprouts of pulmonary arteries	Laryngeal cartilages (derived from the fourth-arch cartilage; originate from lateral plate mesoderm)	Constrictors of pharynx, cricothyroid, levator veli palatini (originates from occipital somites 2 to 4)	Superior laryngeal branch of vagus nerve (X)
6	Ductus arteriosus; roots of definitive pulmonary arteries	Laryngeal cartilages (derived from the sixth-arch cartilage; originate from lateral plate mesoderm)	Intrinsic muscles of larynx (originate from occipital somites 1 and 2)	Recurrent laryngeal branch of vagus nerve (X)

* See Chapter 8 for a thorough discussion of aortic arch artery development.
† See Chapter 13 for a thorough discussion of the cranial nerves.

ossicles of the middle ear: The maxillary cartilage forms the **incus,** and the mandibular cartilage forms the **malleus.** The maxillary cartilage also gives rise to a small bone called the **alisphenoid** located in the orbital wall, which represents a remnant of the old endochondral upper jaw. A small remnant of Meckel's cartilage can be distinguished in the core of the mandible. The maxilla, zygo-matic, temporal squamosa, and most of the mandible are all membrane bones.

The Temporomandibular Joint is a Mammalian Invention. There is a curious reason why the incus and malleus bones of the mammalian middle ear form from the first-arch cartilage. In all jawed vertebrates except mammals, the jaw joint is

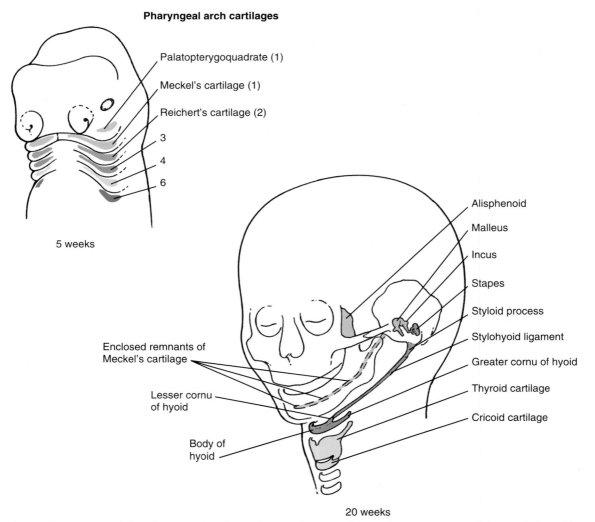

Figure 12–5. Fate of the pharyngeal arch cartilages. These cartilages give rise to a small bone of the orbit, to elements of the jaw skeleton, to the three auditory ossicles, and to the hyoid and laryngeal skeleton.

formed by endochondral bones developing from the maxillary and mandibular cartilages, even though other portions of the jaw may be made of membrane bones. Among the immediate ancestors of mammals, however, a second, novel jaw articulation developed between two membrane bones: the mandible and the temporal squamosa. As this new **temporomandibular joint** became dominant, the bones of the ancient endochondral jaw articulation shifted into the adjacent middle ear and joined with the preexisting stapes to form the unique three-ossicle auditory mechanism of mammals.

There is some dispute as to how the temporomandibular joint develops in the embryo. Some researchers believe that the joint forms within a single mesenchymal condensation that differentiates into temporal and mandibular portions in response to a morphogenetic field. Other workers report that the joint forms from two mesenchymal condensations—a **temporal** or **glenoid blastema** associated with the temporal bone and a **condylar blastema** associated with the mandible—which slowly grow to meet each other. The joint forms between the 7th and 11th weeks, and it is thought that temporomandibular joint malformations may be caused by teratogens acting during this sensitive period.

The Second-Arch Cartilage Has Evolved to Support the Jaw, Tongue, and Larynx; it Also Gives Rise to the Stapes.

After the jaws evolved, the second-arch cartilage was recruited as a bracing element to help support them. This function is still detectable in humans. The human second-arch cartilage, called **Reichert's cartilage,** undergoes endochondral ossification to form the **stapes** of the middle ear, the **styloid process** of the temporal bone, the fibrous **stylohyoid ligament,** and the **lesser horns (cornua)** and upper rim of the **hyoid** bone (see Fig. 12–5). The hyoid bone is stabilized by muscle attachments to the styloid process and mandible and, through its muscular attachments to the larynx and the tongue, serves in both swallowing and vocalization. Reichert's cartilage is formed from neural crest cells derived from the cranial end of the myelencephalon (the caudal subdivision of the rhombencephalon).

The Third Pharyngeal Arch Also Contributes to the Hyoid.

The cartilage of the third arch develops from neural crest cells that originate in the midregion of the myelencephalon. It ossifies endochondrally to form the **greater horns** (cornua) and **lower rim** of the **hyoid** bone (see Fig. 12–5).

The Fourth and Sixth Arches Contribute to the Larynx.

The mesoderm of the fourth and sixth arches together gives rise to the larynx, consisting of the **thyroid, cuneiform, corniculate, arytenoid,** and **cricoid** cartilages (see Fig. 12–5). The results of quail–chick transplantation experiments suggest that these cartilages are formed from lateral plate mesoderm rather than from neural crest. The development of the larynx begins in the fifth week as a pair of mesodermal condensations called the **arytenoid swellings** form in the region of the sixth arch. These condensations begin to chondrify in the early seventh week to form the arytenoid cartilages. The chondrification of the thyroid and cricoid cartilages begins at about the same time, and late in the seventh week the cuneiform and corniculate cartilages begin to form.

The Epiglottis Develops at the Location of the Fourth Arch but May Not Form From Pharyngeal Arch Mesoderm.

The **epiglottal cartilages** do not appear until the fifth month, long after the other pharyngeal arch cartilages have formed. This fact supports the view that the epiglottal cartilages develop from mesenchyme that immigrates into the fourth-arch area long after the arch itself has differentiated. Other workers, however, have reported observing mesodermal condensations within an epiglottal swelling of the fourth arch as early as the sixth week, raising the possibility that the chondrification of this cartilage is merely greatly delayed relative to the other arch cartilages.

THE THIRD AORTIC ARCH ARTERIES GIVE RISE TO VESSELS THAT SUPPLY THE HEAD AND NECK

In human embryos, as in fishes, the arch artery system initially takes the form of a basket-like arrangement of five pairs of arteries that arise from the expansion at the end of the truncus arteriosus called the **aortic sac** and pass through the pharyngeal arches to empty into the paired dorsal aortae (Fig. 12–6). The remodeling of this system to produce the great arteries of the thorax is described in Chapter 8 and Table 12–1.

Arterial blood reaches the head via paired vertebral arteries that form from intersegmental artery anastomoses and via the **common carotid** arteries. The common carotid arteries branch to form the **internal** and **external carotid arteries.** The common carotids and the roots of the internal carotids are derived from the third-arch arteries, whereas the distal portions of the internal carotids are derived from the cranial extensions of the paired dorsal aortae (see also Fig. 8–3). The external carotid arteries sprout de novo from the common carotids. The endothelium of the head vasculature and aortic arch arteries is derived from paraxial mesoderm.

THE PARAXIAL MESODERM OF EACH PHARYNGEAL ARCH GIVES RISE TO A FUNCTIONALLY RELATED MUSCLE GROUP

The musculature of the pharyngeal arches is derived from the paraxial mesoderm of the somitomeres and occipital somites. Although the borders between adjacent somitomeres are difficult to de-

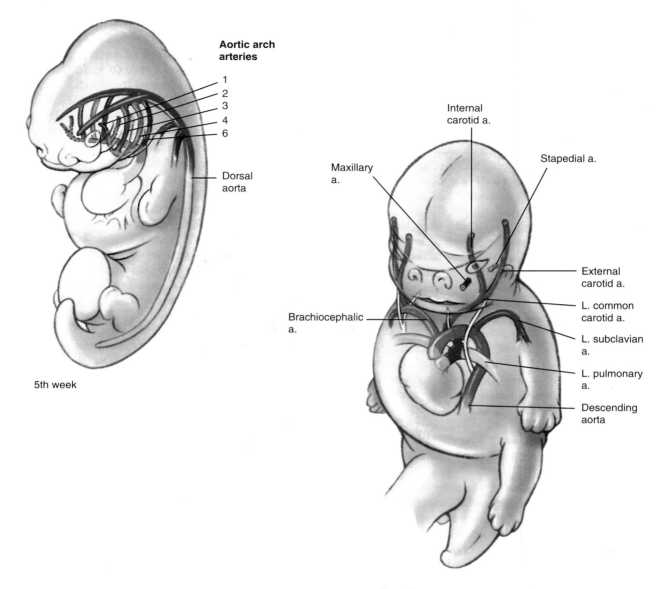

Aortic arch arteries

1
2
3
4
6

Dorsal aorta

5th week

Internal carotid a.

Maxillary a.

Stapedial a.

Brachiocephalic a.

External carotid a.

L. common carotid a.

L. subclavian a.

L. pulmonary a.

Descending aorta

8 weeks

Figure 12–6. Fate of the pharyngeal arch arteries. These arteries are modified to form definitive arteries of the upper thorax, neck, and head (see Ch. 8).

tect, the origin of the premuscle mesoderm in each of the human arches has been fairly reliably pinpointed by studies on experimental animals plus descriptive studies of human embryos. The muscles that form in each arch are innervated by a cranial nerve branch specific to that arch, and each muscle drags its nerve behind it as it migrates. Thus, even though the pharyngeal arch muscles intermingle as

they move to their final locations on the face and neck, the origin of each muscle can be determined from its innervation. Figure 12–7 shows the muscles derived from the pharyngeal arches.

In the first arch, paraxial mesoderm derived from the fourth cranial somitomere gives rise to the **muscles of mastication** (the **temporalis, masseter,** and **medial** and **lateral pterygoids**), as well

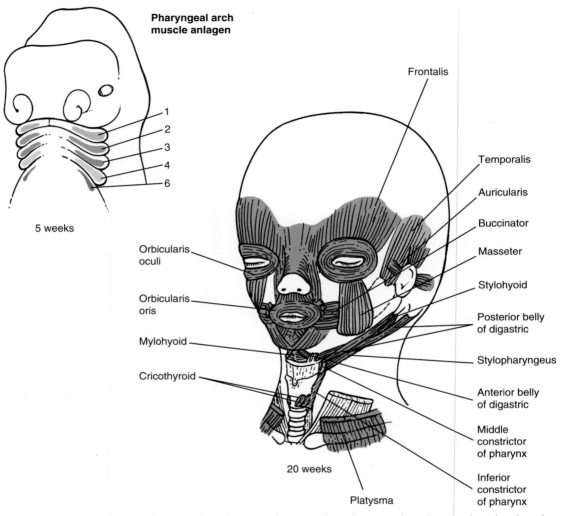

Pharyngeal arch muscle anlagen

1
2
3
4
6

5 weeks

Frontalis

Temporalis

Auricularis

Buccinator

Masseter

Stylohyoid

Posterior belly of digastric

Stylopharyngeus

Anterior belly of digastric

Middle constrictor of pharynx

Inferior constrictor of pharynx

Orbicularis oculi

Orbicularis oris

Mylohyoid

Cricothyroid

20 weeks

Platysma

Figure 12–7. Fate of the pharyngeal arch musculature. The pharyngeal arch muscles develop from paraxial mesoderm derived mainly from cranial somitomeres and occipital somites. The myoblasts of the sixth arch become the intrinsic laryngeal muscles (not shown).

as to the **myelohyoid, anterior belly of the digastric, tensor tympani,** and **tensor veli palatini** muscles (see Fig. 12–7).

In the second arch, paraxial mesoderm from the sixth cranial somitomere gives rise to the **muscles of facial expression,** including the **orbicularis oculi, orbicularis oris, risorius, platysma, auricularis, fronto-occipitalis,** and **buccinator** muscles, as well as to the **posterior belly of the digastric,** the **stylohyoid,** and the **stapedius** muscles. The muscle anlagen of these first and second

arches intermingle in their final locations on the head.

In the third arch, paraxial mesoderm from the seventh somitomere gives rise to a single muscle: the long, slender **stylopharyngeus,** which originates on the styloid process and inserts into the wall of the pharynx. This muscle raises the pharynx during vocalization and swallowing.

Muscles originating in the fourth arch are the **superior, middle,** and **inferior constrictors** of the pharynx, the **cricothyroid,** and the **levator veli**

palatini, which function in vocalization and deglutition. The mesoderm giving rise to these muscles is derived from the second to fourth occipital somites and the first cervical somite.

Paraxial mesoderm derived from the first and second occipital somites becomes associated with the sixth pharyngeal arch to form **intrinsic musculature of the larynx** (see Figs. 12–5 and 12–7). The lateral **cricoarytenoids, thyroarytenoids,** and **vocalis** muscles are thus primarily devoted to the function of vocalization.

A CRANIAL NERVE INNERVATES EACH PHARYNGEAL ARCH

Four cranial nerves arising in the hindbrain supply branches to the pharyngeal arches and their derivatives (Fig. 12–8). (See Ch. 13 for a complete discussion of the 12 cranial nerves.) The maxillary and mandibular swellings of the first arch are innervated, respectively, by the **maxillary** and **mandibular branches** of the **trigeminal** nerve (cranial nerve V). The second arch is innervated by the **facial** nerve (nerve VII); the third arch, by the **glossopharyngeal** nerve (nerve IX); and the fourth and sixth arches, respectively, by the **superior laryngeal** and **recurrent laryngeal** branches of the **vagus** nerve (nerve X).

As discussed in Chapter 13, the various cranial nerves carry different combinations of somatic motor, autonomic, and sensory fibers. In all cases, however, the somatic motor neurons develop in the basal (ventral) columns of the brain, whereas the sensory neurons are located in cranial nerve ganglia. Unlike the sensory neurons of the dorsal ganglia of the spinal cord, which all arise from neural crest cells, some cranial nerve sensory neurons arise from special areas of ectoderm known as **neurogenic ectodermal placodes.** These placodes are discussed in detail in Chapter 13. The remaining cranial nerve sensory cells arise from rhombencephalic neural crest.

The sensory innervation of the ventral side of the face is supplied by the ophthalmic, maxillary, and mandibular divisions of the trigeminal nerve, as would be expected from the fact that the dermis in this region develops from neural crest cells that migrate into the first pharyngeal arch and frontonasal prominence of the face (see later). The sensory innervation of the dorsal side of the head and neck is supplied by the second and third cervical spinal nerves. The sensory innervation to the endodermal derivatives of the pharynx is supplied by cranial nerves V, VII, IX, and X, as described in Figure 12–8.

THE FACE DEVELOPS FROM FIVE FACIAL SWELLINGS

The basic morphology of the face is created between the 4th and 10th weeks by the development and fusion of five prominences: an unpaired **frontonasal process** plus the two **maxillary swellings** and two **mandibular swellings** of the first pharyngeal arches (Fig. 12–9). The spectrum of congenital facial defects known as **facial clefts**—including cleft lip and cleft palate—result from the failure of some of these facial processes to fuse correctly. These relatively common congenital anomalies are discussed in the Clinical Applications section of this chapter.

All five facial swellings appear by the end of the fourth week. During the fifth week, the paired maxillary swellings enlarge and grow ventrally and medially. Simultaneously, a pair of ectodermal thickenings called the **nasal placodes (nasal discs, nasal plates)** appear on the frontonasal process and begin to enlarge (Fig. 12–10; see also Fig. 12–9). In the sixth week, the ectoderm at the center of each nasal placode invaginates to form an oval **nasal pit,** thus dividing the raised rim of the placode into **lateral** and **medial nasal processes** (see Fig. 12–10A). The groove between the lateral nasal process and the adjacent maxillary swelling is called the **nasolacrimal groove.** During the seventh week, the ectoderm at the floor of this groove invaginates into the underlying mesenchyme to form a tube called the **nasolacrimal duct.** This duct is invested by bone during the ossification of the maxilla. After birth, it functions to drain excess tears from the conjunctiva of the eye into the nasal cavity.

During the sixth week, the medial nasal processes migrate toward each other and fuse to form the primordium of the bridge and septum of the nose (see Fig. 12–10A, B). By the end of the sev-

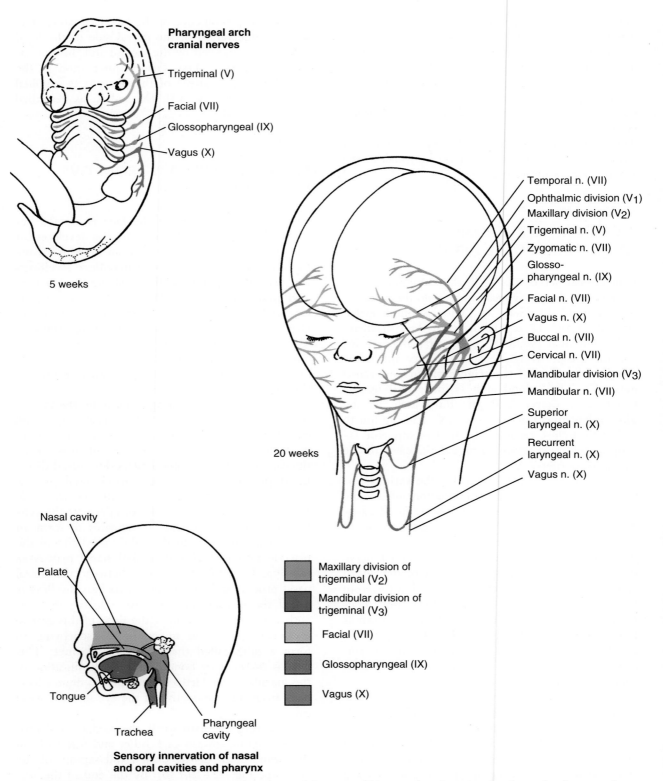

Pharyngeal arch cranial nerves

Trigeminal (V)

Facial (VII)

Glossopharyngeal (IX)

Vagus (X)

5 weeks

Temporal n. (VII)
Ophthalmic division (V$_1$)
Maxillary division (V$_2$)
Trigeminal n. (V)
Zygomatic n. (VII)
Glosso-pharyngeal n. (IX)
Facial n. (VII)
Vagus n. (X)
Buccal n. (VII)
Cervical n. (VII)
Mandibular division (V$_3$)
Mandibular n. (VII)
Superior laryngeal n. (X)
Recurrent laryngeal n. (X)
Vagus n. (X)

20 weeks

Nasal cavity

Palate

Tongue

Trachea

Pharyngeal cavity

Maxillary division of trigeminal (V$_2$)

Mandibular division of trigeminal (V$_3$)

Facial (VII)

Glossopharyngeal (IX)

Vagus (X)

Sensory innervation of nasal and oral cavities and pharynx

Figure 12–8. Fate of the pharyngeal arch cranial nerves. The muscles that develop in each pharyngeal arch are served by the cranial nerve that originally innervates that arch.

A 4th week   **B** 4th week   **C** 5th week

Frontonasal prominence
Nasal placode
Disintegrating buccopharyngeal membrane
Maxillary swelling
Mandibular swelling
2nd pharyngeal arch

Figure 12–9. Origin of the human face and mouth. The face develops from five primordia that appear in the fourth week: the frontonasal prominence, the two maxillary swellings, and the two mandibular swellings. The buccopharyngeal membrane breaks down to form the opening to the oral cavity. (*A, B,* Photos courtesy of Dr. Arnold Tamarin.)

enth week, the inferior tips of the medial nasal processes expand laterally and inferiorly and fuse to form the **intermaxillary process** (see Fig. 12–10*C, D*). The tips of the maxillary swellings grow to meet the intermaxillary process and fuse with it. On the upper lip, the intermaxillary process gives rise to the **philtrum** (see Fig. 12–10*E*).

Although the two mandibular swellings appear to be separated by a fissure midventrally (see Fig. 12–9*A*), they actually form in continuity with each other like the rest of the pharyngeal arches. The transient intermandibular depression is filled in during the fourth and fifth weeks by proliferation of mesenchyme, creating the primordium of the lower lip (see Fig. 12–9*C*). Meanwhile, on day 24, the buccopharyngeal membrane ruptures to form a broad, slitlike embryonic mouth (see Fig. 12–9*C*). The mouth is reduced to its final width during the second month as the fusion of the lateral portions of the maxillary and mandibular swellings creates the cheeks (see Fig. 12–10*D, E*).

The Nasal Passages Are Formed by the Deepening of the Nasal Pits

Figure 12–11 illustrates the process by which the nasal pits give rise to the nasal passages. At the end of the sixth week, the deepening nasal pits

fuse to form a single, enlarged, ectodermal nasal sac lying superoposterior to the intermaxillary process. From the end of the sixth week to the beginning of the seventh week, the floor and posterior wall of the nasal sac proliferate to form a thickened, platelike fin, or keel, of ectoderm separating the nasal sac from the oral cavity. This structure is called the **nasal fin.** Vacuoles develop in the nasal fin and fuse with the nasal sac, thus enlarging the sac and thinning the fin to a thin membrane called the **oronasal membrane,** which separates the sac from the oral cavity. This membrane ruptures during the seventh week to form an opening called the **primitive choana.** The floor of the nasal cavity at this stage is formed by a posterior extension of the intermaxillary process called the **primary palate.**

The Secondary Palate Enlarges the Nasal Cavity, and the Nasal Septum Divides It Into Two Nasal Passages

During the eighth and ninth weeks, the medial walls of the maxillary processes produce a pair of thin medial extensions called the **palatine shelves** (Fig. 12–12*A, B*). At first, these shelves grow downward parallel to the lateral surfaces of the tongue. At the end of the ninth week, however,

Figure 12–10. Development of the face. *A, B,* In the sixth week, the nasal placodes of the frontonasal prominence invaginate to form the nasal pits and the lateral and medial nasal processes. *C, D,* In the seventh week, the medial nasal processes fuse at the midline to form the intermaxillary process. *E,* By the 10th week, the intermaxillary process forms the philtrum of the upper lip. The dotted lines in *B, D,* and *E* represent regions of fusion of facial primordia. (*A, C,* Photos courtesy of Dr. Arnold Tamarin.)

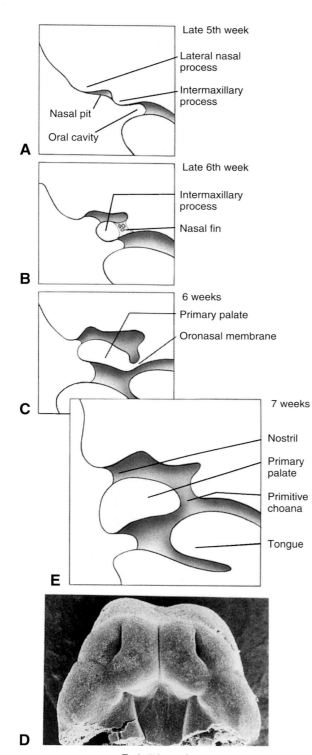

A

Late 5th week

Lateral nasal process

Intermaxillary process

Nasal pit

Oral cavity

B

Late 6th week

Intermaxillary process

Nasal fin

C

6 weeks

Primary palate

Oronasal membrane

E

7 weeks

Nostril

Primary palate

Primitive choana

Tongue

D

Early 7th week

they rotate rapidly upward into a horizontal position and then fuse with each other and with the primary palate to form the **secondary palate** (see Fig. 12–12C, D). The rotation of the palatine shelves has been ascribed to the rapid synthesis and hydration of hyaluronic acid within the extracellular matrix of the shelves, and the alignment of the elevated shelves in a horizontal plane may be determined by the orientation of collagen and mesenchymal cells. Fusion occurs first at the ventral end of the palatine shelves and proceeds dorsally.

Mesenchymal condensations in the ventral portion of the secondary palate undergo endochondral ossification to form the bony **hard palate.** In the dorsal portion of the secondary palate, myogenic mesenchyme condenses to give rise to the musculature of the soft palate.

While the secondary palate is forming, ectoderm and mesoderm of the frontonasal process and the medial nasal processes proliferate to form a midline **nasal septum** that grows down from the roof of the nasal cavity to fuse with the upper surface of the primary and secondary palates along the midline (see Fig. 12–12). The nasal cavity is now divided into two **nasal passages,** which open into the pharynx behind the secondary palate through an opening called the **definitive choana.**

The Postnatal Development of the Air Sinuses Significantly Alters the Relative Sizes of the Face and Cranial Vault

At birth, the ratio of the volume of the facial skeleton to the volume of the cranial vault is about 1:7. During infancy and childhood, this ratio steadily

Figure 12–11. Formation of the nasal cavity and primitive choana. *A, B,* The nasal pits invaginate to form a single nasal cavity separated from the oral cavity by a thick partition called the nasal fin. *C–E,* The nasal fin thins to form the oronasal membrane, which breaks down completely to form the primitive choana. The posterior extension of the intermaxillary process forms the primary palate. (*D,* Photo courtesy of Dr. Arnold Tamarin.)

A 7th week

B 7th week

C 8th week

D 10th week

Figure 12–12. Formation of the secondary palate and nasal septum. The secondary palate forms from palatine shelves that grow medially from the maxillary swellings. During the same period, growth of the nasal septum separates the left and right nasal passages. The palatine shelves at first grow inferiorly on either side of the tongue (*A, B*) but then rapidly rotate upward to meet in the midline (*C*), where they fuse with each other and with the inferior edge of the nasal septum (*D*). (*B*, Photo courtesy of Dr. Arnold Tamarin.)

decreases, mainly as a result of the development of teeth (see Ch. 14) and the growth of the four pairs of **paranasal sinuses: the maxillary, ethmoid, sphenoid,** and **frontal sinuses.** These sinuses develop from invaginations of the nasal cavity that extend into the bones. Two of the sinuses appear during fetal life and the other two after birth.

The *maxillary sinuses* appear during the third fetal month as invaginations of the nasal sac that slowly expand within the maxillary bones. The resulting cavities are small at birth but expand throughout childhood.

The *ethmoid sinuses* appear during the fifth fetal month as invaginations of the middle meatus of the nasal passages (the space underlying the middle nasal concha) and grow into the ethmoid bone. These sinuses do not complete their growth until puberty.

The *sphenoid sinuses* actually represent extensions of the ethmoid sinuses into the sphenoid bones. These extensions first appear in the fifth postnatal month and continue to enlarge throughout infancy and childhood.

The *frontal sinuses* do not appear until the fifth or sixth postnatal year and expand throughout adolescence. Each frontal sinus actually consists of two independent spaces that develop from different sources. One forms by the expansion of the ethmoid sinus into the frontal bone, and the other develops from an independent invagination of the middle meatus of the nasal passage. Because these cavities never coalesce, they drain independently.

THE FIRST PHARYNGEAL CLEFT BECOMES THE EXTERNAL ACOUSTIC MEATUS, AND THE REMAINING THREE CLEFTS NORMALLY DISAPPEAR

As described earlier, the pharyngeal arches are separated by pharyngeal clefts externally and by pharyngeal pouches internally (Fig. 12–13; see also Fig. 12–4). The first pharyngeal cleft and pouch, located between the first and second pharyngeal arches, participate in the formation of the ear: the first cleft becomes the **external acoustic meatus,** and the first pouch expands to form a cavity called the **tubotympanic recess,** which differentiates to become the **tympanic cavity** of the middle ear and the **auditory (eustachian) tube** (see Fig. 12–13). The development of these structures is covered in

more detail in the section Development of the Ears at the end of this chapter.

The remaining three pharyngeal clefts are normally obliterated during development. During the fourth and fifth weeks, the rapidly expanding second pharyngeal arch overgrows these clefts and fuses caudally with the cardiac eminence enclosing the clefts in a transient, ectoderm-lined **lateral cervical sinus** (see Fig. 12–13B, C). This space normally disappears rapidly and completely.

The First Pharyngeal Cleft and the Lateral Cervical Sinus May Form Anomalous Cysts or Fistulae

Infrequently, reduplication of the first pharyngeal cleft results in the formation of an ectoderm-lined **first-cleft sinus** or **cervical aural fistula** located in the tissues inferior or ventral to the external acoustic meatus (Fig. 12–14C). A fully enclosed first-cleft sinus may become apparent as a swelling just inferior or ventral to the auricle or external ear. Alternatively, it may drain to the exterior through a cervical aural fistula, which usually opens into the external auditory canal. Depending

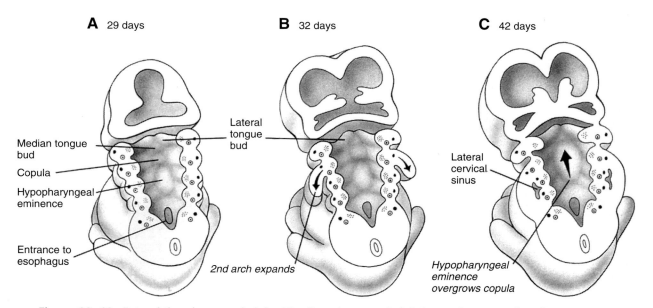

A 29 days   **B** 32 days   **C** 42 days

Median tongue bud

Copula

Hypopharyngeal eminence

Entrance to esophagus

Lateral tongue bud

2nd arch expands

Lateral cervical sinus

Hypopharyngeal eminence overgrows copula

Figure 12–13. Fate of the pharyngeal clefts. The first pharyngeal cleft forms the external auditory meatus. The second pharyngeal arch expands and fuses with the cardiac eminence to cover the remaining pharyngeal clefts, which form the transient lateral cervical sinus.

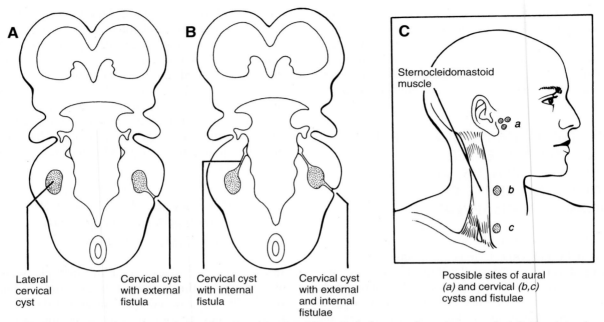

Possible sites of aural (a) and cervical (b,c) cysts and fistulae

Figure 12–14. Abnormal cysts produced by the lateral cervical sinus or first pharyngeal cleft The lateral cervical sinus occasionally persists in the form of an abnormal lateral cervical cyst. A, B, Such cysts may be isolated or may connect to the skin of the neck by an external cervical fistula, or to the pharynx by an internal fistula, or both. C, Lateral cervical cysts are located just medial to the anterior border of the sternocleidomastoid muscle. Anomalous derivatives of the first pharyngeal cleft known as aural cysts may form anterior to the ear.

on its position, a first-cleft cyst or fistula may threaten the facial nerve if it becomes infected and may require resection.

The lateral cervical sinus occasionally persists on one or both sides in the form of a **cervical cyst** located just ventral to the ventral border of the sternocleidomastoid muscle (see Fig. 12–14). A completely enclosed cyst may expand to form a palpable lump as its epithelial lining desquamates or if it becomes infected. Occasionally, the cyst communicates either with the skin via an **external cervical fistula** or with the pharynx via an **internal cervical fistula.** Internal cervical fistulae most commonly open into the embryonic derivative of the second pouch, the palatine tonsil. Less often, they communicate with derivatives of the third pouch (see later). Rarely, a cervical cyst has both internal and external fistulae. Cysts of this type may be diagnosed by the drainage of mucus through the small opening of the external fistula on the neck just medial to the ventral border of the sternocleidomastoid. Cervical cysts are usually

of minor clinical importance but may require resection if they become seriously infected.

THE TONGUE AND THYROID DEVELOP FROM PHARYNGEAL ARCH TISSUE

The Tongue Develops From Pharyngeal Arches 1, 3, and 4 and From Occipital Somite Mesoderm

At the end of the fourth week, the floor of the pharynx consists of the five pharyngeal arches and the intervening pharyngeal pouches. The development of the tongue begins late in the fourth week when the first arch forms a median swelling called the **median tongue bud** or **tuberculum impar** (Fig. 12–15*A*). An additional pair of lateral swellings, the **distal tongue buds,** or **lateral lingual swellings,** develop on the first arch early in the

Figure 12–15. Development of the tongue mucosa from the endoderm of the pharyngeal floor. The mucosa of the anterior two thirds of the tongue develops primarily from the distal tongue buds (lateral lingual swellings) of the first pharyngeal arch, whereas the mucosal lining of the posterior one third of the tongue is formed by overgrowth of the copula of the second arch by the hypopharyngeal eminence of the third and fourth arches. (Photo courtesy of Dr. Arnold Tamarin.)

fifth week and rapidly expand to overgrow the median tongue bud. These swellings continue to grow throughout embryonic and fetal life and form the anterior two thirds of the tongue (see Fig. 12–15B–D).

Late in the fourth week, the second arch develops a midline swelling called the **copula** (see Fig. 12–15A). This swelling is rapidly overgrown during the fifth and sixth weeks by a midline swelling of the third and fourth arches called the **hypopharyngeal eminence,** which gives rise to the posterior one third of the tongue. The hypopharyngeal eminence expands mainly by the growth of third-arch endoderm, whereas the fourth arch contributes only a small region on the most posterior aspect of the tongue (see Fig. 12–15C, D). Thus, the bulk of the tongue mucosa is formed by the first and third arches. Table 12–2 summarizes the developmental origins of the parts of the tongue.

The surface features of the definitive tongue reflect its embryonic origins. The boundary between the first-arch and third-arch contributions—roughly, the boundary between the anterior two thirds and posterior one third of the tongue—is marked by a transverse groove called the **terminal sulcus** (see Fig. 12–15D). The line of fusion between the right and left distal tongue buds is marked by a midline groove, the **median sulcus,** on the anterior two thirds of the tongue. A depression called the **foramen cecum** is visible where the median sulcus intersects the terminal sulcus. As discussed later, this depression is the site of origin of the thyroid gland.

All the muscles of the tongue except the palatoglossus are formed by mesoderm derived from the myotomes of the occipital somites, and the proliferation of this mesoderm is responsible for most of the growth of the tongue primordia. The innervation of the tongue muscles is consonant with their origin: all the muscles except the palatoglossus are innervated by the **hypoglossal nerve** (cranial nerve XII), which is the cranial nerve asso-

Table 12–2

Development of the Tongue From Pharyngeal Arches 1 Through 4 and the Occipital Somites

EMBRYONIC PRECURSOR	INTERMEDIATE STRUCTURE	ADULT STRUCTURE	INNERVATION
Pharyngeal arch 1	Median tongue bud	Overgrown by lateral lingual swellings	Lingual branch (sensory) of mandibular division of trigeminal nerve (V)
	Lateral lingual swellings	Mucosa of anterior two thirds of tongue	Chorda tympani from facial nerve (VII; innervating arch 2) (innervates all taste buds except vallate papillae)
Pharyngeal arch 2	Copula	Overgrown by other structures	
Pharyngeal arch 3	Large, ventral part of hypopharyngeal eminence	Mucosa of most of posterior one third of tongue	Sensory branch of glossopharyngeal nerve (IX) (also supplies vallate papillae)
Pharyngeal arch 4	Small, dorsal part of hypopharyngeal eminence	Mucosa of small, dorsal region of tongue	Sensory fibers of superior laryngeal branch of vagus nerve (X)
Occipital somites	Myoblasts	Intrinsic muscles of tongue	Hypoglossal nerve (XII)
		Palatoglossus muscle	Pharyngeal plexus of vagus nerve (X)

ciated with the occipital somites, whereas the palatoglossus is innervated by the **pharyngeal plexus of the vagus** (nerve X).

The mucosal covering of the tongue is derived from pharyngeal arch endoderm and is innervated by sensory branches of the corresponding four cranial nerves (see Table 12–2). The tongue mucosa is thus innervated by different nerves from those of the tongue musculature. The general sensory receptors on the anterior two thirds of the tongue are supplied by a branch of the mandibular nerve (cranial nerve V_3) called the **lingual nerve.** The taste buds of the anterior two thirds of the tongue are supplied by a special branch of the facial nerve (cranial nerve VII) called the **chorda tympani.** In contrast, the vallate papillae (a row of large taste buds flanking the terminal sulcus) and the general sensory endings over most of the posterior one third of the tongue are supplied by the **glossopharyngeal nerve.** The small area on the most posterior aspect of the tongue that is derived from the fourth pharyngeal arch receives sensory innervation from the **superior laryngeal** branch of the vagus nerve.

The Thyroid Gland Develops From an Invagination of the Tongue Endoderm and Migrates to a Ventrocaudal Location

Figure 12–16 illustrates the embryogenesis of the thyroid gland. The gland primordium first appears in the late fourth week as a small, solid mass of endoderm proliferating at the apex of the foramen cecum on the developing tongue. The thyroid primordium descends through the tissues of the neck at the end of a slender **thyroglossal duct.** The thyroglossal duct breaks down by the end of the fifth week, and the isolated thyroid, now consisting of lateral lobes connected by a well-defined isthmus, continues to descend, reaching its final position just inferior to the cricoid cartilage by the seventh week. Studies on the ability of the embryonic thyroid to incorporate iodine into thyroid hormones and to secrete these hormones into the circulation show that this gland begins to function as early as the 10th to the 12th week in human embryos.

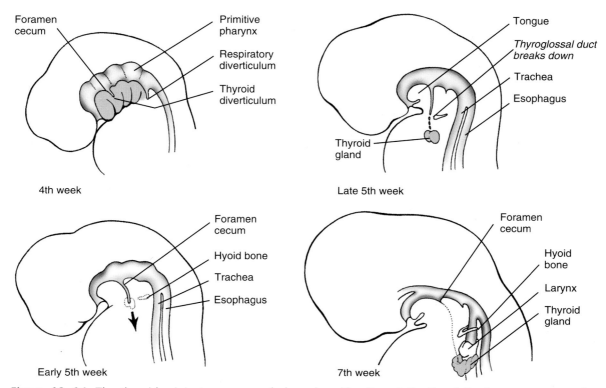

Figure 12–16. The thyroid originates as an endodermal proliferation at the tip of the foramen cecum of the developing tongue and migrates inferiorly to its final site anterior and inferior to the larynx. Until the fifth week, the thyroid remains connected to the foramen cecum by the thyroglossal duct. The gland reaches its final site in the seventh week.

Normally, the only remnant of the thyroglossal duct is the foramen cecum itself. Occasionally, however, a portion of the duct persists either as an enclosed **thyroglossal cyst** or as a **thyroglossal sinus** communicating with the surface of the neck. Rarely, a fragment of the thyroid becomes detached during the descent of the gland and forms a patch of ectopic thyroid tissue, which may be located anywhere along the route of descent.

ALL THE PHARYNGEAL POUCHES GIVE RISE TO IMPORTANT STRUCTURES

Figure 12–17 summarizes the several structures that arise from the pharyngeal pouches. The fate of the first pharyngeal pouch, which differentiates into the tympanic cavity and auditory tube, is discussed in detail in the section Development of the Ear. The genesis of the structures arising from the remaining pharyngeal pouches is illustrated in Figures 12–17 and 12–18.

The Second Pharyngeal Pouch Gives Rise to the Palatine Tonsils

The palatine tonsils arise from the endoderm lining the second pharyngeal pouch (located between the second and third arches) and from the mesoderm of the second pharyngeal membrane and adjacent regions of the first and second arches. Development of these tonsils begins early in the third

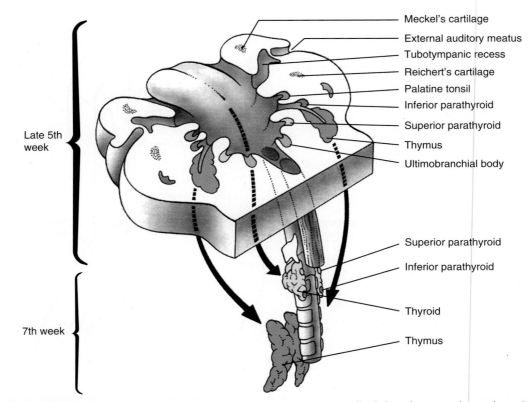

Late 5th
week

7th week

Meckel's cartilage
External auditory meatus
Tubotympanic recess
Reichert's cartilage
Palatine tonsil
Inferior parathyroid
Superior parathyroid
Thymus
Ultimobranchial body

Superior parathyroid
Inferior parathyroid

Thyroid

Thymus

Figure 12–17. Development of the pharyngeal pouch derivatives. All of the pharyngeal pouches give rise to adult structures. These are the tubotympanic recess (pouch 1), the palatine tonsils (pouch 2), the inferior parathyroid glands and thymus (pouch 3), the superior parathyroid glands (pouch 4), and the ultimobranchial (telopharyngeal) body (inferior part of pouch 4 or a hypothetical pouch 5). The parathyroids, thymus primordia, and ultimobranchial bodies separate from the lining of the pharynx and migrate to their definitive locations within the neck and thorax.

month as the epithelium of the second pouch proliferates to form solid endodermal buds, or ledges, growing into the underlying mesoderm, which will give rise to the tonsillar stroma. The central cells of the buds later die and slough, converting the solid buds into hollow **tonsillar crypts,** which are rapidly infiltrated by lymphoid tissue. The definitive lymph follicles of the tonsil do not form until the last three months of prenatal life, however.

Similar lymphatic tonsils, called **pharyngeal tonsils,** develop in association with mucous glands of the pharynx. The major pharyngeal tonsils are the **adenoids,** the **tubal tonsils** (associated with the auditory tubes), and the **lingual tonsils** (associated with the posterior regions of the tongue). Mi-

nor intervening patches of lymphoid tissue also form.

The Thymus Arises From the Third Pharyngeal Pouch and Migrates to a Position Just Dorsal to the Sternum

The two thymic primordia arise at the end of the fourth week in the form of endodermal proliferations at the end of ventral elongations of the third pharyngeal pouches (see Figs. 12–17 and 12–18). These endodermal proliferations form hollow

Parathyroid III (inferior)

Parathyroid IV (superior)

Ultimobranchial body

Thymus

Thyroid

Mid-6th week

6 weeks

7 weeks

Definitive condition

Figure 12–18. Migration of pharyngeal pouch derivatives. The parathyroid glands and the ultimobranchial bodies migrate inferiorly to become embedded in the posterior wall of the thyroid gland. The two parathyroids exchange position as they migrate: parathyroid III becomes the inferior parathyroid, whereas parathyroid IV becomes the superior parathyroid.

tubes that invade the underlying mesoderm and later transform into solid, branching cords. These cords are the primordia of the polyhedral **thymic lobules.** The underlying mesoderm is derived from neural crest (see Experimental Principles section).

Between the fourth and seventh weeks, the thymus glands lose their connections with the pharynx and migrate to their definitive location inferior and ventral to the developing thyroid and just dorsal to the sternum. There they fuse to form a single, bilobate thymus gland. By 12 weeks, each thymic lobule is 0.5 to 2 mm in diameter and has a well-defined cortex and medulla. The whorl-like **Hassall's corpuscles** within the medulla apparently arise from the ectodermal cells of the third pharyngeal cleft, whereas the loosely organized **epithelial reticulum** of the thymus is of endodermal origin. The lobules are supported by mesenchymal septa. Shortly after the thymus forms, it is infiltrated by lymphocytes derived from stem cells in the yolk sac, omentum, and liver. These lymphocytes presumably home on the thymus by a chemotactic mechanism.

The thymus is highly active during the perinatal period and continues to grow throughout childhood, reaching its maximum size at puberty. After puberty, the gland involutes rapidly and is represented only by insignificant fatty vestiges in the adult.

The Parathyroids Arise From Pharyngeal Pouches 3 and 4

The rudiments of the **inferior parathyroid glands (parathyroids III)** form in the dorsal portion of the third pouch early in the fifth week (see Figs. 12–17 and 12–18). They detach from the pharyngeal wall and migrate inferiorly and medially, coming to rest by the seventh week on the dorsal side of the inferior end of the thyroid lobes.

Early in the fifth week, the rudiments of the **superior parathyroid glands (parathyroids IV)** form in the fourth pouch. They detach from the pharynx and migrate inferiorly and medially, coming to rest by the seventh week in a position slightly superior to the inferior parathyroid glands. Thus, the superior parathyroids arise more inferiorly on the pharynx than the inferior parathyroids, and the two glands switch position during their descent; their names reflect their final relative positions.

The Ultimobranchial (Telopharyngeal) Bodies Arise From a Controversial Fifth Pharyngeal Pouch

During the fifth week, a minor invagination appears just caudal to the fourth pharyngeal pouch (see Fig. 12–17). This invagination has been described by many embryologists as a **fifth pharyngeal pouch.** Almost immediately after they appear, these invaginations become populated by epithelial cells, which form the rudiments of the paired **ultimobranchial bodies** (see Fig. 12–18). These rudiments immediately detach from the pharyngeal wall and migrate medially and caudally to implant in the dorsal wall of the thyroid gland, where they differentiate into the calcitonin-producing **C cells (parafollicular cells)** of the thyroid.

The origin of the epithelial cells that form the ultimobranchial bodies are the ectomesenchymal cells of neural crest origin. However, the fourth epibranchial placode has also been implicated in the formation of the inferior and superior parathyroid glands (see Ch. 13 for a discussion of the epibranchial placodes).

THE SALIVARY GLANDS ARISE FROM ECTODERM AND ENDODERM IN THE PHARYNGEAL REGION

Three pairs of salivary glands develop in humans: the **parotid, submandibular,** and **sublingual** glands. The parotid gland develops from a groove-like invagination of ectoderm that forms in the crease between the maxillary and mandibular swellings. This groove differentiates into a tubular duct that sinks into the underlying mesenchyme but maintains a ventral opening at the angle of the primitive mouth. As the cheek portions of the maxillary and mandibular swellings fuse, this opening is transferred to the inner surface of the cheek. The blind dorsal end of the tube differentiates to form the parotid gland, whereas the stem of the tube becomes the parotid duct. Similar invaginations of the endoderm in the floor of the oral cavity and in the paralingual sulci on either side of the tongue give rise to the submandibular and sublingual salivary glands, respectively.

Part Two

Development of the Eyes

Summary

The eyes first appear early in the fourth week in the form of a pair of lateral grooves, the **optic sulci,** which evaginate from the forebrain neural folds and grow toward the surface ectoderm to form the **optic vesicles.** As soon as the expanded tip of the optic vesicle reaches the surface ectoderm, its distal face (called the **retinal disc**) invaginates, transforming the optic vesicle into a goblet-shaped **optic cup** that is attached to the forebrain by a narrower, hollow **optic stalk.** The adjacent surface ectoderm simultaneously thickens to form a **lens placode,** which invaginates and pinches off to become a hollow **lens vesicle** that sits in the optic cup.

The lens vesicle gives rise to the solid **lens** of the eye. Posterior cells of the lens vesicle form long slender anteroposteriorly oriented **primary lens fibers.** Anterior cells of the lens give rise to a simple epithelium covering the face of the lens. This epithelium gives rise to the **secondary lens fibers,** which make up most of the bulk of the mature lens. Blood is supplied to the developing lens and retina by a terminal branch of the ophthalmic artery, called the **hyaloid artery,** which gains access to the interior of the optic globe via a groove called the **choroidal fissure** on the ventral surface of the optic stalk. The portion of the artery that traverses the vitreous body to reach the lens degenerates during fetal life as the lens matures; the remainder of the artery becomes the **central artery of the retina.**

The inner wall of the optic cup (the former optic disc) gives rise to the **neural retina,** whereas the outer wall gives rise to the thin, melanin-containing **pigment retina.** Although the **intraretinal space** separating these two layers is obliterated as the retina develops, the two layers never fuse firmly. The differentiation of the neural retina takes place between the sixth week and the eighth month. Waves of cells are produced by an outer **proliferative layer** next to the intraretinal space and migrate inward to form the cell layers of the mature retina. Axons from the neural retina grow through the optic stalk to the brain, converting the optic stalk to the optic nerve.

As the optic vesicle forms, it is enveloped by a sheath of mesenchyme that is derived in part from neural crest. This sheath differentiates to form the two coverings of the optic globe: the thin inner **choroid** and the fibrous outer **sclera.** This mesenchyme also grows to cover the anterior surface of the developing eye, including the lens. The mesenchyme overlying the developing lens splits into two layers, which enclose a new space called the **anterior chamber.** The external wall of the anterior chamber is continuous with the sclera of the optic globe, and the internal wall is continuous with the choroid of the optic globe. The external wall of the anterior chamber gives rise to the inner layers of the cornea, whereas the outer layer of the cornea is derived from the overlying surface ectoderm. The inner wall of the anterior chamber, overlying the

Development of the Optic Cup, Lens, Cornea, Iris, and Ciliary Body

Formation of the Neural and Pigment Retina and the Optic Nerve

Development of the Extrinsic Ocular Muscles and Eyelids

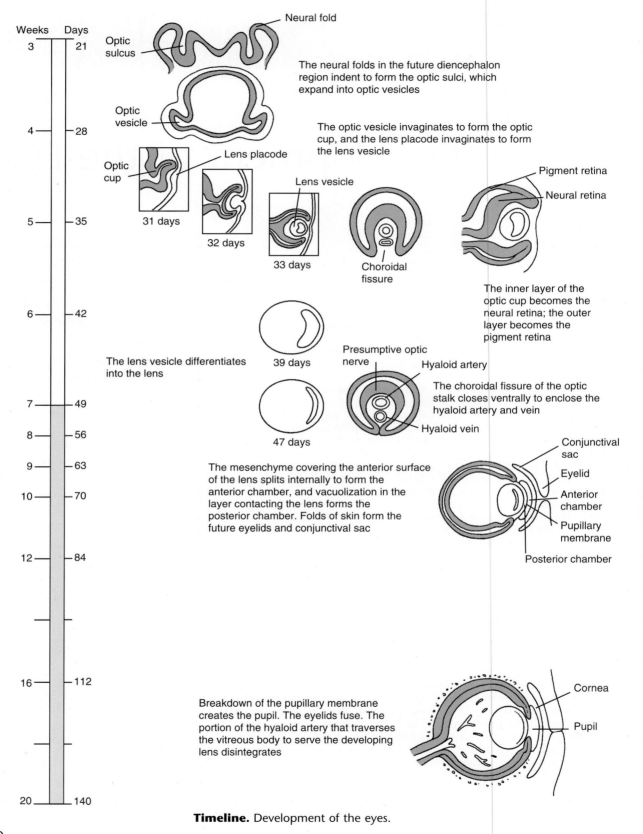

Weeks | **Days**

3 — 21

Optic sulcus

Neural fold

4 — 28

The neural folds in the future diencephalon region indent to form the optic sulci, which expand into optic vesicles

Optic vesicle

The optic vesicle invaginates to form the optic cup, and the lens placode invaginates to form the lens vesicle

Optic cup

Lens placode

31 days

Lens vesicle

32 days

5 — 35

Pigment retina

Neural retina

33 days

Choroidal fissure

The inner layer of the optic cup becomes the neural retina; the outer layer becomes the pigment retina

6 — 42

The lens vesicle differentiates into the lens

39 days

Presumptive optic nerve

Hyaloid artery

The choroidal fissure of the optic stalk closes ventrally to enclose the hyaloid artery and vein

47 days

Hyaloid vein

7 — 49

8 — 56

9 — 63

10 — 70

The mesenchyme covering the anterior surface of the lens splits internally to form the anterior chamber, and vacuolization in the layer contacting the lens forms the posterior chamber. Folds of skin form the future eyelids and conjunctival sac

Conjunctival sac

Eyelid

Anterior chamber

Pupillary membrane

Posterior chamber

12 — 84

16 — 112

Breakdown of the pupillary membrane creates the pupil. The eyelids fuse. The portion of the hyaloid artery that traverses the vitreous body to serve the developing lens disintegrates

Cornea

Pupil

20 — 140

Timeline. Development of the eyes.

lens, is called the **pupillary membrane.** The deep layers of this wall undergo vacuolization to create a new space, the **posterior chamber,** between the lens and the thin remaining pupillary membrane. Early in fetal life, the pupillary membrane breaks down completely to form the **pupil.**

The rim of the optic cup, along with the overlying choroid, differentiates to form the **iris** and the **ciliary body.**

Mesoderm adjacent to the optic globe differenti-ates in the fifth and sixth weeks to form the extrinsic ocular muscles. The origin of this mesoderm is unclear: it is derived either from paraxial mesoderm or from the prechordal plate. The connective tissue components of the extrinsic ocular muscles are derived from neural crest.

The **eyelids** arise as folds of surface ectoderm. The two eyelids are fused from the eighth week to about the fifth month.

THE EYES BEGIN THEIR DEVELOPMENT AS DIVERTICULAE OF THE FOREBRAIN EARLY IN THE FOURTH WEEK

The first morphologic evidence of the eyes is the formation of an **optic primordium** and **optic sulcus** in the future diencephalic region of the prosencephalic (forebrain) neural folds at 22 days (Fig. 12–19A, B). These structures are induced and supported in their initial growth by interactions with the adjacent pharyngeal endoderm and head mesoderm.

By the time the cranial neuropore closes on day 24, the optic primordia have developed into lateral evaginations of the neural tube called **optic vesicles** (see Fig. 12–19C, D). The walls of the optic vesicles are continuous with the neurectoderm of the future brain, and the cavity or **ventricle** within the optic vesicle is continuous with the neural canal. As the optic vesicle forms, it is surrounded by a sheath of mesenchyme that consists partly of neural crest cells that detach from the optic vesicle itself. This sheath begins to form on day 24 and completely envelops the optic vesicle on day 26 (see Fig. 12–19C).

By day 28, the distal face of the optic vesicle (called the **retinal disc**) reaches the surface ectoderm, from which it is separated only by a few mesenchymal cells. On about day 32, the retinal disc invaginates into the expanded tip of the optic vesicle to form a goblet-shaped **optic cup** (Fig. 12–20D–F). Simultaneously, the stem of the optic vesicle narrows to form the hollow **optic stalk.** The lumen of the optic cup remains continuous with the ventricle of the forebrain through the optic stalk. Blood vessels gain access to the interior of the optic cup through a longitudinal groove, the **choroidal (retinal) fissure,** which develops on the ventral surface of the optic stalk (see Fig. 12–22).

The Lens Develops From an Ectodermal Placode That Forms Adjacent to the Optic Cup

As soon as the optic cup reaches the surface ectoderm, the ectoderm apposed to it thickens to form a **lens placode** (see Fig. 12–20). Until recently, the optic cup was thought to induce the lens placode. This view, suggested by the timing of placode formation, was supported by experiments carried out in the early 1900s. More recent experiments, however, give contradicting results. It now seems likely that lens induction can occur in the absence of an optic cup and that it depends on a complex series of interactions with other tissues that takes place before the optic vesicle is formed. Lens induction apparently begins when definitive endoderm first arrives next to the prospective lens ectoderm early in gastrulation. Later in gastrulation, the neural plate may pass inductive signals to the presumptive lens through the plane of the neurectoderm. During embryonic folding, the heart mesoderm also exerts a significant inductive effect when it comes into proximity with the prospective lens.

Even though the optic cup apparently does not induce the lens placode, several experiments indicate that it does influence the growth, differentiation, and maintenance of the developing lens. If the portion of the optic cup in contact with the ectoderm is resected, the lens eventually degenerates, although it continues to develop for a period that depends on how long it had already interacted with the optic cup.

Figure 12–19. Formation of the optic vesicle and optic cup. *A, B,* The optic vesicle begins to form as an evagination of the diencephalic neural folds on day 22, before the cranial neuropore has closed. *C, D,* By day 24, the optic vesicles lie adjacent to the surface ectoderm. *E, F,* During the fifth week, the optic vesicle invaginates to become the optic cup, and the choroidal fissure forms on the inferior surface of the optic cup and stalk. (*A,* From Morriss-Kay G. 1981. Growth and development of pattern in the cranial neural epithelium of rat embryos during neurulation. J Embryol Exp Morphol 65:225. *D,* From Garcia-Porrero JA, Colvee E, Ojeda JL. 1987. Retinal cell death occurs in the absence of retinal disc invagination. Anat Rec 217:395. *F,* From Morse D, McCann PS. 1984. Neurectoderm of the early embryonic rat eye. Invest Ophthalmol Vis Sci 25:899.)

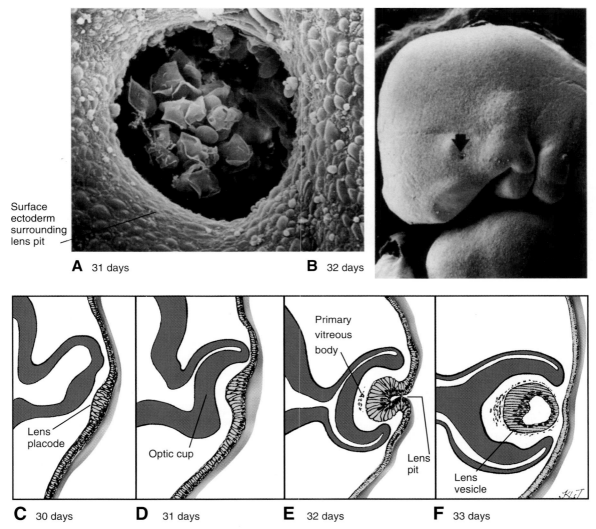

Figure 12–20. Formation of the lens placode and lens vesicle. Contact with the optic cup is necessary for the maintenance and development of the lens placode, although other influences are apparently more important in its induction. *A–E,* During the fifth week, the lens placode begins to invaginate to form the lens pit (arrow in *B*). *E, F,* The invaginating lens placode pinches off to form a lens vesicle enclosed in the optic cup. (*A,* Photo courtesy of Dr. Arnold Tamarin.)

Immediately after the lens placode appears on day 32, it invaginates to form a **lens pit** (see Fig. 12–20*A, B, D*). By day 33, the placode pinches off from the surface ectoderm, becoming a hollow **lens vesicle.** This event coincides with the invagination of the retinal disc, and the newly formed lens vesicle sits within the optic cup. A gelatinous matrix called the **primary vitreous body** is subsequently secreted into the **lentiretinal space** between the lens vesicle and the inner wall of the

expanding optic cup (see Fig. 12–12*E*). The lens vesicle becomes surrounded by a mesenchymal capsule as it forms.

Beginning on day 33, the cells of the posterior (deep) wall of the lens vesicle differentiate to form long, slender, anteroposteriorly oriented **primary lens fibers** (Fig. 12–21; see also Fig 12–20). The elongation of these cells transforms the deep wall of the lens vesicle into a rounded **lens body,** obliterating the cavity of the lens vesicle by the

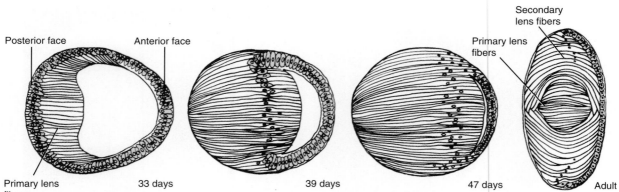

Figure 12–21. Differentiation of the lens. The lens develops rapidly in the fifth to seventh weeks as the cells of its posterior wall elongate and differentiate to form the primary lens fibers. Secondary lens fibers begin to form in the third month.

late seventh week. After the eighth week, the primary lens fibers are augmented by a new population of **secondary lens fibers** that arise from the simple epithelium that differentiates from cells of the anterior wall of the lens vesicle.

The Lens and Retina Are Vascularized by the Hyaloid Branch of the Ophthalmic Artery

As soon as the lens vesicle forms on day 32, it becomes vascularized by a branch of the ophthalmic artery called the **hyaloid artery,** which also vascularizes the developing retina (Fig. 12–22*A*). This artery gains access to the lentiretinal space via the choroidal fissure on the ventral surface of the optic stalk. The lips of the choroidal fissure fuse by day 37, enclosing the hyaloid artery and its accompanying vein in a canal within the ventral wall of the optic stalk (see Fig. 12–22*B–D*). When the lens matures during fetal life and ceases to need a blood supply, the portion of the hyaloid artery that crosses the vitreous body degenerates. Even in the adult, however, the course of this former artery is marked by a conduit through the vitreous body called the **hyaloid canal.** The proximal portion of the hyaloid artery becomes the **central artery of the retina,** which supplies blood to the retina.

The Outer and Inner Walls of the Optic Cup Differentiate Into the Pigment and Neural Retinas, Respectively

The two walls of the optic cup give rise to the two layers of the retina: the thick inner wall of the cup (the former retinal disc) becomes the **neural retina,** which contains the light-receptive **rods** and **cones** plus associated neural processes, and the thin outer wall of the cup becomes the melanin-containing **pigment retina** (Fig. 12–23). These two walls are initially separated by a narrow **intraretinal space.**

Melanin first appears in the cells of the developing pigment retina on day 33. Differentiation of the neural retina begins at the end of the sixth week as the layer of cells adjacent to the intraretinal space (which is homologous to the proliferative neuroepithelium lining the neural tube; see Ch. 4) begins to produce waves of cells that migrate inward toward the vitreous body. By the sixth week, these cells form two cellular embryonic retinal layers: an **outer neuroblastic layer** and an **inner neuroblastic layer.**

By the ninth week, two additional membranes develop to cover the two surfaces of the neural retina. An **external limiting membrane** is interposed between the pigment retina and the proliferative zone of the neural retina, and the in-

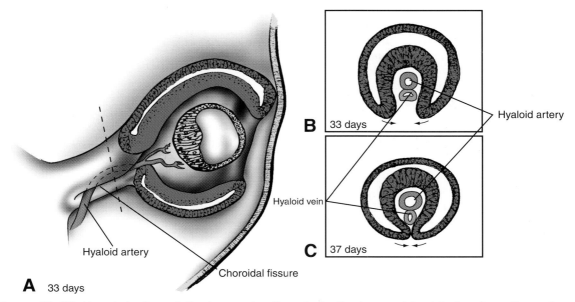

Figure 12–22. Vascularization of the lens and retina. *A,* As the lens vesicle detaches from the surface ectoderm, it becomes vascularized by the hyaloid vessels, which gain access to the lens through the choroidal fissure. *B, C,* During the seventh week, the edges of the choroidal fissure fuse together, enclosing the hyaloid artery and vein in the hyaloid canal. When the lens matures, the vessels serving it degenerate, and the hyaloid artery and vein become the central artery and vein of the retina.

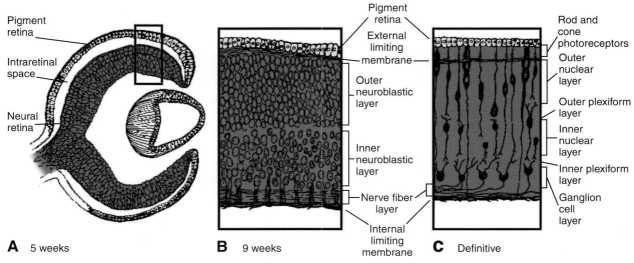

Figure 12–23. Differentiation of the inner layer of the optic cup to form the neural retina. The definitive layers of the neural retina do not develop until late fetal life.

ner surface of the retina is sealed off by an **inner limiting membrane** (see Fig. 12–23B).

The definitive cell layers of the mature neural retina arise from the inner and outer neuroblastic layers. The rods and cones, which form the outermost layer of the mature neural retina, are derived from the outer neuroblastic layer. The inner neuroblastic layer gives rise to the **ganglion cells** and **supporting cells** of the retina. In the sixth week, the ganglion cells sprout axons that emerge onto the inner surface of the retina and grow across it toward the optic stalk. These axons form the definitive **fiber layer** that lines the inner surface of the retina. All the cell layers of the definitive retina are apparent by the eighth month.

Nerve Fibers from the Retina Grow to the Brain Through the Optic Stalk, Transforming It Into the Optic Nerve

The nerve fibers that emerge from the retinal ganglion cells in the sixth week travel through the optic stalk to reach the brain. The stalk lumen is gradually obliterated by the growth of these fibers, and by the eighth week the hollow optic stalk is transformed into the solid **optic nerve** (cranial nerve II). Just before the two optic nerves enter the brain, they join to form an X-shaped structure called the **optic chiasm.** Within the chiasm, about half the fibers from each optic nerve cross over to the contralateral (opposite) side of the brain. The resulting combined bundle of ipsilateral and contralateral fibers on each side then grows back to the lateral geniculate body of the thalamus (see Ch. 13), where the fibers synapse starting in the eighth week. More than 1 million nerve fibers grow from each retina to the brain. The mechanism of axonal pathfinding that allows each of these axons to map to the correct point in the lateral geniculate body is discussed in the Experimental Principles section of Chapter 13.

The intraretinal space between the neural and pigment retinas disappears by the seventh week. The two layers of the retina never fuse firmly, however, and various types of trauma—even a simple blow to the head—can cause **retinal detachment** between them.

The Mesenchymal Capsule of the Optic Vesicle Gives Rise to the Choroid, the Sclera, and the Anterior Chamber

During weeks 6 and 7, the mesenchymal capsule that surrounds the optic cup differentiates into two layers: an inner, pigmented, vascular layer called the **choroid** and an outer, fibrous layer called the **sclera** (Fig. 12–24). The choroid layer is homologous in origin with the pia mater and arachnoid membranes investing the brain (the leptomeninges), and the sclera is homologous with the dura mater. The tough sclera supports and protects the delicate inner structures of the optic globe.

Late in the sixth week, the mesenchyme surrounding the optic cup invades the region between the lens and the surface ectoderm, thus forming a complete mesenchymal jacket around the developing globe. During the seventh week, the mesenchyme overlying the lens splits into two layers that enclose a new cavity called the **anterior chamber of the eye** (see Fig. 12–24C). The anterior (superficial) wall of this chamber is continuous with the sclera of the optic globe, and the posterior (deep) wall is continuous with the choroid.

The Two Inner Layers of the Cornea Form From the Superficial Wall of the Anterior Chamber, and the Third (Outer) Layer Forms From the Overlying Ectoderm. By the eighth week, the superficial wall of the anterior chamber differentiates into two layers: a thin inner epithelium lining the anterior chamber (called the **mesothelium of the anterior chamber**) and, external to it, an **acellular postepithelial layer.** Mesenchymal cells rapidly invade the latter and convert it to a cellular **stromal layer (substantia propria).** The anterior chamber mesothelium and the substantia propria constitute the two deep layers of the cornea, which thus are of mesodermal origin. In contrast, the outer layer of the cornea, called the **anterior epithelium,** is derived from the overlying surface ectoderm.

The Inner Wall of the Anterior Chamber Forms the Pupillary Membrane. When the anterior chamber forms, its thick posterior wall rests directly against the lens. The deep layers of this wall subsequently break down by a process of vac-

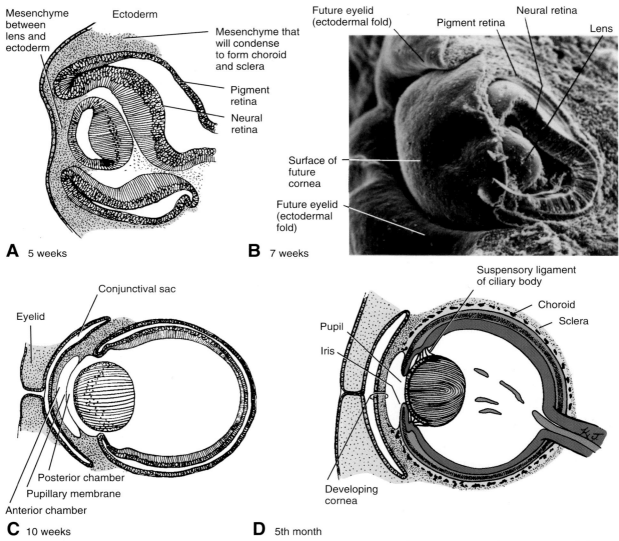

Figure 12–24. Development of the anterior and posterior chambers, the eyelids, and the coverings of the optic globe. *A, B,* Mesenchyme surrounds the developing eyeball (optic globe) between the fifth and seventh weeks to form the choroid and sclera. *C, D,* Vacuolization within this mesenchyme in the seventh week forms the anterior chamber. Shortly thereafter, vacuolization in the layer of mesenchyme immediately anterior to the lens forms the posterior chamber. The pupillary membrane, which initially separates the anterior and posterior chambers, breaks down in early fetal life. The upper and lower eyelids form as folds of surface ectoderm. They fuse together by the end of the eighth week and separate again between the fifth and seventh months.

uolization to create a new space, the **posterior chamber,** between the lens and the thin remaining layer of the wall (see Fig. 12–24C). This thin remaining layer, called the **pupillary membrane,** breaks down early in the fetal period to form the opening called the **pupil** through which the anterior and posterior chambers communicate. On rare occasions, the pupillary membrane fails to break down completely, leaving strands that traverse the pupil. The posterior chamber eventually expands to underlie the iris and part of the ciliary body (see later), as well as the pupil.

The Rim of the Optic Cup and the Overlying Choroidal Mesenchyme Form the Iris and Ciliary Body

At the end of the third month, the anterior rim of the optic cup and its overlying choroidal mesenchyme expand to form a thin ring that projects between the anterior and posterior chambers and overlaps the lens (see Fig. 12–24B). This ring differentiates into the **iris** of the eye. The inner surface of the iris is lined by a thin epithelium that represents the two, fused layers of the optic cup; the remainder of the iris differentiates from choroidal mesoderm. The circumferentially arranged smooth muscle bundles of the **pupillary muscles** in the iris form from neural crest-derived ectomesenchymal cells in the choroid. These muscles act as a diaphragm, controlling the diameter of the pupil and thus the amount of light that enters the eye.

Just posterior to the developing iris, the optic cup and overlying choroid differentiate to form the **ciliary body.** The lens is suspended from the ciliary body by a radial network of elastic fibers called the **suspensory ligament** of the lens. Around the insertions of these fibers, the optic cup epithelia of the ciliary body proliferate to form a ring of highly vascularized, feathery elaborations that are specialized to secrete the fluid that fills the optic globe. Ectomesenchymal cells in the choroid of the ciliary body differentiate to form the smooth muscle bundles of the **ciliary muscle,** which controls the shape and hence the focusing power (accommodation) of the lens. Contraction of this muscle reduces the diameter of the ciliary ring from which the lens is suspended, thus allowing the lens to relax toward its natural spherical shape and providing the greater focusing power needed for near vision.

The Extrinsic Ocular Muscles Develop From Mesenchyme Adjacent to the Optic Cup

The first of the extraocular muscles to appear are the **lateral** and **superior rectus** muscles, which begin to condense adjacent to the mesenchymal sheath of the optic vesicle as early as day 28. Within a few days, the insertions of these muscles on the globe also begin to condense. By the early sixth week, the **superior oblique** muscle appears, followed by the **medial rectus** and the common primordium of the **inferior rectus** and **inferior oblique.** The **trochlea**—the ligamentous pulley for the superior oblique muscle—does not appear until early in the eighth week, at about the same time that the muscle of the upper eyelid, the **levator palpebrae superioris,** is formed by delamination from the superior rectus muscle.

Experiments carried out to determine the origin of the myocytes of the extrinsic ocular muscles and levator palpebrae superioris have yielded ambiguous results. Some data suggest that these muscles arise from paraxial mesoderm; other studies indicate that they arise from prechordal plate mesoderm. These conflicting results may simply reflect the limited precision possible with current transplantation techniques. Alternatively, the muscle precursor cells may change their location during the period before their final migration to the region of the globe, so that differences in the timing of the transplantation experiments could result in divergent findings. It is generally agreed, however, that the connective tissue associated with the extrinsic ocular muscles is derived from neural crest.

The extrinsic ocular muscles are innervated by three cranial nerves: the **oculomotor nerve** (cranial nerve III), the **trochlear nerve** (cranial nerve IV), and the **abducent nerve** (cranial nerve VI). The oculomotor nerve reaches the vicinity of the developing eye early in the fifth week and innervates the levator palpebrae superioris; the superior, inferior, and medial recti; and the inferior oblique. The trochlear and abducent nerves appear at the end of the fifth week and innervate the superior oblique and the lateral rectus, respectively.

THE EYELIDS FORM FROM FOLDS IN THE SURFACE ECTODERM AND ASSOCIATED MESENCHYME

By the sixth week, small folds of ectoderm with a mesenchymal core appear just cranial and caudal to the developing cornea (see Fig. 12–24). These upper and lower eyelid primordia rapidly grow toward each other, meeting and fusing by the eighth week. The space between the fused eyelids and the cornea, which is lined with ectoderm-derived epithelium, is called the **conjunctival sac.** The eyelids separate again between the fifth and seventh months.

The **lacrimal glands** form from invaginations of the ectoderm at the superolateral angles of the conjunctival sacs but do not mature until about 6 weeks after birth. The tear fluid produced by the glands is excreted into the conjunctival sac, where it lubricates the cornea. Excess tear fluid drains through the nasolacrimal duct into the nasal cavity.

12

Part Three

Development of the Ears

Summary

The ear is a composite structure with a complex embryonic origin. The external and middle ears, as mentioned earlier in this chapter, arise from structures of the first and second pharyngeal arches and from the intervening pharyngeal cleft and pouch. The inner ear, in contrast, develops from an epidermal **otic placode** that appears on either side of the head at the level of the future hindbrain. At the end of the third week, this otic placode invaginates and then pinches off to form an **otic vesicle** within the head mesenchyme. The otic vesicle rapidly differentiates into three subdivisions: a slender, dorsal **endolymphatic duct** and **sac,** an expanded central **utricle,** and a tapered ventral **saccule.** From the fourth to the seventh weeks, the utricle differentiates to form the three semicircular canals, and the ventral end of the saccule elongates and coils to form the cochlea. All these otic vesicle derivatives collectively constitute the **membranous labyrinth.** The otic placode also gives rise to the sensory ganglia of the vestibulocochlear nerve (cranial nerve VIII).

From weeks 9 to 23, the mesenchymal condensation that surrounds the membranous labyrinth, called the **otic capsule,** first chondrifies and then ossifies to form a **bony labyrinth** within the petrous part of the temporal bone.

The first pharyngeal pouch lengthens to form the **tubotympanic recess,** which differentiates into the **tympanic cavity** of the middle ear and the **auditory (eustachian) tube.** The cartilages of the first and second pharyngeal arches give rise to the three auditory ossicles. These ossicles develop not in the tympanic cavity itself but rather in the adjacent mesenchyme. The tympanic cavity expands during the last month of gestation to enclose the ossicles. In consequence, the ossicles are sheathed by the endoderm that lines the tympanic cavity.

The **auricle (pinna)** of the external ear develops from six **auricular hillocks,** which appear during the sixth week on the facing edges of the first and second arches. The first pharyngeal cleft lengthens to form the primordium of the external auditory canal. However, the ectoderm lining the canal subsequently proliferates to form a **meatal plug** that completely fills the inner portion of the canal. The inner two thirds of the definitive canal are formed by recanalization of this plug during the 26th week. The tympanic membrane is derived from the pharyngeal membrane that separates the first pharyngeal pouch and cleft. It is therefore a three-layered structure, consisting of an external layer of ectoderm, a mesodermal **fibrous stratum,** and an inner layer of endoderm. The definitive tympanic membrane is formed during the recanalization of the external auditory meatus.

Development of the Membranous Labyrinth, Tympanic Cavity, Auditory Tube, Auditory Ossicles, Outer Ear, and Tympanic Membrane

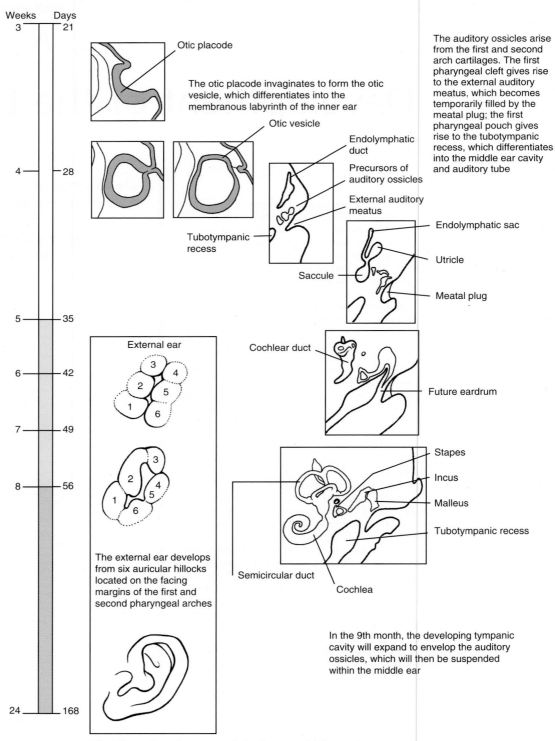

Weeks   Days

3 —— 21

Otic placode

The otic placode invaginates to form the otic vesicle, which differentiates into the membranous labyrinth of the inner ear

Otic vesicle

4 —— 28

Endolymphatic duct

Precursors of auditory ossicles

External auditory meatus

Tubotympanic recess

Saccule

Endolymphatic sac

Utricle

Meatal plug

5 —— 35

External ear

Cochlear duct

6 —— 42

Future eardrum

7 —— 49

Stapes

Incus

8 —— 56

Malleus

Tubotympanic recess

The external ear develops from six auricular hillocks located on the facing margins of the first and second pharyngeal arches

Semicircular duct

Cochlea

The auditory ossicles arise from the first and second arch cartilages. The first pharyngeal cleft gives rise to the external auditory meatus, which becomes temporarily filled by the meatal plug; the first pharyngeal pouch gives rise to the tubotympanic recess, which differentiates into the middle ear cavity and auditory tube

In the 9th month, the developing tympanic cavity will expand to envelop the auditory ossicles, which will then be suspended within the middle ear

24 —— 168

Timeline. Development of the inner, middle, and outer ears.

THE INNER EAR FORMS BY INVAGINATION OF AN OTIC PLACODE IN THE SURFACE ECTODERM OF THE HEAD

Late in the third week, a thickening of the surface ectoderm called the **otic placode** or **otic disc** appears next to the rhombencephalic (hindbrain) region of each neural fold (Fig. 12–25). This placode is the primordium of the membranous labyrinth of the inner ear, including the sensory receptors for hearing and balance, and of the **statoacoustic ganglion** of the **vestibulocochlear nerve** (cranial nerve VIII), which innervates these receptors. The growth of the head causes the otic placode to be translocated caudally to the level of the second pharyngeal arch. During the fourth week, the otic placode gradually invaginates to form first an **otic pit** and then a closed, hollow **otic vesicle** (see Fig. 12–25). A stem of ectoderm briefly connects the otic vesicle to the surface but disintegrates at the end of the fourth week.

The Otic Vesicle Differentiates Into a Dorsal Endolymphatic Sac, an Intermediate Utricle, and a Ventral Saccule

By day 26 of the fourth week, the dorsomedial region of the otic vesicle begins to elongate, forming an **endolymphatic appendage** (Fig. 12–26A, B). Simultaneously, the rest of the otic vesicle differentiates into an expanded **utricle** and a tapered, ventral **saccule**. The endolymphatic appendage elongates over the following week, and its distal portion expands to form an **endolymphatic sac** that is connected to the utricle by a slender **endolymphatic duct** (see Fig. 12–26C).

During the fifth week, the ventral tip of the saccule begins to elongate and coil, forming a **cochlear duct,** which is the primordium of the cochlea (see Fig. 12–26D, E). The connection between the developing cochlea and the saccule constricts to form the **ductus reuniens.** During the seventh week, cells of the cochlear duct differentiate to form the **spiral organ of Corti** (the structure that bears the hair cell receptors responsible for transducing sound vibrations into electrical impulses). The organ of Corti is innervated by the sensory neurons of the **spiral ganglion (cochlear ganglion)** tucked into the coil of the cochlea. The fibers from the spiral ganglion form the **cochlear branch** of the vestibulocochlear nerve, and they synapse in the medial geniculate bodies of the brain (see Ch. 13).

During the seventh week, three flattened diverticulae grow from the utricular portion of the otic vesicle and differentiate sequentially to form the **anterior, posterior,** and **lateral semicircular ducts** (see Fig. 12–26D, E; timeline). A small expansion called the **ampulla** forms at one end of each semicircular duct. The hair cell sensory structures in the ampullae and the utriculus, which are responsible for detecting the accelerations and orientation of the head, are innervated by the **vestibular ganglion** of the vestibulocochlear nerve. The fibers of this ganglion form the **vestibular branch** of the vestibulocochlear nerve.

Beginning in the ninth week, the mesenchyme surrounding the membranous labyrinth chondrifies to form a cartilage called the **otic capsule.** Transplantation experiments have shown that the presence of the otic vesicle is necessary to induce chondrogenesis in this mesenchyme and that the shape of the vesicle controls the morphogenesis of the capsule. During the third to fifth months, the layer of cartilage immediately surrounding the membranous labyrinth undergoes vacuolization to form a cavity somewhat larger than the membranous labyrinth. The membranous labyrinth is suspended in this cavity in a fluid called **perilymph,** and the space between the membranous labyrinth and the walls of the otic capsule is called the **perilymphatic space.** The otic capsule ossifies between 16 and 23 weeks to form the **petrous portion** of the **temporal bone** (Fig. 12–27). Continued ossification later produces the mastoid portion of the temporal bone. The bony enclosure that houses the membranous labyrinth and the perilymph is called the **bony labyrinth.**

THE MIDDLE EAR CAVITY AND AUDITORY TUBE ARE DERIVED FROM THE FIRST PHARYNGEAL POUCH AND ARE LINED BY ENDODERM

As mentioned in part one of this chapter, the first pharyngeal pouch elongates to form a **tubotym-**

A 25 days

B 25 days

Otic pit

Otic placode

C 25 days

Otic pit

Otic vesicle

Programmed cell death

Otic vesicle

ED

D 28 days   **E** 28 days   **F** 28 days

Figure 12–25. Formation of the otic vesicle. *A,* The otic placode appears in the surface ectoderm adjacent to the rhombencephalon late in the third week. *B, C,* By day 25, the placode invaginates to form the otic pit. *D–F,* By the end of the fourth week, continued invagination forms the otic vesicle, which quickly detaches from the surface ectoderm (ED, endolymphatic duct). (*A, F,* From Kikuchi T, Tonosaki A, Takasaka T. 1988. Development of apical-surface structures of mouse otic placode. Acta Otolaryngol 106:200.)

panic recess, which subsequently differentiates to form the expanded **tympanic cavity** of the middle ear and the slender **auditory (eustachian) tube,** which connects the tympanic cavity to the pharynx. During the seventh week, the cartilaginous precursors of the three **auditory ossicles** condense in the mesenchyme of the first and second arches near the tympanic cavity (see Fig. 12–26). As described in part one of this chapter, the cartilage of the mandibular process gives rise to the malleus, the cartilage of the maxillary process to the incus, and the cartilage of the second arch to the stapes. The developing ossicles remain embedded in the mesenchyme adjacent to the tympanic cavity through the eighth month of gestation. Their associated

middle ear muscles—the **tensor tympani** and the **stapedius**—form in the ninth week from first- and second-arch mesenchyme.

During the ninth month of development, the mesenchyme surrounding the auditory ossicles and associated muscles disperses, and the tympanic cavity expands to enclose them (see Fig. 12–26*E*). The endoderm that lines the tympanic cavity therefore jackets the ossicles and also forms transient endodermal mesenteries that suspend the ossicles in the cavity until their definitive supporting ligaments develop.

Meanwhile, the pharyngeal membrane separating the tympanic cavity from the external auditory meatus (derived from the first pharyngeal

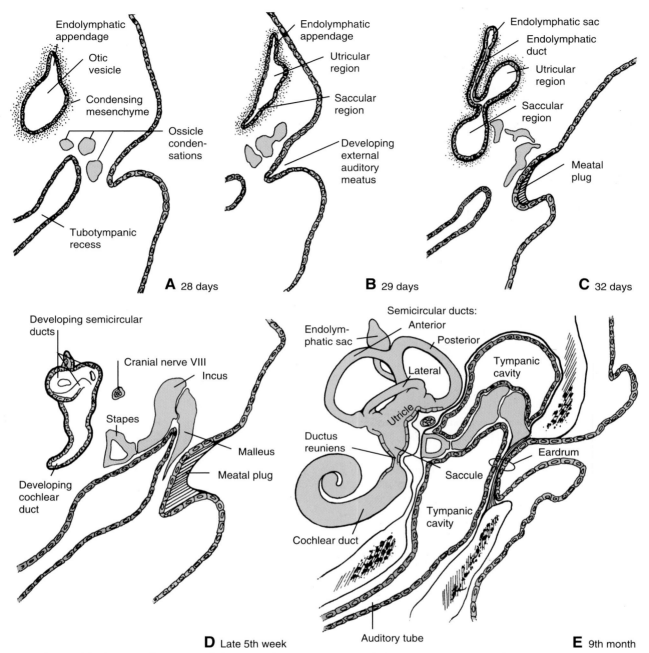

Figure 12–26. Development of the ear. The components of the inner, middle, and outer ears arise in coordination from several embryonic structures. The otic vesicle gives rise to the membranous labyrinth of the inner ear and to the eighth nerve ganglia. *A, B,* The superior end of the otic vesicle forms an endolymphatic appendage, and the body of the vesicle then differentiates into utricular and saccular regions. *C, D,* The endolymphatic appendage elongates to form the endolymphatic sac and duct; the utricle gives rise to the three semicircular ducts; and the inferior end of the saccule elongates and coils to form the cochlear duct. Simultaneously, the three auditory ossicles arise from mesenchymal condensations formed by the first and second pharyngeal arches; the first pharyngeal pouch enlarges to form the tubotympanic recess (the future middle ear cavity), and the first pharyngeal cleft (the future external auditory meatus) becomes filled with a transient meatal plug of ectodermal cells. *E,* Finally, in the ninth month, the tubotympanic cavity expands to enclose the auditory ossicles, forming the functional middle ear cavity. The definitive eardrum represents the first pharyngeal membrane and is thus a three-layered structure comprising ectoderm, mesoderm, and endoderm.

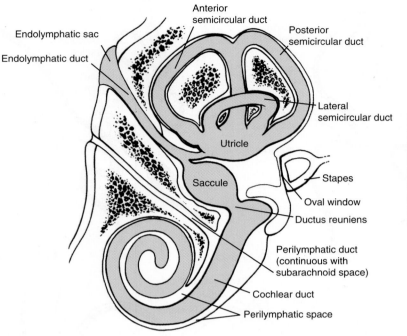

Figure 12-27. The definitive membranous labyrinth is suspended in the fluid-filled perilymphatic space within the bony labyrinth of the petrous portion of the temporal bone. The perilymphatic space is connected to the subarachnoid space by the perilymphatic duct. The membranous labyrinth itself is filled with endolymph.

cleft) develops into the **tympanic membrane** or **eardrum** (see Fig. 12–26E). The tympanic membrane is composed of an outer lining of ectoderm, an inner lining of endoderm, and an intervening mesodermal layer called the **fibrous stratum.** As described below, the definitive ectodermal layer of the tympanic membrane is formed during the process of recanalization that created the definitive external auditory meatus.

A common cause of hearing loss is the development of a small, benign growth in the tympanic cavity called a **cholesteatoma.** Although the origin of these growths is controversial, one popular theory suggests that they develop from small "epidermoid thickenings" of the endodermal lining of the tympanic cavity. These thickenings are thought to form in all normal embryos but only occasionally to persist and then proliferate to form a cholesteatoma.

During the ninth month, the suspended auditory ossicles assume their functional relationships with each other and with the associated structures of the outer, middle, and inner ears. The ventral end of the malleus becomes attached to the eardrum, and the foot plate of the stapes becomes attached to the **oval window,** a small fenestra in the bony labyrinth that is sealed by a portion of the membranous labyrinth (see Figs. 12–26E and 12–27). Sonic vibrations are transmitted from the eardrum to the oval window by the articulated chain of ossicles and from the oval window to the cochlea by the fluid filling the perilymphatic space. The cochlea transduces these vibrations into neural impulses.

During the ninth month, the tympanic cavity expands into the mastoid part of the temporal bone to form the **mastoid antrum.** The **mastoid air cells** in the mastoid portion of the temporal bone do not form until about 2 years of age, when the action of the sternocleidomastoid muscle on the mastoid part of the temporal bone induces the mastoid process to form.

THE EXTERNAL EAR IS DERIVED FROM THE FIRST PHARYNGEAL CLEFT AND THE FIRST AND SECOND PHARYNGEAL ARCHES

The external ear consists of the funnel-shaped **external auditory meatus** and the **auricle (pinna).**

The precursor of the external auditory meatus develops by deepening of the first pharyngeal cleft during the sixth week. However, the ectodermal lining of the deep portion of this tube later proliferates, producing a solid core of tissue called the **meatal plug** that completely fills the medial end of the external auditory meatus by week 26. Canalization of this plug begins almost immediately and produces the medial two thirds of the definitive meatus. The meatus does not achieve its final length until the age of 9 or 10 years.

The auricle develops from three pairs of **auricular hillocks** that arise during the fifth week on the facing edges of the first and second arches (Fig. 12–28). From ventral to dorsal, the hillocks on the first arch are called the **tragus, helix,** and

Early fetus

Late fetus

Newborn

Figure 12–28. Differentiation of the auricle. The auricle develops from six auricular hillocks, which arise on the apposed surfaces of the first and second pharyngeal arches. (*A,* Photo courtesy of Dr. Arnold Tamarin.)

cymba concha, and the hillocks on the second arch are called the antitragus, antihelix, and concha. Except for the tragus, these names reflect the shapes of the resulting portions of the pinna. The tragus is named for the goat's-beard tuft of hair that may grow from it (Greek *tragos*, billy goat). During the seventh week, the auricular hillocks begin to enlarge, differentiate, and fuse to produce the definitive form of the auricle. As the face develops, the auricle is gradually translocated from its original location low on the side of the neck to a more lateral and cranial site.

The absence or abnormal development of one or more of the auricular hillocks may result in malformations of the auricle. A defect that suppresses the growth of all the hillocks results in microtia (small auricle) or anotia (absence of the auricle). Accessory hillocks may also form, producing ectopic auricular tags.

Clinical Applications

Craniofacial Abnormalities

It has been estimated that the various kinds of craniofacial anomalies—including malformations of the frontonasal process, clefting defects, calvarial malformations, and anomalies of the pharyngeal arch derivatives—account for approximately one third of all congenital defects. Most craniofacial anomalies have a multifactorial etiology (see the Clinical Applications section of Ch. 7), although in some types a clear genetic basis can often be demonstrated, for example, in Meckel syndrome (Fig. 12–29), which is inherited as an autosomal recessive trait. A number of teratogens are also known to cause craniofacial malformations. The most clinically significant craniofacial teratogen—and possibly the best studied—is alcohol. Drugs such as hydantoin and Accutane can cause craniofacial anomalies in humans, as can toluene, cigarette smoking, ionizing radiation, and hyperthermia.

The Most Common Cause of Holoprosencephaly May Be Consumption of Alcohol During the Third Week of Pregnancy

Disturbances in the early induction of the forebrain (prosencephalon) can result in a spectrum of anomalies known as holoprosencephaly. Depending on the severity of the condition, the frontonasal process, calvaria (skull vault), and midfacial structures may be deformed, as well as the forebrain itself. The great majority of cases of holoprosencephaly are caused by consumption of alcohol during the period during which the events responsible for forebrain induction take place. Alcohol-induced holoprosencephaly is thought to be the most common cause of congenital mental retardation in the western world. The spectrum of defects typical of holoprosencephaly has also been induced in mice by administering alcohol during the appropriate sensitive period.

Holoprosencephaly is the most dramatic and damaging manifestation of fetal alcohol syndrome, the spectrum of defects that can be caused by consumption of alcohol during pregnancy. It is crucial to realize that alcohol-induced holoprosencephaly is specifically caused during the first month of pregnancy. Consumption of amounts of alcohol as low as 80 g per day during the sensitive period can cause significant defects, and it has been suggested that even a single binge may be teratogenic. Chronic consumption of even quite small amounts of alcohol later in pregnancy can result in other, less destructive effects, such as some degree of growth retardation and minor physical defects. Few women are fully aware that, although it is important to avoid alcohol throughout pregnancy, it is *crucial* to abstain from drinking during the early weeks following any act of intercourse that might have resulted in pregnancy—whether or not the woman knows herself to be

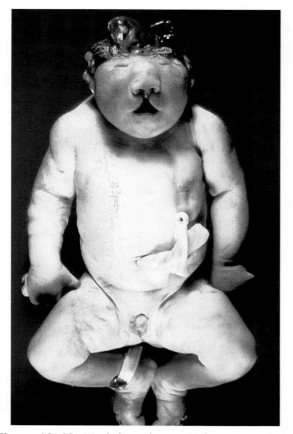

Figure 12–29. Meckel syndrome. Holoprosencephalic defects of the midface, including absence of the olfactory bulbs, are common manifestations of this autosomal recessive syndrome. (Photo courtesy of Children's Hospital Medical Center, Cincinnati, OH.)

Holoprosencephaly and Other Craniofacial Syndromes Have Variable Severity

The forebrain anomalies characteristic of holoprosencephaly result from defective development of the ventromedial forebrain and include defects of the olfactory nerves, olfactory bulbs, olfactory tracts, basal olfactory cortex, and associated structures including the limbic lobe, hippocampus, and mammillary bodies. The corpus callosum is sometimes affected. The hindbrain is usually normal in holoprosencephaly, although exposure to alcohol slightly later in development may cause hindbrain anomalies by interfering with the induction of the hindbrain by the notochordal process.

The typical facial anomalies of a fully developed case of holoprosencephaly include a short, upturned nose, a long upper lip with a deficient philtrum, a highly arched palate, and retrognathia (short, retracted lower jaw). The skull is small (microcephaly), and the brain has abnormalities. Particularly severe cases of holoprosencephaly involve dramatic defects of the facial structures arising from the frontonasal prominence, most notably the nasal placodes. Failure of the medial nasal processes to form results in agenesis of the intermaxillary process (Fig. 12–30A) and the reduction or absence of other midfacial structures, such as the nasal bones, nasal septum, and ethmoid. The consequence may be **cebocephaly** (a single nostril; see Fig. 12–30B) and **hypotelorism** (close-set eyes; see Fig. 12–30C) or **cyclopia** (a single eye; see Fig. 12–30D). Mild cases of holoprosencephaly, on the other hand, are characterized by relatively minimal midface anomalies and by **trigonocephaly,** a triangular skull shape that develops as a result of premature closure (**synostosis**) of the suture between the frontal bones and causes compression of the growing cerebral hemispheres.

A familial condition called **craniofrontonasal dysplasia syndrome** is characterized by a tall, narrow skull shape known as **acrocephaly (tower skull),** which results from premature synostosis of the coronal suture, as well as by **hypertelorism** (wide-set eyes) and clefting of the nose and upper lip. The pathogenesis of this syndrome is not understood. Two other craniofacial syndromes that also involve premature synostosis of cranial sutures are Crouzon and Apert syndromes (Fig. 12–31).

pregnant. It is therefore of paramount importance that appropriate counseling be provided to couples planning to produce a child. Fetal alcohol syndrome is thought to affect as many as 2 in 1000 live-born infants.

Other causes of holoprosencephaly are known. Children with typical defects have been born to mothers who inhaled toluene during early pregnancy, and offspring of diabetic mothers are at increased risk. Holoprosencephaly may also occur with chromosomal anomalies such as trisomies 13, 18, and 21 or single-gene mutations (see Experimental Principles section).

Figure 12–30. Examples of holoprosencephaly. This spectrum of malformations that may occur as a manifestation of fetal alcohol syndrome ranges in severity from minor midfacial defects to extremely devastating malformations. *A,* The intermaxillary process failed to form in this infant *B,* Cebocephaly is a midfacial defect characterized by a single nostril. *C,* The generalized reduction of midface structures in holoprosencephaly may lead to absence of the nose and hypotelorism. *D,* Extreme reduction of midfacial structures may result in cyclopia. (Photos courtesy of Children's Hospital Medical Center, Cincinnati, OH.)

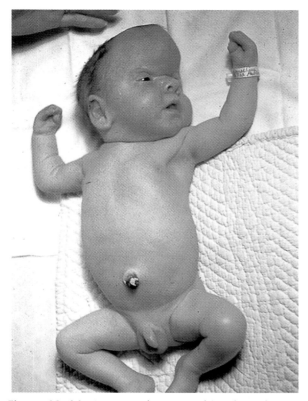

Figure 12–31. Apert syndrome. In this infant, the coronal suture has fused prematurely and the cranium has therefore been forced to adopt a "tower skull" (acrocephalic) shape to accommodate the growing brain. (Photo courtesy of Dr. David Billmire.)

Factors That Disturb the Fusion of the Facial Swellings Result in Clefting Defects

As described in part one of this chapter, the face is created by the growth and fusion of five facial swellings. Complete or partial failure of fusion between any of these swellings results in a **facial cleft,** which may be unilateral or bilateral. The two most common types of facial cleft are **cleft lip** (Figs. 12–32 and 12–33), which results from failure of the maxillary swelling to fuse with the intermaxillary process, and **cleft palate** (see Fig. 12–33), which results from the failure of the two palatine shelves to fuse with each other along the midline. Although cleft lip and cleft palate often occur

together, the two defects differ in their distribution with respect to sex, familial association, race, and geography and therefore probably have different etiologies.

Cleft lip has been ascribed to underdevelopment of the mesenchyme of the maxillary swelling, which would result in inadequate contact of the maxillary swelling with the medial nasal process and intermaxillary process. The resulting cleft may range in length from a minor notch in the vermilion border of the lip just lateral to the philtrum to a cleft that completely separates the lateral lip from the philtrum and nasal cavity. The depth of clefting also varies: some clefts involve just the soft tissue of the lip; others divide the lateral portion of the maxillary bone from the premaxillary portion (the portion bearing the incisors) and from the primary palate. Clefts of this type often result in deformed, absent, or supernumerary teeth.

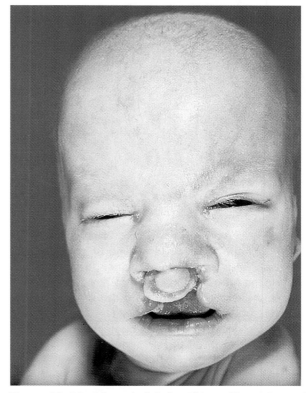

Figure 12–32. Bilateral cleft lip. This malformation results from failure of the medial nasal processes to fuse with the maxillary swellings. (Photo courtesy of Children's Hospital Medical Center, Cincinnati, OH.)

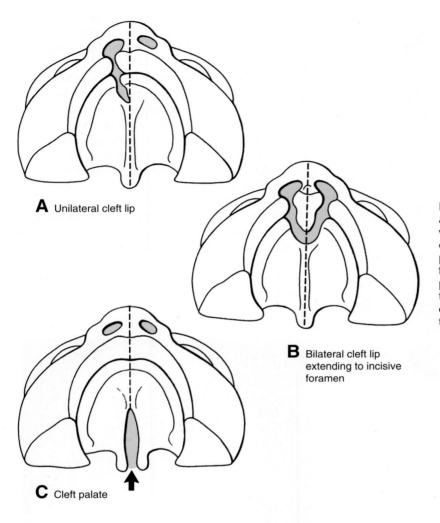

A Unilateral cleft lip

B Bilateral cleft lip extending to incisive foramen

C Cleft palate

Figure 12–33. Cleft lip and cleft palate. *A, B,* Cleft lip. The cleft may involve the lip only or extend posteriorly along one or both edges of the primary palate. *C,* Cleft palate results from failure of the palatine shelves to properly fuse during development of the secondary palate. Cleft lip and cleft palate appear to represent distinct errors of development.

Any of several pathogenetic factors might account for the underdevelopment of the maxillary processes in cleft lip; these include inadequate migration or proliferation of neural crest ectomesenchyme and excessive cell death during the developmental modeling of the maxillary swelling and nasal placode. Although the etiology of the defect is generally multifactorial, a number of common drugs, including the anticonvulsant phenytoin (Dilantin), vitamin A, and some vitamin A analogues, particularly the oral antiacne drug isotretinoin (Accutane), have been shown to induce cleft lip in experimental animals. Vitamin A and its analogues are notorious for their ability to cause facial defects. They apparently have particularly deleterious effects on the development of the frontonasal process mesenchyme and, consequently, on the development of the nasal processes.

In cleft palate, the failure of the palatine shelves to fuse during the 7th to 10th weeks may result from a variety of errors. These include inadequate growth of the palatine shelves, failure of the shelves to elevate at the correct time, an excessively wide head, failure of the shelves to fuse, and secondary rupture after fusion. Cleft palate can therefore result from a wide range of congenital insults and genetic errors. Most cases are multifactorial in etiology, although an X-linked cleft palate

Figure 12–34. An infant with Goldenhar syndrome, exhibiting characteristic hemifacial microsomia anomalies of the ear. These defects apparently are caused by an expanding hematoma of the stapedial artery system. (Photo courtesy of Children's Hospital Medical Center, Cincinnati, OH.)

syndrome has been described. Teratogens such as phenytoin, vitamin A and its analogues, and some corticosteroid anti-inflammatory drugs also can cause cleft palate in sensitive individuals.

Errors in the Development of Pharyngeal Arch and Pouch Derivatives Cause a Great Variety of Facial Anomalies

Not surprisingly, errors in the development of the numerous pharyngeal arch and pouch elements that contribute to the human head and face can cause varied malformations. After cleft lip and cleft palate, the most common group of facial malformations are the defects caused by underdevelopment of the first and second arches, collectively known as **craniofacial microsomia** (*microsomia* is from the Greek for small body). The most com-mon of these defects is a **lateral cleft,** in which incomplete fusion of the maxillary and mandibular processes in the cheek region results in a cleft extending back from the corner of the mouth, occasionally as far as the tragus of the auricle. According to one theory, this malformation arises not from primary nonfusion of the maxillary and mandibular processes but, rather, from secondary ischemic necrosis caused by an expanding hematoma arising from the stapedial artery system. The stapedial artery provides the initial blood supply to this region of the maxillary and mandibular arches.

The group of more extensive deformities known collectively as **hemifacial microsomia** is thought to arise in many cases by the same vascular mechanism. In these deformities, the lateral cleft of the face usually is not large, but the posterior portion of the mandible, the temporomandibular joint, the muscles of mastication, and the outer and middle ear may all be underdeveloped. Figure 12–34 illustrates **Goldenhar syndrome,** a particularly severe member of this group.

The syndromes classified as **mandibulofacial dysostosis** closely resemble the above deformities but arise by very different mechanisms. In these disorders, underdevelopment of the lower face and mandible and associated abnormalities of the palate and external ears result from a deficit of mesenchyme in the first and second pharyngeal arches. This deficit has been explained as resulting from defective migration or proliferation of neural crest cells or, alternatively, from excessive cell death.

Two genetic syndromes involving mandibulofacial dysostosis are Treacher-Collins syndrome and Hallerman-Streif syndrome. It is thought that the former may be an autosomal dominant form and the latter an autosomal recessive form of the same genetic syndrome. Other cases of mandibulofacial dysostosis apparently arise through diverse etiologies. The oral antiacne drug isotretinoin can cause similar abnormalities in humans if administered during the first month of development and also in experimental animals if administered during the comparable period of development (Fig. 12–35). Additional genetic syndromes affecting first and second arch development are discussed in the Experimental Principles section below.

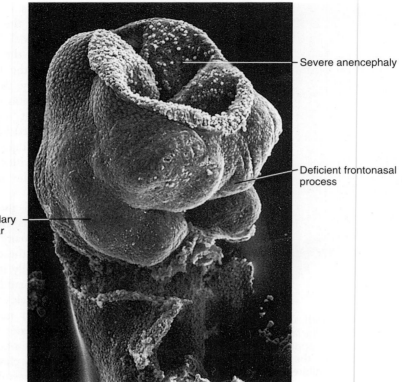

Severe anencephaly

Deficient frontonasal process

No distinction between maxillary and mandibular swellings

Figure 12–35. Mouse embryo treated with the teratogen isotretinoin (an analogue of vitamin A) and exhibiting anencephalic and first arch abnormalities. This drug has been implicated in the formation of malformations of the skull, face, central nervous system, lungs, cardiovascular system, and limbs of human infants born to mothers ingesting it during the first 3 months of pregnancy. (From Irving D, Willhite C, Burk D. 1986. Morphogenesis of isotretinoin-induced microcephaly and micrognathia studied by scanning electron microscopy. Teratology 34:141.)

The complex of congenital malformations known as **DiGeorge syndrome** is characterized by three groups of malformations: (1) minor craniofacial defects, including **micrognathia** (small jaw), low-set ears, auricular abnormalities, cleft palate, and hypertelorism; (2) total or partial agenesis of the derivatives of the third and fourth pharyngeal pouches (the thymus and parathyroid glands); and (3) cardiovascular anomalies, including persistent truncus arteriosus and interrupted aortic arch. This syndrome may be caused by abnormalities of neural crest migration and proliferation occurring during the formation of the third and fourth arches—that is, slightly later in development than for mandibulofacial dysostosis.

The inclusion of cardiac abnormalities is explained by the migration of neural crest cells through the fourth and sixth pharyngeal arches to form the aorticopulmonary septum (see the Experimental Principles section of Ch. 7).

Although some cases of DiGeorge syndrome are associated with partial monosomy of chromosome 22, the syndrome also occurs among offspring of alcoholic women. Experiments have shown that acute administration of alcohol to animals during the period of third- to sixth-arch development can result in a spectrum of anomalies similar to DiGeorge syndrome.

Experimental Principles

Segmental Development of the Head and Neck

Recent Evidence Supports the Theory That the Head Arises From a Series of Highly Modified Segments

One of the most obvious patterns in the developing embryo is the segmental arrangement of the somites. The question immediately arises as to how the head, most of which shows no obvious somitic segmentation, relates to the segmentation of the rest of the axis. Anatomists of the early 19th century postulated that the head develops through simple modification of trunk segments. This idea was soon shown to be untenable, and, in addition, the relation of trunk and/or head segmentation to the segmented pharyngeal arches remained a vexing question. Eventually, the concept of **metamerism** was proposed, describing the origin of the head and trunk from a fundamental pattern of repeating units. It was suggested, however, that this underlying segmentation in the head region has been obscured by an evolutionary process of **cephalization** (head specialization). Data from classic and comparative anatomy were used to propose various schemes of head segmentation, but none was entirely convincing, and the tools were lacking to explore the matter further.

A number of fascinating discoveries involving the cranial somitomeres, the hindbrain rhombomeres, and a series of **homeotic genes** that regulate segmentation in mammals have revived the interest in how the theory of head metamerism might explain head and neck development. It has been possible to show that the segmental development of the somitomeres and rhombomeres may be related to each other and to the expression of homeotic genes and that these events in turn are related to the formation of the pharyngeal arches.

The Cranial Paraxial Mesoderm and the Brain of Vertebrate Embryos Are Transiently Segmented

As described in Chapter 3, the paraxial mesoderm initially differentiates into whorl-like structures called **somitomeres.** Most somitomeres proceed to form somites. The first seven somitomeres, however, never form somites. These somitomeres develop next to the caudal end of the forebrain, the midbrain, and the cranial half of the hindbrain. The four somitomeres that develop next to the caudal half of the hindbrain differentiate to form the four occipital somites.

The neural tube also displays segmentation early in its development (see Chs. 4 and 13). This segmentation is clearest in the hindbrain (rhombencephalon), which is transiently divided into a series of small swellings called **neuromeres** or, more specifically, **rhombomeres.** Nine rhombomeres form in rats, fishes, and humans; eight have been detected in the chick.

In the Chick, the Rhombomeres Are Spatially Related to the First Three Pharyngeal Arches and Their Cranial Nerves

In the chick, each of the first three pharyngeal arches is aligned with two pairs of rhombomeres (Fig. 12–36). Experiments in which the roots of the cranial nerves serving these arches were injected with a fluorescent dye showed, moreover, that the corresponding motor nuclei develop in one pair of the rhombomeres: The motor nuclei of cranial nerve V (serving the first arch) develop in rhombomere 2 (r2); those of cranial nerve VII (serving the second arch) develop in r4; and those of cranial nerve IX (serving the third arch) develop in r6. Furthermore, the motor roots of cranial nerves III through XI initially grow through the cranial portions of the adjacent somitomere. The somitomeres thus appear to guide the growing motor axons of these cranial nerves in the same way that the somites in the neck and trunk guide the motor nerve axons of spinal nerves (see Ch. 5).

Figure 12–36. Stylized depiction of the brain stem showing the spatial relationships of the pharyngeal arches, neuromeres, cranial nerves, cranial nerve motor nuclei, neural crest domains, somitomeres and somites, and *Hox, Eux-1, Pax-2,* and *Krox-20* gene expression. (*Krox-20, Eux-1,* and *Pax-2,* like the *Hox* genes, have been implicated in transcription regulation.) (Data from Lumsden A, Keynes R. 1989. Segmental patterns of neuronal development in the chick hindbrain. Nature [London] 337:424; Wilkinson DG, Bhatt S, Cook M, et al. 1989. Segmental expression of *Hox-2* homeobox-containing genes in the developing mouse hindbrain. Nature [London] 341:405; Jacobson AG. 1992. Somitomeres: mesodermal segments of the head and trunk. In Hanken J, Hall BH [eds]: The Vertebrate Skull. University of Chicago Press, Chicago; and Krumlauf R. 1993. *Hox* genes and pattern formation in the branchial region of the vertebrate TIG 9:106.)

The Developmental Fate of Hindbrain Neural Crest Cells is Determined Before They Leave the Neural Tube

Quail–chick transplantation experiments have shown that the neural crest cells that migrate into each of the pharyngeal arches arise from the adjacent portion of the hindbrain neural tube. Moreover, the developmental fate of these crest cells is determined *before* the cells leave the neural tube. For example, if the presumptive first-arch neural crest of a quail is transplanted to the site of the presumptive second-arch neural crest in a chick, it will migrate into the second arch but will differentiate to produce ectopic first-arch structures, in-

cluding jaw elements and Meckel's cartilage. Surprisingly, even when much of the hindbrain neural crest cells and the dorsal hindbrain are ablated, neural crest cells regenerate at the cut edge of the rhombencephalon. Moreover, the regenerated neural crest migrates into appropriate arches and differentiates into appropriate arch-specific structures. This is in contrast to the situation in the trunk, where the fate of the crest cells is determined largely by the influences they encounter during their migration.

As described earlier in this chapter, each of the first three pharyngeal arches derives its myoblast cells from an adjacent somitomere. The fate of these myoblast cells is not determined while they are in the somitomere. Instead, they are apparently guided to the appropriate pharyngeal arch by a connective tissue substratum laid down by the neural crest cells during their previous migration. Moreover, the differentiation of the myoblasts within the pharyngeal arch apparently is directed by the resident neural crest cells which enclose the somitomere-derived mesodermal core at the cranial, lateral, and caudal perimeters of each pharyngeal arch. In the quail–chick transplantation experiment described above, not only did the quail first-arch neural crest cells form first-arch skeletal elements in the second arch, but also the normal chick myoblast cells of the second arch formed typical first-arch musculature.

Segmentation of the Rhombomeres in Animals Appears to Be Regulated by Growth Factors

As in the case of somite segmentation, fibroblast growth factor appears to play a pivotal role in the segmentation of the hindbrain into rhombomeres. Transiently, with the appearance of rhombomeric segments in chicken embryos, **FGF-3** is first expressed in rhombomeres 4 and 5, but is then quickly expressed only at the **boundaries between adjacent rhombomeres.** FGF-3 expression then disappears in the region of rhombomeric boundaries just before disappearance of the transient morphologic boundaries that demarcate the rhombomeres, suggesting that this growth factor may play a pivotal role in rhombomere segmentation. Interestingly, in transplantation studies, the engraftment of odd-numbered rhombomeres next to even-numbered rhombomeres results in re-expression of FGF-3 at the contiguous boundary between them. In contrast, however, the engraftment of odd-numbered rhombomeres next to odd-numbered rhombomeres or engraftment of even-numbered rhombomeres next to even-numbered rhombomeres fails to stimulate re-expression of FGF-3 at their boundaries.

In addition, it is also quite apparent that each rhombomere is specified by a combinatorial code of *Hox* gene expression similar to that described for the paraxial mesoderm and somites in the trunk (see the Experimental Principles section of Ch. 4). In fact, the anterior expression boundaries of several *Hox* genes coincide exactly with rhombomere boundaries, providing a basis for the unique developmental function of each rhombomere (see Fig. 12–36).

Distinct Functions of *Hox* Genes in Pharyngeal Arch Development Are Revealed by Studies of Gain-of-Function and Loss-of-Function Transgenic Mice

The pattern of expression of a *Hox* gene can be mapped by using a technique called **in situ hybridization,** which localizes the messenger RNA of the gene (Fig. 12–37). When this technique is applied to mouse embryos after the formation of the rhombomeres, a number of *Hox* genes are found to be expressed in different but overlapping domains along the rhombomeres and adjacent paraxial mesoderm (see Fig. 12–36). When the pattern of expression of these *Hox* genes is combined with the patterns of expression of some other kinds of regulatory genes, each rhombomere expresses a unique combination of regulatory genes. This pattern could be responsible for the independent differentiation of each rhombomere.

Knockout of *Hoxa-1* in transgenic mice results in severe alteration of rhombomeres 4 and 5. Rhombomere 4 is significantly reduced, and rhombomere 5 is almost absent. The parts of these rhombomeres that remain fuse with rhombomere 6 to form a single "fourth" rhombomere. As an apparent consequence, the motor nuclei of facial and abducens nerves that normally develop within rhombomeres 4, 5, and 6 (see Fig. 12–36) are not formed.

Targeted disruption of *Hoxa-2*, however, produces a truly dramatic effect. Indeed, the effect can be described as a **homeotic transformation of pharyngeal arch 2 to pharyngeal arch 1.** The resulting mice thus exhibit duplication of first-arch structures. For example, first-arch skeletal elements duplicated in the second arch include the **malleus** and **incus** bones. Interestingly, an additional **atavistic** element appears that corresponds to the reptilian **pterygoquadrate** bone. On the other hand, duplications of first-arch dermal bones such as the **maxillary** and **palatine** bones do not occur. It has been suggested that only neural crest derivatives from the rhombencephalon (mainly from the

Figure 12–37. Expression of (*A*) *Hoxb-5* and (*B*) *Hoxc-8* messenger RNA in adjacent sections of a mouse embryo, visualized using the technique of in situ hybridization. (From Holland PWH, Hogan B. 1988. Spatially restricted patterns of expression of the homeobox-containing gene *Hoxb-5* during mouse embryogenesis. Development 102:159.)

fourth rhombomere) are affected by the mutation. Thus, because dermal bones of the first arch are derived from neural crest cells migrating from the mesencephalon, they are not duplicated by this mutation.

One explanation for effects of the disruption of *Hoxa-2* is that a *Hox*-independent ground pattern drives development of the first pharyngeal arch and underlies development of the second pharyngeal arch. Knockout of the *Hoxa-2* gene in arch 2 thus transforms the overriding *Hoxa-2*-driven developmental program of the second arch to the basic ground pattern-driven program of the first arch. A prediction of this hypothesis is that ectopic expression of *Hoxa-2* in cranial rhombomeres of the metencephalon and mesencephalon (which produce neural crest cells that populate the first arch) will result in duplication of the second arch.

Several Interacting Factors Have Been Implicated in Regulation of *Hox* Gene Expression in Individual Arches and in Craniofacial Development

Disruption of *Hoxa-1* expression in transgenic mice (see earlier) also results in reduction of *Hoxb-1* expression, thereby resulting in deletion of rhombomeres exhibiting rhombomere 4 and rhombomere 5 identity (see earlier). Conversely, in a gain-of-function mutant in which *Hoxa-1* is expressed ectopically, *Hoxb-1* is also expressed, transforming rhombomere 2 to a rhombomere 4 identity. These experiments support the possibility that *Hox* gene expression is, to some extent, interactive, that the expression of one may depend, in part, on expression of another.

In the homozygous **kreisler segmentation mutant** of the mouse, rhombomeres 5 and 6 are transformed to rhombomere 4. Thus, rhombomeres 4 to 7 appear to be replaced by a region of unsegmented neural tube. Structures produced by the second and third pharyngeal arches (respectively populated by neural crest from rhombomeres 4 and 6) are abnormal; the greater horn of the hyoid bone exhibits an accessory process, probably an ectopic second arch structure, the lesser horn of the hyoid. In situ analysis shows that expression patterns of several *Hox* genes and the *Krox-20* gene, which encodes a transcription factor unrelated to the *Hox* genes, are significantly disturbed. For example, during normal development, *Krox-20* is normally expressed first in rhombomere 3, then rhombomeres 3 and 5, and then is finally restricted to rhombomere 5. In the kreisler mutant, *Krox-20* is never expressed in rhombomere 5 and is only weakly expressed in rhombomere 3. The cranial expression boundaries of *Hoxb-3* and *Hoxb-4* are cranialized, from the boundary between rhombomeres 4/5 and 6/7 to 3/4 and 4/5, respectively. The expression domain of the gene encoding **FGF-3** is also cranially displaced and its activity significantly reduced.

All of these results taken together support

the hypothesis that the specific development of each neural crest subpopulation and subsequent differentiation of structures in each pharyngeal arch depend on interactions of unique constellations of elements within each rhombomere. Indeed, many other factors are implicated in the differentiation of the pharyngeal arches, including the transcription factor **Barx1, endothelin-1,** the zygotic gene *m-twist,* the homeobox genes **goosecoid,** *Lim-1,* and genes of the **NK gene family, platelet-derived growth factor,** and the zinc-finger proteins **snail** and **slug.** Recall from Chapter 3 that Lim-1 expression is essential for cranial organization of the primitive streak and development of the entire head.

The *Dlx* Gene Family Plays Important Roles in Craniofacial and Inner Ear Development

The *Dlx* gene family encodes a group of evolutionarily conserved homeobox-containing transcription factors involved in early embryonic patterning. These genes are related to the *distal-less (dll)* gene of *Drosophila.* In humans and in mice there are six members of the *Dlx* gene family: *Dlx1-3* and *Dlx5-7.* Both expression data and findings from mice with targeted mutations in some of these genes have revealed crucial roles for *Dlx* family members in craniofacial and inner ear development (Table 12–3).

Dlx1-3 and *Dlx5-6* are expressed in the first and second branchial arches, as well as parts of the developing brain and, in the case of *Dlx2* and *Dlx5,* the developing limb. Targeted homozygous *Dlx1* or *Dlx2* mutants have a number of defects, including abnormalities or loss of particular first arch splanchnocranial bones (e.g., the proximal part of the ala temporalis, a component of the alisphenoid), and proximal dermatocranial structures (e.g., palatine and pterygoid bones in *Dlx1* and *Dlx2* mutants, and maxillary and squamosal bones in *Dlx2* mutants), and loss of second arch splanchnocranial structures (including the stapes and styloid bone). Although targeted mutations of *Dlx3* are embryonic lethal due to defects in placental development, a human disease, **tricho-dento-osseous syndrome,** has been linked to *Dlx3* muta-

tions, with patients manifesting malformations of the teeth and calavaria.

The autosomal dominant form of another human syndrome called **split hand/split foot malformation** (SHFM; also called lobster-claw deformity) has been linked to mutations in the *Dlx5* gene. Patients with this mutation typically have missing digits and a clawlike appearance of the distal extremities. In addition to deformities in the extremities, some SHFM patients also have craniofacial and other abnormalities. Interestingly, mice with targeted mutations of *Dlx5* have severe craniofacial and inner ear defects. The functions of *Dlx6* and *Dlx7* are still not clear, but their expression patterns are also consistent with a role in craniofacial development.

Retinoic Acid May Play a Role in Normal and Abnormal Development of the Head and Neck

It is clear that **retinoic acid** is a potent craniofacial teratogen, especially affecting arches 1 and 2; this presumptive morphogen has also been implicated in normal differentiation of head and neck structures. Ectopic application of retinoic acid to developing chick embryos, for example, transforms rhombomeres 2/3 to rhombomeres 4/5. Recall from the Experimental Principles section of Chapter 4 that excess retinoic acid results in a caudalization of axial structures in the trunk. In addition, the application of excess retinoic acid inhibits neural crest migration, resulting in hypoplasia of the first three arches. More direct evidence of the role of retinoic acid in normal development, however, is provided by the results of double retinoic acid receptor knockout experiments (see the Experimental Principles section of Ch. 7). These knockouts result in arch-related craniofacial abnormalities. Finally, the mediation of retinoic acid effects by *Hox* genes is supported by the discovery of **retinoic acid response elements** in **enhancers** of *Hoxa-1* and *Hoxa-2.* In addition, knockouts of these elements abolish the normal expression of *Hoxa-1* and *Hoxa-2* in the neural epithelium caudal to the fourth rhombomere.

Table 12–3
Developmental Functions of *Dlx* Genes in Mice and Humans

GENE	CHROMOSOME	PHENOTYPE IN TARGETED MOUSE MUTATION	HUMAN DISEASE
Dlx1	Mouse: 2 Human: 2q32	aberrant cranial neural crest-derived skeletal elements	?
Dlx2	Mouse: 2 Human: 2q32	aberrant cranial neural crest-derived skeletal elements leading to cleft palate; also show altered differentiation of olfactory bulb interneurons	?
Dlx3	Mouse: n.d. Human: 17q21.33-22	early embryonic lethal	tricho-dento-osseous syndrome
Dlx5	Mouse: 6 Human: 7q22	numerous craniofacial and inner ear defects; exencephaly in some null embryos	split-hand/split foot malformation
Dlx6	Mouse: 6 Human: 7q22	?	?
Dlx7l	Mouse: n.d. Human: 17q21.33-22	?	?

Adapted from Kraus P, Lufkin T. 1999. Mammalian Dlx homeobox gene control of craniofacial and inner ear morphogenesis. J Cell Biochem 32:136.

The Unique Specification of Each Neural Crest Subpopulation Occurs Before Migration Into Respective Pharyngeal Arches

Even when rhombencephalic neural crest cells and dorsal regions of the rhombencephalon are ablated, the neural crest cells regenerating from the cut edge of the hindbrain (see earlier) continue to express *Hox* genes unique to their regions of origin. It therefore seems likely that the rhombomere-specific identity of these cells is determined by unique patterns of *Hox* gene expression within these specific segments of the neural tube, before neural crest cell detachment and migration. Support for this possibility is provided by a rhombomere transplantation experiment. In normal chicken embryos, the cranial expression boundary of *Hoxa-2* is at the border between rhombomere 1 and rhombomere 2 (see Fig. 12–36). Therefore, *Hoxa-2* is expressed in both rhombomeres 2 and 4. Uniquely, however, the neural crest cells derived from rhombomere 2 do not express this *Hox* gene once they begin to migrate or within the arch they migrate to—the first pharyngeal arch. In contrast, *Hoxa-2* expression is not downregulated in the neural crest cells

derived from rhombomere 4; they continue to express *Hoxa-2* along their migratory pathway and within the second pharyngeal arch. The likelihood that the difference in *Hoxa-2* expression in these two rhombomere-specific populations of neural crest cells is determined by **prepatterning** within the rhombomere rather than by **influences of the migratory pathway,** was further supported by results of an experiment in which the positions of rhombomere 2 and rhombomere 4 were switched. *Hoxa-2* expression patterns were not altered by the switch in position; *Hoxa-2* gene expression continued to be downregulated in neural crest derived from rhombomere 2 and maintained in neural crest derived from rhombomere 4.

Patterning by neural crest of several pharyngeal pouch derivatives has also been shown to be essential for their normal development. For example, the targeted disruption of *Hoxa-3* in mice results in abnormal development of pharyngeal pouch derivatives received from or patterned by neural crest. These include the thymus and the telopharyngeal (ultimobranchial) bodies. Cell tracing experiments demonstrate, however, that the defects in these structures do not result from disruptions of migration but rather from the inability of the neural crest cells to differentiate or appropriately induce responsive tissues. These mice are athymic and the ultimobranchial (telopharyngeal) bodies are abnormal, thus reflecting the developmental dependence of these structures on a specific neural crest subpopulation.

Members of the Sonic Hedgehog Family Are Required for Normal Forebrain and Craniofacial Development in Mice and Humans

Among other phenotypes (see Ch. 4 and 11), mice with targeted sonic hedgehog (Shh) mutations exhibit cyclopia, the most severe form of holoprosencephaly (see Clinical Applications). As in the case of the interaction between the notochord and ventral spinal cord, Shh expression in the prechordal mesoderm appears to play a key role in the induction of ventral midline structures in the forebrain. These include the optic stalks that normally express *Pax-2* in response to the Shh signal of the prechordal mesoderm. As might be expected (see Ch. 4, Experimental Principles), development of ventral midline structures in the presumptive spinal cord, such as the floor plate and motor columns, is also disrupted. Although the notochord forms in these animals, it rapidly degenerates. Collectively, these findings support a crucial role for Shh in midfacial and forebrain development as well as maintenance of the notochord.

Findings from mice with targeted Shh mutations and from other mouse mutants have also shed light on why particular human craniofacial syndromes are sometimes accompanied by limb and axial defects. As discussed in Chapter 4, sonic hedgehog (Shh) expressed by the notochord induces the medial region of the somite to form the sclerotome. Recall from Chapter 11 that Shh also plays a key role in craniocaudal differentiation of the limb buds. Thus, one might expect that Shh mutations or mutations that mediate Shh activity would have multiple defects involving the limbs, axial skeleton, forebrain, and craniofacial structures. Interestingly, heterozygous *extra-toes* (*Xt*) mice, identified in a series of irradiation experiments, exhibit polysyndactyly in all four limbs as well as an enlarged frontal bone and hydrocephaly. Homozygous *Xt* mice are nonviable and have more severe craniofacial defects including midbrain exen-

cephaly. A human syndrome that shares numerous similarities with the *Xt* phenotype is **Greig cephalopolysyndactyly,** in which patients have polydactyly, an enlarged forehead, and **hypertelorism** (abnormally increased distance between the eyes). Greig cephalopolysyndactyly and the *Xt* phenotype have been linked to deletions or other mutations in the *gli3* gene that encode a transcription factor downstream of Shh, linking this defect to aberrant Shh signaling. Another mouse mutant displaying both limb and craniofacial defects is *doublefoot*, which exhibits extreme polydactyly accompanied by foreshortening of the tibia and fibula, a broad skull, and lack of fission of the maxillary processes. In these mice, another member of the Shh family, **Indian hedgehog (Ihh)** is ectopically expressed in the limb bud mesenchyme and in the visceral arches.

It is now clear that normal Shh signaling depends upon an autoprocessing step that cleaves the molecule into carboxyl and amino terminal fragments. During this process, the carboxyl fragment functions as a cholesterol transferase that covalently links cholesterol to the amino fragment as a lipophilic adduct converting the amino fragment to an active Shh signaling factor. Thus, given the phenotype of the Shh knockout described earlier, it should not be surprising that similar holoprosencephalic malformations occur in pups born to rats treated with inhibitors of cholesterol biosynthesis. Similarly, this relationship between cholesterol and Shh signaling may also explain the occurrence of holoprosencephalic and limb abnormalities in humans suffering from the autosomal recessive disorder Smith-Lemli-Opitz syndrome (SLOS). It is estimated that this autosomal recessive disease, which is characterized by elimination of activity of the last enzyme in the cholesterol pathway, affects about 1 in 9000 births (alive and stillborn).

Deletions in the human homologue for sonic hedgehog **(SHH),** which maps to chromosome 7q36, result in recessive inheritance of holoprosencephaly. In contrast, truncations or amino acid substitutions of SHH result in dominant inheritance of HPE, and mild forms of HPE may occur following translocation at several HPE breakpoints even though the SHH gene itself is not disrupted. These human forms of holoprosencephaly mimic the phenotype that occurs in murine knockouts of Shh.

It has also been suggested that the disruption of other human homologues of the *Drosophila* **segment polarity genes** may result in holoprosencephaly. For example, *Wnt-4* is absent in zebrafish cyclops mutants and missexpression of *Wnt-4* also results in cyclopia in zebrafish.

SUGGESTED READING

Development of the Head and Neck

Ballabio M, Nicolini U, Jowett T, et al. 1989. Maturation of thyroid function in normal human fetuses. Clin Endocrinol 31:565

Ferguson MWJ. 1988. Palate development. Development 103(suppl):41

Friedberg J. 1989. Pharyngeal cleft sinuses and cysts, and other benign neck lesions. Pediatr Clin North Am 36:1451

Gans C. 1987. The neural crest: a spectacular invention. p. 361. In Maderson PFA (ed): Developmental and Evolutionary Aspects of the Neural Crest. John Wiley, New York

Gans C. 1988. Craniofacial growth, evolutionary questions. Development 103(suppl):3

Goeringer GC, Vidic SD. 1987. The embryogenesis and anatomy of Waldeyer's ring. Otolaryngol Clin North Am 20:207

Hengerer AS. 1984. Embryological development of the sinuses. Ear Nose Throat J 63:134

Le Douarin NM, Ziller C, Couly GF. 1993. Patterning of neural crest derivatives in the avian embryo: in vivo and in vitro studies. Dev Biol 159:24

Lobach DF, Haynes BF. 1987. Ontogeny of the human thymus during fetal development. J Clin Immunol 7:81

Margriples U, Laitman JT. 1987. Developmental change in the position of the fetal human larynx. Am J Phys Anthropol 72:463

Marion M, Hinojosa R, Khan AA. 1985. Persistence of the stapedial artery: a histopathologic study. Otolaryngol Head Neck Surg 93:298

Merida-Velasco JA, Garcia-Garcia JD, Espin-Ferra J, Linares J. 1989. Origin of the ultimobranchial body and its colonizing cells in human embryos. Acta Anat 136:325

Muller F, O'Rahilly R, Tucker J. 1985. The human larynx at the end of the embryonic period proper. 2. The laryngeal cavity and the innervation of its lining. Ann Otol Rhinol Laryngol 94:607

Noden DM. 1984. Craniofacial development: new views on old problems. Anat Rec 208:1

Noden DM. 1988. Interactions and fates of avian craniofacial mesenchyme. Development 103(suppl):121

O'Rahilly R. 1978. The timing and sequence of events in the development of the human digestive system and associated structures during the embryonic period proper. Anat Embryol 153:123

O'Rahilly R, Muller F. 1984. The early development of the hypoglossal nerve and occipital somites in staged human embryos. Am J Anat 169:237

O'Rahilly R, Muller F. 1987. Developmental stages in human embryos. Carnegie Inst Wash Publ 637:1

Siefert R, Crist B. 1990. On the differentiation and origin of myoid cells in the avian thymus. Anat Embryol 181:287

Swarts JD, Rood SR, Doyle WJ. 1986. Fetal development of the auditory tube and paratubal musculature. Cleft Palate J 23:289

Tan SS, Morriss-Kay GM. 1986. Analysis of cranial neural crest cell migration and early fates in postimplantation rat chimeras. J Embryol Exp Morphol 98:21

Thorogood P. 1988. The developmental specification of the vertebrate skull. Development 103(suppl):141

Trainer PA, Tam PP. 1995. Cranial paraxial mesoderm and neural crest cells of the mouse embryo: co-distribution in the craniofacial mesenchyme but distinct segregation in branchial arches. Development 121:2569

Van der Linden EJ, Burdi A, de Jonge HJ. 1987. Critical periods in the prenatal morphogenesis of the human lateral pterygoid muscle, the mandibular condyle, the articular disk and medial articular capsule. Am J Orthod Dentofacial Orthop 91:22

von Gaudecker B. 1986. The development of the human thymus microenvironment. p. 1. In Muller-Hermelink HK (ed): The Human Thymus, Histophysiology and Pathology. Springer-Verlag, Berlin

von Gaudecker B. 1988. Development and functional anatomy of the human tonsilla palatina. Acta Otolaryngol (suppl) 454:28

Wachtler F, Jacob M. 1986. Origin and development of the cranial skeletal muscles. Bibl Anat 29:24

Wedden SE, Ralphs JR, Tickle C. 1988. Pattern formation in the facial primordia. Development 103(suppl):31

Wong G, Weinberg S, Symington JM. 1985. Morphology of the developing articular disc of the human temporomandibular joint. J Oral Maxillofac Surg 43:565

Zaw-Tun HA. 1985. Reexamination of the origin and early development of the human larynx. Acta Anat 122:163

Development of the Eyes

Barnstable CJ. 1987. A molecular view of vertebrate retinal development. Mol Neurobiol 1:9

Jacobson AG, Sater AK. 1988. Features of embryonic induction. Development 104:341

O'Rahilly R. 1966. The early development of the eye in staged human embryos. Contrib Embryol Carnegie Inst 38:1

O'Rahilly R. 1983. The timing and sequence of events in the development of the human eye and ear during the embryonic period proper. Anat Embryol 168:87

Noden D. 1983. The role of the neural crest in patterning of avian cranial skeletal, connective, and muscle tissues. Dev Biol 96:144

Saha MS, Spann C, Grainger RM. 1989. Embryonic lens induction: more than meets the optic vesicle. Cell Differ Dev 28:153

Sevel D. 1988. A reappraisal of development of the eyelids. Eye 2:123

Tam P. 1989. Regionalization of the mouse embryonic ectoderm: allocation of prospective ectodermal tissues during gastrulation. Development 107:55

Wachtler F. 1984. The extrinsic ocular muscles in birds are derived from the prechordal plate. Naturwissenschaften 71:379

Development of the Ears

Declau F, Jacob W, Dorrine W, et al. 1989. Early ossification within the human fetal otic capsule: morphological and microanalytical findings. J Laryngol Otol 103:1113

Gilbert P. 1957. The origins and development of the human extrinsic ocular muscles. Contrib Embryol Carnegie Inst 246:61

Mallo M, Gridley T. 1996. Development of the mammalian ear: coordinate regulation of formation of the tympanic ring and the external acoustic meatus. Development 122:173

Marquet JE, DeClau F, De Cock M, et al. 1988. Congenital middle ear malformations. Acta Otorhinolaryngol Belg 42:117

McPhee JR, Van De Water TR. 1986. Epithelial-mesenchymal tissue interactions guiding otic capsule formation: the role of the otocyst. J Embryol Exp Morphol 97:1

Michaels L. 1988. Origin of congenital cholesteatoma from a normally occurring epidermoid rest in the developing middle ear. Int J Pediatr Otorhinolaryngol 15:51

Moro J, Pastor F, Gato A, Barbosa E. 1990. Patterns of epithelial cell death during early development of the human inner ear. Ann Otol Rhinol Laryngol 99:482

O'Rahilly R. 1963. The early development of the otic vesicle in staged human embryos. J Embryol Exp Morphol 11:741

Van De Water TR. 1988. Tissue interactions and cell differentiation: neurone-sensory cell interaction during otic development. Development 103(suppl):185

Van De Water TR. 1980. The morphogenesis of the

middle and the external ear. Birth Defects: Orig Artic Ser 16:147

Clinical Applications

al-Ghamdi S, Freedman A, Just N, et al. 1992. Fourth branchial cleft cyst. J Otolaryngol 21:447

Ali F, Persaud TVN. 1988. Mechanisms of fetal alcohol effects: role of acetaldehyde. Exp Pathol 33:17

Anneren G, Gustafsson J, Sunnegardh J. 1989. DiGeorge syndrome in a child with partial monosomy of chromosome 22. Uppsala J Med Sci 94:47

Bockman DE, Kirby ML. 1985. Neural crest interactions in the development of the immune system. J Immunol 135:766s

Burdi AR, Kusnetz AB, Venes JL, Gebarski SS. 1986. The natural history and pathogenesis of the cranial coronal ring articulations: implications in understanding the pathogenesis of the Crouzon craniostenotic defects. Cleft Palate 23:28

Cozzi F, Myers NA, Piacenti S, et al. 1993. Maturational dysautonomia and facial anomalies associated with esophageal atresia: support for neural crest involvement. J Pediatr Surg 28:798

Ferguson MWJ. 1987. Palate development: mechanisms and malformations. Ir J Med Sci 156:309

Granstrom G, Kullaa-Mikkonen A. 1990. Experimental craniofacial malformations induced by retinoids and resembling branchial arch syndromes. Scand J Plast Reconstr Surg Hand Surg 24:3

Hall BK. 1982. Mandibular morphogenesis and craniofacial malformations. J Craniofac Genet Dev Biol 2:309

Hinojosa R, Green JD, Brecht K, et al. 1996. Otocephalus: histopathology and three-dimensional reconstruction. Otolaryngol Head Neck Surg 114:44

Kirby M. 1989. Plasticity and predetermination of mesencephalic and trunk neural crest transplanted into the region of the cardiac neural crest. Dev Biol 134:402

McNutt TL, Harris C. 1994. Lindane embryotoxicity and differential alteration of cysteine and glutathione levels in rat embryos and visceral yolk sacs. Reprod Toxicol 8:351

Nucci P, Manitto MP, Faiella A, et al. 1994. Balanced translocation (t 2q; 10p) and ocular anomalies. A possible HOX gene defect. Ophthal Gen Z 15:129

Poswillo D. 1988. The aetiology and pathogenesis of craniofacial deformity. Development 103(suppl):207

Pruzansky S, Costaras M, Rollnick BR. 1982. Radiocephalometric findings in a family with craniofrontonasal dysplasia. Birth Defects Orig Artic Ser 18:121

Rutledge JC. 1989. Recent advances in prenatal craniofacial development: report of a conference and review of topics. Pediatr Pathol 9:613

Shean ML, Duester G. 1993. The role of alcohol dehydrogenase in retinoic acid homeostasis and fetal alcohol syndrome. Alcohol Alcohol 2(suppl):51

Slavkin HC. 1993. Rieger syndrome revisited: experimental approaches using pharmacologic and antisense strategies to abrogate EGF and TGF-alpha functions resulting in dysmorphogenesis during embryonic mouse craniofacial morphogenesis (review). Am J Med Genet 47:689

Solazza L, Madaro E, De Gionni PP, et al. 1994. Dermoid cysts of the oral floor. A clinical case report and review of the literature. Minerva Stomatol 43: 171

Sperber GH, Honoré LH, Machin GA. 1989. Microscopic study of holoprosencephalic facial anomalies in trisomy 13 fetuses. Am J Med Genet 32:443

Snodgrass SR. 1994. Cocaine babies: a result of multiple teratogenic influences. J Child Neurol 9:227

Sperber GH, Johnson ES, Honoré L, Machin GA. 1987. Holoprosencephalic synophthalmia (cyclopia) in an 8 week fetus. J Craniofac Genet Dev Biol 7:7

Sulik KK. 1984. Craniofacial defects from genetic and teratogen-induced deficiencies in presomite embryos. Birth Defects Orig Artic Ser 20:79

Sulik KK, Cook CS, Webster WS. 1988. Teratogens and craniofacial malformations: relationships to cell death. Development 103(suppl):213

Sulik KK, Johnston MC, Daft PA, et al. 1986. Fetal alcohol syndrome and DiGeorge anomaly: critical ethanol exposure periods for craniofacial malformations as illustrated in an animal model. Am J Med Genet 2(suppl):97

Sulik KK, Johnston MC, Smiley SJ, et al. 1987. Mandibulofacial dysostosis (Treacher Collins syndrome): a new proposal for pathogenesis. Am J Med Genet 27:359

Taylor LE, Bennett GD, Finnel RH. 1995. Altered gene expression in murine branchial arches following in utero exposure to retinoic acid. J Craniofac Genet Dev Biol 15:13

Van Mierop LHS, Kutsche LM. 1986. Cardiovascular anomalies in DiGeorge syndrome and importance of neural crest as a possible pathogenetic factor. Am J Cardiol 58:133

Walker PJ, Edwards MJ, Petroff V, et al. 1995. Agnathia (severe micrognathia), aglossia and choanal atresia in an infant. J Pediatr Child Health 31:358

Waterson EJ, Murray-Lyon IM. 1990. Preventing alcohol related birth damage: a review. Soc Sci Med 30:349

Webster WS, Lipson AH, Sulik KK. 1988. Interference with gastrulation during the third week of pregnancy as a cause of some facial abnormalities and CNS defects. Am J Med Genet 31:505

Wedden SE. 1987. Epithelial-mesenchymal interactions in the development of chick facial primordia and the target of retinoid action. Development 99:341

West JR, Chen WJ, Pantzis NJ. 1994. Fetal alcohol syndrome: the vulnerability of the developing brain and possible mechanisms of damage. Metab Brain Dis 9:291

Willhite C, Hill RM, Irving D. 1986. Isotretinoin-induced craniofacial malformations in humans and hamsters. J Craniofac Genet Dev Biol 2(suppl):193

Experimental Principles

Akam M. 1989. *Hox* and *HOM:* homologous gene clusters in insects and vertebrates. Cell 57:347

Alberch P, Kollar E. 1988. Strategies of head development: workshop report. Development 103(suppl): 25

Balling R, Mutter G, Gruss P, Kessel M. 1989. Craniofacial abnormalities induced by ectopic expression of the homeobox gene *Hox-1.1* in transgenic mice. Cell 58:337

Barnes JD, Crosbey JL, Jones CM, et al. 1994. Embryonic expression of *Lim-1*, the mouse homolog of *Xenopus XLim-1*, suggest a role in lateral mesoderm differentiation and neurogenesis. Dev Biol 161:168

Belloni E, Muenke M, Roessler E, et al. 1996. Identification of Sonic Hedgehog as a candidate gene responsible for holoprosencephaly. Nat Genet 14: 353

Birgbauer E, Sechrist J, Bronner-Fraser M, et al. 1995. Rhombomeric origins and rostrocaudal reassortment of neural crest cells revealed by intravital miscroscopy. Development 121:935

Chan VY, Tam PPL. 1988. A morphological and experimental study of the mesencephalic neural crest cells in the mouse embryo using wheat germ agglutinin-gold conjugate as the cell marker. Development 102:427

Chiang G, Litingtung Y, Lee E, et al. 1996. Cyclopia and defective axial patterning in mice lacking sonic hedgehog gene function. Nature 383:407

Ciment G, Weston JA. 1985. Segregation of developmental abilities in neural-crest-derived cells: identification of partially restricted intermediate cell types in the branchial arches of avian embryos. Dev Biol 111:73

Couly GF, LeDouarin N. 1987. Mapping of the early neural primordium in quail-chick chimeras. II. The prosencephalic neural plate and neural folds: implications for the genesis of cephalic human congenital abnormalities. Dev Biol 120:198

Cserjesi P, Brown D, Lyons GE, et al. 1995. Expression of the novel basic helix-loop-helix gene *eHAND* in neural crest derivatives and extraembryonic membranes during mouse development. Dev Biol 170: 664

Dean M. 1996. Polarity, proliferation and the hedgehog pathway. Nat Genet 14:245

Dickinson ME, Krumlauf R, McMahon AP. 1994. Evidence for a mitogenic effect of *Wnt-1* in the developing mammalian central nervous system. Development 120:1453

Dolle P, Lufkin T, Krumlauf, et al. 1993. Local alterations of *Krox20* and *Hox* gene expression in the hindbrain suggest lack of rhombomers 4 and 5 in homozygote null *Hoxa-1 (Hoxo-1.6)* mutant embryons. Proc Natl Acad Sci U S A 90:7666

Dony C, Gruss P. 1988. Expression of a murine homeobox gene precedes the induction of c-fos during mesodermal differentiation of P19 teratocarcinoma cells. Differentiation 37:115

Duboule D, Dolle P. 1989. The structural and functional organization of the murine *Hox* gene family resembles that of *Drosophila* homeotic genes. EMBO J 8:1497

Fekete DM. 1999. Development of the vertebrate ear: insights from knockouts and mutants. Trends Neurosci 22:263

Frasch M, Chen X, Lufkin T. 1995. Evolutionary-conserved enhancers direct region-specific expression of the murine *Hoxa-1* and *Hoxa-2* loci in both mice and *Drosophila*. Development 121:957

Fraser S, Keynes R, Lumsden A. 1990. Segmentation in the chick embryo hindbrain is defined by cell lineage restrictions. Nature (London) 344:431

Frohman MA, Martin GR, Cordes SP, et al. 1993. Altered rhombomere-specific gene expression and hyoid bone differentiation in the mouse segmentation mutant, kreisler (kr). Development 117:925

Gaunt SJ, Blum M, De Robertis EM. 1993. Expression of the mouse goosecoid gene during mid-embryogenesis may mark mesenchymal cell lineages in the developing head, limbs and body wall. Development 117:769

Gaunt SJ, Sharpe PT, Duboule D. 1988. Spatially restricted domains of homeo-gene transcripts in mouse embryos: relation to a segmented body plan. Development 103(suppl):169

Gendron-Maguire M, Mallo M, Zhang M, et al. 1993. *Hoxa-2* mutant mice exhibit homeotic transformation of skeletal elements derived from cranial neural crest. Cell 75:1317

Goodrich ES. 1930. Studies on the Structure and Development of Vertebrates. Macmillan, London

Hanneman EH, Trevarrow B, Metcalfe W, et al. 1988. Segmental pattern of development of the hindbrain and spinal cord of the zebrafish embryo. Development 103(suppl):49

Hart P, Krumlauf R. 1991. Deciphering the *Hox* code: clues to patterning branchial regions of the head. Cell 66:1075

Holland PWH. 1988. Homeobox genes and the human head. Development 103(suppl):117

Hopwood ND, Pluck A, Gurdon JB. 1989. A *Xenopus* mRNA related to *Drosophila* twist is expressed in response to induction in the mesoderm and the neural crest. Cell 59:893

Hunt P, Ferretti P, Krumlauf F, et al. 1995. Restoration of normal *Hox* code and branchial arch morphogenesis after extensive deletion of hindbrain neural crest. Dev Biol 168:584

Irving D, Willhite C, Burk D. 1986. Morphogenesis of isotretinoin-induced microcephaly and micrognathia studied by scanning electron microscopy. Teratology 34:141

Jacobson AG. 1988. Somitomeres: mesodermal segments of vertebrate embryos. Development 104(suppl):209

Jacobson AG. 1993. Somitomeres: mesodermal segments

of the head and trunk. In Hanken J, Hall BH (eds): The Skull. University of Chicago Press, Chicago

Jeffs P, Jaques K, Osmund M. 1992. Cell death in cranial neural crest development. Anat Embryol 185:583

Jefferies RPS. 1986. The Ancestry of the Vertebrates. Cambridge University Press, Cambridge

Kessel M, Balling R, Gruss P. 1990. Variations of cervical vertebrae after expression of a *Hox 1.1* transgene in mice. Cell 61:301

Kessel M, Gruss P. 1990. Murine developmental control genes. Science 249:374

Kraus P, Lufkin T. 1999. Mammalian Dlx homeobox gene control of craniofacial and inner ear morphogenesis. J Cell Biochem 32–33:133

Kurtani SC, Eichele G. 1993. Rhombomere transplantation repatterns the segmental organization of cranial nerves and reveals cell-autonomous expression of a homeodomain protein. Development 117:105

Krumlauf R. 1993. Mouse *Hox* genetic functions. Curr Opin Genet Devel 3:621

Krumlauf R. 1993. *Hox* genes and pattern formation in the branchial region of the vertebrate head. Trends Genet 9:106

Krumlauf R. 1994. *Hox* genes in vertebrate development. Cell 78:191

Krumlauf R, Marshall H, Studer M, et al. *Hox* homeobox genes and regionilization of the nervous system. J Neurobiol 124:1328

LeDouarin N, Smith J. 1988. Development of the peripheral nervous system from the neural crest. Annu Rev Cell Biol 4:375

Lee YM, Osumi-Yamashita N, Ninomiya Y, et al. 1995. Retinoic acid stage dependently alters the migration pattern and identity of hindbrain neural crest cells. Development 121:825

Leonard L, Horton C, Maden M, et al. 1995. Anteriorization of CRABP-1 expression by retinoic acid in the developing mouse central nervous system and its relationship to teratogenesis. Dev Biol 168:514

Lewis J. 1989. Genes and segmentation. Nature (London) 341:382

Lohnes D, Mark M, Mendelsohn C, et al. 1995. Developmental roles of the retinoic acid receptors. J Steroid Biochem Mol Biol 53:475

Lonai P, Orr-Urtreger A. 1990. Homeogenes in mammalian development and the evolution of the cranium and the central nervous system. FASEB J 4:1436

Lumsden A, Keynes R. 1989. Segmental patterns of neuronal development in the chick hindbrain. Nature (London) 337:424

Lumsden A, Sprawson N, Graham A. 1991. Segmental origin and migration of neural crest cells in the hindbrain region of the chick embryo. Development 113:1281

Lyn S, Giguere V. 1994. Localization of CRABP-I and CRABP-II mRNA in the early mouse embryo by whole-mount in situ hybridization: implications for teratogenesis and neural development. Dev Dynam 199:280

Maden M, Horton C, Graham A, et al. 1992. Domains of cellular retinoic acid-binding protein I (CRABPI) expression in the hindbrain and neural crest of the mouse embryo. Mech Dev 37:13

Mahmood R, Flanders KC, Morriss-Kay GM. 1992. Interactions between retinoids and TGF-βs in mouse morphogenesis. Development 116:67

Mahmood R, Kiefer P, Guthrie S, et al. 1995. Multiple roles for FGF-3 during cranial neural development in the chicken. Development 121:1399

Manley NR, Cappecchi MR. 1995. The role of Hoxa-3 in mouse thymus and thyroid development. Development 121:1989

Mark M, Lufkin T, Vonesch JL, et al. 1993. Two rhombomers are altered in Hoxa-1 mutant mice. Development 119:39

Marshall H, Nonchev S, Sham MH, et al. 1992. Retinoic acid alters hindbrain Hox code and induces transformation of rhombomeres 2/3 into a 4/5 identity. Nature 360:737

McKay IJ, Muchamore I, Krumlauf R, et al. 1994 The kreisler mouse: a hindbrain segmentation mutant that lacks two rhombomeres. Development 120: 2199

Meier S. 1979. Development of the chick mesoblast: formation of the embryonic axis and establishment of the metameric pattern. Dev Biol 73:25

Meier S. 1981. Development of the chick embryo mesoblast: morphogenesis of the prechordal plate and cranial segments. Dev Biol 83:49

Mendelsohn C, Lohnes D, Decimo D, et al. 1994. Function of the retinoic acid receptors (RARs) during development (II). Multiple abnormalities at various stages of organogenesis in RAR double mutants. Development 120:2749

Moore G, Ivens A, Chambers J, et al. 1988. The application of molecular genetics to detection of craniofacial abnormality. Development 103(suppl):233

Moro Balbas JA, Gato A, Alonso Revuelta MI, et al. 1993. Retinoic acid induces changes in the rhomboencephalic neural crest cells migration and extracellular matrix composition in chick embryos. Teratology 48:197

Morrison-Graham K, Schatteman GC, Bork T, et al. 1992. A PDGF receptor mutation in the mouse (Patch) perturbs the development of a nonneuronal subset of neural crest-derived cells. Development 115:133

Nieto MA, Sechrist J, Wilkinson DG, et al. 1995. Relationship between spatially restricted Krox-20 gene expression in branchial neural crest and segmentation of the chick embryo hindbrain. EMBO J 14: 1697

Murphy P, Davidson D, Hill RE. 1989. Segment-specific expression of a homeobox-containing gene in the mouse hindbrain. Nature (London) 341:156

Noden D. 1980. The migration and cytodifferentiation of cranial neural crest cells. p. 3. In Pratt RM, Christiansen RL (eds): Current Research Trends in Prenatal Craniofacial Development. Elsevier/North-Holland, New York

Noden DM. 1986. Patterning of avian craniofacial muscles. Dev Biol 116:347

Noden D. 1988. Interactions and fates of avian craniofacial mesenchyme. Development 103(suppl):121

Ohuchi H, Yoshioka H, Tanaka A, et al. 1994. Involvement of androgen-induced growth factor (FGF-8) gene in mouse embryogenesis and morphogenesis. Biochem Biophys Res Comm 204:882

Osumi-Yamashita N, Ninomiya Y, Doi H, et al. 1994. The contribution of both forebrain and midbrain crest cells to the mesenchyme in the frontonasal mass of mouse embryos. Dev Biol 164:409

Pannese M, Polo C, Andreazzoli M, et al. 1995. The Xenophus homolog of Otx2 is a maternal homeobox gene that demarcates and specifies anterior body regions. Development 121:707

Popperl H, Bienz M, Studer M, et al. 1995. Segmental expression of Hoxb-1 is controlled by a highly conserved autoregulatory loop dependent upon exd/pbx. Cell 81:1031

Porter JA, Young KE, Beachy PA. 1996. Cholesterol modification of hedgehog signalling proteins in animal development. Science 274:255

Prince V, Lumsden A. 1994. Hoxa-2 expression in normal and transposed rhombomeres: independent regulation in the neural tube and neural crest. Development 120:911

Qiu M, Bulfone A, Martinez S, et al. 1995. Null mutation of Dlx-2 results in abnormal morphogenesis of proximal first and second branchial arch derivatives and abnormal differentiation in the forebrain. Genes Dev 9:2523

Raju K, Tang S, Dube ID, et al. 1993. Characterization and developmental expression of Tlx-1, the murine homolog of HOX11. Mech Dev 44:51

Rijli FM, Mark M, Lakkaraju S, et al. 1993. A homeotic transformation is generated in the rostral branchial region of the head by disruption of Hoxa-2, which acts like a selector gene. Cell 75:1333

Reid L. 1990. From gradients to axes, from morphogenesis to differentiation. Cell 63:875

Robinson GW, Mahon KA. 1994. Differential and overlapping expression domains of Dlx-2 and Dlx-3 suggest distinct roles for Distal-less homeobox genes in craniofacial development. Mech Dev 48: 199

Roessler E, Belloni E, Gaudenz K, et al. 1996. Mutations in the human Sonic Hedgehog gene cause holoprosencephaly. Nat Gen 14:357

Ruiz JC, Robertson EJ. 1994. The expression of the receptor-protein tyrosine kinase gene, eck, is highly restricted during early mouse development. Mech Dev 46:87

Schneider RA, Hu D, Helms JA. 1999. From head to toe: conservation of molecular signals regulating limb and craniofacial morphogenesis. Cell Tissue Res 296:103

Sechrist J, Scheron T, Bronner-Fraser M. 1994. Rhombomere rotation reveals that multiple mechanisms contribute to the segmental pattern of hindbrain neural crest migration. Development 120:1777

Sechrist J, Serbedzija GN, Scherson T, et al. 1993. Segmental migration of the hindbrain neural crest does not arise from its segmental generation. Development 189:691

Sham MH, Vesque C, Nonchev S, et al. 1993. The zinc finger gene *Krox20* regulates *HoxB2 (Hox 2.8)* during hindbrain segmentation. Cell 72:183

Shawlot W, Behringer R. 1995. Requirement for *Lim1* in head organization function. Nature 374:425

Shum L, Sakakura Y, Bringas P Jr, et al. 1993. EGF abrogation-induced fusilliform dysmorphogenesis of Meckel's cartilage during embryonic mouse mandibula morphogenesis in vitro. Development 118:903

Simeone A, Acampora D, Arcioni L, et al. 1990. Sequential activation of *HOX2* homeobox genes by retinoic acid in human embryonal carcinoma cells. Nature (London) 346:763

Simeone A, Avantaggiato V, Moroni MC, et al. 1995. Retinoic acid induces stage-specific antero-posterior transformation of rostral central nervous system. Mech Dev 51:83

Stadler HS, Solursh M. 1994. Characterization of the homeobox-containing gene *GH6* identifies novel regions of homeobox gene expression in the developing chick embryo. Dev Biol 161:251

Stoetzel C, Weber B, Bourgeois P, et al. 1995. Dorsoventral and rostro-caudal sequential expression of *M-twist* in the postimplantation murine embryo. Mech Dev 51:251

Studer M, Popperl H, Marshall H, et al. 1994. Role of conserved retinoic acid response element in rhombomere restriction of *Hoxb-1*. Science 265:1728

Tan S, Morriss-Kay G. 1985. The development and distribution of the cranial neural crest in the rat embryo. Cell Tissue Res 240:403

Tissier-Seta JP, Mucchielli ML, Mark M, et al. 1995. *Barxl*, a new mouse homeodomain transcription factor expressed in cranio-facial ectomesenchyme and the stomach. Mech Dev 51:3

Tongiori E, Bernhardt RR, Zinn K, et al. 1995. Tenascin-C mRNA is expressed in cranial neural crest cells, in some placodal derivatives, and in discrete domains of the embryonic zebrafish brain. J Neurobiol 28:391

Trainor PA, Pam PP. 1995. Cranial paraxial mesoderm and neural crest cells of the mouse embryo: co-distribution of the cranio-facial mesenchyme but distinct segregation in branchial arches. Development 121:2569

Treisman JE. 1999. A conserved blueprint for the eye? Bioessays 21:843

Tsuzuki, Takahashi M, Asai N, et al. 1995. Spatial and temporal expression of the rat proto-oncogene product in embryonic, infant and adult rat tissues. Oncogene 10:191

Tuckett F, Lim L, Morriss-Kay G. 1985. The ontogenesis of cranial neuromeres in the rat embryo. I. A scanning electron microscope and kinetic study. J Embryol Exp Morphol 87:215

Wawersik, Maas RL. 2000. Vertebrate eye development as modeled in Drosophila. Hum Mol Genet 9:917

Wedden SE, Ralphs JR, Tickle C. 1988. Pattern formation in the facial primordia. Development 103(suppl):31

Wilkinson DG, Bhatt S, Charvier P, et al. 1989. Segment-specific expression of a zinc-finger gene in the developing nervous system of the mouse. Nature (London) 337:461

Wilkinson DG, Bhatt S, Cook M, et al. 1989. Segmental expression of *Hox-2* homeobox-containing genes in the developing mouse hindbrain. Nature (London) 341:405

Willhite CC, Hill RM, Irving D. 1986. Isotretinoin-induced craniofacial malformations in human and hamsters. J Craniofac Genet Dev Biol 2(suppl): 193

Zhang M, Kim HJ, Marshall H, et al. 1994. Ectopic *Hoxa-1* induces rhombomere transformation in mouse hindbrain. Development 120:2431

13

Development of the Brain and Cranial Nerves

Summary

Even before neurulation begins, the primordia of the three **primary brain vesicles**—the **prosencephalon, mesencephalon,** and **rhombencephalon**—are visible as broadenings in the neural plate. During the fifth week, the prosencephalon subdivides into a **telencephalon** and a **diencephalon,** and the rhombencephalon subdivides into a **metencephalon** and a **myelencephalon;** thus, along with the mesencephalon, creating five **secondary brain vesicles.** During this period the brain is also transiently divided into smaller segments called **neuromeres.**

The primordial brain undergoes flexion at three points. The forebrain folds back under the rest of the brain at the **mesencephalic (cranial) flexure.** Ventral folding also occurs at a **cervical flexure** between the myelencephalon and the spinal cord. Reverse, dorsal bending at the **pontine flexure** in the region of the future pons folds the metencephalon back against the myelencephalon.

The cytodifferentiation of the neural tube begins in the rhombencephalon at the end of the fourth week. As described in Chapter 4, the neural tube neuroepithelium proliferates to produce, in succession, the neuroblasts, glioblasts, and ependyma of the central nervous system. The neuroblasts migrate peripherally to establish a **mantle zone,** the precursor of the gray matter. In the regions of the spinal cord and brain stem, the mantle zone immediately overlies the **ventricular zone** of proliferating neuroepithelium, and the growing neuronal fibers establish a **marginal zone** (the future white matter) peripheral to the mantle zone. In the higher centers of the brain, including the cerebellum and cerebral hemispheres, the pattern of cytodifferentiation is more complex.

The mantle zone of the brain stem, like that of the spinal cord, is organized into a pair of **ventral (basal) columns** (or **plates**) and a pair of **dorsal (alar) columns** (or **plates**). Laterally, the two columns are separated by a groove called the **sulcus limitans;** dorsally and ventrally, they are separated by thinnings of the neural tissue called, respectively, the **roof plate** and the **floor plate.**

The nuclei of the 3rd to 12th cranial nerves are located in the brain stem. Some of these cranial nerves are motor, some are sensory, and some are mixed, and therefore some of them arise from more than one nucleus. The cranial nerve motor nuclei develop from the brain stem basal plates, and the associational nuclei develop from the brain stem alar plates. The brain stem cranial nerve nuclei are organized into seven columns, which correspond to the types of function they subserve. From ventromedial to dorsolateral, the three basal columns contain **somatic efferent, branchial efferent,** and **visceral efferent** motor neurons, and

Development of the Regions of the Brain

Organization of the Cranial Nerves and Their Nuclei and Ganglia

Cytodifferentiation in the Brain

Development of the Ventricular System

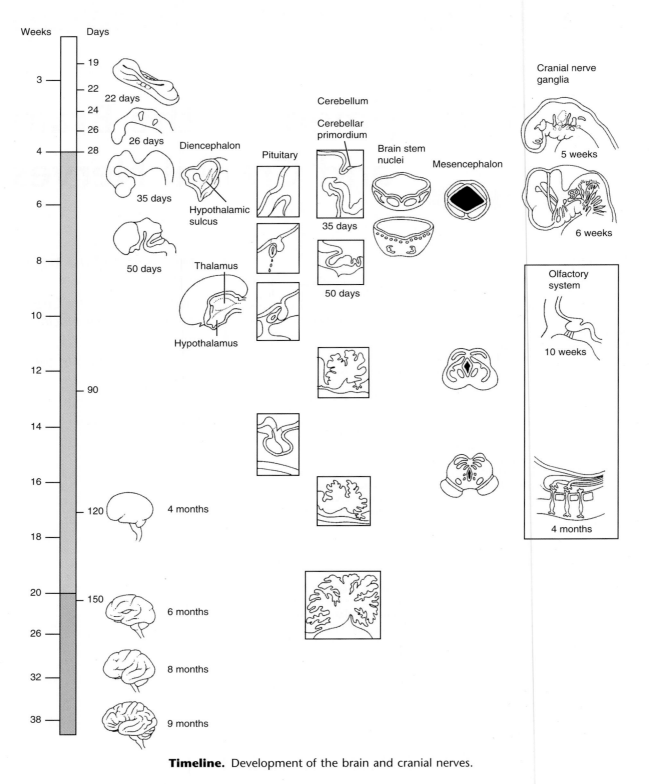

Timeline. Development of the brain and cranial nerves.

the four alar columns contain **visceral afferent, special visceral afferent** (subserving the special sense of taste), **general afferent,** and **special somatic afferent** (subserving the special senses of hearing and balance) associational neurons.

As in the spinal cord, the peripheral neurons of the sensory and autonomic (parasympathetic) cranial nerve pathways reside in ganglia located outside the central nervous system. Cranial nerve parasympathetic ganglia are derived from neural crest. Some cranial nerve sensory ganglia develop from neural crest, but some are derived partly or entirely from **ectodermal placodes.**

The myelencephalon gives rise to the **medulla oblongata,** which is the portion of the brain most similar in organization to the spinal cord. The metencephalon gives rise to the **pons,** an expansion that consists mainly of the massive white matter tracts serving the cerebellum, and to the **cerebellum.** The cerebellum arises from the dorsal **rhombic lips** of the metencephalic alar plates, which flank the expanded roof plate in this region. A specialized process of cytodifferentiation in the cerebellum gives rise to the gray matter of the **cerebellar cortex,** as well as to internal **basal nuclei.** The cerebellum controls posture, balance, and the smooth execution of movements.

The mesencephalon contains nuclei of three cranial nerves as well as various other structures. In particular, the alar plates give rise to the **superior** and **inferior colliculi,** which are visible as round protuberances on the dorsal surface of the midbrain. The superior colliculi control ocular reflexes; the inferior colliculi serve as relays in the auditory pathway.

The forebrain has no basal plates. The alar plates of the diencephalon are divided into a dorsal portion and a ventral portion by a deep groove called the **hypothalamic sulcus.** The **hypothalamic swelling** ventral to this groove differentiates into the nuclei collectively known as the **hypothalamus,** the most prominent function of which is to control visceral activities such as heart rate and pituitary secretion. Dorsal to the hypothalamic sulcus, the large **thalamic swelling** gives rise to the **thalamus,** which serves as a relay center, processing information from subcortical structures before passing it to the cerebral cortex. Finally, a dorsal swelling, the **epithalamus,** gives rise to a few diminutive structures, including the pineal gland.

A ventral outpouching of the diencephalic floor plate, called the **infundibulum,** differentiates to form the **posterior pituitary.** A matching diverticulum of the stomodeal roof, called **Rathke's pouch,** grows to meet the infundibulum and becomes the **anterior pituitary.** Diencephalic outpouchings also form the eyes, as discussed in Chapter 12.

The two **cerebral hemispheres** arise as lateral outpouchings of the telencephalon and grow rapidly to cover the diencephalon and mesencephalon. The hemispheres are joined by the cranial **lamina terminalis** (representing the zone of closure of the cranial neuropore) and by fiber tracts called **commissures,** particularly the massive **corpus callosum.** The layered cellular architecture of the cerebral cortex arises by a complex mechanism. The **olfactory bulbs** and **olfactory tracts** arise from the cranial telencephalon and synapse with the primary olfactory neurosensory cells, which differentiate in the nasal placodes.

The expanded **primitive ventricles** formed by the neural canal in the secondary brain vesicles give rise to the ventricular system of the brain. The cerebrospinal fluid that fills the ventricle system is produced mainly by secretory **choroid plexuses** in the lateral, third, and fourth ventricles, which are formed by the ependyma and overlying vascular pia. The third ventricle also contains specialized ependymal secretory structures called **circumventricular organs.**

THE THREE PRIMARY BRAIN VESICLES SUBDIVIDE TO FORM FIVE SECONDARY BRAIN VESICLES

Chapters 3 and 4 describe how the central nervous system (CNS) arises as a neural plate from the ectoderm of the germ disc and folds to form the neural tube. The presumptive brain is visible as the broad cranial portion of the neural plate. The quail–chick transplantation system (described in the Experimental Principles section of Ch. 5) has been used to discover which parts of the neural folds give rise to which parts of the brain. In these experiments, a small portion of chick neural fold is replaced with the homologous portion from a quail, and the structures developing from the quail cells are identified on the basis of their prominent nucleoli (see Fig. 5–11).

Even on day 19, before neurulation begins, the three major divisions of the brain—the **prosencephalon (forebrain), mesencephalon (midbrain),** and **rhombencephalon (hindbrain)**—are demarcated by indentations in the neural folds. The future eyes appear as outpouchings from the forebrain neural folds by day 22 (see Ch. 12). Neurulation begins on day 22, and the cranial neuropore closes on day 24. The three brain divisions are then marked by expansions of the neural tube called **primary brain vesicles** (Fig. 13–1*A, B*).

By day 21, an additional series of narrow swellings called **neuromeres** becomes apparent in the future brain (see Fig. 13–1*B*). At least six neu-

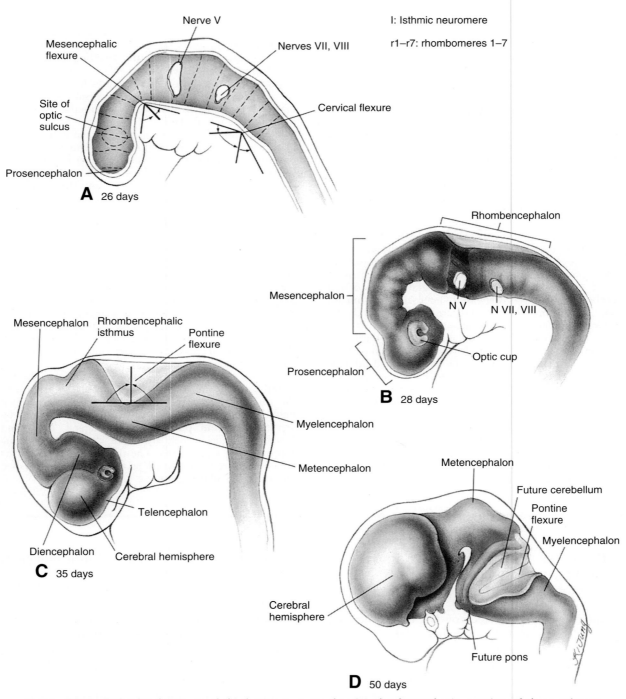

Figure 13–1. Early development of the brain. *A, B,* By day 26, the future brain consists of three primary brain vesicles (the prosencephalon, the mesencephalon, and the rhombencephalon between the bending at the mesencephalic and cervical flexures. *C, D,* Further subdivision of the brain vesicles creates five secondary vesicles: the enlarged mesencephalon, the metencephalon and myelencephalon (that arise from the rhombencephalon), and the diencephalon and telencephalon (that arise from the prosencephalon). The cerebral hemispheres appear and expand rapidly. The pontine flexure folds the metencephalon back against the myelencephalon.

romeres may form in the presumptive prosenceph-alon (P1 to P6), one (M1) in the presumptive mesencephalon, and nine in the presumptive rhombencephalon. The nine hindbrain segments consist of a single **isthmic segment,** occupying the constricted isthmic region of the rhombencepha-lon, and eight **rhombomeres,** numbered r1 through r8. The neuromeres are transient struc-tures and become indistinguishable by the early sixth week. Their possible relation with the seg-mentation of the paraxial mesoderm and pharyn-geal arches is discussed in the Experimental Princi-ples section of Chapter 12.

During the fifth week, the mesencephalon enlarges and the prosencephalon and rhomben-cephalon each subdivide into two portions, thus converting the three primary brain vesicles into five **secondary brain vesicles** (see Fig. 13–1*C*). The prosencephalon divides into a cranial **telen-cephalon** ("end-brain") and a caudal **diencephalon** ("between-brain"). The rhombencephalon divides into a cranial **metencephalon** ("behind-brain") and a caudal **myelencephalon** ("medulla-brain"). Within each of the brain vesicles, the neural canal is expanded into a cavity called a **primitive ventri-cle.** These primitive ventricles will become the de-finitive ventricles of the mature brain (see Fig. 13–15). The rhombencephalon cavity becomes the **fourth ventricle,** the mesencephalon cavity be-comes the cerebral **aqueduct (of Sylvius),** the di-encephalon cavity becomes the **third ventricle,** and the telencephalon cavity becomes the paired **lateral ventricles** of the cerebral hemispheres. Af-ter the closure of the caudal neuropore, the devel-oping brain ventricles and the central canal of the spinal cord (see Ch. 4) are filled with **cerebro-spinal fluid,** a specialized dialysate of blood plasma.

The Brain Folds at The Mesencephalic, Cervical, and Pontine Flexures

Between the fourth and eighth weeks, the brain tube folds sharply at three locations (see Fig. 13–1). The first of these folds to develop is the **mes-encephalic flexure (cranial flexure)** in the midbrain region (see Ch. 6). The prosencephalon rotates ventrally and then posteriorly around this hinge during the fourth and fifth weeks until it is folded back under the mesencephalon. Ventral flexion begins during the fifth week at the **cervical flexure** between the myelencephalon and the spi-nal cord and continues through the eighth week. The development of the cranial and cervical flex-ures is closely related to the craniocaudal folding of the embryonic disc (see Ch. 6).

During the fifth week, reverse, dorsal flexion begins at the location of the developing pons. By the eighth week, the deepening of this **pontine flexure** has folded the metencephalon (including the developing cerebellum) back onto the myelen-cephalon. The pontine flexure may form as a result of differential growth in the ventral part of the metencephalon.

THE FUNDAMENTAL ORGANIZATION OF THE BRAIN STEM AND CRANIAL NERVES IS SIMILAR TO THAT OF THE SPINAL CORD AND SPINAL NERVES

For purposes of description, the brain can be di-vided into two parts: the **brain stem,** which repre-sents the cranial continuation of the spinal cord and is similar to it in organization, and the **higher centers,** which are extremely specialized and retain little trace of a spinal cord-like organization. The brain stem consists of the myelencephalon, the metencephalon derivative called the **pons,** and the mesencephalon. The higher centers consist of the cerebellum (derived from the metencephalon) and the forebrain.

The Brain Stem Is Initially Organized Into Basal and Alar Columns

As described in Chapter 4, the neurons of the developing spinal cord aggregate to form four plates or cell columns: two **basal (ventral) col-umns** and two **alar (dorsal) columns.** The basal columns contain the somatic and visceral motor neurons, and the alar columns contain the associa-tion neurons that synapse with *afferent* (incoming) fibers from the sensory neurons of the dorsal root ganglia. The axon of an association neuron may synapse with motor neurons on the same (ipsilateral) or opposite (contralateral) side of the cord, forming a reflex arc, or may ascend to the brain. The outgoing (*efferent*) motor neuron fibers exit via the ventral roots.

This fundamental pattern of alar columns, basal columns, dorsal sensory roots, and ventral motor roots is detectable in the brain stem and cranial nerves, although the pattern is more elaborate in the brain stem. It is also altered during development as some groups of neurons migrate away from their site of origin to establish a nucleus elsewhere. The primitive pattern is much less easy to detect in the forebrain. Basal plates are entirely lacking in the forebrain. The diencephalon has alar plates, but it is not clear whether the gray matter of the telencephalon represents alar plates.

The Early Differentiation of the Brain Stem Is Similar to That of the Spinal Cord

In the brain stem, as in the spinal cord, all the cell types of the CNS except the microglia are produced by the neuroepithelium lining the neural canal (see Ch. 4). An initial wave of proliferation produces the neuroblasts, which migrate peripherally. As neuroblast production tapers off, a second wave produces the glioblasts, which also migrate peripherally and differentiate to form astrocytes and oligodendrocytes. The layer of neuroepithelium lining the neural canal then differentiates to form the ependyma (see Fig. 4–16).

The neuroblasts aggregate to form a **mantle zone** surrounding the proliferating neuroepithelium, which is then called the **ventricular zone.** Neuronal fibers produced by the mantle neurons form a **marginal zone** external to the mantle layer. The mantle layer gives rise to the **gray matter** of the CNS, whereas the marginal layer gives rise to the **white matter,** so called because of the whitish color imparted by the fatty myelin sheaths that wrap around many of the nerve fibers. In the CNS, these sheaths are formed by oligodendrocytes rather than by Schwann cells. The marginal layer contains the nerve fibers entering and leaving the CNS as well as the fiber tracts coursing to higher or lower levels in the CNS.

The differentiation of the neural tube begins in the region of the rhombencephalon. Because this portion of the brain stem contains most of the cranial nerve nuclei, its morphogenesis will now be described.

THE WALLS OF THE RHOMBENCEPHALON SPLAY APART TO FORM A TROUGHLIKE FOURTH VENTRICLE WITH A THIN ROOF PLATE

The roof and floor plates of the spinal cord are narrow and lie at the bottom of deep grooves. In the rhombencephalon, in contrast, the walls of the neural tube splay open dorsally so that the roof plate is stretched and widened and the alar and basal plates lie nearly parallel to each other in an oblique plane (Fig. 13–2). The rhombencephalic neural canal (future fourth ventricle) is diamond shaped in dorsal view, with the widest point located at the pontine flexure. The dorsal margin of the alar plate, from which the roof plate arises, is called the **rhombic lip.** Cranial to the pontine flexure, the rhombic lip is thickened and laps over onto the roof of the neural canal. This metencephalic portion of the rhombic lip will give rise to the cerebellum.

The thin rhombencephalic roof plate consists mainly of a layer of ependyma and is covered by a well-vascularized layer of pia mater called the **tela choroidea.** On either side of the midline, the pia and ependyma form a zone of minute, finger-like structures projecting into the fourth ventricle. This zone, called a **choroid plexus,** is specialized to secrete cerebrospinal fluid. Similar choroid plexuses develop in the ventricles of the forebrain. Cerebrospinal fluid circulates constantly through the central canal of the spinal cord and the ventricles of the brain and also through the subarachnoid space surrounding the CNS, from which it is reabsorbed into the blood. The fluid gains access to the subarachnoid space via three holes that open in the roof plate of the fourth ventricle: a single **median aperture (foramen of Magendie)** and two **lateral apertures (foramina of Luschka).**

THE CRANIAL NERVE NUCLEI APPEAR IN THE BRAIN STEM DURING THE FIFTH WEEK

All of the 12 cranial nerves except the first (olfactory) and second (optic) arise from nuclei located

Figure 13–2. Early differentiation of the rhombencephalon. The roof plate in the rhombencephalic region forms a wide, transparent membrane over the fourth ventricle. The basal and alar columns give rise to the motor and associational nuclei, respectively, of most of the cranial nerves, as well as to other structures. Extensions of the alar columns also migrate ventrally to form pontine and olivary nuclei.

in the brain stem. These nuclei are among the earliest structures to develop in the brain. The basal plates of the rhombencephalon are the first neuronal aggregations in the CNS. By day 28, all the brain stem cranial nerve motor nuclei are distinguishable. As in the spinal cord, the alar plates of the brain stem form somewhat later than the basal plates, appearing in the middle of the fifth week. The cranial nerve associational nuclei are all distinguishable by the end of the fifth week. Figure 13–5 (see later) illustrates the development of the cranial nerves.

The Cranial Nerves Are Motor, Sensory, or Mixed

Although the cranial nerves show homologies to spinal nerves, they are much less uniform in composition. Three cranial nerves are exclusively sensory (I, II, and VIII); four are exclusively motor (IV, VI, XI, and XII); one is mixed sensory and motor (V); one is motor and parasympathetic (III); and three include sensory, motor, and parasympathetic fibers (VII, IX, and X). The motor and sensory fibers of the cranial nerves nevertheless bear the same basic relation to the cell columns of the brain that the ventral and dorsal roots bear to the cell columns of the spinal cord. Table 13–1 summarizes the relations of the cranial nerves to the subdivisions of the brain.

The Cranial Nerve Nuclei of the Brain Stem Are Organized Into Seven Columns on the Basis of Function

In the same way that the basal plates of the spinal cord are organized into somatic motor and autonomic motor columns (see Ch. 4), the basal and alar cranial nerve nuclei of the brain stem are organized into seven columns that subserve particular functions. Although seven columns form, some textbooks described only six functions, three motor and three sensory. These are as follows:

Motor functions (basal columns)

1. *Somatic efferent* neurons in the brain innervate the extrinsic ocular muscles and the muscles of the tongue.
2. *Branchial efferent* (sometimes called *special visceral efferent*) neurons serve the striated muscles derived from the pharyngeal arches. The motor nucleus of the accessory nerve (XI) is considered to be branchial efferent because it forms part of this column, even though the trapezius and sternocleidomastoid muscles that it innervates are not derived from branchial arch mesoderm.
3. *Visceral efferent* (sometimes called *general visceral*

Table 13–1
Location of the Cranial Nerve Nuclei

BRAIN REGION	ASSOCIATED CRANIAL NERVES
Telencephalon	Olfactory (I)
Diencephalon	Optic (II)
Mesencephalon	Oculomotor (III)
Metencephalon	Trochlear (IV) (Arises in the metencephalon but is later displaced into the mesencephalon)
	Trigeminal (V) (The trigeminal sensory nuclei arise in the metencephalon and myelencephalon but are later displaced partly into the mesencephalon. The trigeminal motor nucleus arises in the metencephalon and remains there.)
	Abducens (VI)
	Facial (VII)
	Vestibulocochlear (VIII)
Myelencephalon	Glossopharyngeal (IX)
	Vagus (X)
	Accessory (XI)
	Hypoglossal (XII)

efferent) neurons serve the parasympathetic pathways innervating the sphincter pupillae and ciliary muscles of the eyes and (via the vagus nerve) the smooth muscle and glands of the thoracic, abdominal, and pelvic viscera, including the heart, the airways, and the salivary glands.

Sensory functions (alar columns)

4. *Visceral afferent* association neurons receive impulses via the vagus nerve from sensory receptors in the walls of the thoracic, abdominal, and pelvic viscera (referred to as interoceptive sensory receptors).
5. *General afferent* association neurons in the brain subserve "general sensation" (touch, temperature, pain, etc.) over the head and neck as well as for the mucosa of the oral and nasal cavities and the pharynx.
6. *Special afferent* association neurons subserve the special senses. This function is sometimes sub-

divided into two functions—special visceral afferent (taste) and special somatic afferent (hearing and balance)—to match the two columns of special afferent nuclei that develop in the brain stem.

Figure 13–3 shows the arrangement of the seven columns of basal and alar cranial nerve nuclei in the brain stem. In the rhombencephalon, the columns are initially laid out in a rough plane from ventromedial to dorsolateral. Only two of the columns penetrate into the mesencephalon. Starting with the most ventromedial, the three basal (motor) columns are as follows:

1. The *somatic efferent* column consists of the nucleus of the hypoglossal nerve (XII) in the caudal rhombencephalon, the nucleus of nerve VI more cranially in the rhombencephalon, and the nuclei of nerves IV and III in the mesencephalon.
2. The *branchial efferent* column contains three nuclei serving nerves V, VII, and IX through XI and is confined to the rhombencephalon. The

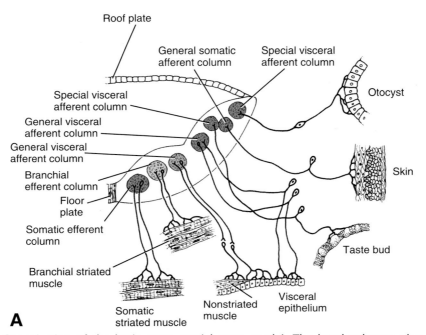

Figure 13–3. Organization of the brain stem cranial nerve nuclei. The basal columns give rise to motor (efferent) cranial nerve nuclei and the alar columns to associational (afferent) cranial nerve nuclei. These nuclei can be grouped into seven discontinuous columns, each subserving a specific type of function. *A,* Idealized organization of the brain stem cranial nerve nuclei into seven columns.

Illustration continued on following page

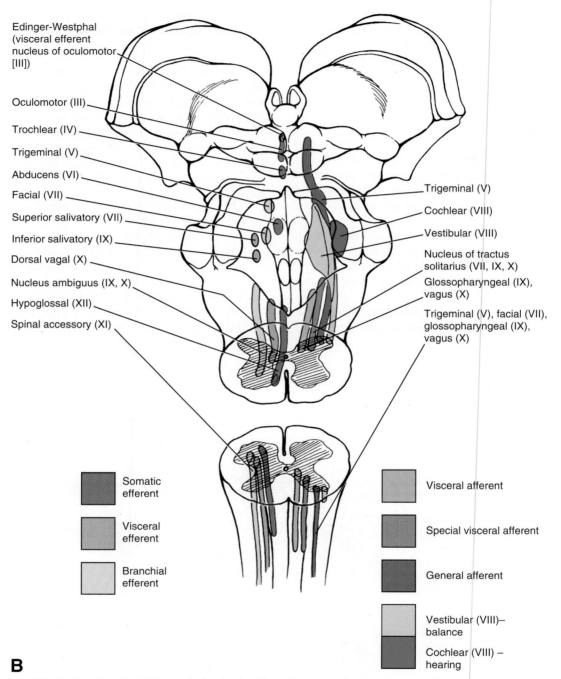

Edinger-Westphal
(visceral efferent
nucleus of oculomotor
[III])

Oculomotor (III)

Trochlear (IV)

Trigeminal (V)

Abducens (VI)

Facial (VII)

Superior salivatory (VII)

Inferior salivatory (IX)

Dorsal vagal (X)

Nucleus ambiguus (IX, X)

Hypoglossal (XII)

Spinal accessory (XI)

Trigeminal (V)

Cochlear (VIII)

Vestibular (VIII)

Nucleus of tractus
solitarius (VII, IX, X)

Glossopharyngeal (IX),
vagus (X)

Trigeminal (V), facial (VII),
glossopharyngeal (IX),
vagus (X)

Somatic
efferent

Visceral
efferent

Branchial
efferent

Visceral afferent

Special visceral afferent

General afferent

Vestibular (VIII)–
balance

Cochlear (VIII) –
hearing

B

Figure 13–3. *Continued. B,* View of the brain stem showing the locations of the cranial nerve nuclei making up the seven columns. The efferent nuclei are shown on the left and the afferent nuclei on the right. (*A,* Modified from Williams PL, Warwick R, Dyson M, Bannister LH. 1989. Gray's Anatomy. Churchill Livingstone, Edinburgh.)

branchial efferent nuclei serving nerves V and VII are located cranially in the rhombencephalon; caudally, the elongated **nucleus ambiguus** supplies branchial efferent fibers for nerves IX, X, and XI.

3. The *visceral efferent* column includes two nuclei located in the rhombencephalon. The **salivatory nuclei** innervate the salivary and lacrimal glands via nerves VII and IX. Just caudal to this nucleus is the **dorsal nucleus of the vagus,** which contains preganglionic parasympathetic neurons innervating the viscera. The Edinger-Westphal nucleus (III) is located in the mesencephalon.

From ventromedial to dorsolateral, the four alar (associational) columns are as follows:

1. The general *visceral afferent* column consists of the nucleus that receives interoceptive information via the glossopharyngeal (IX) and vagus nerve (X).
2. The first *special afferent* column (sometimes called the *special visceral afferent column*) consists of the **nucleus of the tractus solitarius,** which receives taste impulses via the facial (VII), glossopharyngeal (IX), and vagus (X) nerves.
3. The *general afferent* column consists of the neurons that receive impulses of general sensation from areas of the face served by the trigeminal (V) and facial (VII) nerves and from the oral, nasal, and pharyngeal and laryngeal cavities (V, IX, and X).
4. The second *special afferent* column (sometimes called the *special somatic afferent column*) consists of the **cochlear** and **vestibular nuclei,** which subserve the special senses of balance and hearing.

Some Brain Stem Nuclei Migrate After They Form

Not all of the nuclei that develop within the basal and alar columns remain where they form. The branchial efferent nucleus of the facial nerve, for example, travels first dorsocundally and then ventrally to arrive at a location deeper than would be expected on the basis of its function. The nucleus ambiguus also migrates, as do some of the noncranial nerve nuclei of the rhombencephalon, such as the **olivary** and **pontine nuclei,** which arise from the alar plate but migrate to a ventral posi-

tion (see Fig. 13–2). As CNS neurons migrate, they "reel out" their axons behind them; thus, the path of a nucleus can be reconstructed by tracing its axons.

PARASYMPATHETIC AND SENSORY GANGLIA DEVELOP IN ASSOCIATION WITH SOME CRANIAL NERVES

As in the rest of the body, the peripheral neurons of the cranial nerve sensory and parasympathetic pathways are housed in ganglia that lie outside the CNS. Like the rest of the autonomic system, the cranial parasympathetic system consists of two-neuron pathways: the central neuron of each pathway resides in a CNS nucleus, and the peripheral neuron resides in a ganglion. The cranial sensory and parasympathetic ganglia appear during the end of the fourth week and beginning of the fifth week (Table 13–2; see also Fig. 13–5). The cranial nerve sensory ganglia are comparable to the dorsal root ganglia of the spinal cord. The cranial nerve parasympathetic ganglia can be divided into two groups: the ganglia associated with the vagus nerve, which are located in the walls of the visceral organs (gut, heart, lungs, pelvic organs, etc; see Ch. 5), and the parasympathetic ganglia of cranial nerves III, VII, and IX, which innervate structures in the head. The head receives sympathetic innervation via nerves from the cervical chain ganglia (see Ch. 5).

Cranial Nerve Parasympathetic Ganglia Arise From the Neural Crest of the Brain

The origin of the neural crest cells giving rise to the various cranial nerve parasympathetic ganglia has been determined by using quail–chick chimera experiments. Each ganglion arises from neural crest located at roughly the same level as the corresponding brain stem nucleus (Figs. 13–4 and 13–5A; see also Fig. 12–8). Thus, the **ciliary ganglion** of the oculomotor nerve (III) is formed by neural crest arising in the caudal part of the diencephalon and the cranial part of the mesencephalon; the **sphenopalatine** and **submandibular ganglia** of the facial nerve (VII) are formed by neural

Table 13–2
Origins of the Neurons in the Cranial Nerve Ganglia

CRANIAL NERVE	GANGLION AND TYPE	ORIGIN OF NEURONS
Olfactory (I)	Olfactory epithelium (primary neurons of the olfactory pathway) (special afferent)	Nasal placode
Oculomotor (III)	Ciliary ganglion (visceral efferent)	Neural crest of the caudal diencephalon and cranial mesencephalon
Trigeminal (V)	Trigeminal ganglion (general afferent)	Neural crest of the caudal diencephalon and cranial mesencephalon; trigeminal placode
Facial (VII)	Superior ganglion of nerve VII (general and special afferent)	Rhombencephalic neural crest; 1st epibranchial placode
	Inferior (geniculate) ganglion of nerve VII (general and special afferent)	1st epibranchial placode
	Sphenopalatine ganglion (visceral efferent)	Rhombencephalic neural crest
	Submandibular ganglion (visceral efferent)	Rhombencephalic neural crest
Vestibulocochlear (VIII)	Acoustic (cochlear) ganglion (special afferent)	Otic placode
	Vestibular ganglion (special afferent)	Otic placode plus some contribution from neural crest
Glossopharyngeal (IX)	Superior ganglion (general and special afferent)	Rhombencephalic neural crest
	Inferior (petrosal) ganglion (general and special afferent)	2nd epibranchial placodes
	Otic ganglion (visceral efferent)	Rhombencephalic neural crest
Vagus (X)	Superior ganglion (general afferent)	Rhombencephalic neural crest
	Inferior (nodose) ganglion (general and special afferent)	3rd and 4th epibranchial placodes
	Vagal parasympathetic (enteric) ganglia (visceral efferent)	Rhombencephalic neural crest

crest cells that migrate from the cranial end of the rhombencephalon; and the **otic ganglion** of the glossopharyngeal nerve (IX) as well as the enteric ganglia served by the vagus nerve are derived from neural crest originating in the caudal portion of the rhombencephalon (see Ch. 5).

Cranial Nerve Sensory Ganglia Are Derived Partly From Neural Crest and Partly From Ectodermal Placodes

Quail–chick chimera experiments have shown that the cranial nerve sensory ganglia have a dual origin (see Fig. 13–5A–C). Some are formed from neural crest in the same way as the dorsal root ganglia of the spinal nerves, but others are derived partially or exclusively from **ectodermal placodes.** Three of these placodes—the nasal, lens, and otic placodes—were discussed in Chapter 12. In addition, a series of four **epibranchial placodes** develop as ectodermal thickenings just dorsal to the four pharyngeal clefts, and a more diffuse **trigeminal placode** develops in the area between the epibranchial placodes and the otic placode. In the chick, the epibranchial placodes give rise to neuronal precursors at a stage equivalent to the end of the fourth week in humans.

As discussed later in this chapter, the nasal placodes give rise to the primary neurosensory cells of the olfactory epithelium, and the axons of these cells form the olfactory nerve (I). With some

Figure 13–4. Scanning elecron micrograph showing neural crest cells migrating over the surface of the neural fold in the region of the future brain. In the brain region, the crest cells detach and begin to migrate, whereas the neural folds are still broadly open. In the spinal cord region, in contrast, the neural crest detaches as the folds fuse together along the midline. (From Tan SS, Morriss-Kay G. 1985. The development and distribution of the cranial neural crest in the rat embryo. Cell Tissue Res 240:403.)

exceptions, the remaining cranial nerve sensory ganglia show a regular stratification with respect to their origin: the ganglia (or portions of ganglia) that lie closest to the brain are derived from neural crest, whereas the neurons of ganglia (or portions thereof) lying farther from the brain are formed by placode cells. The supporting cells of all cranial nerve sensory ganglia, however, are derived from neural crest.

The **trigeminal (semilunar) ganglion** of cranial nerve V has a mixed origin: the proximal portion arises mainly from diencephalic and mesencephalic neural crest, whereas the neurons of the distal portion arise mainly from the diffuse trigeminal placode. The sensory ganglia associated with the second, third, fourth, and sixth pharyngeal arches are derived from the corresponding epibranchial placodes and from neural crest. Each of these nerves has both a proximal and a distal sensory ganglion. In general, the proximal-distal rule given earlier holds for these ganglia. The combined **superior ganglion** of nerves IX and X is formed by rhombencephalic neural crest, whereas the neurons of the **inferior (petrosal) ganglion** of nerve IX are derived from the second epibranchial placode and those of the **inferior (nodose) ganglion** of nerve X are derived from the third and fourth epibranchial placodes. The **superior combined ganglion** of nerves VII and VIII is derived from both the first epibranchial placode and the rhombencephalic neural crest, but the neurons of the **inferior (geniculate) ganglion** of nerve VII are derived exclusively from the first epibranchial placode. As mentioned in Chapter 12, the distal ganglia of cranial nerve VIII—the **vestibular ganglion** and the **cochlear ganglion**—differentiate from the otic placode.

THE RHOMBENCEPHALON GIVES RISE TO THE MEDULLA OBLONGATA, THE PONS, AND THE CEREBELLUM

The Medulla Oblongata Serves Mainly as a Relay Center Between the Spinal Cord and the Rest of the Brain

The myelencephalon differentiates to form the **medulla oblongata,** which is the portion of the brain most similar to the spinal cord. In addition to housing most of the cranial nerve nuclei, the medulla serves as a relay center between the spinal cord and the higher brain centers and also contains centers and nerve networks that regulate respiration, the heartbeat, reflex movements, and a number of other functions.

The Pons Is Composed Largely of White Matter Tracts That Serve the Cerebellum

The metencephalon gives rise to two structures: the **pons,** which functions mainly to relay signals between the spinal cord and the cerebral and cerebellar cortices, and the **cerebellum,** which is a center for balance and postural control. The pons (named after the Latin word for bridge) consists mainly of massive fiber tracts that relay information between the cerebrum, the cerebellum, and the spinal cord (Fig. 13–6). These tracts arise primarily from the marginal layer of the basal columns of the metencephalon. In addition, ventrally located **pontine nuclei** relay input from the cerebrum to the cerebellum (see Fig. 13–2).

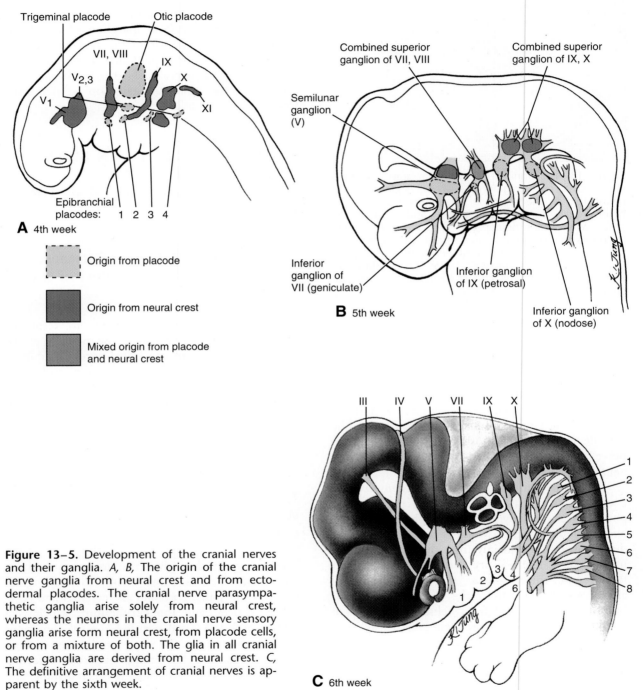

A 4th week

☐ Origin from placode

■ Origin from neural crest

▨ Mixed origin from placode and neural crest

Trigeminal placode
Otic placode
VII, VIII
IX
X
$V_{2,3}$
V_1
XI
Epibranchial placodes: 1 2 3 4

B 5th week

Combined superior ganglion of VII, VIII
Combined superior ganglion of IX, X
Semilunar ganglion (V)
Inferior ganglion of VII (geniculate)
Inferior ganglion of IX (petrosal)
Inferior ganglion of X (nodose)

C 6th week

III IV V VII IX X
1 2 3 4 5 6 7 8
1 2 3 4 6

Figure 13–5. Development of the cranial nerves and their ganglia. *A, B,* The origin of the cranial nerve ganglia from neural crest and from ectodermal placodes. The cranial nerve parasympathetic ganglia arise solely from neural crest, whereas the neurons in the cranial nerve sensory ganglia arise form neural crest, from placode cells, or from a mixture of both. The glia in all cranial nerve ganglia are derived from neural crest. *C,* The definitive arrangement of cranial nerves is apparent by the sixth week.

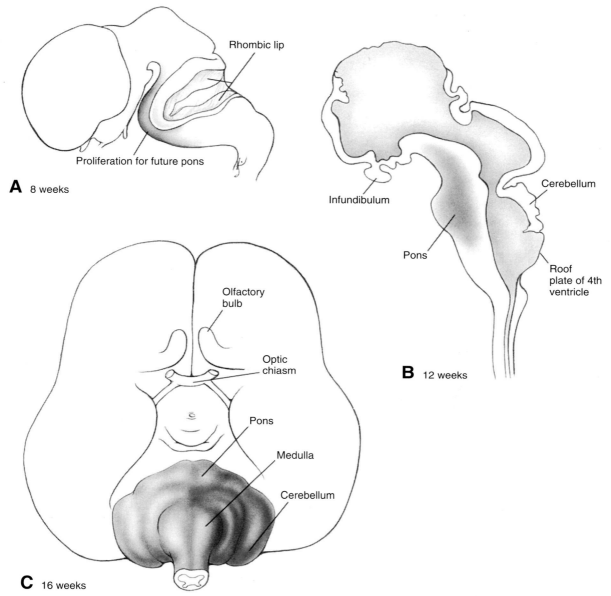

Figure 13–6. *A–C,* Development of the pons. The pons is formed by proliferation of cell and fiber tracts on the ventral side of the metencephalon.

The Cerebellum Is a Specialization of the Metencephalic Alar Plates

The cerebellum is derived largely from the rhombic lips of the metencephalon. It begins to develop at the end of the sixth week and continues to grow after birth, although its gross morphology is similar in the newborn and the adult.

The metencephalic rhombic lips thicken at the end of the sixth week to produce a pair of **cerebellar plates (cerebellar primordia)** (Fig. 13–7; see also Fig. 13–2). By the second month, the cranial portions of the growing rhombic lips meet across the midline, forming a single primordium that covers the fourth ventricle. This primordium initially bulges only into the fourth ventricle

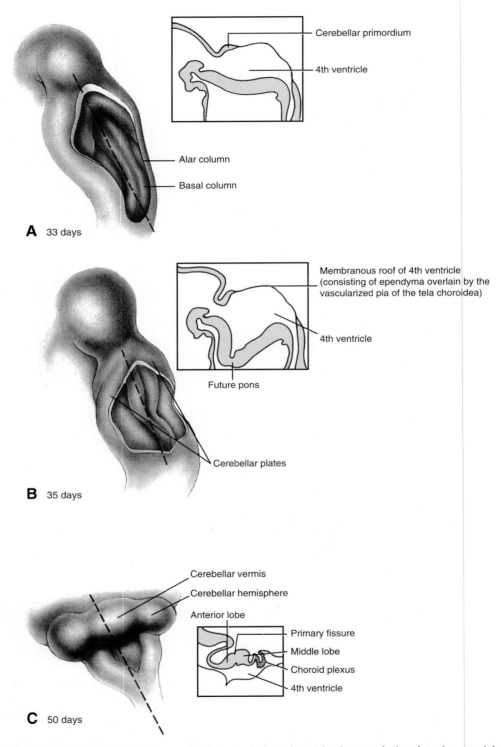

Figure 13–7. Development of the cerebellum and the choroid plexus of the fourth ventricle. *A, B,* Proliferation of cells in the rhombic lips of the metencephalon forms the cerebellar plates. *C,* Further growth creates two lateral cerebellar hemispheres and a central vermis. The primary fissure appears and divides the cerebellum into anterior and middle lobes. A choroid plexus develops in the roof plate of the fourth ventricle.

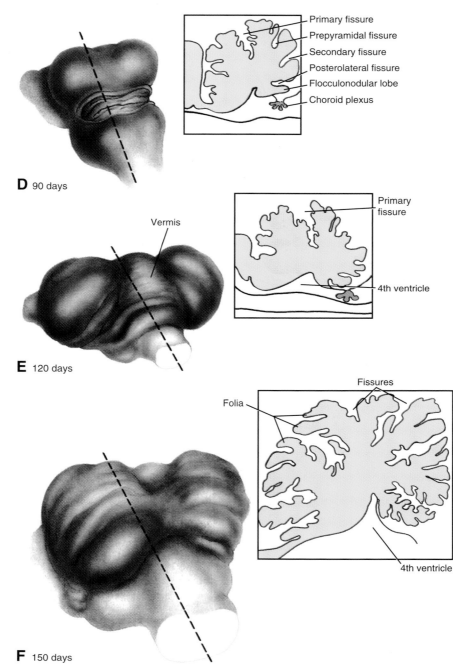

D 90 days

Primary fissure
Prepyramidal fissure
Secondary fissure
Posterolateral fissure
Flocculonodular lobe
Choroid plexus

Vermis

Primary fissure

4th ventricle

E 120 days

Fissures
Folia

4th ventricle

F 150 days

Figure 13–7. *Continued. D–F,* Continued fissuration subdivides the expanding cerebellum into further lobes and then, starting in the third month, into lobules and folia. This process greatly increases the area of the cerebellar cortex.

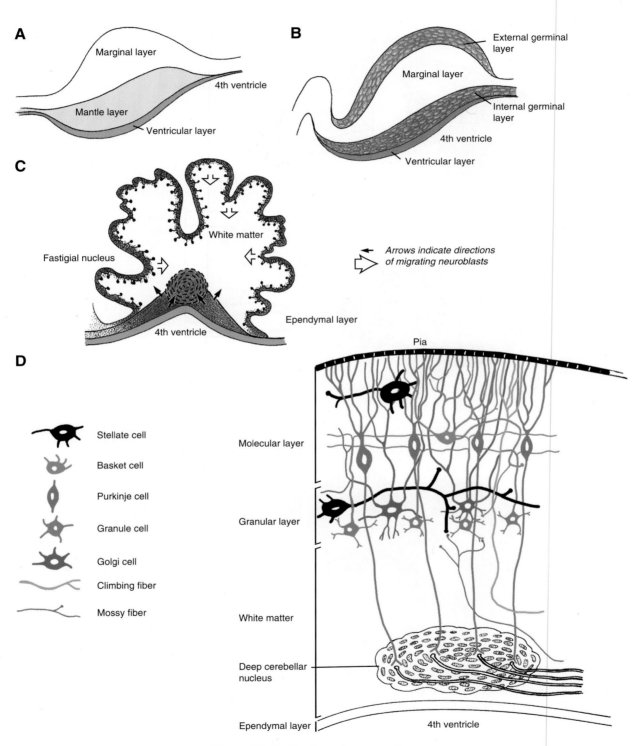

A

Marginal layer

4th ventricle

Mantle layer

Ventricular layer

B

External germinal layer

Marginal layer

Internal germinal layer

4th ventricle

Ventricular layer

C

White matter

Fastigial nucleus

Ependymal layer

4th ventricle

Arrows indicate directions of migrating neuroblasts

D

Pia

Stellate cell

Basket cell

Purkinje cell

Granule cell

Golgi cell

Climbing fiber

Mossy fiber

Molecular layer

Granular layer

White matter

Deep cerebellar nucleus

Ependymal layer

4th ventricle

Figure 13–8. *See legend on opposite page*

and does not protrude dorsally. By the middle of the third month, however, the growing cerebellum begins to bulge dorsally, forming a dumbbell-shaped swelling at the cranial end of the rhombencephalon.

At this stage, the developing cerebellum is separated into cranial and caudal portions by a transverse groove called the **posterolateral fissure.** The caudal portion, consisting of a pair of **flocculonodular lobes,** represents the most primitive part of the cerebellum. The larger cranial portion consists of a narrow median swelling called the **vermis** connecting a pair of broad **cerebellar hemispheres.** This cranial portion grows much faster than the flocculonodular lobes and becomes the dominant component of the mature cerebellum.

The cerebellar vermis and hemispheres undergo an intricate process of transverse folding as they develop. The major **primary fissure** deepens by the end of the third month and divides the vermis and hemispheres into a cranial **anterior lobe** and a caudal **middle lobe** (see Fig. 13–7C, D). These lobes are further divided into a number of **lobules** by the development of additional transverse fissures (starting with the **secondary** and **prepyramidal fissures**), and the surface of the lobules is thrown into closely packed, leaflike transverse gyri called **folia.** These processes of fissuration and foliation continue throughout embryonic and fetal life and have the result of vastly increasing the surface area of the cerebellar cortex (see Fig. 13–7E, F).

The Gray Matter of the Cerebellar Nuclei and Cortex Is Produced by Two Proliferative Zones

The cerebellum has two types of gray matter: a group of internal **deep cerebellar nuclei** and an external **cerebellar cortex.** Four deep nuclei form on each side: the **dentate, globose, emboliform,** and **fastigial nuclei.** All the input to the cerebellar cortex is relayed through these nuclei. The cerebellar cortex has an extremely regular cytoarchitecture that is similar over the entire cerebellum. The cell types of the cortex are arranged in layers.

The deep nuclei and cortex of the cerebellum are produced by a complex process of differentiation (Fig. 13–8). As elsewhere in the neural tube, the neuroepithelium of the metencephalic rhombic lips undergoes an initial proliferation to produce ventricular, mantle, and marginal layers (see Fig. 13–8A). However, in the third month, a second layer of proliferating cells appears in the most superficial layer of the marginal zone. The ventricular proliferating layer is now called the **internal germinal layer,** and the new layer is called the **external germinal layer** (or, sometimes, the **external granular layer**) (see Fig. 13–8B).

Starting in the fourth month, the internal and external germinal layers undergo highly regulated cell divisions that produce the various populations of cerebellar neuroblasts. The internal germinal layer gives rise to the **primitive nuclear neuroblasts,** which migrate to form the cerebellar nuclei (see Fig. 13–8C). In addition, this layer produces two types of neuroblasts that migrate to the cortex: the **primitive Purkinje neuroblasts,** which differentiate to form the Purkinje cells, and the **Golgi neuroblasts,** which differentiate to form the Golgi cells. As each primitive Purkinje neuroblast migrates toward the cortex, it reels out an axon that maintains synaptic contact with neuroblasts in the developing cerebellar nuclei. These axons will constitute the only efferents of the mature cerebellar cortex. The Purkinje cells form a distinct **Purkinje cell layer** just underlying the external germinal layer.

The external germinal layer undergoes three waves of proliferation to produce, in succession,

Figure 13–8. Cytodifferentiation of the cerebellum. A, During the second month, the cranial regions of the rhombic lips form typical ventricular, mantle, and marginal zones. B, During the third month, neuroblasts are produced by proliferation both in an internal germinal layer adjacent to the ventricular zone and in a novel external germinal layer that forms in the most peripheral region of the marginal layer. C, D, Neuroblasts produced by the external germinal layer migrate inward or remain in place to form basket neuroblasts, granule neuroblasts, and stellate neuroblasts. Neuroblasts produced by the internal germinal layer include the Purkinje neuroblasts, which migrate outward, and the nuclear neuroblasts, which form the deep cerebellar nuclei. (Modified from Williams PL, Warwick R, Dyson M, Bannister LH. 1989. Gray's Anatomy. Churchill Livingstone, Edinburgh.)

the three remaining neuroblast populations of the cerebellar cortex: the **basket neuroblasts,** the **granule neuroblasts,** and the **stellate neuroblasts** (see Fig. 13–8*D*). The granule neuroblasts and some of the basket and stellate neuroblasts are displaced to a location deep to the Purkinje cells, where they form the **granular layer** of the definitive cortex. The mechanism of this displacement is unclear (see the Clinical Applications section at the end of this chapter). The remaining basket and stellate cells remain superficial to or closely associated with the Purkinje cells and form the **molecular layer** of the definitive cortex.

As the waves of neurogenesis subside, the germinal layers produce the glioblasts of the cerebellum, which differentiate into astrocytes (including the specialized cerebellar Bergmann cells) and oligodendrocytes. There is little doubt that both of the germinal layers participate in producing the cerebellar glia, although there is controversy regarding the origin of specific glial subpopulations and the time of their formation.

THE MESENCEPHALON IS PRIMARILY A RELAY CENTER BUT ALSO CONTAINS CRANIAL NERVE NUCLEI, VISUAL AND AUDITORY CENTERS, AND OTHER STRUCTURES

Much of the mesencephalon is composed of white matter, principally the massive tracts that connect the forebrain with the hindbrain and spinal cord. The midbrain also contains a number of important neuronal centers, including four cranial nerve nuclei.

The Midbrain Contains Nuclei of Three Cranial Nerves, but Only the Oculomotor Nuclei Originate in the Midbrain

As mentioned earlier, the motor nuclei of the oculomotor (III) and trochlear (IV) nuclei are located in the mesencephalon, as is a portion of the sensory nucleus of the trigeminal nerve (V) called the **mesencephalic trigeminal nucleus** (Fig. 13–9).

Of these nuclei, however, only the two serving the oculomotor nerve arise from mesencephalic neuroblasts; the trochlear and mesencephalic trigeminal nuclei originate in the metencephalon and are secondarily displaced into the mesencephalon. The two nuclei of the oculomotor nerve are the somatic motor **oculomotor nucleus,** which controls the movements of all but the superior oblique and lateral rectus extrinsic ocular muscles, and the general visceral efferent **Edinger-Westphal nucleus,** which supplies parasympathetic pathways to the pupillary constrictor and the ciliary muscles of the globe.

The Superior and Inferior Colliculi Develop From Alar Plate Neuroblasts That Migrate Into the Mesencephalic Roof Plate

The **superior** and **inferior colliculi** are visible as four prominent swellings on the dorsal surface of the midbrain. The superior colliculi receive fibers from the retinas and mediate ocular reflexes. The inferior colliculi, in contrast, form part of the perceptual pathway by which information from the cochlea is relayed to the auditory areas of the cerebral hemispheres. The colliculi are formed by mesencephalic alar plate cells that proliferate and migrate medially into the roof plate (see Fig. 13–9). The roof plate thickening produced by these cells is subsequently divided by a midline groove into a pair of lateral **corpora bigemina,** which are later subdivided into inferior and superior colliculi by a transverse groove. The synapses in the superior colliculi form precise spatial maps of the corresponding sensory fields. The mechanisms responsible for this kind of precise neuronal mapping are discussed in the Experimental Principles section of this chapter.

The Midbrain Neural Canal Forms the Narrow Cerebral Aqueduct

During development, the primitive ventricle of the mesencephalon becomes the narrow **cerebral aqueduct** (see Fig. 13–9). The cerebrospinal fluid produced by the choroid plexuses of the forebrain normally flows through the cerebral aqueduct to

Figure 13–9. Development of the mesencephalon. *A, B,* A shallow longitudinal groove develops on the dorsal surface of the mesencephalon between weeks 6 and 12, creating the corpora bigemina. *C,* Over the next month, a transverse groove subdivides these swellings to produce the superior and inferior colliculi. The mesencephalic alar columns form the stratified nuclear layers of the colliculi, the periaqueductal gray matter, and the substantia nigra. The mesencephalic basal columns form the red nuclei.

reach the fourth ventricle. However, various conditions can cause the aqueduct to become blocked during fetal life. Obstruction of the flow of cerebrospinal fluid through the aqueduct results in the congenital condition called **hydrocephalus,** in which the third and lateral ventricles are swollen with fluid, the cerebral cortex is abnormally thin, and the sutures of the skull are forced apart (Fig. 13–10).

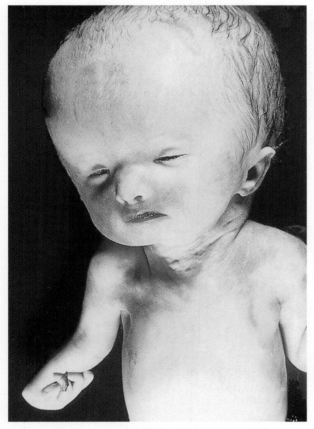

Figure 13–10. Hydrocephaly. Obstruction of the cerebral aqueduct causes the developing forebrain ventricles to become swollen with cerebrospinal fluid. Infants born with this condition may be retarded. However, incipient hydrocephaly can now be detected in utero using ultrasonography and can be corrected by inserting a pressure valve that allows the excess cerebrospinal fluid to vent into the amniotic cavity. (Photo courtesy of Children's Hospital Medical Center, Cincinnati, OH.)

THE MOST EVOLUTIONARILY ADVANCED AND COMPLEX STRUCTURES OF THE BRAIN ARISE FROM THE PROSENCEPHALON

The prosencephalon consists of two secondary brain vesicles, the diencephalon and the telencephalon. The walls of the diencephalon differentiate to form a number of neuronal centers and tracts, described later. In addition, the roof plate, floor plate, and ependyma of the diencephalon give rise to several specialized structures through mechanisms that are relatively unique. These structures include the **choroid plexus** and **circumventricular organs,** the **posterior lobe of the pituitary gland (neurohypophysis),** and the **optic vesicles.** The origin of the optic cups from the diencephalic neural folds was described in Chapter 12.

The telencephalon gives rise to the **cerebral hemispheres** and to the commissures and other structures that join them. It also forms the **olfactory bulbs** and **olfactory tracts,** which, along with the olfactory centers and tracts of the cerebral hemispheres, collectively constitute the **rhinencephalon** ("nose-brain").

THE DIENCEPHALIC ALAR PLATE FORMS THE THALAMUS, HYPOTHALAMUS, AND EPITHALAMUS

As mentioned earlier, the walls of the diencephalon are formed by alar plates; basal plates are lacking. These plates form three embryonic swellings: the **thalamus, hypothalamus,** and **epithalamus** (Fig. 13–11). The thalamus and hypothalamus differentiate to form complexes of nuclei that serve a diverse range of functions. The thalamus acts primarily as the relay center for the cerebral cortex: It receives all the information (sensory and other) projecting to the cortex from subcortical structures, processes it as necessary, and relays it to the appropriate cortical area(s). Within the thalamus, the sense of sight is handled by the **lateral geniculate body** and the sense of hearing by the **medial geniculate body.** The hypothalamus regulates the endocrine activity of the pituitary as well as many

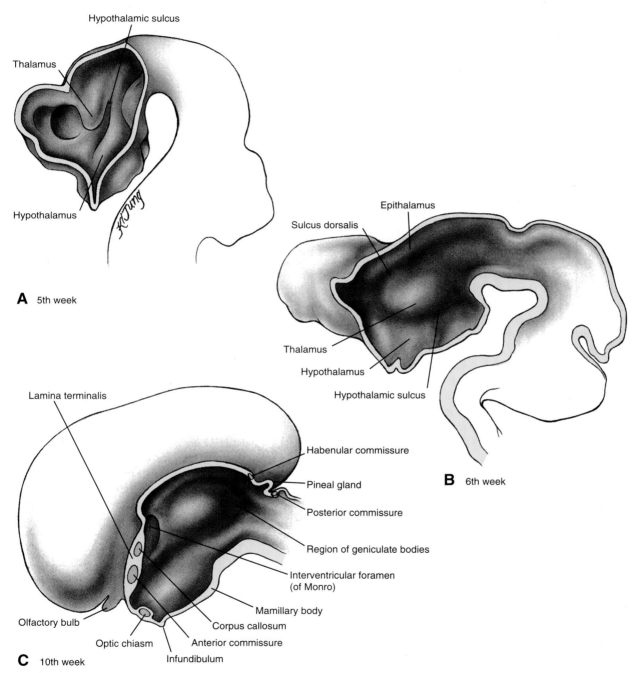

Thalamus

Hypothalamic sulcus

Hypothalamus

A 5th week

Sulcus dorsalis

Epithalamus

Thalamus

Hypothalamus

Hypothalamic sulcus

B 6th week

Lamina terminalis

Habenular commissure

Pineal gland

Posterior commissure

Region of geniculate bodies

Interventricular foramen (of Monro)

Mamillary body

Corpus callosum

Olfactory bulb

Optic chiasm

Anterior commissure

Infundibulum

C 10th week

Figure 13–11. Development of the diencephalon. *A,* The thalamus and hypothalamus become demarcated by a hypothalamic sulcus during the fifth week. *B,* By the end of the sixth week, the thalamus is clearly differentiated from the more dorsal epithalamus by a shallow groove called the sulcus dorsalis. *C,* By 10 weeks, additional specializations of the diencephalon are apparent, including the mamillary body, the pineal gland, and the posterior lobe of the pituitary. The optic sulci, the posterior and habenular commissures, and the geniculate bodies are also specializations of the diencephalon.

autonomic responses. It participates in the limbic system, which controls emotion and coordinates emotional state with the appropriate visceral responses. The hypothalamus also controls the level of arousal of the brain (sleep and waking). The small epithalamus gives rise to a few miscellaneous structures described later.

At the end of the fifth week, the thalamus and hypothalamus are visible as swellings on the inner surface of the diencephalic neural canal, separated by a deep groove called the **hypothalamic sulcus** (see Fig. 13–11*A*). The thalamus grows disproportionately after the seventh week and becomes the largest element of the diencephalon. The two thalami usually meet and fuse across the third ventricle at one or more points called **interthalamic adhesions** (Fig. 13–12).

By the end of the sixth week, a shallow groove called the **sulcus dorsalis** separates the thalamus from the epithalamic swelling, which forms in the dorsal rim of the diencephalic wall and the adjoining roof plate (see Fig. 13–11*B, C*). The epithalamic roof plate evaginates to form a midline diverticulum that differentiates into the endocrine **pineal gland.** The epithalamus also forms a neural structure called the **trigonium habenulae** (including the **nucleus habenulae**) and two small commissures, the **posterior** and **habenular commissures.** The growth of the thalamus eventually obliterates the sulcus dorsalis and displaces the epithalamic structures dorsally.

Retinal fibers from the optic cup project to the lateral geniculate bodies. As described in Chapter 12, the nerve fibers from the retina grow back through the optic nerve to the diencephalon. Just before they enter the brain, nerve fibers growing from both eyes meet to form the **optic chiasm,** a joint structure in which some of the fibers from each side cross over to the other side (decussate). The resulting bundles of ipsilateral and contralateral fibers then project back to the lateral geniculate bodies, where they synapse to form a map of the visual field. The mechanisms of axonal pathfinding that are thought to result in this precise mapping are discussed in the Experimental Principles section at the end of this chapter. Not all retinal fibers project to the lateral geniculate bodies; as mentioned earlier, some of them terminate in the superior colliculus, where they mediate ocular reflex control.

The Diencephalic Roof Plate and Ependyma Form the Choroid Plexus and Circumventricular Organs of the Third Ventricle

Cranial to the epithalamus, the diencephalic roof plate remains epithelial in character. This portion of the roof plate differentiates along with the overlying pia to form the paired choroid plexuses of the third ventricle. Elsewhere in the third ventricle, the ependyma forms a number of unique secretory structures that add specific metabolites and neuropeptides to the cerebrospinal fluid. These structures, collectively known as the **circumventricular organs,** include the **subfornical organ,** the **organum vasculosum of the lamina terminalis,** and the **subcommissural organ.**

The Pituitary Is Formed by the Diencephalon and by Rathke's Pouch

During the third week, a diverticulum called the **infundibulum** develops in the floor of the third ventricle and grows ventrally toward the stomodeum (Fig. 13–13; see also Fig. 13–11*C*). Simultaneously, an ectodermal placode appears in the roof of the stomodeum and invaginates to form a diverticulum called **Rathke's pouch,** which grows dorsally toward the infundibulum. Rathke's pouch eventually loses its connection with the stomodeum and forms a discrete sac that is appressed to the cranial surface of the infundibulum. This sac differentiates to form the **adenohypophysis** of the pituitary. The cells of its anterior surface give rise to the **anterior lobe** proper of the pituitary, and a small group of cells on the posterior surface of the pouch form the functionally distinct **pars intermedia.** Meanwhile, the distal portion of the infundibulum differentiates to form the **posterior pituitary (neurohypophysis).** The lumen of the infundibulum is obliterated by this process, but a small proximal pit, the **infundibular recess,** persists in the floor of the third ventricle.

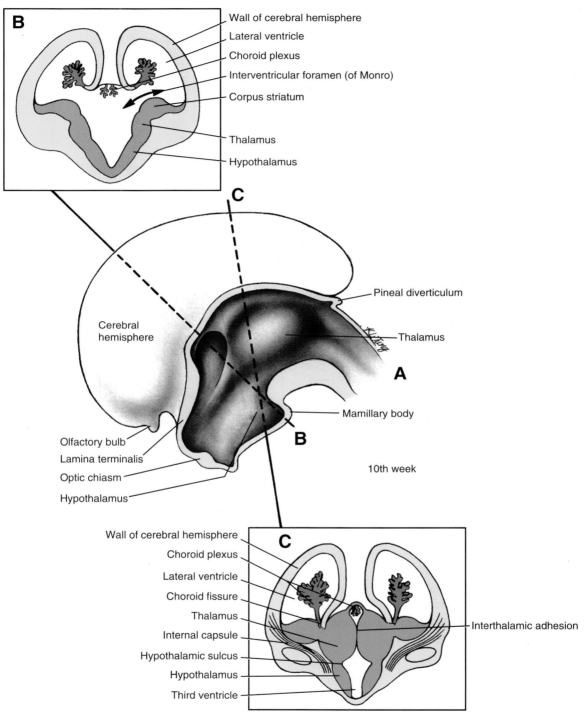

Figure 13–12. Development of the cerebral hemispheres and lateral ventricles. The lateral ventricle in each hemisphere communicates with the third ventricle through an interventricular foramen (of Monro). The choroid fissure running the length of each lateral ventricle contains a choroid plexus, which produces cerebrospinal fluid. The fibers growing to and from the cerebral cortex form the massive fiber bundle called the internal capsule. The thalami function primarily as relay centers that process information destined for the cerebral hemispheres. The growing thalami meet across the third ventricle, forming the interthalamic adhesion.

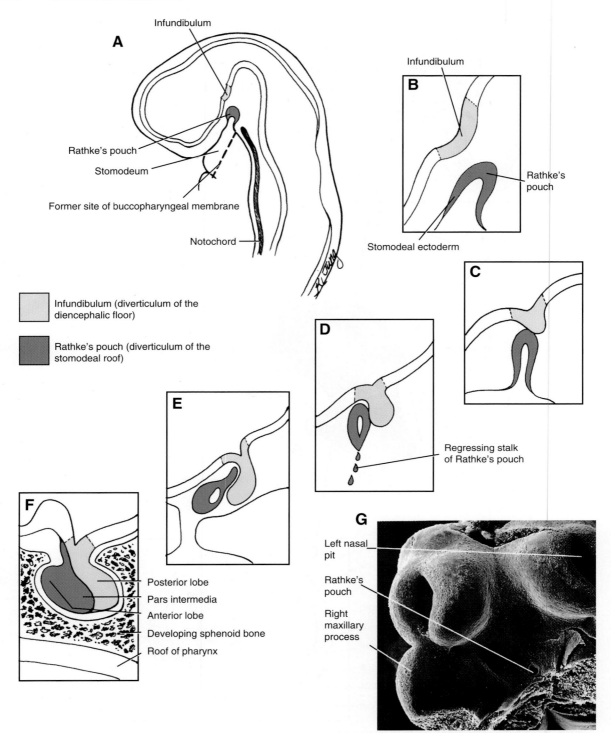

A

Infundibulum

Rathke's pouch

Stomodeum

Former site of buccopharyngeal membrane

Notochord

B

Infundibulum

Rathke's pouch

Stomodeal ectoderm

Infundibulum (diverticulum of the diencephalic floor)

Rathke's pouch (diverticulum of the stomodeal roof)

C

D

Regressing stalk of Rathke's pouch

E

F

Posterior lobe

Pars intermedia

Anterior lobe

Developing sphenoid bone

Roof of pharynx

G

Left nasal pit

Rathke's pouch

Right maxillary process

Figure 13–13. *A–F,* Development of the pituitary. The pituitary gland is a compound structure. The posterior lobe forms from a diverticulum of the diencephalic floor called the infundibulum, whereas the anterior lobe and pars intermedia form from an evagination of the ectodermal roof of the stomodeum called Rathke's pouch. Rathke's pouch detaches from the stomodeum and becomes associated with the developing posterior pituitary. *G,* Scanning electron micrograph of the roof of the embryonic oral cavity, showing the opening to Rathke's pouch. (*G,* Photo courtesy of Dr. Arnold Tamarin.)

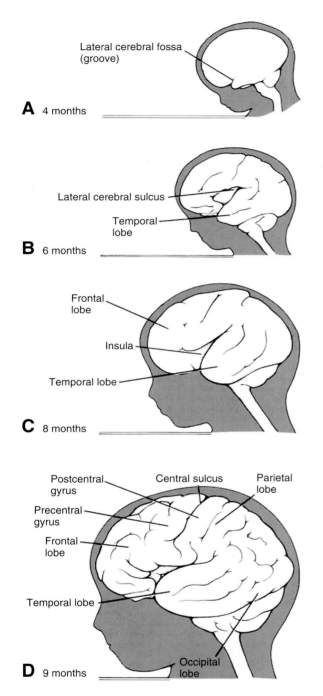

A 4 months
Lateral cerebral fossa (groove)

B 6 months
Lateral cerebral sulcus
Temporal lobe

C 8 months
Frontal lobe
Insula
Temporal lobe

D 9 months
Postcentral gyrus
Central sulcus
Parietal lobe
Precentral gyrus
Frontal lobe
Temporal lobe
Occipital lobe

THE TELENCEPHALON FORMS THE CEREBRAL HEMISPHERES, THEIR CONNECTING COMMISSURES, AND THE OLFACTORY BULBS AND TRACTS

The Cerebral Hemispheres Arise as Lateral Diverticulae of the Telencephalon

The cerebral hemispheres first appear on day 32 as a pair of bubble-like outgrowths of the telencephalon. By 16 weeks, the rapidly growing hemispheres are oval and have expanded back to cover the diencephalon. The thin roof and lateral walls of each hemisphere represent the future **cerebral cortex** (Fig. 13–14*A*). The floor is thicker and contains a neuronal aggregation called the **corpus striatum,** which will give rise to two of the three **basal nuclei** of the cerebral hemispheres (the third is contributed by the diencephalon) (see Fig. 13–12*B*). As the growing hemispheres press against the walls of the diencephalon, the meningeal layers that originally separate the two structures disappear, so that the neural tissue of the thalami becomes continuous with that of the floor of the cerebral hemispheres. This former border is eventually crossed by a massive fiber bundle called the **internal capsule,** which passes through the corpus striatum and carries fibers from the thalamus to the cerebral cortex as well as from the cerebral cortex to lower regions of the brain and spinal cord (see Fig. 13–12*C*).

The cerebral hemispheres are initially smooth-walled. Like the cerebellar cortex, however, the cerebral cortex folds into an increasingly complex pattern of lobes and gyri as the hemi-

Figure 13–14. Growth and folding of the cerebral hemispheres during fetal life. Growth of the cerebral hemispheres is continuous throughout embryonic and fetal development and continues after birth. *A, B,* In the fourth month, the formation of the narrow lateral cerebral fossa delineates the temporal lobe of the cerebral hemisphere. By the sixth month, additional clefts delineate the frontal, parietal, and occipital lobes. *C, D,* Additional sulci and gyri form throughout the remainder of fetal life.

spheres grow. This process begins in the fourth month with the appearance of a small indentation called the **lateral cerebral fossa** in the lateral wall of the hemisphere (see Fig. 13–14*A, B*). The caudal end of the lengthening hemisphere curves ventrally and then grows forward across this fossa, creating the **temporal lobe** of the cerebral hemisphere and converting the fossa into a deep cleft called the **lateral cerebral sulcus.** The portion of the cerebral cortex that originally forms the medial floor of the fossa is covered by the temporal lobe and is called the **insula.**

By the sixth month, several other cerebral sulci have appeared. These include the **central sulcus,** which separates the frontal and parietal lobes, and the **occipital sulcus,** which demarcates the occipital lobe. The detailed pattern of gyri that ultimately forms on the cerebral hemispheres varies somewhat from individual to individual.

A Choroid Plexus Forms in the Choroid Fissure of the Lateral Ventricles

Each cerebral hemisphere contains a diverticulum of the telencephalic primitive ventricle called the **lateral ventricle.** The lateral ventricle initially occupies most of the volume of the hemisphere but is progressively constricted by the thickening of the cortex. However, along the line between the floor and the medial wall of the hemisphere, the cerebral wall does not thicken but instead remains thin and epithelial. This zone forms a longitudinal groove in the ventricle; the groove is called the **choroid fissure** (see Fig. 13–12*C*). A choroid plexus develops along the choroid fissure. As shown in Figure 13–15, the lateral ventricle extends the whole length of the hemisphere, reaching anteriorly into the frontal lobe and, at its posterior end, curving around to occupy the temporal lobe.

The opening between each lateral ventricle and the third ventricle persists as the **interventricular foramen (foramen of Monro).**

The Cytodifferentiation of the Cerebral Cortex Is Complex

The neuroepithelium of the cerebral hemispheres is initially much like that of other parts of the neural tube. Studies on cerebral histogenesis have shown, however, that the process of proliferation, migration, and differentiation by which the mature cortex is produced is unique. The details of this process vary from place to place in the cortex and are not fully understood. To summarize roughly, the proliferating cells of the ventricular layer undergo a series of regulated divisions to produce waves of neuroblasts, which migrate peripherally and establish the layers of the cortex. In general, however, the cortical layers are laid down in a

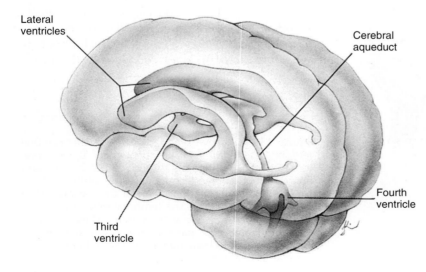

Lateral
ventricles

Cerebral
aqueduct

Third
ventricle

Fourth
ventricle

Figure 13–15. The cerebral ventricles. The expansions of the neural canal in the primary and secondary brain vesicles and cerebral hemispheres give rise to the cerebral ventricles. The ventricle system consists of the lateral ventricles in the cerebral hemispheres, the third ventricle in the diencephalon, the narrow cerebral aqueduct (of Sylvius) in the mesencephalon, and the fourth ventricle in the rhombencephalon.

sequence from *deep* to *superficial:* that is, the neurons of each wave migrate through the preceding layers to establish a more superficial layer. As the production of neuroblasts tapers off, the ventricular layer gives rise to the various kinds of glioblasts and then to the ependyma.

Let us now examine the process in more detail (Fig. 13–16). The first neuroblasts produced in the ventricular layer form neuronal fibers, which grow out of the ventricular layer to form a thin, superficial **marginal zone.** This thin fiber layer immediately underlies the developing pia and remains the most superficial layer of the cortex. Many of these neuroblasts then migrate outward to form an **intermediate zone,** which is intercalated between the ventricular layer and the marginal zone. Some of the cells from the intermediate zone, plus new neuroblasts produced in the ventricular layer, then migrate outward to form a transient lamina called the **cortical plate** between the intermediate zone and the marginal zone. At this point, the ventricular zone gradually ceases to produce neuroblasts, and neuroblast production is taken over by a layer of proliferating cells between the ventricular and intermediate layers, called the **subventricular zone.** Neuroblasts from the subventricular zone migrate peripherally through the intermediate zone to establish a **subplate** layer just deep to the cortical plate. Some of these neurons then migrate through the earlier generations of neuroblasts in the cortical plate to establish outer laminae within the cortical plate. Together, the cortical plate and subplate give rise to the cerebral cortex. The cerebral cortex is made up of several cell layers, which vary in number from three in the phylogenetically oldest parts to about six in the dominant **neocortex.** The intermediate layer, meanwhile, has become relatively devoid of neuroblast cell bodies and differentiates into the **white matter** of the cerebral hemispheres. It must be clearly understood that the sequence and timing of these events vary considerably in different regions of the hemispheres.

The Olfactory Bulbs and Olfactory Tracts Are Derived From the Cranial Telencephalon

As described in Chapter 12, the nasal placodes appear at the end of the fourth week. Very early, some cells in the nasal placode differentiate to form the **primary neurosensory cells** of the fu-

VZ: ventricular zone

MZ: marginal zone

IZ: intermediate zone

CP: cortical plate

SZ: subventricular zone

SP: subplate layer

EL: ependymal layer

WM: white matter

NC: neocortex

ML: molecular layer

Figure 13–16. Cytodifferentiation of the cerebral neocortex. Although the timing of neuroblast formation varies widely in different regions of the cerebral hemispheres, the general scheme illustrated here is typical for all regions. See text for explanation.

ture olfactory epithelium. At the end of the fifth week, these cells sprout axons that cross the short distance to penetrate the most cranial end of the telencephalon (Fig. 13–17*A*). The subsequent ossification of the ethmoid bone around these axons creates the perforated cribriform plates.

In the sixth week, as the nasal pits differentiate to form the epithelium of the nasal passages, the area at the tip of each cerebral hemisphere where the axons of the primary neurosensory cells synapse begins to form an outgrowth called the **olfactory bulb** (Fig. 13–18; see also Fig. 13–17).

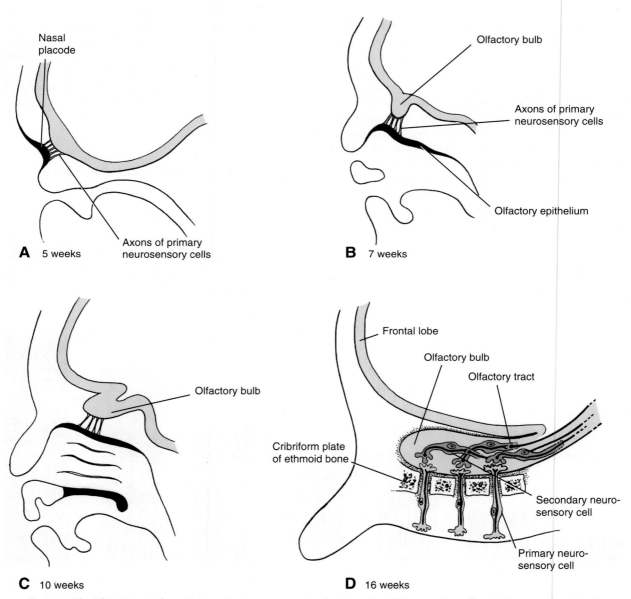

Figure 13–17. Formation of the olfactory tract. *A,* During the fifth week, cells of the nasal placode differentiate into the primary neurosensory cells of the olfactory tract and produce axons that grow into the presumptive olfactory bulb of the adjacent telencephalon and synapse there with secondary neurons. *B–D,* As development continues, the elongating axons of the secondary olfactory neurons in the olfactory bulb produce the olfactory tract.

The cells in the olfactory bulb that synapse with the axons of the primary sensory neurons differentiate to become the secondary sensory neurons of the olfactory pathways. The axons of these cells synapse in the olfactory centers of the cerebral hemispheres. As the changing proportions of the face and brain lengthen the distance between the olfactory bulbs and their point of origin on the hemispheres, the axons of the secondary olfactory neurons lengthen to form stalklike CNS **olfactory tracts.** Traditionally, the olfactory tract and bulb together are referred to as the **olfactory nerve.**

The Telencephalon Produces the Commissures That Connect the Cerebral Hemispheres

The commissures that connect the right and left cerebral hemispheres form from a thickening at the cranial end of the telencephalon, which represents the zone of final neuropore closure. This area can be divided into a dorsal **commissural plate** and a ventral **lamina terminalis.**

The first fiber tract to develop in the commissural plate is the **anterior commissure,** which forms during the seventh week and interconnects the olfactory bulbs and olfactory centers of the two hemispheres (Fig. 13–18). During the ninth week, the **hippocampal** or **fornix commissure** forms between the right and left hippocampi (a phylogenetically old portion of the cerebral hemisphere that is located adjacent to the choroid fissure). A few days later, the massive, arched **corpus callosum** begins to form, linking together the right and left neocortices along their entire length. The most anterior part of the corpus callosum appears first, and its posterior extension (the **splenium**) forms later in fetal life.

MOST OF THE GROWTH OF THE BRAIN TAKES PLACE AFTER BIRTH

At birth, the brain is about 25 percent of its adult volume. Some of the postnatal growth of the brain is due to increase in the size of neuronal cell bodies and to the proliferation of neuronal processes. Most of this growth, however, results from the myelination of nerve fibers.

Neuronal Histogenesis Is Regulated by Multiple Factors and by Cell-Cell Interactions

The manner in which the 10 billion to 1 trillion neurons of the human brain become organized and interconnected is a problem of daunting complexity. Not only do the neurons themselves proliferate, migrate, and differentiate according to a precise pattern, but also their cell processes display awesome pathfinding abilities. The cellular and molecular mechanisms that control these processes have become the subject of intense scientific interest. Because the neuronal architecture of the cerebellar cortex is extremely regular and well understood, the cerebellum is a favored object for research on neuronal differentiation. Studies performed by using a series of mouse strains with specific cerebellar ataxias are described in the Clinical Applications section of this chapter.

Research has focused on the mechanisms by which a family of proteins called **neurotrophins** control the survival, differentiation and synaptic function of various types of neurons. This family of proteins includes **nerve growth factor** (NGF), **brain-derived neurotrophic factor** (BDNF; mentioned in chapter 4 in the context of neural crest migration), **neurotrophin-3** (NT-3), and **neurotrophin-4/5** (NT-4/5). Neurotrophins, released by target neurons, promote the survival of discrete subpopulations of neurons. Neurotrophins also regulate neuronal differentiation and mediate neurite morphology. These activities result from specific interactions with a family of cell surface high-affinity receptors, called trkA, trkB, and trkC, and a low-affinity receptor, p75. The different combinations of neurotrophins and their receptors elicit diverse but specific responses and are central regulators of the structure and function of the nervous system during development and in adulthood. Determining how these proteins function could lead to an understanding not only of congenital defects of nervous system histogenesis but also of the involutional changes that occur with aging. Furthermore, neurotrophins and agents that influence neurotrophin receptor function are being explored for their therapeutic value in CNS injuries and neurodegenerative diseases.

Other growth factors mentioned in previous chapters also influence neuronal growth, differenti-

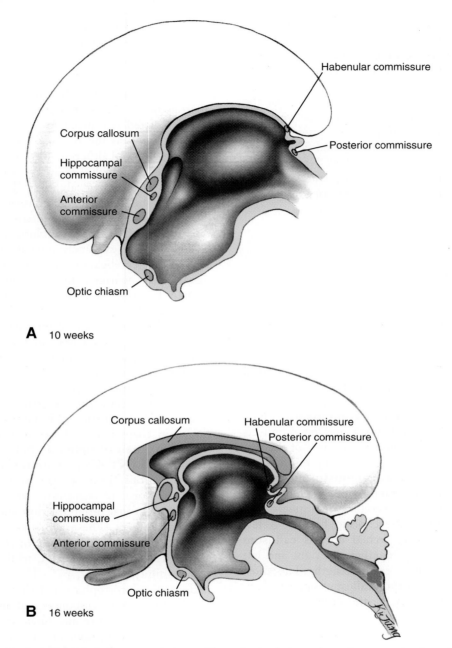

Figure 13–18. Formation of the commissures. The telencephalon gives rise to commissural tracts that integrate the activities of the left and right cerebral hemispheres. These include the anterior and hippocampal commissures and the corpus callosum. The small posterior and habenular commissures arise from the epithalamus.

ation, and survival. For example, epidermal growth factor, members of the fibroblast growth factor family, and insulin-like growth factors all promote neuronal survival and neurite outgrowth. Some of these effects are exerted directly, whereas others are mediated by glial cells, including astrocytes and oligodendrocytes in the CNS and Schwann cells in the PNS. Furthermore, the activities of many of these factors depend on interactions with extracellular matrix components secreted by glial cells. Matrix proteins such as **laminin, fibronectin,** and **collagen,** and proteoglycans such as **heparin sulfate** and **chondroitin sulfate** have each been shown to have dramatic effects on neurite outgrowth.

Sex steroids are also known to influence both the organization and the functioning of the brain. It has been demonstrated, for example, that the number of neurons in a nucleus of the medial preoptic area of the rat brain is determined partly by the level of circulating male sex steroids.

Clinical Applications

Cellular and Molecular Basis for Congenital Malformations of Cerebral Cortex

The human cerebral cortex is subject to a variety of developmental disorders that result from abnormal cell migration, differentiation, survival, or proliferation. The most severe of these abnormalities are obvious in early development, but some do not manifest themselves until later in life. Collectively, these syndromes have an incidence of 1 in every 100,000 live births. Diagnosis can be made from gross specimens or by magnetic resonance imaging (MRI), computed tomography (CT), or ultrasonography.

Classical lissencephaly is a condition that results from incomplete neuronal migration to cerebral cortex during the third and fourth months of gestation. Brains from patients with lissencephaly have a smoothened cerebral surface due to a combination of **pachygyria** (broad, thick gyri), **agyria** (lack of gyri), and widespread neuronal **heterotopia** (cells in aberrant positions compared with those of normal brain). Enlarged ventricles and malformation of the corpus callosum are also common. As newborns, these patients often appear normal but sometimes have apnea, poor feeding, or hypotonia. Patients typically later develop seizures, profound mental retardation, and mild spastic quadriplegia.

Subcortical band heterotopia (SBH) is also believed to result from aberrant migration of differentiating neuroepithelial cells. These patients have bilateral circumferential and symmetric ribbons of gray matter located just beneath the cortex and separated from it by a thin band of white matter. Seizures, mild mental retardation, and some behavioral abnormalities are often evident

from birth. However, intelligence can be normal and seizures may begin later in life. A related syndrome, **X-linked lissencephaly and SBH** also occurs when homozygous males have lissencephaly, whereas heterozygous females have SBH.

Recent studies have identified two genes that are linked to lissencephaly and SBH. One, *LIS1*, maps to chromosome 17p13 and encodes a protein that functions as a regulatory subunit of platelet-activating factor acetylhydrolase. Studies of mice with targeted *Lis-1* mutations suggest that this protein is necessary for normal pyramidal cell migration and neurite outgrowth. Another gene, called *doublecortin*, is located on the X chromosome and is mutated in patients with X-linked lissencephaly and SBH. The protein product of *doublecortin* is highly expressed in fetal neurons and their precursors during cortical development. Interestingly, both the doublecortin protein and platelet-activating factor acetylhydrolase are associated with microtubules, suggesting that they mediate cell migration through interactions with the cytoskeleton.

Cellular and Molecular Basis of Congenital Cerebellar Malformations

The human cerebellum is also subject to a variety of developmental disorders, including **hypoplasias** (underdevelopment), **dysplasias** (abnormal tissue development), and heterotopias. A number of these disorders cause characteristic **cerebellar ataxias** (disruptions of coordination).

Mercury poisoning may result in focal damage to the granular layer of the cerebellum and ataxia in humans. Many cerebellar anomalies, however, are caused by chromosomal anomalies and single-gene mutations. Trisomy 13, for example, is typified by gross brain abnormalities that affect the cerebellum and cerebrum. In the cerebellum, the vermis is hypoplastic and neurons are heterotopically located in the white matter. Cerebellar dysplasia, usually of the vermis, is also characteristic of trisomy 18, and Down syndrome (trisomy 21) may involve abnormalities of the Purkinje and granule cell layers. A variety of chromosome deletion syndromes, including 5p- (**cri du chat**), 13q-, and 4p-, also may cause cerebellar anomalies.

Many cerebellar ataxias are acquired through autosomal recessive inheritance. One of the most common human ataxia syndromes is **Friedreich's ataxia**, which affects the dorsal root ganglia, spinal cord, and cerebellum. It is characterized by clumsy gait, ataxia of the upper limbs, and dysarthria (disturbed speech articulation). Other autosomal recessive cerebellar ataxia syndromes are **Joubert syndrome, Gillespie syndrome, Marinesco-Sjögren syndrome, and Dandy-Walker syndrome. Paine syndrome** is a cerebellar ataxia that is inherited as an X-linked recessive trait. Two forms of autosomal dominant cerebellar ataxia syndromes have been mapped to human chromosomes 6p and 12q. Many of these heritable recessive syndromes also cause such dramatic cerebellar malformations that they can be diagnosed by CT, MRI, or ultrasonography.

The mutations that cause some of the recessive heritable cerebellar ataxias are known to affect the metabolism of mucopolysaccharides, lipids, and amino acids. In the cerebellum, these mutations cause effects such as a deficiency of Purkinje cells (mucopolysaccharidosis III), abnormal accumulation of lipid (juvenile gangliosidosis), and reduced myelin formation (phenylketonuria). The disorder called **olivopontocerebellar atrophy** seems in some cases to be caused by a deficiency in the excitatory neurotransmitter glutamate, resulting in turn from a deficiency in the enzyme glutamate dehydrogenase.

Insight Into the Cause of Cerebellar Defects Has Been Gained by Studying Mouse Mutants With Cerebellar Ataxias

A more detailed understanding of the cellular and molecular mechanisms that cause various cerebellar anomalies has been gained by research on a series of mouse mutants that display a broad array of cerebellar ataxias. The strange gaits of many of these mouse mutants can be correlated with defects in cerebellar cytoarchitecture. For example, the high-stepping, broad-based gait of the "stumbler" mutant is apparently caused by defects in Purkinje cells. The "meander tail" mutant also has Purkinje cell deficits, but only in the anterior lobe of the cerebellum. The "vibrator" mouse displays a rapid postural tremor caused by progressive degeneration of cerebellar neurons. This phenotype has been linked to mutations in the gene encoding phosphatidylinositol transfer protein alpha. "Tottering" and "leaner" mice exhibit symptoms of ataxia and epilepsy, which are likely due to mutations in the calcium channel alpha(1A) subunit gene. In humans, mutations in this gene have been linked to familial hemiplegic migraine, episodic ataxia type 2 and chronic spinocerebellar ataxia type 6.

In Vitro Studies Have Revealed a Basis for Cerebellar Pathogenesis in the "Weaver" Mutant

Normally, the granule cell neuroblasts that arise in the external germinal layer of the developing cerebellum produce bipolar processes and then migrate inward to populate the granule layer, reeling out an axon behind them as they travel. In the homozygous recessive "weaver" mutant (*wv/wv*), the granule cells fail to produce processes, fail to migrate, and then die prematurely.

Evidence from in vitro studies on explants of developing cerebellum indicates that granule cells make a special "migration junction" with astrocyte processes that is essential for normal migration and synapse formation. These junctions are easy to see in explants of normal cerebellum but do not form in explants of "weaver" mutant cerebellum. A series of experiments was carried out in which wild-type and weaver astrocytes and neurons were mixed in vitro. It was found that wild-type neurons interact normally with weaver astrocytes but that weaver granule cells do not form junctions with wild-type astrocytes and do not migrate along astrocyte processes. Thus, the weaver mutation apparently affects the granule cell and not the astrocytes.

Studies of "Staggerer"–Wild-Type Chimeras Suggest a Mechanism for the Numerical Matching of Purkinje and Granule Cells

In the normal cerebellum, the number of granule cells is precisely matched to the number of Purkinje cells. This matching is accomplished by a process of **histogenetic cell death,** by which the great overabundance of granule cell neuroblasts initially produced by the external germinal layer is reduced to the correct number. Various experiments have indicated that this process is automatically controlled by the number of Purkinje cells: Apparently, granule cells die unless they make contact with the dendritic arbor of a Purkinje cell.

This model was tested by using "staggerer"–wild-type chimeras made by aggregating eight-cell "staggerer" embryos with wild-type embryos and then reinserting them into the uterus of a pseudopregnant mother. This technique results in the birth of animals with widely different numbers of normal and wild-type Purkinje cells. Examination revealed a linear relationship between the number of granule cells and the number of wild-type Purkinje cells, confirming the hypothesis that granule cell survival depends on the presence of appropriate Purkinje cell targets.

In-Situ Hybridization and Gene Targeting Implicate the *Wnt* Family in Cerebellar Development

A **proto-oncogene** is a normal gene that can become a tumor-promoting *oncogene* if it mutates or if its expression is disturbed. The clinical interest of these genes is obvious. Moreover, many proto-oncogenes have proved to be important regulators of cell proliferation and differentiation. By using the technique of in situ hybridization, the proto-oncogene *Wnt-1 (int-1)* has been shown to be expressed in the developing central nervous system. In the neural plate, messenger RNA for this gene is localized predominantly in the presumptive mesencephalon and metencephalon. Later in development, the expression of the gene extends caudally to include the myelencephalon and spinal cord. The gene is also expressed to a minor degree in adult mouse spermatids. Interestingly, mice homozygous for the recessive mutation swaying (*sw*) have been shown to harbor a deletion of a single base pair within the *Wnt-1* locus. These mice also exhibit malformation of the anterior cerebellum and are characterized by ataxia and hypertonia (extreme tension of the muscles).

To investigate the role of this gene, mutants in which the gene was nonfunctional were produced by using gene-targeting technology. Embryos homozygous for this nonfunctional "null allele" usually die in utero or shortly after birth, and those that survive are severely ataxic. Examination of animals that died in utero or soon after birth showed that the mesencephalon and cerebellum were completely absent. One animal that survived to adulthood did have the caudal part of the cerebellum, suggesting that differences in the penetrance of the null allele may be regulated by a craniocaudal gradient (see the Experimental Principles sections of Chs. 11 and 12).

Significant midbrain or cerebellar defects are exhibited by transgenic mice homozygous for a targeted deletion of the engrailed-1 or engrailed-2 homeobox gene, respectively, providing evidence for the functional interaction between engrailed and *Wnt*. In other studies, however, the expression of *Wnt-3* does not appear to be affected by the targeted deletion of the engrailed-2 homeobox gene. The cerebellar ataxias displayed by the various strains of mice described in this section resemble some human cerebellar ataxias, although direct comparisons are not currently justified. Nevertheless, it is clear that the investigation of such mutants will lead to new insights into the regulation of neuronal proliferation, pathfinding, and synaptogenesis in the human cerebellum.

Experimental Principles

Spatial Targeting of the Retinal Axons in the Lateral Geniculate Bodies

The Retinal Ganglion Neurons Form a Precise Map of the Visual Field When They Synapse in the Lateral Geniculate Bodies

As described in this chapter and in Chapter 12, the ganglion cells of the retina (the secondary sensory neurons of the visual pathway) produce axons that grow back through the optic nerves to synapse in the lateral geniculate bodies (Fig. 13–19). At the optic chiasm, half the axons from each retina decussate (cross over to the other side) and join the contralateral optic tract, which proceeds to the lateral geniculate body. Specifically, the fibers from the *nasal* half of each retina decussate, whereas the axons from the temporal (lateral) half do not (Fig. 13–20).

In the mature lateral geniculate body, the target neurons are arranged so that they form a map that is correlated with the spatial arrangement of the secondary neurons in the retinas. Each retinal axon courses to the correct region in the geniculate body and synapses with the correct target neurons, thus generally reproducing in the geniculate bodies the spatial information from the retinas. A similar feat is accomplished by the axons of the lateral geniculate body neurons (the tertiary neurons of the visual pathway), which grow back to map onto the **primary visual cortex** in the occipital lobe of the cerebral cortex. By means of these neural maps, a representation of the visual world is transmitted to the cortex, which integrates the right and left visual fields and interprets the image.

Precise visual maps are reproduced by the targeting of specific populations of secondary retinal neurons to the superior colliculus of the mammalian tectum. Recall from the Descriptive Embryology section of this chapter that the superior colliculus, along with other regions of the tectum, including the inferior colliculi, integrates visual, auditory, and somatosensory information and coordinates reflex responses to movement, sound, and somatic sensation. The question of how this mapping is achieved is of interest not only in itself but also because similar spatial maps are a common feature in the CNS. A number of experimental approaches have begun to shed light on the intri-

cate puzzle of how the visual field maps are formed. Most of these studies have been carried out on the retinal axons either of mammals or of amphibians such as the clawed frog *Xenopus*. (In amphibians, fish, reptiles, and birds, the retinal axons grow directly into the tectum of the midbrain.) Basically, the visual map is created in two steps. First, a number of cues guide the growing retinal axons to the correct spot in the lateral geniculate body, where they synapse to form a rough map. These initial, somewhat indiscriminate synapses are then modified by pruning and, possibly, by secondary axonal reconnection to form a highly "tuned" map. The cues that control this secondary tuning process may be different from the ones involved in the initial axonal pathfinding.

The Growth Cones of the Retinal Ganglion Cells Respond to Cues That Tell Them Which Way to Grow and When to Turn

As described in Chapter 5, the **growth cone** at the tip of the axon is the structure responsible for

Figure 13–19. Organization of neurons in the retina and optic nerve. The photoreceptor cells, the rods and cones, form the deepest layer of the neural retina (the layer furthest from the vitreous humor). The information from the rods and cones is gathered by a layer of short primary visual neurons, which synapse in the retina with the secondary visual neurons. The axons of these secondary neurons traverse the surface of the retina and then travel via the optic nerve to the brain.

Secondary visual neuron on temporal side of retina–*projects to ipsilateral side of brain*

Secondary visual neuron on nasal side of retina–*projects to contralateral side of brain*

Pathway of temporal secondary neurons

Pathway of tertiary neurons

Pathway of nasal secondary neurons (decussating at the chiasm)

Pathway of tertiary neurons

Lateral geniculate body

Primary visual cortex

Figure 13–20. Path of visual impulses from the retina. The secondary neurons of the visual pathway undergo partial decussation across the optic chiasm so that each visual cortex receives the information from the contralateral visual field. As shown, the axons from the nasal half of each retina cross over in the chiasm to enter the contralateral visual tract, whereas axons from the temporal half of each retina enter the ipsilateral visual tract. These secondary axons synapse in the lateral geniculate bodies with the tertiary neurons of the visual pathway, which project to the primary visual cortex in the occipital lobe. The synapses in the lateral geniculate bodies and the visual cortex are arranged so as to form a spatial map of the visual field.

pathfinding (Fig. 13–21). The first task of the retinal ganglion cell growth cones, after they enter the fiber layer that lines the retina, is to grow to the site of the optic disc and then turn sharply and enter the optic stalk (see Fig. 13–19). Outgrowth of retinal ganglion cell (RGC) axons and guidance of their growth cones to the optic disc appears to require interaction with radial glia endfeet within the inner layer of the neural retina and associated cell adhe-

sion and extracellular matrix molecules. Indeed, many such substrate-associated factors appear to play a role in activity and behavior of RGC growth cones, including **laminin, L1, axonin-1,** and **N-CAM.** In addition, the survival of RGCs within the retina may be supported by **trophic factors,** including a factor produced by pigment epithelial cells. Other trophic factors that support survival of RGCs include BDNF and neurotrophin 4/5.

Figure 13–21. Comparison of a growth cone with relatively simple morphology (*A*) with one of more complex morphology (*B*) exhibiting numerous filopodia and lamellipodia. (From Roberts A, Taylor JSH. 1983. A study of the growth cones of developing embryonic sensory neurites. J Embryol Exp Morphol 75:31.)

Directional growth by RGC growth cones to the optic disc is probably also regulated by their repulsion from inappropriate regions such as the outer layer of the neural retina. Several repulsive factors have been described that result in "collapse" of the growth cone with loss or slowing of its locomotor activity. One such factor, a protein called **RAGS** (for "*r*epulsive *a*xon *g*uidance *s*ignal"), exhibits significant homology to ligands for receptor tyrosine kinases. In addition, various extracellular matrix molecules such as **tenascin** have also been shown to slow the growth of outgrowing retinal growth cones (see later). Whenever the growth cone reaches a "decision point" such as the optic disc, its morphology changes from a simple tapered cone to a complex, actively pleomorphic structure that puts out numerous cell processes called filopodia (Latin *filum*, thread, + Greek *pous*, foot) and lamellipodia (Latin *lamella*, plate, leaf, + Greek *pous*, foot) (see Fig. 13–21*B*). The filopodia, especially, have been implicated in the sensing and transducing of environmental signals that guide the growth cone to its target. For example, in in vitro experiments, growth cones from *Xenopus* spinal neurons turn to grow in the direction of higher glutamate concentration. Before turning, however, the growth cones develop more filopodia on the side facing the glutamate source. Thus, the morphologic complexity of the growth cone at decision points appears to reflect the response of the growth cone to the environmental signals that determine its behavior. The retinal axon growth cones change back to a simple, tapered shape once they have plunged into the optic stalk, but they become complex again when they reach the optic chiasm (where they must decide whether to decussate) and again when they reach the thalamus.

Experiments with *Xenopus* embryos indicate that it is the growth cone itself and not the neuronal cell body that senses and responds to cues. If an eye is removed from a *Xenopus* embryo after the retinal axons have begun to grow, the growth cones continue to make the correct decisions even though their cell body is gone.

Both Local Factors and Diffusing Signal Molecules Appear to Guide the Growth Cones

Experiments with a **neonatal ocular retardation mutant mouse** provide inferential evidence that targets of the retinal axons within the central nervous system may emit targeting cues that can "attract" retinal growth cones from ectopic sites. When embryonic retinas are implanted on the ventrolateral brain stem or along the course of the internal capsule (before innervation of the lateral geniculate bodies by the endogenous retinas), the axons emitted from the ectopic retina innervate the lateral geniculate bodies and other optic nuclei, even crossing to innervate their contralateral targets. The laminin-related protein **netrin-1** appears to serve as a **neurotropic factor** in the guidance of retinal axon growth cones to their targets in the optic tectum. Immunocytochemical findings demonstrate that expression of **neogenin,** a netrin-1 receptor, within subpopulations of retinal neurons, is correlated with the outgrowth of these retinal axons. Conversely, cessation of neogenin expression is correlated with their final targeting in the optic tectum. Similarly, **netrin-1** and **netrin-2** have been implicated in the guidance of **commissural axons** in the spinal cord along a circumferential pathway from the dorsal spinal cord to ventral floor plate cells. In this case, the netrin-1 receptor expressed by these neurons is a transmembrane protein related to neogenin called **DCC (deleted in colorectal cancer).** (As suggested by its name, allelic deletions of the gene encoding DCC on human chromosome 18q have implicated this member of the immunoglobulin superfamily as a **tumor suppressor** in 70 percent of human colorectal cancers. Recall similar relationships between developmental regulation and tumor suppression discussed in Chapters 3, 4, 10, 12, and 14.) Nonetheless, it is also likely that local factors such as melanin pigment, preexisting fiber tracts, and neural cell adhesion molecules must participate in guiding the axons during normal development of the visual pathway.

For example, as the growth cones turn at the optic disc and then travel through the optic stalk, they establish an orderly spatial relationship among the retinal axons that to some degree matches their points of origin in the retina. This organization probably reflects an active response to locational cues rather than being simply a mechanical consequence of the site of origin of the axon. For example, if the presumptive optic tract of a *Xenopus* embryo is rotated by 90 degrees while the retinal growth cones are migrating through it, the growth cones will respond by rotating 90 degrees to compensate.

One factor in the optic stalk that appears to influence the arrangement of axons is the presence of the pigment melanin in the peripheral pigment layer of the stalk. Axons growing into the optic stalk seem to avoid this pigment layer. In ocular albinos of numerous species, many axons go to the wrong side of the brain, resulting in targeting anomalies that degrade visual acuity and may alter the visible morphology of the lateral geniculate bodies. The conclusion that the retinal axons are pigmentophobic is supported by the observation that in albino rats and Siamese cats the first, pioneering axons to enter the optic stalk sometimes grow through areas that normally contain pigment

and that are otherwise avoided. And although the regulatory mechanism has not been diciphered, compensation for the inverted image produced by the lens of the eye on the retina appears to be achieved by inversion of dorsal and ventral fibers within the optic nerve.

The growth of ipsilaterally targeting axons from the optic nerve back into the optic tract also seems to depend in part on the presence of the axons from the opposite eye that normally cross over in the optic chiasm to join the ipsilateral fibers. If the opposite eye is removed in a mouse embryo, so that these decussating fibers never develop, the ipsilaterally targeting fibers of the remaining eye pause for unusually long periods within the chiasm. Indeed, the behavior of axonal growth cones in the region of the optic chiasm has been a subject of considerable interest given the importance of an axon's decision to cross over or to remain on the ipsilateral side. First, as the growth cones approach the region of the optic chiasm, they enter a part of the optic stalk similar in organization to the neural tube. Axons in this region become more closely associated with the pial surface of the nerve before entering the chiasm. Once they move into the region of the chiasm, they move in bursts with intermittent pauses before "deciding" to cross or to remain on the ipsilateral side.

Structures at the chiasm that are thought to play a role in this **saltatory behavior** of the growth cone and the "decision" to cross or to remain ipsilateral include (1) a small **midline V-shaped array of neurons** that express the cell adhesion molecule L1 (a member of the immunoglobulin superfamily) and the cell surface molecule CD44, and (2) a **midline glial palisade.** Retinal axons never enter the neuronal array; those that cross to the contralateral side turn just at its anterior border. Both ipsilateral and contralateral axons, however, enter the glial palisade before "deciding" whether to cross or not.

Apparently, the ability of a growth cone to interpret the environmental cues that direct it to cross to the other side at this decision point depends on its ability to express a protein called **GAP-43.** In knockout mice deficient in GAP-43, retinal axons become trapped within the chiasm for extended periods but then finally recover to enter the appropriate tracts. Thus GAP-43 does not seem to be required for growth or turning but rather may be involved in amplification of signals to the axon and soma of the RGC.

Finally, effective targeting of secondary retinal ganglion cell growth cones requires expression of a **"stop signal"** within the lateral geniculate bodies and superior colliculi. Many possible signals have been described, including members of the **collapsin/semaphorin family, RAGS** (see earlier), and a serine proteinase called **ERASE.** Immunocytochemical and in situ hybridization studies have shown that the large extracellular matrix glycoprotein **tenascin** may also play a role in inhibiting growth cone migration at their appropriate targets. For example, it appears that tenascin is abundant in the mouse tectum and is only weakly expressed within the retina, the optic nerve, and the optic tracts and that it is produced by radial glial cells

throughout embryonic development. It has been suggested that tenascin may slow the migration of retinal growth cones as they approach their target, and that the growth cones may then facilitate development of arborization and stabilize the resulting synapses.

Factors Other Than Environmental Signals Also Play a Role in the Targeting of the Retinal Axons

Various findings indicate that the targeting of the retinal axons to the lateral geniculate bodies and the subsequent formation of synaptic connections cannot be explained solely on the basis of soluble and local environmental signals. For example, the

Figure 13–22. A "tract-tracing" technique used to show the projection of secondary retinal neurons to a particular locus in the optic tract. The use of dyes to analyze the arrangement of the axons projected by distant neurons is a time-honored neurobiologic technique. In this example, a crystal of the carbocyanine dye DiI was inserted into the optic tract of a 16.5-day mouse embryo at a site caudal to the optic chiasm. After the dye had time to diffuse along the axons, the ipsilateral *A* and contralateral *B* retinas were mounted flat on a microscope slide and examined with a fluorescence microscope to determine which of the axons were back-filled with dye. The back-filled axons can be assumed to represent the axon population that projects to the site of the crystal in the optic tract. In the ipsilateral retina *A*, secondary neurons located mainly in the ventrotemporal crescent project to the site of the crystal, whereas in the contralateral *B*, neurons from all areas project to this site. This pattern is characteristic of the adult retina. Fibers from the ipsilateral and contralateral retinas are intermingled in the optic tract at the site of the crystal. (From Colello RJ, Guillery RW. 1990. The early development of retinal ganglion cells with uncrossed axons in the mouse: retinal position and axomal course. Development 108:515.)

cue that induces the retinal fibers from the nasal half of each retina to decussate at the optic chiasm apparently involves more than their position within the optic nerve and hence more than their response to the ambient signal molecules. Experiments in which nerve fibers arriving at the chiasm were backfilled with fluorescent dyes have shown that many of the fibers that are destined to decussate are intermingled with fibers from the lateral half of the retina that are destined to remain ipsilateral (Fig. 13–22).

Several studies indicate that feedback in the form of neural impulses from the retina is important in tuning the visual map. An ingenious experiment has been used to show that this is not the case in all systems, however. In this experiment, an eye from an embryo axolotl salamander was transplanted to a mutant "eyeless" axolotl embryo before the retinal axons grew out. This chimeric axolotl was then grafted to the flank of a California newt so that the animals shared a common blood supply. California newts produce a toxin called **tetrodotoxin** to which the newt itself is immune but which blocks all neural activity in the axolotl "Siamese" twin. Despite the absence of all neural activity, the transplanted retinal axons of the axolotl grew to their normal targets in the brain. Refinement of the visual map, however, depends as much on the retraction of axons from inappropriate targets as it does on the growth of axons to appropriate targets (see later). If has been demonstrated in several vertebrate and invertebrate systems that the final pattern of synaptic connections depends on the frequency and duration of impulse activity. Indeed, when electrical activity is inhibited within the mammalian visual system, axons are not retracted from inappropriate targets. Moreover, it has been demonstrated in cultured neurons that neurite retraction depends on the density of voltage-activated calcium channels following stimulation.

There is evidence that both the timing of axonal outgrowth and positional predetermination of retinal neurons influence axonal targeting, although experimental alteration of either of these factors does not completely disrupt normal targeting. Some studies suggest that competitive interactions among axons may play a role, but other studies suggest the opposite. In any case, it is apparent that the process of retinal axonal path finding is complex and probably involves several overlapping, redundant control systems.

It is also becoming clear that the visual system is extensively modified by processes such as death of neurons and rearrangement of axons as it is being formed. Recall the effects of impulse activity on neurite retraction above. This type of control is called **developmental regulation.** As in other areas of the nervous system, far more neurons are initially produced than survive in the mature system. It is estimated that three to four million ganglion cells arise in the human retina, for example, but only just over a million survive in the adult. Many of the original synaptic connections made by these cells are eliminated by a pruning process that participates in tuning the visual maps in the geniculate body and superior colliculus.

SUGGESTED READING

Descriptive Embryology

Bossy J. 1980. Development of olfactory and related structures in staged human embryos. Anat Embryol 161:225

Brunjes PC, Frazier LL. 1986. Maturation and plasticity in the olfactory system of vertebrates. Brain Res Rev 11:1

Couly G, Le Douarin NM. 1988. The fate map of the cephalic neural primordium at the presomitic to the 3-somite stage in the avian embryo. Development 103(suppl):101

D'Amico-Martel A. 1982. Temporal patterns of neurogenesis in avian cranial sensory and autonomic ganglia. Am J Anat 163:351

D'Amico-Martel A. 1983. Contributions of placodal and neural crest cells to avian cranial peripheral ganglia. Am J Anat 166:445

Davies AM. 1990. NGF synthesis and NGF receptor expression in the embryonic mouse trigeminal system. J Physiol (Paris) 84:100

Davies AM, Lumsden A. 1990. Ontogeny of the somatosensory system: origins and early development of primary sensory neurons. Annu Rev Neurosci 13:61

Didier YR, Gilbert W. 1990. Pioneer neurons in the

mouse trigeminal sensory system. Proc Natl Acad Sci U S A 87:923

Fontaine-Perus J, Chanconie M, Le Douarin NM. 1988. Developmental potentialities in the nonneuronal population of quail sensory ganglia. Dev Biol 128:359

Friedman WJ, Greene LA. 1999. Neurotrophin signaling via Trks and p75. Exp Cell Res 253:131

Gilbert MS. 1935. Some factors influencing the early development of the mammalian hypophysis. Anat Rec 62:337

Gorski RA. 1988. Sexual differentiation of the brain: mechanisms and implications for neuroscience. p. 256. In Easter SS et al (eds): Message to Mind. Sinauer Associates, Sunderland, MA

Herrup K. 1987. Roles of cell lineage in the developing mammalian brain. Curr Top Dev Biol 21:65

Hinrichsen K, Mestres P, Jacob HJ. 1986. Morphological aspects of the pharyngeal hypophysis in human embryos. Acta Morphol Neerl-Scand 24:235

Jacobson AG. 1981. Morphogenesis of the neural plate and tube. p. 233. In Connally TJ, Brinkley LL, Carlson BM (eds): Morphogenesis and Pattern Formation. Raven Press, New York

Jacobson M. 1984. Cell lineage analysis of neural induction: origins of cells forming the induced nervous system. Dev Biol 102:122

Jacobson M. 1985. Clonal analysis and cell lineages of the vertebrate central nervous system. Annu Rev Neurosci 8:71

Katz DM. 1990. Trophic regulation of nodose ganglion cell development: evidence for an expanded role of nerve growth factor during embryogenesis in the rat. Exp Neurol 110:1

Katz MJ. 1983. Ontophyletics of the nervous system: development of the corpus callosum and the evolution of axon tracts. Proc Natl Acad Sci U S A 80:5936

Le Douarin N, Fontaine-Perus J, Couly G. 1986. Cephalic ectodermal placodes and neurogenesis. Trends Neurosci 9:175

Lefebve PP, Leprince P, Weber T, et al. 1990. Neuronotrophic effect of developing otic vesicle on cochleo-vestibular neurons: evidence for nerve growth factor involvement. Brain Res 507:254

Lemire RJ, Loeser JD, Leech RW, Alvord EC. 1975. Normal and Abnormal Development of the Human Nervous System. Harper & Row, Hagerstown, MD

McKay RDG. 1989. The origins of cellular diversity in the mammalian central nervous system. Cell 58:815

Morriss-Kay G, Tuckett F. 1987. Fluidity of the neural epithelium during forebrain formation in rat embryos. J Cell Sci 8:433

Müller F, O'Rahilly R. 1980. The early development of the nervous system in staged insectivore and primate embryos. J Comp Neurol 193:741

Müller F, O'Rahilly R. 1986. The development of the human brain and the closure of the rostral neuropore at stage 11. Anat Embryol 175:205

Müller F, O'Rahilly R. 1986. The development of the human brain from a closed neural tube at stage 13. Anat Embryol 177:203

Müller F, O'Rahilly R. 1988. The first appearance of the future cerebral hemispheres of the human embryo at stage 14. Anat Embryol 177:495

Müller F, O'Rahilly R. 1989. The human brain at stage 17, including the appearance of the future olfactory bulb and the amygdaloid nuclei. Anat Embryol 180:353

Nichols DH. 1986. Formation and distribution of neural crest mesenchyme to the first pharyngeal arch region of the mouse embryo. Am J Anat 176:221

Noden D. 1984. Craniofacial development: new views on old problems. Anat Rec 208:1

Noden D. 1986. Origins and patterning of craniofacial mesenchymal tissues. J Craniofac Genet Dev Biol 2(suppl): 15

Northcutt RG, Gans C. 1983. The genesis of neural crest and epidermal placodes: a reinterpretation of vertebrate origins. Q Rev Biol 58:1

O'Rahilly R, Gardner E. 1971. The timing and sequence of events in the development of the human nervous system during the embryonic period proper. Z Anat Entwicklungsgesch 134:1

O'Rahilly R, Müller F. 1981. The first appearance of the human nervous system at stage 8. Acta Embryol 163:1

O'Rahilly R, Müller F. 1984. The early development of the hypoglossal nerve and occipital somites in staged human embryos. Am J Anat 169:237

O'Rahilly R, Müller F. 1984. Embryonic length and cerebral landmarks in staged human embryos. Anat Rec 209:265

O'Rahilly R, Müller F. 1986. The meninges in human development. J Neuropathol Exp Neurol 45:588

Rakic P. 1984. Organizing principles for development of primate cerebral cortex. p. 21. In Sharma SC (ed): Organizing Principles of Neural Development. Plenum Press, New York

Rakic P. 1984. Emergence of neuronal and glial cell lineages in primate brain. p. 29. In Black IB (ed): Cellular and Molecular Biology of Neural Development. Plenum Press, New York

Rubenstein JLR, Martinez S, Shinamura K, Puelles L. 1994. The embryonic forebrain: the prosomeric model. Science 266:576

Sakai Y. 1987. Neurulation in the mouse. I. The ontogenesis of neural segments and the determination of topographical regions in a central nervous system. Anat Rec 218:450

Schoenwolf G. 1982. On the morphogenesis of the early rudiments of the developing central nervous system. Scanning Electron Microsc 1:289

Sidman RL, Rakic P. 1973. Neuronal migration, with special reference to developing human brain: a review. Brain Res 62:1

Tam P. 1989. Regionalization of the mouse embryonic ectoderm: allocation of prospective ectodermal tissues during gastrulation. Development 107:55

Tan SS, Morriss-Kay G. 1985. The development and

distribution of the cranial neural crest in the rat embryo. Cell Tissue Res 240:403

Van de Water TR. 1988. Tissue interactions and cell differentiation: neuron-sensory cell interaction during otic development. Development 103(suppl): 185

Walicke PA. 1989. Novel neurotrophic factors, receptors, and oncogenes. Annu Rev Neurosci 12:103

Williams RW, Herrup K. 1988. The control of neuron cell number. Annu Rev Neurosci 11:423

Wilson-Pauwels L, Akesson EJ, Stewart PA. 1988. Cranial Nerves: Anatomy and Clinical Comments. BC Decker Inc, Toronto

Windle W. 1970. Development of neural elements in human embryos of four to seven weeks gestation. Exp Neurol (suppl 5):44

Clinical Applications

Caddy KWT, Sidman RL, Eicher EM. 1981. Stumbler, a new mutant mouse with cerebellar disease. Brain Res 208:251

Chou SM, Gilbert EF, Chun RWM, et al. 1990. Infantile olivopontocerebellar atrophy with spinal muscular atrophy (infantile OPCA + SMA). Clin Neuropathol 9:21

Clarkson TW. 1993. Mercury: major issues in environmental health. Environ Health Perspect 100:31

Cowan WM, Fawcett JW, O'Leary DDM, Standfield BB. 1984. Regressive events in neurogenesis. Science 225:1258

des Portes V, Pinard JM, Billuart P, et al. 1998. A novel CNS gene required for neuronal migration and involved in X-linked subcortical laminar heterotopia and lissencephaly syndrome. Cell 92:51

Fleck MW, Hirotsune S, Gambello MJ, et al. 2000. Hippocampal abnormalities and enhanced excitability in a murine model of human lissencephaly. J Neurosci 20:2439

Fletcher CF, Lutz CM, O'Sullivan TN, et al. 1996. Absence epilepsy in tottering mutant mice is associated with calcium channel defects. Cell 87:607

Francis F, Koulakoff A, Boucher D, et al. 1999. Doublecortin is a developmentally regulated, microtubule-associated protein expressed in migrating and differentiating neurons. Neuron 23:247

Gasser UE, Hatten ME. 1990. Neuron-glia interactions of rat hippocampal cell in vitro: glial-guided neuronal migration and neuronal regulation of glial differentiation. J Neurosci 10:1276

Gleeson JG, Allen KM, Fox JW, et al. 1998. Doublecortin, a brain-specific gene mutated in human X-linked lissencephaly and double cortex syndrome, encodes a putative signaling protein. Cell 92:63

Gleeson JG, Lin PT, Flanagan LA, Walsh CA. 1999. Doublecortin is a microtubule-associated protein and is expressed widely by migrating neurons. Neuron 23:257

Gouw LG, Digre KB, Harris CP, et al. 1994. Autosomal dominant cerebellar ataxia with retinal degenera-

tion: clinical neuropathological and genetic analysis of a large kindred. Neurology 44:1441

Hamilton BA, Smith DJ, Mueller KL, et al. 1997. The vibrator mutation causes neurodegeneration via reduced expression of PITP alpha: positional complementation cloning and extragenic suppression. Neuron 18:711

Hanks M, Wurst W, Anson-Cartwright L, et al. 1995. Rescue of the En-1 mutant phenotype by replacement of En-1 by En-2. Science 269:679

Harding BN, Dunger DB, Grant DB, Erdohazi M. 1988. Familial olivopontocerebellar atrophy with neonatal onset: a recessively inherited syndrome with systemic and biochemical abnormalities. J Neurol Neurosurg Psychiatry 51:385

Hatten ME. 1990. Riding the glial monorail: a common mechanism for glial-guided neuronal migration in different regions of the mammalian brain. Trends Neurosci 13:179

Hatten ME, Liem RKH, Mason CA. 1984. Defects in specific associations between astroglia and neurons occur in microcultures of weaver mouse cerebellar cells. J Neurosci 4:1163

Hatten ME, Liem RKH, Mason CA. 1986. Weaver mouse cerebellar granule neurons fail to migrate on wild-type astroglial processes in vitro. J Neurosci 6:2676

Hattori M, Adachi H, Tsujimoto M, et al. 1994. Miller-Dieker lissencephaly gene encodes a subunit of brain platelet-activating factor acetylhydrolase. Nature 370:216

Herrup K, Sunter K. 1987. Numerical matching during cerebellar development: quantitative analysis of granule cell death in staggerer mouse chimeras. J Neurosci 7:829

Hirotsune S, Fleck MW, Gambello MJ, et al. 1998. Graded reduction of Pafah1b1 (Lis1) activity results in neuronal migration defects and early embryonic lethality. Nat Genet 19:333

Isaacs KR, Abbott LC. 1992. Development of the paramedian lobule of the cerebellum in wild-type and tottering mice. Dev Neurosci 14:386

Kumar D. 1986. Genetic aspects of congenital cerebellar ataxia. Indian J Pediatr 53:761

Leone M, Brignolio F, Rosso MG, et al. 1990. Friedrich's ataxia: a descriptive epidemiological study in an Italian population. Clin Genet 38:161

Mason CA, Edmonson JC, Hatten ME. 1988. The extending astroglial process: development of glial cell shape, the growing tip, and interactions with neurons. J Neurosci 8:3124

McMahon AP, Bradley A. 1990. The Wnt-1(int-1) protooncogene is required for development of a large region of the mouse brain. Cell 62:1073

Salinas PC, Fletcher C, Copeland NG, et al. 1994. Maintenance of Wnt-3 expression in Purkinje cells of the mouse cerebellum depends on interactions with granule cells. Development 120:1277

Sapir T, Elbaum M, Reiner O. 1997. Reduction of microtubule catastrophe events by LIS1, platelet-activating factor acetylhydrolase subunit. EMBO J 16:6977

Schiller F. 1995. Staggering gait in medical history. Ann Neurol 37:127

Sidman RL, Conover CS, Carson JH. 1985. Shiverer gene maps near the distal end of chromosome 18 in the house mouse. Cytogenet Cell Genet 39:241

Sidman RL, Green MC, Appel SH. 1965. Catalog of the Neurological Mutants of the Mouse. Harvard University Press, Cambridge, MA

Sidman RL, Willinger M, Margolis DM. 1983. Mouse weaver mutation affects granule cell neurite growth *in vitro*. Birth Defects Orig Artic Ser 19: 189

Sonmez E, Herrup K. 1984. Role of staggerer gene in determining cell number in cerebellar cortex. II. Granule cell death and persistence of external granule cell layer in young mouse chimeras. Dev Brain Res 12:271

Superneau D, Wertelecki W, Zellweger H. 1985. Letter to the editor: the Marinesco-Sjögren syndrome described a quarter of a century before Marinesco. Am J Genet 22:647

Sussman DJ, Klingensmith J, Salinas P, et al. 1994. Isolation and characterization of a mouse homolog of the *Drosophila* segment polarity gene dishevelled. Dev Biol 166:73

Thomas KR, Capecchi MR. 1990. Targeted disruption of the murine *int-1* proto-oncogene resulting in severe abnormalities in midbrain and cerebellar development. Nature (London) 346:847

Thomas KR, Musci TS, Neumann PE, Capecchi MR. 1991. Swaying is a mutant allele of the proto-oncogene *Wnt-1*. Cell 67:969

Weimar WR, Lane PW, Sidman RL. 1982. Vibrator (*vb*): a spinocerebellar system degeneration with autosomal recessive inheritance in mice. Brain Res 251:357

Wurst W, Auerbach AB, Joyner AL. 1994. Multiple developmental defects in Engrailed-1 mutant mice: an early mid-hindbrain deletion and patterning defects in forelimbs and sternum. Development 120:2065

Experimental Principles

Beazley LD, Dunlop SA, Chelvanyagam DK, Ross WM. 1995. Wiring up the visual system. Clin Exp Pharmacol Physiol 22:550

Beccera SP, Palmer I, Kumar A, et al. 1995. Unique changes of ganglion cell growth cone behavior following cell adhesion molecule perturbations: a time-lapse study of the living retina. J Biol Chem 268:23148

Brittis PA, Lemmon V, Rutishauser U, Silver J. 1995. Unique changes of ganglion cell growth cone behavior following cell adhesion molecule perturbations: a time-lapse study of the living retina. Mol Cell Neurosci 6:433

Bovolenta P, Dodd J. 1990. Guidance of commissural growth cones at the floor plate in embryonic rat spinal cord. Development 109:435

Buettner HM. 1995. Computer simulation of nerve growth cone filopodial dynamics for visualization and analysis. Cell Motil Cytoskeleton 32:187

Burden-Gulley SM, Payne HR, Lemmon V. 1995. Growth cones are actively influenced by substrate-bound adhesion molecules. J Neurosci 15:4370

Calof AL, Campanero MR, O'Rear JJ, et al. 1994. Domain-specific activation of neuronal migration and neurite outgrowth-promoting activities of laminin. Neuron 13:117

Caubit X, Riou JF, Coulon J, et al. 1994. Tenascin expression in the developing, adult and regenerating caudal spinal cord in the urodele amphibians. Int J Dev Biol 38:661

Chien CB, Rosenthal DE, Harris WA, Holt CE1. 1993. Navigational errors made by growth cones without filopodia in the embryonic *Xenopus* brain. Neuron 11:237

Cohen A, Bray GM, Aquayo AJ. 1994. Neurotrophin-4/5 (NT-4/5) increases adult rat retinal ganglion cell survival and neurite outgrowth in vitro. J Neurobiol 25:953

Colello RJ, Guillery RW. 1990. The early development of retinal ganglion cells with uncrossed axons in the mouse: retinal position and axonal course. Development 108:515

Colello RJ, Guillery RW. 1992. Observations on the early development of the optic nerve and tract of the mouse. J Comp Neurol 317:357

Constantine-Paton M. 1990. Patterned activity, synaptic convergence, and the NMDA receptor in developing visual pathways. Annu Rev Neurosci 13:129

Cook JE. 1991. Correlated activity in the CNS: a role on every time scale? Trends Neurosci 14:397

Drescher U, Dremoser C, Handwerker C et al. 1995. In vitro guidance of retinal ganglion cell axons by RAGs, a 25 kDa tectal protein related to ligands for Egh receptor tyrosine kinases. Cell 87:359

Fraser SE, Murray BA, Chuong CM, Edelman GM. 1984. Alteration of the retinotectal map in *Xenopus* by antibodies to neural cell adhesion molecules. Proc Natl Acad Sci U S A 81:4222

Godement P. 1994. Specific guidance and modulation of growth cone motility during in vivo development. J Physiol (Paris) 88:259

Godement P, Salaun J, Mason C. 1990. Retinal axon pathfinding in the optic chiasm: divergence of crossed and uncrossed fibers. Neuron 5:173

Godement P, Wang LC, Mason CA. 1994. Retinal axon divergence in the optic chiasm: dynamics of growth cone behavior at the midline. J Neurosi 14:7024

Goldberg DJ, Wu DY. 1995. Inhibition of formation of filopodia after axotomy by inhibitors of protein tyrosine kinases. J Neurobiol 27:553

Goodman CS, Shatz CJ. 1993. Developmental mechanisms that generate precise patterns of neuronal connectivity. Cell 72 (suppl):77

Goshima Y, Nakamura F, Strittmatter P, Strittmatter SM. 1995. Collapsin-induced growth cone collapse mediated by an intracellular protein related to UNC-33. Nature 376:509

Gottmann K, Lux HD. 1995. Growth cone calcium ion channels: properties, clustering, and functional roles (review). Perspect Dev Neurobiol 2:371

Guillery RW. 1974. Visual pathways in albinos. Sci Am 230:44

Halfter W, Yip YP, Yip JW. 1994. Axonin 1 is expressed primarily in subclasses of avian sensory neurons during outgrowth. Brain Res 78:87

Hankin MH, Lagenaur CF. 1994. Cell adhesion molecules in the early developing mouse retina: retinal neurons show preferential outgrowth in vitro on L1 but not N-CAM. J Neurobiol 25:472

Harris WA. 1984. Axonal pathfinding in the absence of normal pathways and impulse activity. J Neurosci 4:1153

Harris WA. 1986. Homing behavior of axons in the embryonic vertebrate brain. Nature (London) 320: 266

Harris WA. 1989. Local positional cues in the neuroepithelium guide retinal axons in embryonic *Xenopus* brain. Nature (London) 339:218

Harris WA, Holt CE. 1990. Early events in the embryogenesis of the vertebrate visual system. Annu Rev Neurosci 13:155

Harris WA, Holt C, Bonhoeffer F. 1987. Retinal axons with and without their somata, growing to and arborizing in the tectum of *Xenopus* embryos: a time-lapse video study of single fibers *in vivo*. Development 101:123

Heidemann SR, Buxbaum RE. 1991. Growth cone motility (review). Curr Opin Neurobiol 1:339

Johnson JK, Casagrande VA. 1993. Prenatal development of axon outgrowth and connectivity in the ferret visual system. Vis Neurosi 10:117

Kater SB, Rehder V. 1995. The sensory-motor role of growth cone filopedia (review). Curr Opin J Neurobiol 5:68

Kater SB, Shibata A. 1994. The unique and shared properties of neuronal growth cones that enable navigation and specific pathfinding (review). J Physiol (Paris) 88:155

Kolodkin AL, Matthes DJ, Goodman CS. 1993. The semaphorin genes encode a family of transmembrane and secreted growth cone guidance molecules. Cell 75:1389

Lin CH, Forscher P. 1993. Cytoskeletal remodeling during growth cone-target interactions. J Cell Biol 121:1369

Lund RD, Hankin MH. 1995. Pathfinding by retinal ganglion cell axons: transplantation studies in genetically and surgically blind mice. J Comp Neurol 356:481

Marcus RC, Blazeski R, Godement P, Mason CA. 1995. Retinal axon divergence in the optic chiasm: uncrossed axons diverge from crossed axons within a midline glial specialization. J Neurosci 14:3716

Neely MD, Nicholls JG. 1995. Electrical activity,

growth cone motility and the cytoskeleton. J Exp Biol 198:1433

O'Leary DD, Heffner CD, Kutka L, et al. 1991. A target-derived chemoattractant controls the development of the corticopontine projection by a novel mechanism of axon targeting. Development (suppl) 2:123

O'Leary DDM, Fawcett JW, Cowan WM. 1986. Topographic targeting errors in the retinocollicular projection and their elimination by selective ganglion cell death. J Neurosci 6:3692

O'Rahilly R. 1983. The timing and sequence of events in the development of the human eye and ear during the embryonic period proper. Anat Embryol 168:87

O'Rourke NA, Fraser SE. 1990. Dynamic changes in optic fiber terminal arbors lead to retinotopic map formation: an in vivo confocal microscopic study. Neuron 5:159

Pallas SL, Roe AW, Sur M. 1990. Visual projections induced into the auditory pathway of ferrets. I. Novel inputs to primary auditory cortex (AI) from the LP/pulvinar complex and the topography of the MGN-AI projection. J Comp Neurol 298:50

Panni MK, Atkinson J, Lund RD. 1994. Evidence for trophic role of brain-derived neurotrophic factor in transplanted embryonic retinae. Brain Res Dev 81:325

Perez RG, Halfter W. 1994. Tenascin protein and mRNA in the avian visual system: distribution and potential contribution to retinotectal development (review). Perspect Dev Neurobiol 2:75

Provis JM, Penfold PL. 1988. Cell death and the elimination of retinal axons during development. Prog Neurobiol 3:331

Puschel AW, Adams RH, Betz H. 1995. Murine semaphorin D/collapsin is a member of a diverse gene family and creates domains inhibitory for axonal extension. Neuron 14:941

Rader C, Stoeckli ET, Ziegler U et al. 1993. Cell-cell adhesion by homophilic interaction of the neuronal recognition molecule axonin-1. Eur J Biochem 214:133

Rakic P. 1981. Development of visual centers in the primate brain depends on binocular competition before birth. Science 214:928

Rakic P, Riley KP. 1983. Regulation of axon number in primate optic nerve by prenatal binocular competition. Nature (London) 305:135

Ramoa AS, Campbell G, Shatz C. 1989. Retinal ganglion B (beta) cells project transiently to the superior colliculis during development. Proc Natl Acad Sci U S A 86:2061

Roberts CW, Sonder AM, Lumsden A, Korsmeyer SJ. 1995. Development expression of *Hox11* and specification of splenic cell fate. Am J Pathol 146:1089

Sandib M, Rao Y, Siu CH. 1994. The homophilic binding site of the neural cell adhesion molecule NCAM is directly involved in promoting neurite outgrowth from cultured neural retinal cells. J Biol Chem 269:14841

Shatz C. 1990. Competitive interactions between retinal ganglion cells during prenatal development. J Neurobiol 21:197

Shatz CJ, Sretavan DW. 1986. Interactions between retinal ganglion cells during the development of the mammalian visual system. Annu Rev Neurosci 9:171

Sheffield JB, Krasnopolsky V, Dehlinger E. 1994. Inhibition of retinal growth cone activity by specific metalloproteinase inhibitors in vitro. Dev Dynam 200:79

Silver J, Poston M, Rutishauser U. 1987. Axon pathway boundaries in the developing brain. I. Cellular and molecular determinants that separate the optic and olfactory projections. J Neurosci 7:2264

Silver J, Sapiro J. 1981. Axonal guidance during development of the optic nerve: the role of pigmented epithelia and other factors. J Comp Neurol 202:521

Simon DK, O'Leary DM. 1990. Limited topographic specificity in the targeting and branching of mammalian retinal axons. Dev Biol 137:125

Simon H, Gurthrie S, Lumsden A. 1994. Rebulation of SC1/Dm-GRASP during the migration of motor neurons in the chick embryo brain stem. J Neurobiol 25:1129

Sperry RW. 1963. Chemoaffinity in the orderly growth of nerve fiber patterns and connections. Proc Natl Acad Sci U S A 50:703

Sretavan DW. 1990. Specific routing of retinal ganglion cell axons at the mammalian optic chiasm during embryonic development. J Neurosci 10:1995

Sretavan DW, Feng L, Pure E, Reichert LF. 1994. Embryonic neurons of the developing optic chiasm express L1 qand CD44, cell surface molecules with opposing effects on retinal axon growth. Neuron 12:957

Sretavan DW, Reichardt LF. 1993. Time-lapse video analysis of retinal ganglion cell axon pathfinding at the mammalian optic chiasm: growth cone guidance using intrinsic chiasm cues. Neuron 10:761

Stier H, Schlosshauer B. 1995. Axonal guidance in the chicken retina. Devel 121:1433

Stoecki ET, Landmesser LT. 1995. Axonin-1, Nr-CAM, and Ng-CAM play different roles in the in vivo guidance of chick commissural neurons. Neuron 14:1165

Strittmatter SM, Igarashi M, Fishman MC. 1994. Gap-43 amino terminal peptides modulate growth cone morphology and neurite outgrowth. J Neurosci 14:5503

Strittmatter SM, Fankhauser C, Huang PL, et al. 1995. Neuronal pathfinding is abnormal in mice lacking the neuronal growth cone protein GAP-43. Cell 80:445

Sur M, Garraghty PE, Roe AW. 1988. Experimentally induced visual projections into auditory thalamus and cortex. Science 242:1437

Sur M, Pallas SL, Roe AW. 1990. Cross-modal plasticity in cortical development: differentiation and specification of sensory neocortex. Trends Neurosci 13:227

Vaughan L, Weber P, D'Alessandri L, et al. 1994. Tenascin-contactin/F11 interactions: a clue for a developmental role? Perspect Dev Neurobiol 2:43

Walsh C, Guillery R. 1984. Fiber order in the pathways from the eye to the brain. Trends Neurosci 7:208

Webster MJ, Shatz C, Kliot M, Silver J. 1988. Abnormal pigmentation and unusual morphogenesis of the optic stalk may be correlated with retinal axon misguidance in embryonic siamese cats. J Comp Neurol 269:592

Williams RW, Rakic P. 1985. Dispersion of growing axons within the optic nerve of the embryonic monkey. Proc Natl Acad Sci U S A 82:3906

Wizenmann A, Thies E, Klostermann S, et al. 1993. Appearance of target-specific guidance information for regenerating axons after CNS lesions. Neuron 11:975

Zhao X, Siu CH. 1995. Colocalization of the homophilic binding site and the neuritogenic activity of the cell adhesion molecule L1 to its second Ig-like domain. J Biol Chem 270:29413

Zheng JQ, Felder M, Conner JA, Poo MM. 1994. Turning of the nerve growth cones induced by neurotransmitters (see comments). Nature 368:140

Zheng JQ, Wan JJ, Poo MM. 1996. Essential role of filopodia in chemotactic turning of nerve growth cone induced by glutamate gradient. J Neurosci 16:1140

14

Development of the Integumentary System

Summary

The skin, or integument, consists of two layers: the **epidermis** and the **dermis.** The epidermis is formed primarily by the embryonic surface ectoderm, although it is also colonized by **melanocytes** (pigment cells) from the neural crest and by **Langerhans cells,** which are immune cells of bone marrow origin. In addition, it contains pressure-sensing **Merkel cells,** which may or may not arise outside the epidermis. The dermis is a mesodermal tissue. It is derived mainly from the somatopleuric layer of the lateral plate mesoderm but also, in part, from the dermatome subdivisions of the somites.

Just after neurulation, the ectoderm, which originally is a single cell thick, proliferates to produce an outer layer of simple squamous epithelium called the **periderm.** The inner layer of proliferating cells is now called the **basal layer.** In the 11th week, the basal layer produces a new **intermediate layer** between itself and the periderm. The basal stem cell layer is now called the **stratum germinativum;** this layer will continue to produce all the cells of the epidermis throughout life. By the 21st week, the intermediate layer is replaced by the definitive three layers of the outer epidermis: the inner **stratum spinosum,** the middle **stratum granulosum,** and the outer **stratum corneum,** or **horny layer.** The cells of these layers are called **keratinocytes** because they contain the **keratin** proteins characteristic of the epidermis. The layers of the epidermis represent a maturation series: keratinocytes produced by the stratum germinativum differentiate as they pass outward to form the two intermediate layers and the flattened, dead, keratin-filled mature keratinocytes of the horny layer, which are finally sloughed from the surface of the skin. As the definitive epidermis develops, the overlying periderm is gradually shed into the amniotic fluid.

The dermis contains most of the tissues and structures of the skin, including blood vessels, nerves, muscle bundles, and most of the sensory structures. The superficial layer of the dermis develops projections called **dermal papillae,** which interdigitate with downward projections of the epidermis called **epidermal ridges.**

The skin gives rise to a number of specialized structures, including hair, nails, and a variety of epidermal glands. The ectodermal placodes discussed in the preceding two chapters can also be regarded as skin derivatives. **Hair follicles** originate as rodlike downgrowths of the stratum germinativum into the dermis. The club-shaped base of each hair follicle is indented by a hillock of dermis called the **dermal papilla,** and the hair shaft is produced by the **germinal matrix** of ectoderm that overlies this dermal papilla. The various types of epidermal glands also

Development of the Skin, Hair, Epidermal Glands, Nails, and Teeth

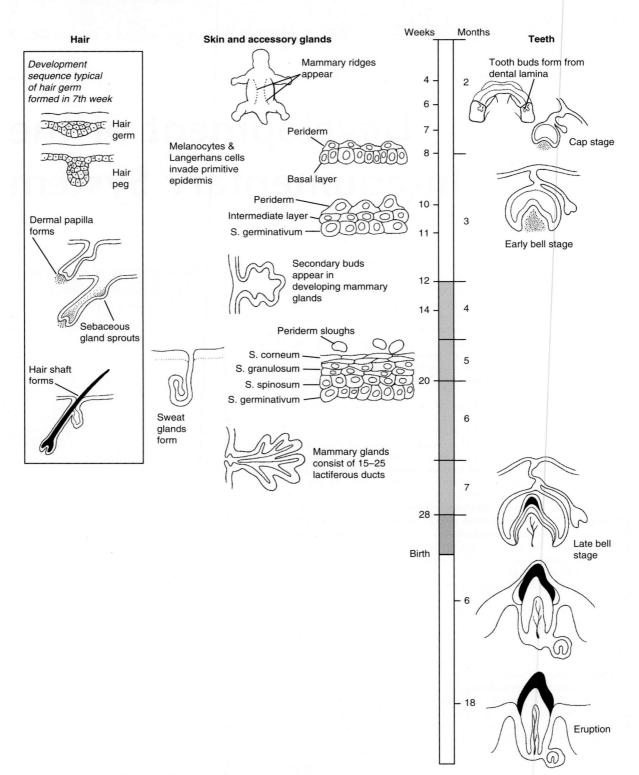

Hair

Development sequence typical of hair germ formed in 7th week

Hair germ

Hair peg

Dermal papilla forms

Sebaceous gland sprouts

Hair shaft forms

Skin and accessory glands

Mammary ridges appear

Periderm

Melanocytes & Langerhans cells invade primitive epidermis

Basal layer

Periderm

Intermediate layer

S. germinativum

Secondary buds appear in developing mammary glands

Periderm sloughs

S. corneum

S. granulosum

S. spinosum

S. germinativum

Sweat glands form

Mammary glands consist of 15–25 lactiferous ducts

Weeks   Months

4   2

6

7

8

10

11   3

12

14   4

5

20

6

28

7

Birth

6

18

Teeth

Tooth buds form from dental lamina

Cap stage

Early bell stage

Late bell stage

Eruption

Timeline. Development of the integument and integumentary derivatives.

arise as diverticula of the epidermis. Some bud from the neck of a hair follicle; others bud directly downward from the stratum germinativum. The four principal types of epidermal glands are the **sebaceous glands,** which secrete the oily sebum that lubricates the skin and hair; the **apocrine glands,** found in the axillae, pubic region, and other specific areas of skin that secrete odorous substances; the **sweat glands;** and the **mammary glands.** The primordia of the fingernails and toenails arise on the palmar and plantar surfaces of the digits and then migrate around to the dorsal side. The nail plate grows from a specialized stratum germinativum located in the **nail fold** of epidermis that overlaps the proximal end of the nail primordium.

The first sign of tooth development is the formation of a U-shaped epidermal ridge called the **dental lamina** along the crest of the upper and lower jaws. Twenty downgrowths from the dental lamina combine with underlying concentrations of neural crest-derived mesenchyme to form the **tooth buds** of the primary (deciduous) teeth. The secondary, permanent teeth are formed by secondary tooth buds that sprout from these primary buds. Soon after each tooth bud forms, its mesenchymal component forms a hillock-like **dental papilla** that indents the overlying dental lamina tissue. This stage of dental development is called the **cap stage** because the dental lamina sits on the papilla like a cap. By the 10th week, the dental lamina becomes a bell-shaped structure that completely covers the dental papilla. During this **bell stage,** the cells of the inner epithelium of the dental lamina differentiate into enamel-producing **ameloblasts,** which begin to secrete radially arranged prisms of enamel between themselves and the underlying papilla. The outermost cells of the papilla differentiate into **odontoblasts,** which secrete the dentin of the tooth. The inner cells of the dental papilla give rise to the tooth pulp. Nerves and blood vessels gain access to the pulp through the tips of the tooth roots.

THE SURFACE ECTODERM GIVES RISE TO MOST CELLS OF THE EPIDERMIS, AND MESODERM GIVES RISE TO THE DERMIS

The Ectoderm First Produces an External Layer of Periderm and Then Differentiates Into the Definitive Four-Layered Epidermis

The ectoderm covering of the embryo is initially a single cell thick. Just after neurulation, in the fourth week, the surface ectoderm proliferates to form a new outer layer of simple squamous epithelium called the **periderm** (Fig. 14–1A). The underlying layer of proliferating cells is now called the **basal layer.** The cells of the periderm are gradually sloughed into the amniotic fluid. The periderm is normally shed completely by the 21st week, but in some fetuses it persists until birth, forming a "shell" or "cocoon" around the newborn infant, which is removed by the physician or shed spontaneously during the first weeks of life. These babies are called **collodion babies.**

In the 11th week, proliferation of the basal layer produces a new **intermediate layer** just deep to the periderm (see Fig. 14–1B). This layer is the forerunner of the outer layers of the mature epidermis, and the basal layer, now called the **germinative layer** or **stratum germinativum,** constitutes the layer of stem cells that will continue to replenish the epidermis throughout life. The cells of the intermediate layer contain the **keratin proteins** characteristic of differentiated epidermis and therefore are called **keratinocytes.**

During the early part of the fifth month, at about the time the periderm is shed, the intermediate layer is replaced by the three definitive layers of keratinocytes: the inner **stratum spinosum,** the middle **stratum granulosum,** and the outer **stratum corneum,** or **horny layer** (Fig. 14–2). This transformation, which involves **apoptosis,** or **programmed cell death,** begins at the cranial end of the fetus and proceeds caudally. The layers of the epidermis represent a maturational series: presumptive keratinocytes are constantly produced by the stratum germinativum, differentiate as they pass outward to the stratum corneum, and finally are sloughed from the surface of the skin.

The stem cells of the stratum germinativum are the only dividing cells of the epidermis. They contain a dispersed network of keratin filaments and are connected by cell-to-cell membrane junctions called **desmosomes.** As cells produced in the stratum germinativum move into the overlying, four-to-eight-cell-thick stratum spinosum, they begin to manufacture large amounts of two keratin proteins and also of **envelope proteins** that cover the inner surface of the plasma membrane. Production of keratins and envelope proteins ceases as the cells move into the stratum granulosum, but a

A

8 weeks

B

11 weeks

Figure 14–1. Differentiation of the ecto-derm into the primitive epidermis. *A,* Be-tween 8 and 9 weeks, the surface ecto-derm has begun to proliferate to form a periderm layer (P). The proliferating layer is now called the basal layer (B). *B,* By week 11, the basal layer (B) produces an intermediate layer (I) while a complete but irregular outer layer of periderm (P) is still apparent. (From Holbrook KA, Dale BA, Smith LT, et al. 1987. Markers of adult skin expressed in the skin of the first trimester fetus. Curr Probl Dermatol 16:94.)

protein called **filagrin** is produced that helps to bundle the keratin filaments within the cell. In addition, the enzyme **transglutaminase** crosslinks the envelope proteins. Finally, lytic enzymes are released within the cell, metabolic activity ceases, and the resulting flattened, scalelike, terminally dif-ferentiated keratinocytes enter the stratum cor-neum.

Many Factors Regulate the Production and Differentiation of Epidermal Cells

The "decision" of a cell in the stratum germinati-vum to remain in the pool of proliferating cells or to move into the stratum spinosum and begin dif-ferentiating is regulated by a number of interacting agents, including several growth factors. Epidermal

growth factor, transforming growth factor-α, trans-forming growth factor-β, keratin growth factor, calcium, retinoic acid, BIG, a ligand for ECK (a member of the EPH receptor tyrosine kinase fam-ily) and the interleukin cytokines IL-1α and IL-6 all appear to play essential and distinct roles in maintaining the balance between proliferation and differentiation in the stratum germinativum. Some of these factors have been mentioned in previous chapters in connection with other roles they play in development. Transcriptional factors, which reg-ulate the expression of specific genes, also play a role in the regulation of keratinocyte differentia-tion.

Not surprisingly, imbalances in this complex dynamic control system can result in disorders of skin proliferation. For example, excessive levels of transforming growth factor-α, which appears to be an autoregulator of epidermal proliferation because

17 weeks

24 weeks

Adult

Figure 14–2. Differentiation of the mature epidermis. The periderm (P) is sloughed during the fourth month and normally is absent by week 21. The definitive epidermal layers, including the stratum spinosum, stratum granulosum, and stratum corneum, begin to develop during the fifth month. (From Foster C, Bertram JF, Holbrook KA. 1988. Morphometric and statistical analyses describing the in utero growth of human epidermis. Anat Rec 222:201.)

cells of the stratum granulosum. As a consequence, the keratinocytes do not mature properly and cannot be sloughed from the surface of the stratum corneum.

Gorlin syndrome (nevoid basal cell carcinoma syndrome [NBCCS]) is an autosomal dominant disorder occurring in about 1:50,00 to 1:100,000 individuals. NBCCS maps to chromosome 9q22.3, and in addition to developmental anomalies consistent with disruption of the sonic hedgehog signaling pathway (see Experimental Principles section of Ch. 4), the syndrome is also characterized by predisposition to several cancers including **basal cell carcinoma (BCC).** This latter finding supports the view that *PTCH* is a **tumor suppressor gene.** Non-neoplastic disorders of epidermal derivatives also characterize NBCCS including **odontogenic keratocysts** and **pathognomonic dyskeratotic pitting** of the hands and feet. The odontogenic keratocysts, or jaw cysts, arise from the **dental lamina** (see later). Both **sporadic** and **hereditary** forms of BCCs occur in humans, but this phenotype is variable (age of onset and frequency), suggesting that other modifier genes or environmental factors such as exposure to sunlight may play a role in their pathogenesis.

Melanocytes, Langerhans Cells, and Merkel Cells Appear in the Fetal Epidermis

In addition to keratinocytes, the epidermis contains a few types of less abundant cells, including melanocytes, Langerhans cells, and Merkel cells. As mentioned in Chapter 4, the pigment cells, or **melanocytes,** of the skin differentiate from neural crest cells that detach from the neural tube in the sixth week and migrate to the developing epidermis. Although morphologic and histochemical studies do not detect melanocytes in the human epidermis until the 10th to 11th weeks, studies using monoclonal antibodies directed against antigens characteristic of melanocyte precursors have identified these cells in the epidermis as early as the sixth to seventh weeks (Fig. 14–3A). Thus, it may take neural crest cells only a few days to a week to migrate to the epidermis. Melanocytes are also found in the dermis during fetal life, but at least the vast majority of these are probably in

it is produced by keratinocytes themselves, can result in **psoriasis** and other hyperproliferative skin diseases. It has been hypothesized that overproduction of this substance can also lead to cancer. Transforming growth factor-β may be involved in arresting proliferation once a cell has begun to differentiate into a mature keratinocyte. CD8+ T cells may act as effectors in pathology of psoriatic lesions.

A number of heritable disorders result in excessive keratinization of the skin. For example, infants suffering from **lamellar ichthyosis** have skin that scales off in flakes, sometimes over the whole body. These infants require special care but are usually viable. **Harlequin fetuses,** in contrast, have rigid, deeply cracked skin and usually die shortly after birth. These babies suffer from a defect in the mechanism that bundles keratin fibers in the

Figure 14–3. Specialized cells of the epidermis. *A,* Melanocytes (M) first appear in the embryonic epidermis during the sixth and seventh weeks. *B,* Langerhans cells (L) migrate into the epidermis from the bone marrow starting in the seventh week. F = hair follicle. (*A,* From Holbrook KA. 1988. Structural abnormalities of the epidermally derived appendages in skin from patients with ectodermal dysplasia: insight into developmental errors. Birth Defects Orig Artic Ser 24:15. *B,* From Foster C, Holbrook KA. 1989. Ontogeny of Langerhans cells in human embryonic and fetal skin: cell densities and phenotypic expression relative to epidermal growth. Am J Anat 1984:157.)

transit to the epidermis. Recall from the Experimental Principles section of Chapter 5 that c-kit ligand and c-kit receptor play a pivotal role in migration of melanocytes to the skin.

The density of melanocytes increases during fetal life, reaching a peak of about 2300 cells/mm³ at the end of the third month, after which it drops to the final value of about 800 cells/mm³. Melanocytes represent between 5 and 10 percent of the cells of the epidermis in the adult. In the 10th week, many melanocytes become associated with the developing hair follicles (see later), where they function to donate pigment to the hairs.

Melanocytes function as a sunscreen, protecting the deeper layers of the skin from solar radiation, which can cause not only sunburn but also, in the long run, cancer. Unfortunately, melanocytes themselves are relatively likely to produce tumors. Most of these remain benign, but sometimes they give rise to the highly malignant type of cancer called **melanoma.**

The **Langerhans cells** are the macrophage immune cells of the skin, functioning both in contact sensitivity (allergic skin reactions) and in immune surveillance against invading microorganisms. They arise in the bone marrow and first appear in the epidermis by the seventh week (see Fig. 14–3*B*). Langerhans cells continue to migrate into the epidermis throughout life.

Merkel cells are pressure-detecting mechanoreceptors. In humans, they are found only in the thick skin of the palmar or plantar (foot sole) regions.

They lie at the base of the epidermis and are associated with underlying nerve endings in the dermis. Although the origin of these cells is not clear, they contain keratin and form desmosomes with adjacent keratinocytes; therefore, they may represent a modified type of keratinocyte. They appear in the fourth to sixth months.

THE DERMIS IS DERIVED FROM BOTH THE DERMATOMES AND THE SOMATOPLEURIC MESODERM

The dermis or **corium**—the layer of skin that underlies the epidermis and contains blood vessels, hair follicles, nerve endings, sensory receptors, and so forth—is a mesodermal tissue with a dual embryonic origin. Most of it is derived from the somatopleuric layer of the lateral plate mesoderm, but part of it is derived from the dermatomal divisions of the somites. During the third month, the outer layer of the developing dermis proliferates to form ridgelike **dermal papillae** that protrude into the overlying epidermis (Fig. 14–4). The intervening protrusions of the epidermis into the dermis are called **epidermal ridges.** This superficial region of the dermis is called the **papillary layer,** whereas the thick underlying layer of dense, irreg-

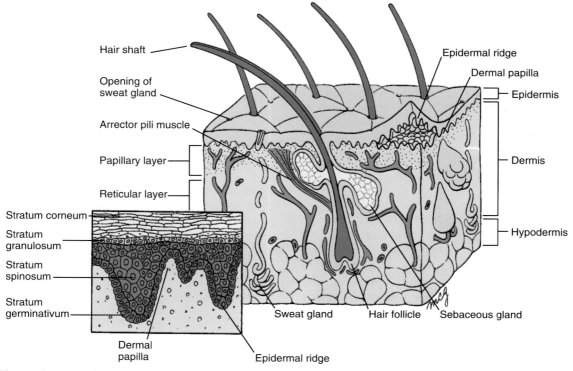

Figure 14–4. Definitive organization of the dermis and epidermis. The patterns of interdigitating dermal papillae and epidermal ridges first develop during the third month. Sebaceous glands develop from the epidermal lining of the hair follicles, appearing about 1 month after a given hair bud is formed. (Modified from Williams PL, Warwick R, Dyson M, Bannister LH. 1989. Gray's Anatomy. Churchill Livingstone, Edinburgh.)

ular connective tissue is called the **reticular layer.** The dermis is underlain by subcutaneous fatty connective tissue called the **hypodermis (subcorium).** The dermis differentiates to its definitive form in the second and third trimesters, although it is thin at birth and thickens progressively through infancy and childhood.

The pattern of external ridges and grooves produced in the skin by the dermal papillae varies from one part of the body to another. The palmar and plantar surfaces of the hands and feet carry a familiar pattern of whorls and loops; the eyelids have a diamond-shaped pattern, and the ridges on the upper surface of the trunk resemble a cobweb. The first skin ridges to appear are the whorls on the palmar and plantar surfaces of the digits, which develop in the 11th and 12th weeks. The entire system of surface patterns is established early in the fifth month of fetal life. Thereafter, each patch

of skin retains its characteristic pattern even if it is transplanted to a different part of the body.

Blood vessels form within the subcutaneous mesenchyme, deep to the developing dermis, in the fourth week. These branch to form a single layer of vessels in the dermis by the late sixth week and two parallel planes of vessels by the eighth week. Branches of these vessels follow nerves within the dermis and enter the papillary layer to become associated with the hair follicles. These branches may disappear and reappear during different stages of hair follicle differentiation.

It is estimated that the skin of the neonate contains 20 times more blood vessels than it needs to support its own metabolism. This excess is required for thermoregulation in the neonate. Much of the definitive vasculature of the skin develops in the first few weeks after birth.

THE INTEGUMENT PRODUCES SPECIALIZED STRUCTURES INCLUDING HAIR, EPIDERMAL GLANDS, AND NAILS

The skin contains a large number of specialized structures, including the hair; the sebaceous, sweat, and mammary glands; the nails of the fingers and toes; and the teeth. In addition, the ectodermal placodes discussed in the preceding two chapters can be regarded as skin derivatives.

Hair Follicles Are Formed by the Epidermis and Dermis Together

Hair follicles first appear at the end of the second month on the eyebrows, eyelids, upper lip, and chin. Hair follicles do not appear in other regions until the fourth month. Most, if not all, hair follicles are present by the fifth month, and it is believed that novel hair follicles do not form after birth. About 5 million hair follicles develop in both males and females. The differences between the two sexes in the distribution of various kinds of hairs is caused by the different concentrations of circulating sex steroid hormones.

The hair follicle first appears as a small concentration of ectodermal cells called a **hair germ** in the basal layer of the primitive, two-layered epidermis (Fig. 14–5*A*). Hair germs are thought to be induced by the underlying dermis. The hair germ proliferates to form a rodlike **hair peg** that pushes down into the dermis (see Fig. 14–5*B–F*). Within the dermis, the tip of the hair peg expands, forming a **bulbous hair peg,** and the dermis cells just beneath the tip of the bulb proliferate to form a small hillock called the **dermal papilla.** About 4 weeks after the hair germ begins to grow, the dermal papilla invaginates into the expanded base of the hair bulb (see Fig. 14–5*D, E*). Except in the case of the eyebrows and eyelashes, the dermal root sheath of the follicle becomes associated with a bundle of smooth muscle cells called the **arrector pili** muscle, which functions to erect the hair (making goose flesh) (see Fig. 14–4).

The layer of proliferating ectoderm that overlies the dermal papilla in the base of the hair bulb becomes the **germinal matrix.** The germinal matrix is responsible for producing the hair shaft (see Fig. 14–5*D–F*): proliferation of the germinal matrix produces cells that undergo a specialized process of keratinization and are added to the base of the hair shaft. The growing hair shaft is thus pushed outward through the follicular canal. If the hair is to be colored, the maturing keratinocytes incorporate pigment produced by the melanocytes of the hair bulb. The epidermal cells lining the follicular canal constitute the **inner** and **outer epidermal root sheaths.**

The first generation of hairs formed are fine and unpigmented and are called **lanugo.** These hairs first appear during the 12th week. They are mostly shed before birth and are replaced by coarser hairs during the perinatal period. At puberty, the rising levels of sex hormones cause the fine body hair to be replaced by coarser hairs on some parts of the body: the axilla and pubis of both sexes and the face and (in some races) the chest and back of males.

Sebaceous, Sweat, and Apocrine Glands Are Produced by Downgrowths of the Epidermis

Several types of glands are produced by downgrowth of the epidermis. Three types of glands—the sebaceous glands, apocrine glands, and sweat glands—are widespread over the body. The milk-producing mammary glands represent a specialized type of epidermal gland.

The **sebaceous glands** produce the oily **sebum** that lubricates the skin and hair. Over most of the body, these glands form as diverticula of the hair follicle shafts, budding from the side of the epidermal root sheath about 4 weeks after the hair germ begins to elongate. In some areas of hairless skin—such as the glans penis of males and the labia minora of females—sebaceous glands develop as independent downgrowths of epidermis. The bud grows into the dermis tissue and branches to form a small system of ducts ending in expanded secretory acini (alveoli) (see Fig. 14–4). The acini secrete by a **holocrine** mechanism; that is, entire secretory cells that are filled with vesicles of secretory products break down and are shed. The basal layer of the acinar epidermis consists of proliferating stem cells that constantly renew the supply of maturing secretory cells.

Figure 14–5. Development of the hair follicle. *A,* Hair germ at 80 days. *B,* Elongating hair germ later in the first trimester. *C,* Hair peg in the second trimester. *D–F,* Development of the follicle base from the elongated hair peg stage to the bulbous hair peg stage. The dermal papilla (DP) invaginates into the base of the developing follicle, inducing the germinal matrix (GM). In *F,* the hair shaft can be seen growing up the center of the follicle, and the inner and outer epidermal root sheaths (IRS and ORS) are differentiating. *G,* Scanning electron micrograph of the undersurface of the developing epidermis, showing hair germs (HG), hair pegs (HP), and bulbous hair pegs (BHP) growing into what originally was the dermis. (From Holbrook KA. 1988. Structural abnormalities of the epidermally derived appendages in skin from patients with ectodermal dysplasia: insight into developmental errors. Birth Defects Orig Artic Ser 24:15. Photographs courtesy of Dr. Karen Holbrook.)

Mature sebaceous glands are present on the face by 6 months of development. Sebaceous glands are highly active in the fetus, and the sebum they produce combines with desquamating epidermal cells and remnants of the periderm to form a waterproof protective coating for the fetus called the **vernix caseosa.** After birth, the sebaceous glands become relatively inactive, but at puberty they again begin to secrete large quantities of sebum in response to the surge in circulating sex steroids.

The **apocrine glands** are highly coiled, unbranched glands that develop in association with hair follicles. They initially form over most of the body, but in the later months of fetal development they are lost except in certain areas, such as the axillae, mons pubis, prepuce, scrotum, and labia minora. They begin to secrete at puberty, produc-

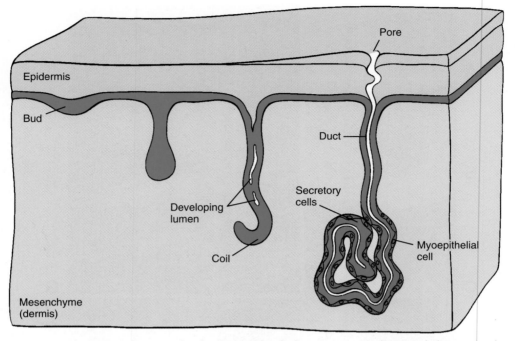

Figure 14–6. Development of sweat glands. Sweat glands first appear as elongated downgrowths of the epidermis at about 20 weeks. The outer cells of the downgrowth develop into a layer of smooth muscle, whereas the inner cells become the secretory cells of the gland.

ing a complex mix of substances that are modified by bacterial activity into odorous compounds. These compounds may function primarily in social and sexual communication. The secretory cells lining the deep half of the gland secrete their products by an **apocrine** mechanism: small portions of cytoplasm containing secretory vesicles pinch off and are released into the lumen of the gland.

The **sweat glands** first appear at about 20 weeks as buds of stratum germinativum that grow down into the underlying dermis to form unbranched, highly coiled glands (Fig. 14–6). The central cells degenerate to form the gland lumen, and the peripheral cells differentiate into an inner layer of secretory cells and an outer layer of **myoepithelial cells,** which are innervated by sympathetic fibers and contract to expel sweat from the gland (see Fig. 14–6). The secretory cells secrete fluid directly across the plasma membrane (**eccrine** secretion). Sweat glands form over the entire body surface except for a few areas such as the nipples. Large sweat glands develop as buds of the epithelial root sheath of hair follicles, superficial to the buds of sebaceous glands, in the axilla and areola.

Sweat glands fail to develop in the X-linked genetic disorder **hypohidrotic ectodermal dysplasia.** Infants with this disorder are vulnerable to potentially lethal hyperpyrexia (extremely high fever). The disease is also associated with abnormal dermal papillae. An apparently homologous condition in the mouse can be "cured" by administering epidermal growth factor after birth.

The Mammary Glands Are Modified Apocrine Glands That Arise Along Mammary Ridges on Either Side of the Body

In the fourth week, a pair of epidermal thickenings called the **mammary ridges** develop along either side of the body from the area of the future axilla to the future inguinal region and medial thigh (Fig. 14–7). In humans, these ridges normally disappear except at the site of the breasts. The remnant of the mammary ridge produces the **primary bud** of the mammary gland in the fifth week (see

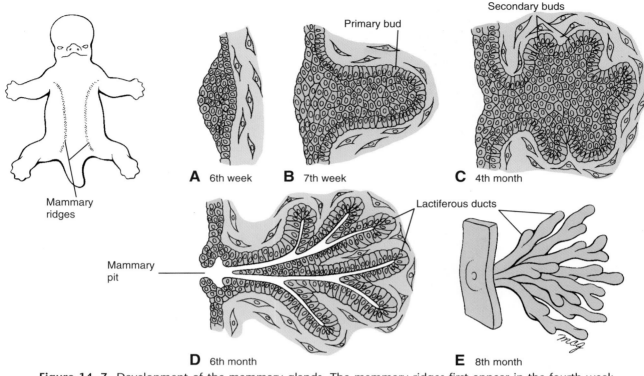

Figure 14–7. Development of the mammary glands. The mammary ridges first appear in the fourth week as thickened lines of epidermis that extend from the thorax to the medial thigh. *A, B,* In the region of the future mammary glands, the mammary ridge ectoderm begins to proliferate in the fifth week to form the primary mammary buds. *C, D,* Secondary buds form during the third month and become canalized to form lactiferous ducts during the last 3 months of fetal life. *E,* Organization of lactiferous ducts around the developing nipple in the eighth month.

Fig. 14–7*A, B*). This bud grows down into the underlying dermis. In the tenth week, the primary bud begins to branch, and by the 12th week, several **secondary buds** have formed (see Fig. 14–7*C*). These buds lengthen and branch throughout the remainder of gestation, and the resulting ducts canalize by the coalescence of small lumina (see Fig. 14–7*D, E*). At birth, the mammary glands consist of 15 to 25 **lactiferous ducts,** which open onto a small superficial depression called the **mammary pit** (see Fig. 14–7*D, E*). Proliferation of the underlying mesoderm usually converts this pit to an everted nipple within a few weeks after birth, although occasionally the nipple remains depressed **(inverted nipple).** The skin surrounding the nipple also proliferates to form the areola.

It is not very infrequent for one or more supernumerary nipples **(polythelia)** or supernumerary breasts **(polymastia)** to form along the line of the mammary ridges. The most common location is just below the normal breast. Supernumerary nipples are about as common in males as in females. More rarely, an ectopic nipple forms off the line of the mammary ridge as a consequence of migration of mammary tissue. Supernumerary breasts are often discovered at puberty or during pregnancy, when they enlarge or even lactate in response to stimulatory hormones.

The Fingernails and Toenails Form From Epidermis on the Palmar and Plantar Surfaces of the Digits

The nail anlagen first appear as epidermal thickenings on the palmar and plantar surfaces of the tips of the digits (Fig. 14–8*A*). These thickenings form

A

12 weeks

B

12–14 weeks

C

16 weeks

Figure 14–8. Sequence of scanning electron micrographs showing the development of the nails between 12 and 16 weeks. *A,* At first, the surface of the nail bed is covered with periderm. *B,* The margin of the dorsal nail fold (arrow) is clearly defined by 12 to 14 weeks. *C,* The nail plate is apparent by 16 weeks. (From Holbrook KA. 1988. Structural abnormalities of the epidermally derived appendages in skin from patients with ectodermal dysplasia: insight into developmental errors. Birth Defects Orig Artic Ser 24:15.)

at about 10 weeks on the fingers and at about 14 weeks on the toes. Almost immediately, the nail anlagen migrate to the dorsal surface of the digits, dragging branches of the palmar and plantar nerves along with them. On the dorsal surface, the nail anlage forms a shallow depression called the **primary nail field,** which is surrounded laterally and proximally by ectodermal **nail folds** (see Fig. 14–8*A,* *B*). The stratum germinativum of the proximal nail fold proliferates to become the **formative zone,** or **root,** that produces the horny **nail plate** (see Fig. 14–8*C*). Like a hair, the nail plate is made of compressed keratinocytes. A thin layer of epidermis called the **eponychium** initially covers the nail plate, but this layer normally degenerates except at the nail base. The growing nails reach the tips of the fingers by the eighth month and the tips of the toes by birth.

THE TEETH ARE FORMED BY ECTODERM AND NEURAL CREST–DERIVED MESENCHYME

In the sixth week, a U-shaped ridge of epidermis called the **dental lamina** appears on the upper and lower jaws (Fig. 14–9*A*). In the seventh week, 10 centers of epidermal cell proliferation develop at intervals on each dental lamina and grow down into the underlying mesenchyme. A concentration of mesenchyme appears under and around each of these 20 ingrowths. The composite structure consisting of the dental lamina ingrowth and the mesenchymal concentration is called a **tooth bud** (see Fig. 14–9*A*).

Experiments in which dental laminae and mesenchymal concentrations have been cultured with and without each other have shown that tooth development requires both components. Moreover, the concentration of mesenchymal tissue actually consists of neural crest–derived cells migrating from the caudal region of the mesencephalon and the cranial region of the metencephalon. These neural crest cells may be guided by signals (including a variety of extracellular matrix molecules) generated by the presumptive centers of tooth development in the epidermis.

It was also suggested at one point that the tooth buds are induced by the sensory branch of the trigeminal nerve that reaches the site of each

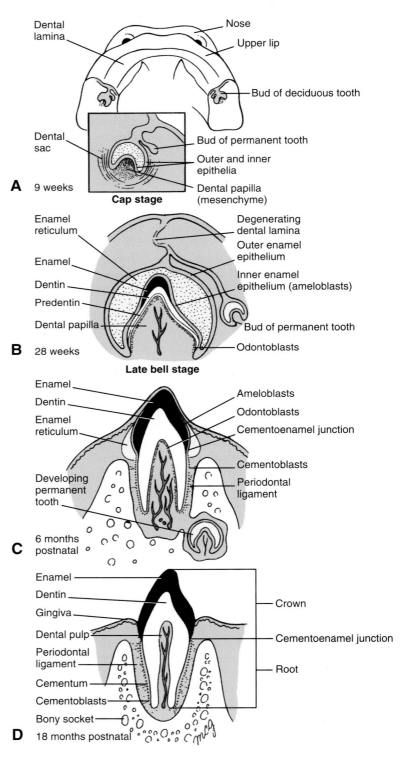

Figure 14–9. *A–D,* Development and eruption of the primary dentition. Notice that the ectodermal dental lamina gives rise to the enamel organ, which secretes the enamel of the tooth, whereas the neural crest cells that initially form the dental papilla differentiate into the odontoblasts, which secrete the dentin.

presumptive tooth bud just before the tooth bud forms. However, experiments in which the epidermal and mesenchymal precursors of the tooth buds were cultured with and without the trigeminal ganglion demonstrated that tooth development depends only on the ectodermal and mesenchymal precursors.

During the eighth week, instructive influences from the epidermis cause the mesenchymal condensation to invade the base of the dental lamina ingrowth, forming a hillock-shaped mesenchymal **dental papilla** (see Fig. 14–9A). This stage of tooth development is called the **cap stage** because the dental lamina invests the top of the papilla like a cap. The mesenchyme surrounding the papilla and its dental lamina cap condenses to form an enclosure called the **dental sac** (see Fig. 14–9A). By 10 weeks, the dental papilla has deeply invaginated the dental lamina and constitutes the core of the developing tooth. This is called the **bell stage** of tooth development, because the dental lamina looks like a bell resting over the dental papilla (see Fig. 14–9B).

During the bell stage, the outermost cells of the dental papilla become organized into a layer just adjacent to the inner enamel epithelium. These cells differentiate into the **odontoblasts,** which will produce the dentin of the teeth (see Fig. 14–9B). In the seventh month, these cells begin to secrete the nonmineralized matrix of the dentin, called **predentin,** which later progressively calcifies to form **dentin.** Production of predentin begins at the junction with the inner enamel epithelium and moves inward. The odontoblasts migrate inward as the dentin matrix is laid down, but they spin out behind them long cell processes **(odontoblastic processes)** that extend through the thickness of the dentin. The inner mesenchyme of the dental papilla becomes the tooth pulp.

During the bell stage, the dental lamina differentiates to form the **enamel organ,** which will produce the enamel layer of the tooth. First, the dental lamina becomes a three-layered structure, consisting of an **inner enamel epithelium** overlying the dental papilla; a middle **enamel epithelium,** or **stellate reticulum** of star-shaped cells, dispersed in an extracellular layer; and an **outer enamel epithelium.** As soon as mineralized dentin is formed, cells of the inner epithelium differentiate into enamel-producing **ameloblasts** and begin to secrete rod-shaped enamel prisms between them-

selves and the underlying dentin (see Fig. 14–9B, C). It is thought that previous production of mineralized dentin is necessary for the induction of enamel secretion by the ameloblasts.

The 20 tooth buds give rise directly to the **primary (deciduous** or **milk) teeth,** consisting in each half-jaw of two incisors, one canine, and two premolars. Early in the bell stage, however, the dental lamina superficial to each tooth bud produces a small diverticulum that migrates to the base of the primary tooth bud and becomes the bud of the **secondary (permanent)** tooth that will replace it (see Fig. 14–9C). The buds of the permanent molars, which do not have a deciduous precursor, arise during postnatal life from a pencil-like extension of the dental lamina that burrows back into the posterior jaw from the hindmost primary tooth buds. The full human dentition consists of 32 teeth, including three molars, but the third molars (wisdom teeth) often fail to develop or to erupt.

The roots of the teeth begin to form in late fetal and early postnatal life. At the base of the tooth crown, the confluence of the inner and outer enamel epithelia elongate to form the **epithelial root sheath** (see Fig. 14–9D). The mesenchyme just internal to the epithelial sheath differentiates into odontoblasts, which produce dentin. Each root contains a narrow canal of dental pulp by which nerves and blood vessels enter the tooth (see Fig. 14–9D).

The tooth roots are enclosed in extensions of the mesenchymal dental sac. The inner cells of this portion of the dental sac differentiate into **cementoblasts,** which secrete a layer of **cementum** to cover the dentin of the root. At the neck of the tooth root, the cementum meets the enamel at a **cementoenamel junction** (see Fig. 14–9C, D). The outermost cells of the dental sac participate in bone formation as the jaws ossify and also form the **periodontal ligament** that holds the tooth to its bony socket, or **alveolus.**

Experimental studies suggest that the formation of the primary teeth is enhanced by vitamin D_3 and that the specific morphology of each tooth crown is regulated by interactions with the surrounding mesenchyme. The eruption of the primary teeth, starting at about 6 months after birth, is due to the lengthening of the tooth roots. Mandibular teeth usually erupt earlier than the corresponding maxillary teeth. The primary dentition is usually fully erupted by 2 years. Between approximately age 6 and 8 years, the primary teeth begin to be shed and are replaced by the permanent teeth.

The formation of enamel or dentin is affected by a number of congenital disorders, such as **amelogenesis imperfecta** and **dentinogenesis**

imperfecta. Studies show that these disorders are caused by mutations in regulatory or structural genes involved in the synthesis of enamel or dentin. A combination of genetic, molecular, and developmental studies promises to bring rapid advances in the diagnosis and treatment of these conditions.

SUGGESTED READING

Barnhill RL, Wolf JE. 1987. Angiogenesis and the skin. J Am Acad Dermatol 16:1226

Biggs PJ, Wooster R, Ford D, et al. 1995. Familial cylindromatosis (turban tumor syndrome) gene localized to chromosome 16q12–q13: evidence for its role as a tumor suppressor gene. Nat Genet 11:441

Blecher SR, Kapalanga J, LaLonde D. 1990. Induction of sweat glands by epidermal growth factor in murine X-linked anhidrotic ectodermal dysplasia. Nature (London) 345:542

Byrne C, Tainsky M, Fuchs E. 1994. Programming gene expression in developing epidermis. Development 120:2369

Chang JC, Smith LR, Froning KJ, et al. 1995. CD8+ T-cells in psoriatic lesions preferentially use T-cell receptor V beta 3 and/or V beta 13.1 genes. Ann N Y Acad Sci 756:370

Chiego DJ Jr. 1995. The early distribution and possible role of nerves during odontogenesis. Int J Dev Biol 39:191

Epstein EH Jr. 1993. The morbid cutaneous anatomy of the human genome. Arch Dermatol 129:1417

Foster C, Bertram JF, Holbrook KA. 1988. Morphometric and statistical analyses describing the *in utero* growth of human epidermis. Anat Rec 222:201

Foster C, Holbrook KA. 1989. Ontogeny of Langerhans cells in human embryonic and fetal skin: cell densities and phenotypic expression relative to epidermal growth. Am J Anat 184:157

French LE, Chonn A, Ducrest D, et al. 1993. Murine clusterin: molecular cloning and mRNA localization of a gene associated with epithelial differentiation processes during embryogenesis. J Cell Biol 122:1119

Fuchs E. 1990. Epidermal differentiation: the bare essentials. J Cell Biol 111:2807

Gans C. 1988. Craniofacial growth, evolutionary questions. Development 103(suppl):3

Hahn H, Wicking C, Zaphiropoulos PG, et al. 1996. Mutations of the human homolog of Drosophila patched in the nevoid basal cell carcinoma syndrome. Cell. 85:841

Heikinheimo K. 1994. Stage-specific expression of decapentaplegic-Vg-related genes 2, 4, and 6 (bone morphogenetic proteins 2, 4, and 6) during human tooth development. J Dent Res 73:590

Helder MN, Ozkaynak E, Sampath KT, et al. 1995. Expression pattern of osteogenic protein-1 (bone morphogenetic protein-7) in human and mouse development. J Histochem Cytochem 43:1035

Holbrook K. 1989. Biologic structure and function: perspectives on morphologic approaches to the study of the granular layer keratinocyte. J Invest Dermatol 92:84S

Holbrook KA. 1988. Structural abnormalities of the epidermally derived appendages in skin from patients with ectodermal dysplasia: insight into developmental errors. Birth Defects Orig Artic Ser 24:15

Holbrook KA, Dale BA, Smith LT, et al. 1987. Markers of adult skin expressed in the skin of the first trimester fetus. Curr Probl Dermatol 16:94

Holbrook K, Smith LT. 1981. Ultrastructural aspects of human skin during the embryonic, fetal, premature, neonatal, and adult periods of life. Birth Defects Orig Artic Ser 17:9

Holbrook KA, Underwood RA, Vogel AM, et al. 1989. The appearance, density, and distribution of melanocytes in human embryonic and fetal skin revealed by the anti-melanoma monoclonal antibody, HMB-45. Anat Embryol 180:443

Holbrook K, Vogel AM, Underwood RA, Foster CA. 1988. Melanocytes in human embryonic and fetal skin: a review and new findings. Pigment Cell Res 1(suppl):6

Johnson CL, Holbrook KA. 1989. Development of human embryonic and fetal dermal vasculature. J Invest Dermatol 93:10s

Kollar EJ. 1981. Tooth development and dental patterning. p. 87. In Connelly TJ, Brinkley LL, Carlson BM (eds): Morphogenesis and Pattern Formation. Raven Press, New York

Krey AK, Moshell AN, Dayton DH, et al. 1987. Morphogenesis and malformations of the skin. NICHD/NIADDK Research Workshop. J Invest Dermatol 88:464

Lumsden AGS. 1988. Spatial organization of the epithelium and the role of neural crest cells in the initiation of the mammalian tooth germ. Development 103(suppl):155

Lumsden AGS, Buchanan JAG. 1986. An experimental study of timing and topography of early tooth development in the mouse embryo with an analysis of the role of innervation. Arch Oral Biol 31:301

Mina M, Kollar EJ. 1987. The induction of odontogenesis in nondental mesenchyme combined with early murine mandibular arch epithelium. Arch Oral Biol 32:123

Moore K. 1988. The Developing Human. WB Saunders, Philadelphia

Moynahan EJ. 1974. The developmental biology of the skin. p. 526. In Davis JA, Dobbing J (ed): Scientific Foundations of Paediatrics. WB Saunders, Philadelphia

Newman M. 1988. Supernumerary nipples. Am Fam Physician 38:183

Nieukoop PD, Johnen AG, Albers B. 1985. The Epigenetic Nature of Early Chordate Development. p. 249. Cambridge University Press, Cambridge

Niswander L, Martin GR. 1992. Egf-4 expression during gastrulation, myogenesis, limb and tooth development in the mouse. Development 114:755

Nordlund J. 1986. The lives of pigment cells. Dermatol Clin 4:407

Nordlund JJ, Abdel-Malek ZA, Boissy R, Rheins LA. 1989. Pigment cell biology: an historical review. J Invest Dermatol 92:53S

Pablos JL, Everett ET, Harley R et al. 1995. Transforming growth factor-β 1 and collagen gene expression during postnatal skin development and fibrosis in tight skin mouse. Lab Invest 72:670

Perkins T, Trickler DP, Shklar G. 1988. Improvement of dental development in osteopetrotic mice by maternal vitamin D_3 sulfate administration. J Craniofac Genet Dev Biol 8:83

Polakowska RR, Haake AR. 1994. Apoptosis: the skin from a new perspective. Death Differ 1:19

Price ML, Griffiths WAD. 1985. Normal body hair—a review. Clin Exp Dermatol 10:87

Ranta R. 1986. A review of tooth formation in children with cleft lip/palate. Am J Orthod Dentofac Orthop 90:11

Salinas CF. 1981. Orodental findings and genetic disorders. Birth Defects Orig Artic Ser 18:79

Sasaki S, Shimokawa H. 1995. The amelogenin gene. Int J Dev Biol 39:127

Satokata I, Maas R. 1994. Msx1 deficient mice exhibit cleft palate and abnormalities of craniofacial and tooth development, Nat Genet 6:348

Scott G, Ewing J, Ryan D, Abboud C. 1994. Stem cell factor regulates human melanocyte-matrix interactions. Pigment Cell Res 7:44

Slavkin HC. 1987. Gene regulation in the development of oral tissues. J Dent Res 67:1142

Slavkin HC, MacDougall M, Zeichner-David M, et al. 1988. Molecular determinants of cranial neural crest-derived odontogenic ectomesenchyme during dentinogenesis. Am J Med Genet 4:7

Slootweg PJ, de Weger RA. 1994. Immunohistochemical demonstration of bcl-2 protein in human tooth germs. Arch Oral Biol 39:545

Smith LT, Holbrook KA. 1986. Embryogenesis of the dermis in human skin. Pediatr Dermatol 3:271

Spritz RA, Ho L, Strunk KM. 1994. Inhibition of proliferation of human melanocytes by a KIT antisense oligodeoxynucleotide: implications for human piebaldism and mouse dominant white spotting (W). J Invest Dermatol 103:148

Takahashi J, Ikeda T. 1995. Molecular cloning and expression of rat and mouse B16 gene: implications on organogenesis. Oncogene 11:879

Turner EP. 1974. The growth and development of the teeth. p. 420. In Davis JA, Dobbing J (eds): Scientific Foundations of Paediatrics. WB Saunders, Philadelphia

van Oostrom CT, de Vries A, Verbeek, SJ, et al. 1994. Cloning and characterization of the mouse XPAC gene. Nucleic Acids Res 22:11

15

Fetal Development and the Fetus as Patient

Summary

The gestation period of humans from fertilization to birth is usually 266 days or 38 weeks. The period between the end of the third through the eighth week constitutes the **embryonic period,** during which most of the major organ systems are formed. The remainder of gestation constitutes the **fetal period,** which is devoted mainly to the maturation of organ systems and to growth. For convenience, the 9-month gestation period is divided into three 3-month **trimesters.** It is not yet possible to keep alive fetuses born before 22 weeks, and fetuses born before 28 weeks have grave difficulty in surviving, mainly because of the immaturity of the lungs (see Ch. 6).

From the end of the third week until birth, the fetus receives nutrients and eliminates its metabolic wastes via the **placenta,** an organ that has both maternal and fetal components. The mature placenta consists of a mass of feathery fetal **villi** that project into an **intervillous space** lined with fetal syncytiotrophoblast and filled with maternal blood. The fetal blood in the villus vessels exchanges materials with the maternal blood across the villus wall. Exchange of nutrients is not the only function of the placenta, however; the organ also secretes a plethora of hormones, including the sex steroids that maintain pregnancy. Maternal antibodies cross the placenta to enter the fetus, where they provide protection against fetal and neonatal infections. However, teratogenic compounds and some microorganisms also can cross the placenta. The placenta grows along with the fetus; at birth it weighs about one sixth as much as the fetus.

Development of the placenta begins when the implanting blastocyst induces the **decidual reaction** in the maternal endometrium, causing the endometrium to become a nutrient-packed, highly vascular tissue called the **decidua.** By the second month, the growing embryo begins to bulge into the uterine lumen. The protruding side of the embryo is covered with a thin capsule of decidua called the **decidua capsularis,** which later disintegrates as the fetus fills the womb. The decidua underlying the embedded **embryonic** pole of the embryo—the pole at which the embryonic disc and connecting stalk are attached—is called the **decidua basalis,** which forms the maternal face of the developing placenta. The remainder of the maternal decidua is called the **decidua parietalis.**

As described in Chapter 2, the intervillous space of the placenta originates as lacunae within the syncytiotrophoblast, which anastomose with maternal capillaries and become filled with maternal blood at about 10 weeks. **Stem villi** grow from the fetal chorion into these spaces (see Ch. 2). Each villus has a core of extraembryonic mesoderm con-

Timeline. Fetal development.

taining blood vessels and a two-layered outer skin of cytotrophoblast and syncytiotrophoblast. Villi originally cover the entire chorion, but by the end of the third month they are restricted to the area of the embryonic pole, which becomes the site of the mature placenta. This part of the chorion is called the **chorion frondosum;** the remaining, smooth chorion is the **chorion laeve.** The villi continue to grow and branch throughout gestation. The intervillous space is subdivided into 15 to 25 partially separated compartments, called **cotyledons,** by wedgelike walls of tissue called **placental septae** that grow inward from the maternal face of the placenta.

Human twins formed by the splitting of a single early embryo (monozygotic twins) may share fetal membranes to varying degrees. In contrast, twins formed by the fertilization of two oocytes (dizygotic twins) always implant separately and develop independent sets of fetal membranes.

Advances in the safety and sophistication of techniques for sampling fetal tissues and the use of novel imaging techniques to examine the fetus are rapidly providing new approaches to the prenatal diagnosis and treatment of congenital disorders. As more is learned about the molecular biology and molecular genetics of development, it may become possible to devise treatments to correct developmental deficiencies such as the absence of sweat glands or lung surfactant. Moreover, the development of **gene therapy** techniques (see the Experimental Principles section of Ch. 1) may make it possible to correct many heritable disorders at the genetic level in utero.

The increasing ability to diagnose and treat diseases in utero and in very premature infants raises ethical and legal questions that require thoughtful debate. Questions of this nature have always arisen at the forefront of new medical techniques. What is somewhat unusual in this case is the extreme speed with which both our understanding of human developmental biology and our clinical practice are advancing and the fact that the decisions and solutions to the resulting medical questions affect a new category of patient: the unborn fetus.

DURING THE FETAL PERIOD, THE EMBRYONIC ORGAN SYSTEMS MATURE AND THE FETUS GROWS

Most of the preceding text has concentrated on the **embryonic period,** from the late third through the eighth week, the period during which the organs and systems of the body are formed. The succeeding **fetal period,** from 8 weeks to birth at about 38 weeks, is devoted to the maturation of these organ systems and to growth. The fetus grows from 8 g at 8 weeks to about 3400 g at birth, a 425-fold increase. Most of this weight is put on in the third trimester (7 to 9 months), although the fetus grows in length mainly in the second trimester (4 to 6 months). The growth of the fetus is accompanied by drastic changes in proportion: at 9 weeks, the head of the fetus represents about half of its **crown-rump length** (the "sitting height" of the fetus), whereas at birth it represents about one fourth of the crown-rump length.

Although all the organ systems are present by 8 weeks, few of them are functional. The most prominent exceptions are the heart and blood vessels, which begin to circulate blood during the fourth week. Even so, the reconfiguration of the fetal circulatory system described in Chapter 8 is not complete until 3 months. The sensory systems also lag. The auditory ossicles are not free to vibrate until just before birth, for example, and, although the neural retina of the eye differentiates during the third and fourth months, the eyelids remain closed until 5 to 7 months, and the eyes cannot focus properly until several weeks after birth.

A number of organs do not finish maturing until after birth. The most obvious example is the reproductive system and associated sexual characteristics, which, as in most animals, do not finish developing until the individual is old enough to be likely to reproduce successfully. In humans, a relatively large number of other organs are also immature at birth. This accounts for the prolonged helpless infancy of humans compared with many mammals. The most slowly maturing organ of humans, and the one that largely sets the pace of infancy and childhood, is the brain. The cerebrum and cerebellum are both quite immature at birth.

Chorion laeve

Chorion frondosum

Decidua capsularis

Decidua basalis

Decidua capsularis

Decidua parietalis

8 weeks

4 weeks

12 weeks

20 weeks

Figure 15–1. Development of the chorion and decidua during the first 5 months. The decidua is divided into three portions: the decidua capsularis overlying the growing conceptus, the decidua basalis underlying the placenta, and the decidua parietalis lining the remainder of the uterus.

FETAL LIFE IS SUPPORTED BY THE PLACENTA, AN ORGAN WITH MATERNAL AND FETAL COMPONENTS

The Placental Tissues Are Derived From the Maternal Decidua Basalis and the Fetal Chorion

As the blastocyst implants, it stimulates a response in the uterine endometrium called the **decidual reaction.** The cells of the endometrial **stroma** (the fleshy layer of endometrial tissue that underlies the endometrial epithelium lining the uterine cavity) accumulate lipid and glycogen and are then called **decidual cells.** The stroma thickens and becomes more highly vascularized, and the endometrium as a whole is then called the **decidua.**

Late in the embryonic period, the **abembryonic** side of the growing embryo (the side opposite to the **embryonic** pole where the germ disc and connecting stalk attach) begins to bulge into the uterine cavity (Fig. 15–1). This protruding portion of the embryo is covered by a thin capsule of endometrium called the **decidua capsularis.** The embedded, embryonic pole of the embryo is underlain by a zone of decidua called the **decidua basalis,** which will participate in forming the mature placenta. The remaining areas of decidua are called the **decidua parietalis.** In the third month, as the growing fetus begins to fill the womb, the decidua capsularis is pressed against the decidua parietalis, and in the fifth and sixth months the decidua capsularis disintegrates.

Development of the uteroplacental circulatory system begins late in the second week as cavities called **trophoblastic lacunae** form in the syncytiotrophoblast of the chorion and anastomose with maternal capillaries. At the end of the third week, fetal blood vessels begin to form in the connecting stalk and extraembryonic mesoderm. Meanwhile, as described in Chapter 2, the extraembryonic mesoderm lining the chorionic cavity proliferates to form **tertiary stem villi** that project into the trophoblastic lacunae that become blood-filled after 10 weeks. By the end of the fourth week, tertiary stem villi cover the entire chorion. It is becoming more apparent that hypoxia, or lower tissue oxygen content in the decidua, is critical for normal trophoblast invasion.

The Villi Disappear From the Chorion Laeve and Lengthen in the Chorion Frondosum

As the embryo begins to bulge into the uterine lumen during the second month, the villi on the protruding, abembryonic side of the chorion disappear (see Fig. 15–1). This region of the chorion is now called the **smooth chorion,** or **chorion laeve,** whereas the portion of the chorion associated with the decidua basalis retains its villi and is called the **chorion frondosum** (from Latin *frondosus,* leafy).

The placental villi continue to grow during most of the remainder of gestation. Starting in the ninth week, the tertiary stem villi lengthen by the formation of terminal **mesenchymal villi,** which originate as sprouts of syncytiotrophoblast (**trophoblastic sprouts**) similar in cross section to primary stem villi (see Ch. 2) (Fig. 15–2). These terminal extensions of the tertiary stem villi reach their maximum length in the 16th week and are called **immature intermediate villi.** The cells of the cytotrophoblastic layer become more dispersed in these villi, leaving gaps in that layer of the villus wall.

Starting near the end of the second trimester, the tertiary stem villi also form numerous slender side branches called **mature intermediate villi.** The first-formed mature intermediate villi finish forming by week 32 and then begin to produce small, nodule-like secondary branches called **terminal villi.** These terminal villi complete the structure of the **placental villous tree.** It has been suggested that the terminal villi are formed not by active outgrowth of the syncytiotrophoblast but rather by coiled and folded villous capillaries that bulge against the villus wall.

Because the **intervillous space** into which the villi project is formed from trophoblastic lacunae that grow and coalesce, it is lined on both sides with syncytiotrophoblast (see Fig. 15–2). The maternal face of the placenta, called the **basal plate,** consists of this syncytiotrophoblast lining plus a supporting layer of decidua basalis. On the

Figure 15–2. Development of the placenta. (From Castellucci M, Scheper M, Scheffen I, et al. 1990. The development of the human villous tree. Anat Embryol 181:117.)

fetal side, the layers of the chorion form the **chorionic plate** of the placenta.

The Placenta Is Subdivided Into Cotyledons by the Wedgelike Placental Septa

During the fourth and fifth months, wedgelike walls of decidual tissue called **placental (decidual) septa** grow into the intervillous space from the maternal side of the placenta, separating the villi into 15 to 25 groups called **cotyledons** (see Fig. 15–2). Because the placental septa do not fuse with the chorionic plate, maternal blood can flow freely from one cotyledon to another.

RESPIRATORY GASES, NUTRIENTS, WASTE PRODUCTS, AND ANTIBODIES ARE EXCHANGED BETWEEN MATERNAL AND FETAL BLOOD IN THE PLACENTA

Maternal blood enters the intervillous spaces of the placenta through about 100 **spiral arteries,** bathes the villi, and leaves again via **endometrial veins.** The placenta contains approximately 150 mL of maternal blood, and this volume is replaced about three or four times per minute. Nutrients and oxygen pass from the maternal blood across the cell layers of the villus into the fetal blood, and waste products such as carbon dioxide, urea, uric acid, and bilirubin (a breakdown product of hemoglobin) reciprocally pass from the fetal blood to the maternal blood.

Maternal proteins are endocytosed and degraded by the trophoblast unless bound to receptors (e.g., IgG, Transcobalamin II). Antibodies cross the placenta to enter the fetal circulation, and in this way the mother gives the fetus limited passive immunity against a variety of infections, such as diphtheria and measles. These antibodies persist in the infant's blood for several months after birth, guarding the infant against infectious diseases until its own immune system matures.

Erythroblastosis Fetalis Is Caused by the Passage of Anti-Rh Antibodies from an Rh− Mother to an Rh+ Fetus

There is one fairly common instance in which the transfer of antibodies from the mother to the fetus is not beneficial: when the antibodies are directed against an Rh factor on the fetal red blood cells and cause hemolysis (dissolution) of the fetal red blood cells. The **Rh factors** are a group of genetically determined surface molecules that are present on the plasma membrane of red blood cells in most, but not all, individuals. Individuals whose blood cells carry an Rh factor are **Rh+**; individuals whose blood cells lack one are Rh−; Rh factors provoke a strong immune response in Rh− individuals. If an Rh− mother carries an Rh+ fetus and fetal blood leaks into the maternal circulation, the mother will manufacture antibodies against the fetal red blood cells. Significant leaks of fetal blood across the placenta into the maternal circulation normally occur only at birth, so the resulting antibodies do not form in time to harm the fetus that first induces them. However, if the same mother bears a second Rh+ fetus, her anti-Rh antibodies can cross the placenta and destroy fetal red blood cells, causing anemia in the fetus and newborn. This condition is called **hemolytic disease of the newborn** or **erythroblastosis fetalis.** The latter name comes from the fact that the destruction of red blood cells stimulates a compensatory production of large numbers of immature nucleated fetal red blood cells called **erythroblasts.** Another, sometimes fatal, consequence of the disease is **hydrops**—the accumulation of water in the fetus. Moreover, the destruction of red blood cells releases large amounts of bilirubin (a breakdown product of hemoglobin) into the fetal circulation. This substance can be deposited in the developing brain, leading to cerebral damage and, in some cases, to death.

The effects of erythroblastosis fetalis can be prevented by giving transfusions of Rh− blood to the fetus in utero and to the newborn, so that the maternal antibodies find fewer cells to destroy. A more economical preventive approach is to administer anti-Rh antibodies to the Rh− mother immediately after the birth of each Rh+ baby. These antibodies destroy the fetal Rh⁺ red blood cells in her circulation before they stimulate her own immune system; this prevents her from manufacturing anti-Rh antibodies.

The Placenta Also Allows the Passage of Some Viral and Bacterial Pathogens

Although the placenta is fairly impermeable to microorganisms, a number of viruses and bacteria can cross it and infect the fetus. Because the fetus has no functioning immune system and relies solely on maternal antibodies for protection, it is often inept at fighting infections. Therefore, a disease that is mild in the mother may damage or kill the fetus. Viruses that can cross the placenta and infect the fetus include rubella virus (the agent of rubella or German measles), varicella-zoster virus (the agent of varicella or chickenpox), cytomegalovirus (the agent of mononucleosis), and coxsackievirus (the agent of various diseases, usually mild, in the adult). Cytomegalovirus causes one of the most common viral infections of the fetus. If this virus infects the embryo early in development, it may induce abortion; infection occurring later may cause a wide range of congenital abnormalities, including blindness, microcephaly, and mental retardation. One bacterium that has recently come to unpleasant prominence as a cause of congenital infections in American children is *Treponema pallidum*, the agent of syphilis. The incidence of syphilis among Americans has increased steadily since the 1950s, and the bacterium readily crosses the placenta.

HIV Can Be Transmitted Across the Placenta, During Parturition, or in Breast Milk

Human immunodeficiency virus (HIV) is the agent of human immune deficiency syndrome (AIDS) and related syndromes. This virus can sometimes cross the placenta from an infected mother to infect the unborn fetus. It is important to note that 25–40 percent of babies are HIV positive if their mothers are HIV positive and untreated with anti-HIV therapies. This difference is related to whether the placenta has specific co-receptors for specific strains of HIV and whether the placenta expresses active virus. It is commonly transmitted during the birth process or in the mother's milk during breast-feeding. Infants infected perinatally with HIV may appear to be healthy at birth, but they usually come down with AIDS by the time they are 3 years old. As in adults, the disease slowly destroys a crucial component of the immune system and leaves the infant vulnerable to repeated infections. Parotid gland infections, diarrhea, bronchitis, and chronic middle ear infections are common in infants with AIDS. Pneumonia caused by the protozoan *Pneumocystis carinii*, a characteristic infection of adults with AIDS, is a particularly alarming symptom in infants: the mean survival time of infants diagnosed with AIDS and *Pneumocystis carinii* pneumonia is 1 to 3 months. HIV-1 infection is also correlated with an increased rate of low birthweight, intrauterine fetal death, and preterm birth.

The incidence of transmission of HIV from mother to infant in the United States was estimated to be 1.5:1000 population in 1989; the incidence in the state of New York for that year was estimated as 5.8:1000. In the late 1980s, about 1800 HIV-infected infants were born per year in the United States. However, the World Health Organization estimated that by the year 2000, 10 million infants worldwide would have acquired HIV from their mothers.

Teratogens Reach the Fetus by Crossing the Placenta

Many previous chapters have alluded to the role of teratogens in causing various specific congenital abnormalities (see, in particular, the Clinical Applications sections of Chs. 7, 11, and 12). Other teratogens may not cause a specific malformation but may nevertheless result in **intrauterine growth restriction (IUGR).** Teratogens reach the fetus by crossing the placenta.

It is not always easy to identify a compound as a teratogen. Two approaches are used: **epidemiologic studies,** which attempt to relate antenatal exposure to a suspect compound with the occurrence of various congenital anomalies; and studies in which the compound is administered to pregnant experimental animals and the offspring are checked for abnormalities. It is often difficult to gather enough epidemiologic data to yield a clear result, however, and findings from animal studies are not necessarily applicable to humans. These difficulties are compounded by the complicated nature of teratogenesis. As discussed in previous chapters, most congenital deformities are multifactorial in etiology: that is, their pathogenesis depends on the genetic makeup of the individual as well as on exposure to the teratogen. An identical dose of a teratogen may cause severe anomalies in one individual and have no effect on another. In addition, malformations of a given structure can usually be caused only during the **sensitive period,** when that structure is undergoing morphogenesis. The timeline illustrations at the beginning of each chapter in this book generally define the sensitive periods of the corresponding tissues and organ systems. Because the major events of organogenesis take place during the first 8 weeks of development, that is the period during which the fetus is most vulnerable to teratogens.

Many therapeutic drugs are known to be teratogenic; these include retinoids (vitamin A and analogues), the anticoagulant warfarin, the anticonvulsants trimethadione and phenytoin, and a number of the chemotherapeutic agents used to treat cancer. Most teratogenic drugs exert their main effects during the embryonic period. However, care must be exercised in administering certain anesthetics and other drugs even late in pregnancy or at term, because they may endanger the health of the fetus.

Some recreational drugs are also teratogenic; these include tobacco, alcohol, and cocaine. The manifestations of fetal alcohol syndrome were described in the Clinical Applications section of Chapter 12. Cocaine, ingested by alarming numbers of pregnant women (the drug affected 300,000 to 400,000 newborns in 1990 in the United States), readily crosses the placenta and may cause addiction in the developing fetus. In some of the major cities of the United States, as many as 20 percent of babies are born to mothers who abuse cocaine. Unfortunately, fetal cocaine addiction may have permanent effects on the individual, although studies suggest that early intervention with intensive emotional and educational support in the first few years of life may be helpful.

Pregnant women who use cocaine have higher frequencies of fetal morbidity (disease) and mortality (death) than pregnant women who do not. Cocaine use is associated not only with low birthweight but also with some specific developmental anomalies, including infarction of the cerebral cortex and a variety of cardiovascular malformations. It is often difficult to isolate cocaine as the teratogen responsible for a given effect, however, because women who abuse cocaine often abuse other drugs as well, including marijuana, alcohol, tobacco, and heroin.

Children of cocaine-abusing mothers may be born premature as well as addicted: cocaine-using mothers have a very high frequency of **preterm labor.** Preterm labor occurs in 25 percent of women who test positive for cocaine on a urine test at admission to the hospital for labor and delivery but in only 8 percent of women who do not test positive for cocaine at admission. Two mechanisms have been proposed by which cocaine could cause preterm labor. On the one hand, cocaine, which is a potent constrictor of blood vessels, may cause abruption of the placental membranes (premature separation of the placenta from the uterus) by partly shutting off the flow of blood to the placenta. Oxidant stress is associated with preterm labor, and in vitro antioxidants can protect against membrane damage. On the other hand, there is evidence that cocaine directly affects the contractility of the uterine myometrium (muscle layer), perhaps making it hypersensitive to signals that initiate labor.

THE PLACENTA PRODUCES STEROID AND PROTEIN HORMONES AND PROSTAGLANDINS

The placenta is an extremely prolific producer of hormones. Two of its major products are the steroid hormones **progesterone** and **estrogen,** which are responsible for maintaining the pregnant state and preventing spontaneous abortion or preterm labor. As discussed in Chapter 1, the corpus luteum produces progesterone and estrogen during the first weeks of pregnancy. By the 11th week, however, the corpus luteum degenerates and the placenta assumes its role.

During the first 2 months of pregnancy, the

syncytiotrophoblast of the placenta produces the glycoprotein hormone **human chorionic gonadotropin,** which supports the secretory activity of the corpus luteum. Because this hormone is produced only by fetal tissue and is excreted in the mother's urine, it is used as the basis for pregnancy tests. However, it is also produced abundantly by hydatidiform moles (see the Clinical Applications section of Ch. 2), and persistence of the hormone beyond 2 months of gestation may indicate a molar pregnancy.

The placenta produces an extremely wide range of other protein hormones, including, to name a few, placental lactogen (hPL), human chorionic thyrotropin, human chorionic corticotropin, insulin-like growth factors, prolactin, relaxin, corticotropin-releasing hormone, and endothelin. In fact, it is becoming increasingly clear that the placenta makes many of the hormones also manufactured by the hypothalamus and pituitary.

Human placental lactogen is another important hormone produced by the placenta. hPL converts the mother from being principally a carbohydrate user to being a fatty acid user, thus sparing carbohydrates for the conceptus.

In addition, placental membranes synthesize **prostaglandins,** a family of compounds that perform a range of functions in various tissues of the body. Placental prostaglandins appear to be intimately involved in the maintenance of pregnancy and onset of labor. The signal that initiates labor seems to be a reduction in the ratio of progesterone to estrogen, but the effect of this signal may be mediated by an elevation in the levels of prostaglandins produced by the placenta.

THE PRODUCTION AND RESORPTION OF AMNIOTIC FLUID ARE NORMALLY IN CLOSE BALANCE

As described in Chapter 6, embryonic folding transforms the amnion from a small bubble on the dorsal side of the germ disc to a sac that completely encloses the embryo. By the eighth week, the expanding amniotic sac completely fills the old chorionic cavity and fuses with the chorion. The expansion of the amnion is due largely to an increase in the amount of **amniotic fluid.** The volume of amniotic fluid increases through the seventh month and then decreases somewhat in the last two months. At birth the volume of amniotic fluid is typically about 1 L.

Amniotic fluid, which is very similar to blood plasma in composition, is initially produced by the transport of fluid across the amniotic membrane itself. After about 16 weeks, fetal urine also makes an important contribution to the amniotic fluid. If the fetus does not excrete urine—either because of bilateral renal agenesis (absence of both kidneys; see the Clinical Applications section of Ch. 6) or because the lower urinary tract is obstructed (obstructive uropathy; see the Clinical Applications section of Ch. 10, and later in this chapter)—the volume of amniotic fluid will be too low (the condition called **oligohydramnios),** and the amniotic cavity, in consequence, will be too small. A small amniotic cavity can cramp the growth of the fetus and cause various congenital malformations, notably pulmonary hypoplasia (discussed in the Clinical Applications section of Ch. 6).

Because amniotic fluid is constantly produced, it must also be constantly resorbed. This is accomplished mainly by the fetal gut, which absorbs the fluid drunk by the fetus. Excess fluid is then returned to the maternal circulation via the placenta. Malformations that make it impossible for the fetus to drink—for example, esophageal atresia or anencephaly (see the Clinical Applications sections of Chs. 4 and 6)—result in an overabundance of amniotic fluid, a condition called **hydramnios** or **polyhydramnios.**

THE DEGREE TO WHICH MONOZYGOTIC TWINS SHARE FETAL MEMBRANES INDICATES THE STAGE AT WHICH THEY SEPARATED

Twins that form by the splitting of a single original embryo are called **monozygotic,** or **identical,** twins. These twins share an identical genetic makeup and therefore look alike as they grow up. **Dizygotic,** or **fraternal,** twins, in contrast, arise from separate oocytes produced during the same menstrual cycle. Dizygotic twin embryos implant separately and develop separate fetal membranes (amnion, chorion, and placenta). Monozygotic twins, in contrast, may share none, some, or all of their fetal membranes, depending on how late in development the original embryo splits to form twins.

If the splitting occurred during cleavage—for example, if the two blastomeres produced by the first cleavage division become separated—the monozygotic twin blastomeres will implant separately, like dizygotic twin blastomeres, and will not share fetal membranes (Fig. 15–3). Alternatively, if the twins are formed by splitting of the inner cell mass within the blastocyst, they will occupy the same chorion but will be enclosed by separate amnions and will use separate placentae, each placenta developing around the connecting stalk of its respective embryo (see Fig. 15–3). Finally, if the twins are formed by splitting of a bilaminar germ disc, they will occupy the same amnion (see Fig. 15–3).

Because fetal membranes fuse when they are forced together by the growth of the fetus, it may not be immediately obvious whether the membranous septum separating a pair of twins represents just amniotic membranes (meaning that the twins share a chorion) or fused amnions and chorions (meaning that the twins originally did not share fetal membranes). The clue is the thickness and opacity of the septum: Amniotic membranes are thin and almost transparent, whereas chorionic membranes are thicker and somewhat opaque.

Chorionic Vessels in the Placentae of Monozygotic Twins May Become Connected and May Cause Problems for the Fetuses

Monozygotic placentae usually become connected by anastomosis of chorionic vessels, usually arteries. This shared circulation usually poses no problem, but if one twin dies late in gestation or if the blood pressure of one twin drops significantly, the remaining twin is at risk. If one twin dies, the other twin may be killed by an **embolism** (blocked blood vessel) caused by bits of tissue that break off in the dead twin and enter the shared circulation. If the blood pressure of one twin falls sharply, the other twin may suffer heart failure as its heart attempts to fill both circulatory systems at once.

In the past, the only treatment for these situations was to wait until the healthy twin was old enough to have a chance of surviving outside the womb and then to perform a cesarean section. Surgical techniques are being developed, however, that may allow routine removal of the dead or diseased twin, allowing the other twin to develop normally. This procedure is technically difficult, however, because fetal operations have a tendency to induce preterm labor.

MODERN DIAGNOSTIC TECHNIQUES MAKE IT POSSIBLE TO ASSESS THE HEALTH OF THE UNBORN

Three diagnostic techniques have begun to revolutionize the diagnosis of embryonic and fetal malformations and genetic diseases. These are **amniocentesis, chorionic villus sampling,** and **ultrasonography.**

In Amniocentesis, Amniotic Fluid Is Aspirated and Examined

In amniocentesis, amniotic fluid is aspirated from the amniotic cavity (usually between 14 and 16 weeks gestation) through a needle inserted via the abdominal wall and is examined for various clues to fetal disease. Amniotic fluid contains metabolic byproducts of the fetus as well as cells sloughed from the fetus (possibly the lungs) and amniotic membrane. The protein α-fetoprotein, for example, is a useful indicator. Elevated levels of this protein may indicate the presence of an open neural tube defect, such as anencephaly, or other open defects such as gastroschisis. Fetal cells in the amniotic fluid can be cultured and karyotyped to determine the sex of the fetus and to detect chromosomal anomalies. The technique of Southern blotting (see the Clinical Applications section of Ch. 1) can be used to screen the genome for the presence or absence of specific mutations that cause heritable diseases. Amniocentesis has limitations early in gestation, however, both because it is difficult to perform when the volume of amniotic fluid is small and because a small sample may not yield enough cells for Southern blotting.

Dizygotic twins

Monozygotic twins

Splitting occurs at 2-cell stage

Splitting in early blastocyst yields two inner cell masses

Later splitting yields two embryos from one inner cell mass

Separate amnions, chorions, and placentae

Separate amnions; common chorion and placenta

Common amnion, chorion, and placenta

Figure 15–3. Uterine disposition of various types of twins. The degree to which monozygotic twins share placental membranes depends on the stage of development at which the originally single embryo separates: If the splitting occurs at the two-cell stage of cleavage, the twins will develop as separately as dizygotic twins; if the splitting yields a blastocyst with two inner cell masses, then the embryos will share a single chorion and placenta but occupy separate amnions; if the splitting occurs after the formation of the inner cell mass, the embryos will occupy a single amnion.

Chorionic Villus Sampling Yields Larger Cell Samples Than Amniocentesis

In chorionic villus sampling, a small sample of tissue (10–40 mg) is removed from the chorion by a catheter inserted through the cervix or with a needle inserted through the abdominal wall. This tissue may be directly karyotyped or karyotyped after culture. Chorionic villus sampling can be performed early in gestation and yields enough tissue for Southern blotting. A complication of this technique, however, is that maternal tissue may be mistaken for fetal tissue. This error could lead to an incorrect diagnosis or sex determination and, in the worst case, could lead to a decision to abort a fetus that was actually normal. This risk is avoided by growing cells from the sample in culture and comparing them with fetal cells obtained by amniocentesis. This use of chorionic villus sampling or amniocentesis is usually recommended for mothers older than 35 years.

Ultrasonography Can Be Used to View the Fetus In Utero

In ultrasonography, the inside of the body is scanned with a beam of ultrasound (sound with a frequency of 3 to 10 MHz), and a computer is used to analyze the pattern of returning echoes. Because tissues of different density reflect sound differently, revealing tissue interfaces, the pattern of echoes can be used to decipher the inner structure of the body. The quality of the images yielded by ultrasonography is rapidly improving, and it is now possible to visualize the structure of the developing fetus and to identify many malformations. Ultrasonography is also now used to guide the needles or catheters used for amniocentesis and chorionic villus sampling. These procedures were formerly performed unguided, with a higher consequent risk of piercing the fetus. There is as yet no evidence that ultrasound harms fetal tissues.

Various types of "display modes," or ways of analyzing and displaying ultrasound data, are used, each with particular advantages. **M-mode** ultrasonography shows the changes in position of a structure with time. **B-mode** ultrasonography (such as **two-dimensional echocardiography)** shows the anatomy of a two-dimensional plane of scanning and can be performed in real time. **Doppler ultrasonography** yields flow information and can be used to study the pattern of flow within the heart and developing blood vessels. The miniaturization of ultrasound electronics has led to the development of **endosonography,** in which a miniature ultrasound probe is inserted into a body orifice such as the vagina and is thus brought close to the structure of interest, permitting a higher resolution image.

Real-time B-mode ultrasonography is the type most often used to examine the fetus. A wide variety of fetal anomalies can be seen and diagnosed by this technique, including craniofacial defects, limb anomalies, diaphragmatic hernias, caudal dysgenesis syndromes, teratomas, spina bifida, and renal agenesis (Fig. 15–4). Abnormalities of the fetal heart and heartbeat can be analyzed.

IMPROVING TECHNIQUES OF FETAL DIAGNOSIS AND SURGERY POSE NEW QUESTIONS FOR PARENT AND PHYSICIAN

If amniocentesis or chorionic villus sampling reveals that a fetus has a significant genetic anomaly, should the fetus be aborted? If ultrasonography shows a malformation serious enough to kill or deform the fetus, should corrective fetal surgery be attempted? The answers to these questions involve many factors, including (1) the risk to the mother of continuing the pregnancy, (2) the availability of surgeons and resources for fetal surgery, (3) the risk of the operation to the fetus and the mother, (4) the severity of the anomaly or disease, and (5) the advantage of correcting the defect in utero instead of after birth.

A wide range of fetal anomalies could potentially be corrected operatively. For example, a diaphragmatic hernia that would result in pulmonary hypoplasia (see the Clinical Applications section of Ch. 6) has been corrected by opening the uterus, restoring the herniated viscera to the abdominal cavity, and repairing the fetal diaphragm (Fig. 15–5). Hydrocephalus caused by stenosis of the cerebral aqueduct of Sylvius (see Ch. 13) can be corrected by inserting a ventriculoamniotic shunt

Figure 15–4. Cystic hygroma detected by ultrasound. *A,* Ultrasound scan showing the fetus in the uterine cavity. The smaller circular structure (long arrows) is the fetal skull: the large, thin-walled, cushion-like structure posterior to it (short arrows) is a cystic hygroma in the cervical region. *B,* The stillborn fetus. (Photos courtesy of Dr. Tariq Siddiqi.)

through the skull into the forebrain ventricle. This shunt has a one-way pressure valve that allows excess cerebrospinal fluid to vent into the amniotic cavity. The brain is then free to develop normally. Obstructive uropathy (constriction of the lower urinary tract, which prevents the urine produced by the kidneys from escaping) results in oligohydramnios and consequent fetal malformations, including pulmonary hypoplasia and defects of the face and limbs (see the Clinical Applications section of Ch. 6), and also in damage to the developing kidneys because of the backpressure of urine in the kidney tubules. Repair of the obstruction prevents these problems.

The anomalies in these examples would all cause death or major malformation if left uncorrected until birth. What about the case of a defect, such as cleft lip, which is not life-threatening? Cleft lips are routinely repaired after birth, but the result is not perfect; it has been argued that correction in utero would prevent scarring and give a cosmetically perfect result. Is the potential value of this outcome to parents and child worth the risk and expense of the procedure? These are questions under current debate.

Gene Therapy of the Fetus May Be Possible

As discussed above, modern techniques such as amniocentesis, chorionic villus sampling, and Southern blotting make it possible to detect mutations and chromosomal anomalies in the fetus. Is

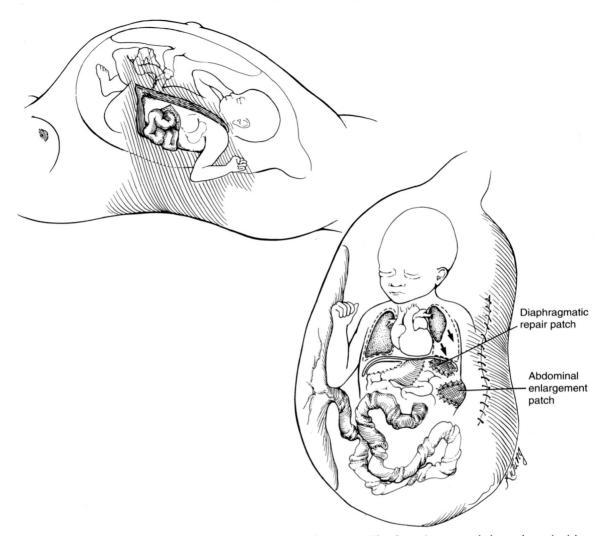

Figure 15–5. Repair of a diaphragmatic hernia by fetal surgery. The fetus is exposed through an incision in the uterine and abdominal walls. The fetal viscera are retracted from the left pleural cavity, and the hole in the diaphragm is repaired with a Gore-Tex patch. The left lung now has room to grow normally. Because the fetal abdominal cavity is too small for the restored viscera, a second Gore-Tex enlargement patch is placed in the fetal abdominal wall. (Modified from Harrison MR, Adzik NS, Longaker MT, et al. 1990. Successful repair in utero of a fetal diaphragmatic hernia after removal of herniated viscera from the left thorax. N Engl J Med 322:1582.)

there any way to correct these errors at the genetic level before birth so that development can be normal? The answer to this question is: Possibly yes.

The technique of insertional mutagenesis has been used successfully to cure genetic diseases in experimental animals, for example, in mice with a dominant mutation that impairs normal blood cell differentiation and causes anemia. In this experi-

ment, primitive hematopoietic (blood cell-producing) stem cells were removed from a mutant mouse and the wild-type, normal gene was introduced (transfected) into these cells via a retrovirus vector. The "cured" stem cells were then introduced back into the mutant mouse, which in the meantime had been subjected to high-dose irradiation to destroy all its hematopoietic stem cells. The "cured" stem cells repopulated the mouse's bone marrow and proceeded to produce genetically normal blood cells.

Not all genetic diseases are good candidates for gene therapy. It has been suggested that a candidate disease should meet the following criteria: (1) it should be a recessive disease caused by the absence of a normally functioning copy of the gene; (2) its gene should be amenable to cloning; (3) its gene should encode a single polypeptide; (4) the polypeptide should not require either a specific cellular environment or precise regulation to be expressed and perform its function; (5) it should be cured if the polypeptide is expressed by a cell type other than the affected tissue; and (6) it should be feasible to insert the gene into a tissue that can safely be removed from and then replaced into the body. These sound like daunting criteria, but in fact a long list of genetic diseases apparently meet them, including adenosine deaminase deficiency, argininosuccinic aciduria, citrullinemia, Gaucher disease type I, phenylketonuria, and some autoimmune diseases.

It may be feasible to apply the technique of gene therapy to correct some of the human genetic blood diseases by using a procedure called **fetal liver transplant.** In a preliminary experiment, this procedure was used to treat fetuses that were diagnosed with diseases that severely cripple the white blood cells of the immune system (such as the disease suffered by the "boy in the bubble") or with thalassemia (a blood disease caused by a genetic error that prevents the synthesis of a protein involved in the production of hemoglobin). In these cases, cells from the fetal liver (the first major hematopoietic organ) were obtained from normal aborted fetuses and were infused via an ultrasound-guided needle into the umbilical vein of the affected fetus. These cells successfully colonized the liver of the developing fetus and proceeded to manufacture the missing protein, alleviating the disease. It is easy to transplant cells from one fetus to another because the immature fetal immune system does not reject foreign tissue. It is also possible to utilize umbilical cord blood for transplants such as these because this is an excellent source of hematopoietic stem cells. Moreover, because in some disorders there may be advantages to using gene therapy to correct an infant's own cells, the infant's own umbilical cord may provide cells that can be appropriately transfected, grown up, and

reintroduced without rejection. Advantages of the use of cord blood (compared with bone marrow or fetal liver), include (1) lack of discomfort during collection, (2) high recovery of viable stem cells, (3) rapid expansion of stem cells in culture, (4) high rate of recovery of viable stem cells after **cryopreservation,** (5) reduced graft vs host disease, and (6) efficiency of transfection with "corrected" genes. Umbilical cord blood has already been used in many human patients to treat diseases potentially curable with bone marrow transplants, including **severe combined immunodeficiency.**

THE FIELD OF HUMAN DEVELOPMENTAL BIOLOGY IS ADVANCING AT A DAZZLING RATE

The fields of embryology and genetics have made steady progress since the days of Brooks, Whitman, Spemann, and Mangold in the early 20th century. Our understanding of animal and plant development began to make much more rapid strides, however, as the disciplines of embryology, genetics, biochemistry, and cytology began to merge into the science that in the early 1950s Paul Weiss first called **developmental biology.** Many of the advances of the last half century have led to an understanding of fundamental developmental mechanisms and have established the conceptual framework for modern developmental biology.

More recently, the study of mammalian development (including the genetics and development of humans) has made impressive progress. The project of mapping the entire human genome is now complete; the location of virtually every human gene will be known. Recombinant DNA technology, antisense agents, and transgenic techniques are rapidly leading to an understanding of the genomic control of development and of the pathogenesis of many human congenital anomalies.

These advances, along with the findings of previous decades, have begun to answer the questions of how the development of humans and other mammals is regulated on the molecular level. It is especially exciting to witness our emerging understanding of the significance of master genes, such as the *Hox* genes and other well-conserved regulator genes that play a key role in morphogenesis, especially in autism. These insights, in turn, have made it feasible to address the clinical correction of human congenital abnormalities. Optimism in this area is also supported by the staggering development of sophisticated technology, including computers, diagnostic techniques, and fe-

tal surgical methods. This explosive increase in our understanding of human development will produce countless practical applications over the next 10 to 20 years. We must carefully consider how this knowledge can be applied so that suffering can be alleviated.

SUGGESTED READING

Almici C, Carlo-Stella C, Wagner JE, Rizzoli V. 1995. Umbilical cord blood as a source of hematopoietic stem cells: from research to clinical application. Hematologica 80:473

Bernischke K, Driscoll SG. 1967. The placenta in multiple pregnancy. Handb Pathol Histol 7:187

Bordignon C, Notarangelo LD, Nobili N, et al. 1995. Gene therapy in peripheral blood lymphocytes and bone marrow for ADA-immunodeficient patients. Science 270:470

Brambati B, Tului L, Simoni G, Travi M. 1991. Genetic diagnosis before the eighth gestational week. Obstet Gynecol 77:318

Brundin P, Bjorklund A, Lindvall O. 1990. Practical aspects of the use of human fetal brain tissue for intracerebral grafting. Prog Brain Res 82:707

Burton DJ, Filly RA. 1991. Sonographic analysis of the amniotic band syndrome. AJR 156:555

Caldwell MB, Rodgers MF. 1991. Epidemiology of pediatric HIV infection. Pediatr Clin North Am 38:1

Castellucci M, Scheper M, Scheffen I, et al. 1990. The development of the human villous tree. Anat Embryol 181:117

Champetier J, Yver R, Tomasella T. 1989. Functional anatomy of the liver of the human fetus: applications of ultrasonography. Surg Radiol Anat 11:53

Chiriboga CA, Vibbert M, Malouf R, et al. 1995. Neurological correlates of fetal cocaine exposure: transient hypertonia of infancy and early childhood. Pediatrics 96:1070

Christ JE. 1990. Plastic surgery for the fetus. Plast Reconstr Surg 86:1238

Crombleholme TM, Langer JC, Harrison MR, Zanjani ED. 1991. Transplantation of fetal cells. Am J Obstet Gynecol 164:218

Dado DV, Kernahan DA, Gianopoulos JG. 1990. Intrauterine repair of cleft lip: what's involved. Plast Reconstr Surg 85:461

Dick JE, Magli MC, Huszar D, et al. 1985. Introduction of a selectable gene into primitive stem cells capable of long-term reconstitution of the hemopoietic system of W/W^v mice. Cell 42:71

Doran TA. 1990. Chorionic villus sampling as the primary diagnostic tool in prenatal diagnosis. J Reprod Med 35:935

Dunbar CE, Emmons RV. 1994. Gene transfer into

hematopoietic progenitor and stem cells: progress and problems. Stem Cells 12:563

Editorial. 1990. Editorial comments. J Am Osteopathol Assoc 90:970

European Collaborative Study. 1991. Children born to women with HIV-1 infection: natural history and risk of transmission. Lancet 337:253

Evans MI. 1989. Fetal surgery in the 1990s. Am J Dis Child 143:1431

Evans RG (ed). Council on Scientific Affairs. 1991. Medical diagnostic ultrasound instrumentation and clinical interpretation. Report of the Ultrasonography Task-force. JAMA 265:1155

Fox DA. 1995. Biological therapies: a novel approach to the treatment of autoimmune disease. Am J Med 99:82

Goldsmith MF. 1988. Anencephalic organ donor program suspended; Loma Linda report expected to detail findings. JAMA 260:1671

Gwinn M, Pappaioanou M, George JR, et al. 1990. Prevalence of HIV infection in childbearing women in the United States. JAMA 265:1704

Hallock GG. 1990. In defense of intrauterine repair of cleft lip. Plast Reconstr Surg 86:801

Hanania EG, Kavanagh J, Hortobagyi G, et al. 1995. Recent advances in the application of gene therapy to human disease. Am J Med 99:537

Harrison MR, Adzik NS, Longaker MT, et al. 1990. Successful repair in utero of a fetal diaphragmatic hernia after removal of herniated viscera from the left thorax. N Engl J Med 322:1582

Hepper PG. 1995. Human fetal behavior and maternal cocaine use: a longitudinal study. Neurotoxicology 16:139

Holloway M. 1990. Experimental surgery may feed ethical debates. Sci Am 263:46

Jones KL, Bernischke K. 1983. The developmental pathogenesis of structural defects: the contribution of monozygotic twins. Semin Perinatol 7:239

Jones SA, Challis JRG. 1990. Effects of corticotropin releasing hormone and adenocorticotropin on prostaglandin output by human placenta and fetal membranes. Gynecol Obstet Invest 29:165

Kaplan P, Normandin J, Wilson GN, et al. 1990. Malformations and minor anomalies in children whose mothers had prenatal diagnosis: comparison between CVS and amniocentesis. Am J Med Genet 37:366

Karson EM. 1990. Prospects for gene therapy. Biol Reprod 42:39

Kohn DB, Weinberg KI, Nolta JA, et al. 1995. Engraftment of gene modified umbilical cord blood cells in neonates with adenosine deaminase deficiency. Nat Med 1:1017

Kumar RM, Uduman SA, Khurranna AK. 1995. Impact of maternal HIV-1 infection on perinatal outcome. Int J Gynecol Obstet 49:137

Leach RE, Ory SJ. 1989. Modern management of ectopic pregnancy. J Reprod Med 34:324

Livingston RA, Hutton N, Halsey NA, et al. 1995. Human immunodeficiency virus-specific IgA in infants born to human immunodeficiency virus-seropositive women. Arch Pediatr Adol Med 149:503

Lipshultz SE, Frassica JJ, Orav EJ. 1991. Cardiovascular abnormalities in infants prenatally exposed to cocaine. J Pediatr 118:44

Longaker MT, Golbus MS, Filly R, et al. 1991. Maternal outcome after open fetal surgery. A review of the first 17 human cases. JAMA 265:737

Lu L, Shen RN, Broxmeyer HE. 1996. Stem cells from bone marrow, umbilical cord blood and peripheral blood for clinical application: current status and future application. [Review]. Crit Rev Oncol-Hemat 22:61

Luebke HJ, Reiser CA, Pauli RM. 1990. Fetal disruptions: assessment of frequency, heterogeneity, and embryological mechanisms in a population referred to a community-based stillbirth assessment program. Am J Med Genet 36:56

Marshall E. 1995. Gene therapy's growing pains. Science 269:1050

Moore KL. 1988. The Developing Human. Clinically Oriented Embryology. WB Saunders, Philadelphia

Olsen GD. 1995. Potential mechanisms of cocaine-induced developmental neurotoxicity: a minireview. Neurotoxicology 16:159

Orrell RW, Lilford RJ. 1990. Chorionic villus sampling and rare side effects: will a randomised controlled trial detect them? Int J Gynecol Obstet 32:29

Peabody JL, Emery JR, Aswal S. 1989. Experience with anencephalic infants as prospective organ donors. N Engl J Med 321:344

Quinn NP. 1990. The clinical application of cell grafting techniques in patients with Parkinson's disease. Prog Brain Res 82:619

Ray JG. 1995. Lues-lues: maternal and fetal considerations of syphilis. Obstet Gynecol Surv 50:845

Reynolds DW, Stagno S, Alford CA. 1986. Congenital cytomegalovirus infection. p. 93. In Sever JL, Brent RL (eds): Teratogen Update: Environmentally Induced Birth Defect Risks. Alan R Liss, New York

Rosenfeld MA, Chu CS, Seth P, et al. 1994. Gene transfer to freshly isolated human respiratory epithelial cells in vitro using replication-deficient adenovirus containing the human cystic fibrosis transmembrane conductance regulator cDNA. Hum Gene Ther 5:331

Rothenberg LS. 1990. The anencephalic neonate and brain death: an international review of medical, ethical, and legal issues. Transplant Proc 22:1037

Sachs ES, Jahoda MGJ, Los FJ, et al. 1990. Interpretation of chromosome mosaicism and discrepancies in chorionic villous studies. Am J Med Genet 37:268

Santulli TV. 1990. Fetal echocardiography: assessment of cardiovascular anatomy and function. Clin Perinatol 17:911

Schlesinger C, Raabe G, Ngo T, Miller K. 1990. Discordant findings in chorionic villus direct preparation and long term culture—mosaicism in the fetus. Prenatal Diagn 10:609–612

Slavkin HC. 1995. Molecular biology experimental strategies for craniofacial-oral-dental dysmorphology. Connect Tissue Res 32:233

Snodgrass SR. 1994. Cocaine babies: a result of multiple teratogenic influences. J Child Neurol 9:227

Stolar CJH. 1990. Repair in utero of a fetal diaphragmatic hernia. N Engl J Med 323:1279

Taylor BJ, Chadduck WM, Kletzel M, et al. 1990. Anencephalic infants as organ donors: the medical, legal, moral, and economic issues. J Arkansas Med Soc 87:184

Thompson MW. 1986. Genetics in Medicine. 4th ed. WB Saunders, Philadelphia

Touraine JL, Raudrant D, Royo C, et al. 1991. In utero transplantation of hemopoietic stem cells in humans. Transplant Proc 23:1706

Wapner RJ, Jackson L. 1988. Chorionic villus sampling. Clin Obstet Gynecol 31:328

Ward H. 1990. Review of the development and current status of techniques for monitoring embryonic and fetal development in the first trimester of pregnancy. Am J Med Genet 35:157

Warwick R, Williams PL. 1990. Gray's Anatomy. 36th ed. Churchill Livingstone, Edinburgh

Werler MM, Pober BR, Holmes LB. 1986. Smoking and pregnancy. p. 131. In Sever JL, Brent RL (eds): Teratogen Update: Environmentally Induced Birth Defect Risks. Alan R Liss, New York

Glossary

A

Abdominal foregut Segment of the gastrointestinal tract that is vascularized by the celiac trunk; includes the abdominal esophagus, stomach, and upper half of the duodenum.

Abducent nerve (VI) Possesses only motor functions and innervates the lateral rectus muscles of the eyeball.

Abembryonic Away from the embryo.

Achrodolichomelia Disproportionately large hands and feet.

Acoustic (cochlear) ganglion of nerve VIII Neurons of this ganglion (serving special sense of hearing) arise from ectoderm within the otic placode.

Adactyly Absence of all the digits on a limb.

Adenohypophysis Anterior lobe of the pituitary formed by invagination of stomodeal ectoderm (Rathke's pouch); produces small peptide hormones including prolactin, luteinizing hormone, and follicle-stimulating hormone in response to blood-borne releasing factors produced by the hypothalamus.

Alar (dorsal) columns Pair of columns of the spinal cord and brain stem formed by gray matter of the dorsal regions of the neural tube; cells give rise to association neurons.

Alisphenoid bone Bone of the orbit that arises from the palatopterygoquadrate bar.

Allantois Ventral diverticulum of the hindgut that becomes a superior extension of the primitive urogenital sinus after partitioning of the cloaca; forms the urachus or median umbilical ligament.

Alveolus See **Mature alveoli**.

Alveolus (of tooth) Bony socket of the tooth formed by mesenchyme of the dental sac; teeth are anchored to it by the periodontal ligament.

Ambisexual stage (also **Indifferent phase**) Course of genital development in male and female embryos is virtually identical until the seventh week.

Amelia Absence of one or more limbs.

Ameloblasts Ectodermal cells that differentiate from the inner enamel epithelium; secrete the enamel of the tooth.

Amnioblasts Cells differentiated from epiblast cells that form the amniotic membrane.

Amniocentesis Aspiration of amniotic fluid for analysis, usually through a needle inserted into the amnion via the abdominal wall; typically done between 14 and 16 weeks of gestation.

Amnion (amniotic cavity) Appears on day 8 as fluid begins to collect between epiblast cells; eventually fills with amniotic fluid for protection and space for growth of embryo and fetus.

Amniotic fluid Dialysate of blood, first secreted by the amniotic membrane; by 16 weeks of gestation fetal urine is a major contributor to volume.

Amniotic membrane Surrounds the amnion; inner layer is composed of amnioblasts while the outer layer is extraembryonic somatopleuric mesoderm.

Ampulla Structures that form at tips of bifurcating ureteric buds; ultimately induce the metanephric intermediate mesoderm to form nephrons.

Anal membrane Formed at about 7 weeks, along with the urogenital membrane, as the cloacal membrane is divided by the urorectal septum.

Anal pit (proctodeum) Ectoderm-lined invagination formed by proliferation of mesenchyme surrounding the anal membrane; forms the lower one third of the anorectal canal.

Anencephaly Anomaly caused by failure of the neuropore to close; brain may be completely missing or reduced to an exposed dorsal mass of undifferentiated neural tissue.

Angioblastic cords Short blind-ended cords formed as angiocysts coalesce.

Angioblastic plexuses Formed as angioblastic cords coalesce into complex interconnected vascular networks.

Angioblasts Vessel-forming cells that may arise from any kind of mesoderm except prechordal plate mesoderm.

Angiocysts Vesicles formed by angioblasts during the process of vasculogenesis.

Angiogenesis Mechanism whereby pre-existing vessels lengthen or branch by sprouting.

Anterior cardinal veins Bilaterally symmetric, paired veins that drain blood from the head and neck into their respective common cardinal veins during early fourth week; distal ends give rise to internal jugular veins; proximal right end becomes the superior vena cava.

Anterior commissure Fiber tract that develops within the lamina terminalis at the most cranial end of the telencephalon to connect olfactory centers in the left and right cerebral hemispheres.

Anterior lobe (of the pituitary) See **Adenohypophysis**.

Anti-müllerian hormone (AMH) Member of the TGF-β family; produced by pre-Sertoli cells following expression of the sex-determining region of the Y chromosome; causes regression of the paramesonephric ducts (also termed **Müllerian-inhibiting substance [MIS]**).

Aortic arches   Paired arteries derived from arteries surrounding the pharynx of piscine progenitors; correspond to arches 1, 2, 3, 4, and 6 of the ancestral fish but have become highly modified to form the great vessels of the thorax.

Aortic sac   Aortic arches (2, 3, 4, and 6) sprout from this most distal specialization of the truncus arteriosus; forms part of the arch of the aorta and the brachiocephalic artery.

Aortic valve   See **Semilunar valves.**

Apical ectodermal ridge   Thickening at the distal end of the limb bud that induces underlying mesodermal core to grow distally; type of segment produced from the mesodermal core depends on a *HOX* gene combinatorial code.

Apocrine glands   Coiled glands that develop with hair follicles; later lost except in the regions of the mons pubis, axilla, prepuce, scrotum, and labia minora; at puberty they produce complex secretions modified by bacterial activity into odorous compounds that may function in social and sexual communication.

Appendix epididymis   Small remnant of the degenerate cranial end of the mesonephric duct in males.

Appendix testis   Small remnant of the proximal end of the paramesonephric duct in males.

Arrector pili muscle   Smooth muscle within the papillary layer of the dermis attached to the dermal root sheath of the hair follicle; raises the hair shaft, causing "goose flesh."

Ascending aorta   Most proximal segment of the aorta derived from the truncus arteriosus.

Association neurons   Cells of the dorsal column that develop to interconnect the motor neurons of the ventral columns with neuronal processes.

Associational nuclei (of the cranial nerves)   Neuronal concentrations formed by gray matter of the alar columns of the brain stem; serve cranial nerves V, VII, VIII, IX, and X.

Astrocytes   Neuroglial cells of the central nervous system; one of many kinds of non-neuronal "supporting" cells of the central nervous system; formed by glioblasts arising from cells of the ventricular layer of the neural tube.

Atrioventricular node (AVN)   Secondary pacemaker region within the superior endocardial cushion that receives impulses from the sinoatrial node (SAN) to regulate beating of the ventricles.

Atrioventricular sulcus   Constriction that demarcates the primitive atrium and primitive ventricle in the third week.

Atrioventricular (AV) valves   Prevent backflow into the atria during systole; their cusps, chordae tendineae, and papillary muscles are sculpted from ventricular muscle; two-cusped AV valve of the left ventricle is the **bicuspid (mitral) valve;** three-cusped AV valve of the right ventricle is the **tricuspid valve.**

Auditory ossicles   Three small bones (incus, malleus, and stapes) suspended in the middle ear in mammals to transduce vibrations from the eardrum to the oval window of the cochlea.

Aural (auricular) cysts and fistulae   May be formed as regions of the first pharyngeal cleft are enclosed during formation of the external auditory meatus; may drain into the external auditory meatus or preauricular region via an auricular fistula.

Autonomic nervous system   Composed of two-neuron pathways that constitute the sympathetic and parasympathetic nervous systems; systems operate "autonomously" to effect contractions of smooth muscle and glands throughout the body.

Axis arteries   Central arteries of the limbs derived from the seventh intersegmental arteries (upper limb) and fifth lumbar intersegmental arteries (lower limb).

Axon   Processes that usually conduct impulses away from the neuronal cell body; usually synapse with other neurons or with effector organs.

B

Basal (ventral) columns   Pair of columns of the spinal cord and brain stem formed by gray matter of the ventral regions of the neural tube; cells give rise to somatic motor neurons.

Basal layer (of the dermis)   Underlying layer of the periderm consisting of proliferating cells; gives rise to the germinative layer of the mature epidermis.

Basal nuclei (of the cerebral hemispheres)   Heterogeneous nuclear masses located subcortically within the cerebral hemispheres; include the amygdaloid body, caudate, and lentiform nuclei.

Basket neuroblasts   Neuroblasts of the cerebellar cortex; formed during the initial wave of neuroblast production by the external germinal layer of the cerebellum.

Bell stage (of tooth)   Stage of tooth development attained by 10 weeks when the dental papilla invaginates deeply into the core of the bud of the developing tooth.

Bicuspid (mitral) valve   See **Atrioventricular valves.**

Bilaminar germ disc   Embryo following differentiation of the epiblast and hypoblast.

Bladder   Arises from the primitive urogenital sinus; formed as an anterior division of the cloaca by the urorectal septum.

Blood islands   Cysts of angioblasts containing hemoblasts; coalesce to form blood vessels in the yolk sac and also form the coronary vasculature.

Bone collar   Arises by ossification of the periphery of the shaft of long bones from the primary ossification center.

Bony socket (of tooth)   See **Alveolus (of tooth).**

Bowman's capsule   Distal, thin-walled expansion of the renal vesicle that surrounds the glomerulus to form the renal corpuscle.

Brachial plexus   Mixture of ventral primary rami of

spinal nerves C5 to T1; innervates the upper extremity.

Brain stem Cranial extension of the spinal cord; includes the myelencephalon, pons of the metencephalon, and mesencephalon.

Branchial arches Gill bars of fish; homologous structures of humans are pharyngeal arches.

Branchial efferent Refers to motor nuclei and pathways innervating striated muscles derived from pharyngeal (branchial) arch mesoderm (cranial nerves V, VII, IX, and X).

Broad ligament (of uterus) Formed as peritoneal folds are swept toward the midline of the pelvic cavity as the paramesonephric ducts zipper together to form the superior vagina and uterus.

Bronchial bud First three branchings of respiratory diverticulum are primary, secondary, and tertiary bronchial buds that respectively form the primary bronchi, lung lobes, and bronchopulmonary segments.

Buccopharyngeal membrane Region of fusion of epiblast and hypoblast apparent early in the third week; breaks down in the fourth week, opening the oral cavity to the pharynx.

Bulbourethral glands Endodermal diverticula of the pelvic urethra in the male that form just interior to the prostate between weeks 10 and 12; formed under the influence of dihydrotestosterone.

Bulbous hair peg Formed from a rod-like hair peg as the dermal papilla invaginates into its tip.

Bulboventricular sulcus Constriction that demarcates the superior end of the primitive ventricle (presumptive left ventricle) and inferior end of the bulbus cordis (presumptive right ventricle) in the third week.

Bulbus cordis Segment of primitive heart tube that is first apparent at the end of the third week; inferior end forms much of the **right ventricle;** superior end forms an outflow channel, the **conotruncus,** which then forms the proximal **conus cordis** and distal **truncus arteriosus,** which later divides into ascending aorta and pulmonary trunk.

Bundle of His Specialized myocytes that comprise a conduction pathway that carries impulses from the atrioventricular node to the ventricles; right and left branches serve the right and left ventricles, respectively.

C

Calvaria Dermal bones that constitute the cranial vault, skull cap, or roof of the skull.

Cap stage (of tooth development) Is initiated as neural crest-derived mesenchymal dental papillae invade the tooth buds in the eighth week.

Cardiac jelly Acellular secretion of the myocardium that plays a central role in septation of the heart and formation of the atrioventricular canals but later disappears.

Cardinal system of veins Drains the head and neck, body wall, and extremities of the embryo; consists of anterior and posterior cardinal veins; posterior cardinals are replaced by subcardinal and supracardinal veins during the second month.

Cardiogenic area Forms between the septum transversum and neural plate on day 19; cardiogenic angioblasts coalesce into vascular cords and later into lateral endocardial tubes; lateral endocardial tubes fold and fuse to form the primitive heart tube.

Cartilage Dense avascular connective tissue containing chondrocyte surrounded by an extracellular matrix (mainly collagen type II and proteoglycans).

Caudal and cranial neuropores Openings produced by the initial formation of the neural tube; as the neural tube closes, both become progressively smaller, closing on day 24 and day 26, respectively.

Cementoblasts Cells that differentiate from the inner layer of mesenchyme of the dental sac adjacent to the tooth root; secrete a layer of cementum to cover the tooth root dentin.

Cementoenamel junction Region at the neck of the tooth root that marks the boundary between cementum of the root and enamel of the crown.

Cementum Mineralized secretion (modified bone) of the cementoblasts that covers the dentin of the tooth root.

Central canal (of spinal cord) Arises from the neural canal; formed within the neural tube during neurulation; contains cerebrospinal fluid and is continuous with the brain ventricles.

Central sulcus Groove within the cerebrum separating frontal and parietal lobes.

Central tendon of the diaphragm Forms as the diaphragm differentiates and myoblasts of the septum transversum migrate into its periphery and into pleuroperitoneal membranes.

Cephalocaudal folding Stiff dorsal midline structures (notochord, neural plate, and somites) overgrow cranial and caudal ends of the embryo; both flexible ends fold sharply under to form three-dimensional vertebrate form.

Cerebellar hemispheres Formed by the cerebellar primordia of the rhombic lips; connected by the vermis.

Cerebellar nuclei (dentate, globose, emboliform, fastigial) Pairs of neuronal nuclei of the cerebellum formed by the internal granular layer; relay all cerebellar input.

Cerebellar primordia (plates) Lateral swellings of the rhombic lips; give rise to the cerebellar hemispheres.

Cerebellum Higher center formed by alar plates of the metencephalon; controls posture, balance, and smooth execution of movements.

Cerebral aqueduct Formed from narrowing of primitive ventricle of mesencephalon; transports cerebrospinal fluid produced by the choroid plexuses to the fourth ventricle; constriction may result in hydrocephalus.

Cerebral cortex   Multilayered stratum of gray matter within the cerebrum; formed by the differentiation of the cortical plate and subplate during cytodifferentiation of the cerebral hemispheres.

Cerebral hemispheres   Bubble-like outpouchings of the telencephalon; first appear at day 32 and expand rapidly to cover the diencephalon; initially smooth walled but begin to form folds (gyri) separated by grooves (sulci) in the fourth month that continue to form throughout fetal life; most evolutionarily advanced part of the brain.

Cerebrospinal fluid   Produced by the choroid plexuses of the lateral, third, and fourth ventricles; intraventricular pressure is maintained through a balance between synthesis and reabsorption through venous plexuses within the spinal cord and cranial sinuses; supports and protects the brain and spinal cord.

Cervical cysts   Produced by enclosure of the second, third, and fourth pharyngeal clefts by overgrowth of the second arch; typically transitory lateral cervical sinus does not disappear; may drain to the skin through an external cervical fistula; typically drains to the palatine tonsil through an internal cervical fistula.

Cervical flexure   Second of three flexures that develop between the fifth and eighth weeks to bend the brain ventrally at the junction between the spinal cord and the myelencephalon.

Cervical nephrotomes   Primitive excretory structures that arise in the cervical intermediate mesoderm during the early part of the fourth week; nonfunctional.

Chain ganglion (also **Sympathetic chain ganglion**)   Formed as neural crest cells collect on both sides of the developing spinal cord at almost every level; contain peripheral neurons of the sympathetic nervous system.

Chemoaffinity hypothesis   Axonal growth cones exhibit differential adherence to molecules specifically distributed within the extracellular matrix.

Chondrification   Process by which dense mesenchymal precursors of the skeleton are converted into cartilage.

Chondrocranium   Endochondral enclosure composing skulls of protochordates and early fishes; most primitive part of the skull in humans; now composes bones of the skull base.

Chondrocytes   Cells that differentiate from dense condensation of lateral plate mesoderm; form the bones of limbs in response to growth factors.

Chorda tympani   Branch of the facial nerve that carries special afferent fibers innervating taste buds on the anterior two thirds of the tongue.

Chordae tendineae   See **Atrioventricular valves.**

Chorion   Outermost fetal membrane consisting of three kinds of tissues: syncytiotrophoblast, cytotrophoblast, and extraembryonic somatopleuric mesoderm.

Chorion frondosum   Region of the chorionic wall that becomes associated with the decidua basalis; in the region of implantation retains its "leaf-like" chorionic villi.

Chorion laeve   Abembryonic wall of the chorion loses its chorionic villi during the second month to become smooth walled.

Chorionic cavity   Separates the embryo with its attached amnion and yolk sac from the chorion; by the end of the eighth week growth of the amniotic cavity obliterates it as layers of amniotic membrane and chorion loosely fuse together.

Chorionic villous sampling   A small amount of tissue is removed from the chorion via a catheter inserted through the cervix or a needle inserted via the abdominal wall.

Choroid plexus   Specialization of ependyma and vasculature that produces cerebrospinal fluid within the lateral, third, and fourth ventricles.

Ciliary ganglion   Parasympathetic ganglion of the third cranial nerve; contains peripheral neurons of the parasympathetic pathway innervating the sphincter pupillae muscle of the iris and smooth muscles of the ciliary body.

Circumventricular organs   Specializations of the third ventricle ependyma; include the subfornical organ, organum vasculosum of the lamina terminalis, and median eminence; may secrete material from the nervous tissues or vasculature into the cerebrospinal fluid.

Clitoris   Arises from the genital tubercle in females.

Cloacal folds   Develop in both male and female embryos just lateral to the cloacal membrane early in the fifth week; later divide into anterior urethral (urogenital) folds and posterior anal folds.

Cloacal membrane   Caudal membrane that disintegrates in the seventh week to form the inferior boundary of the urinary system and gastrointestinal tract.

Coagulation plug   A fibrin coagulum that forms at the site of the invading blastocyst in the endometrial lining of the uterus.

Cochlear ganglion (VIII)   See **Acoustic ganglion.**

Collecting tubules (ducts)   One to three million develop within the metanephroi from the last 10 or 11 generations of branchings of the ureteric buds.

Collodion baby   Baby is born with a persistent periderm "cocoon" that may slough after birth or may be removed by the physician.

Combined superior ganglion of cranial nerves VII and VIII   Contain sensory neurons derived from both the neural crest of the rhombencephalon and ectoderm from the first epibranchial placode; serve taste and general sensory functions (cranial nerve VII) and balance and hearing (cranial nerve VIII).

Common cardinal veins   Short vessel segments that drain blood into the right and left horns of the sinus venosus, respectively; the confluence of the anterior and posterior cardinal veins.

Compaction   Polarization and adhesion of blastomeres within the morula maximizing cell-to-cell contact; facilitated by cytoskeletal and cytomuscular elements.

Conduction system Myocytes within the developing heart tube develop a more rapid rate of depolarization to produce two pacemaker regions, the sinoatrial node (regulating atrial rhythm) and atrioventricular node connected by a myocardial conduction pathway to coordinate ventricular rhythmicity via the bundle of His; a primitive conduction system develops as early as day 22.

Connecting stalk A broad mass of extraembryonic somatopleuric mesoderm connecting the amnion to the cytotrophoblast that later forms the umbilical cord.

Conotruncus Region of the bulbus cordis that forms the conus cordis and the truncus arteriosus.

Contact guidance theory Axonal growth cones are guided by physical characteristics of the extracellular matrix.

Conus cordis Segment of the outflow tract that is derived from the conotruncus and remodeled to form outflow regions (conus arteriosus or infundibulum) of the definitive right ventricle and part of the left ventricle.

Copula Median swelling of the second pharyngeal arch is overgrown by the hypopharyngeal eminence of the third and fourth arches.

Cornua of the hyoid Greater and lesser horns of the hyoid that provide attachment sites for muscles and the stylohyoid ligament; lesser cornua and upper rim of the hyoid are derived from the second pharyngeal arch cartilage (Reichert's cartilage); lower rim and greater cornua are derived from the third arch cartilage.

Coronary sinus Vestige of the left horn of the sinus venosus that completely detaches from the left anterior cardinal vein; in conjunction with cardiac veins, forms venous system that will drain the myocardium.

Coronary sulcus (of the phallus) A shallow depression that demarcates the glans from the shaft.

Coronary vessels Form from epicardium as subepicardial plexuses fuse with sprouts of the aorta and coronary sinus; form the coronary arteries and coronary veins, respectively.

Corpora bigemina Longitudinal swellings of the mesencephalon that are precursors of the inferior and superior colliculi.

Corpus callosum Large fiber tract that connects the neocortices of the left and right cerebral hemispheres.

Corpus striatum Neuronal aggregations within the floor of the cerebral hemispheres; form some of the basal nuclei of the cerebrum.

Cortical plate See **Cerebral cortex.**

Cortical sex cords (secondary) Secondary sex cords at the cortex of the developing genital ridges surround the primordial germ cells in the female gonad to become follicle cells.

Cotyledons Formed during the fourth and fifth months as placental septa grow into the intervillous space, separating the villi into 15 to 25 groups.

Cranial (mesencephalic) flexure Initial flexure of the brain; bends the prosencephalon ventrally between the fourth and eighth weeks of development in the region of the mesencephalon.

Cranial nerve sensory ganglia Comparable to the dorsal root ganglia of the spinal cord; form in association with cranial nerves V, VII, VIII, IX, and X; contain peripheral sensory neuronal cell bodies that receive input from sensory organs in the head and pharynx for relay to associational nuclei within the brain stem.

Cranial nerves Twelve pairs develop in humans in association with the brain stem; serve diverse functions; motor, sensory, somatic, or mixed; mainly innervate structures and tissues of the head and pharynx; vagus nerve (X) provides parasympathetic preganglionic fibers to thoracic and abdominal viscera.

Cranial (rostral) neuropore See **Caudal and cranial neuropores.**

Cribriform plate (of the ethmoid bone) Perforated bone formed from ossification around fibers from the developing olfactory bulbs.

Cricoid cartilage Complete cartilaginous ring at the base of the larynx that may be derived from cartilage arising within sixth pharyngeal arch.

Crista terminalis Ridge of tissue that demarcates the boundary between the sinus venarum (definitive atrium) and right primitive atrium (right auricle); contains a conduction pathway connecting the sinoatrial node and atrioventricular node.

Crown (of the tooth) Covered with enamel and extends into the jaw to the level of the cementoenamel junction.

Crura of the diaphragm Muscular bands formed of condensed mesenchyme that attach to vertebral bodies L1 to L3 (on the right) and L1 and L2 (on the left).

Cumulus expansion Following ovulatory stimulus cumulus cells secrete a hyaluronic acid-rich extracellular matrix; resultant mucoid mass adheres to the oocyte during ovulation and may aid in transport of the cumulus-oocyte complex into the oviduct.

Cystic diverticulum Endodermal outgrowth that appears about day 26 just inferior to the hepatic diverticulum on the ventral wall of the duodenum; forms the gallbladder, cystic duct, and part of the common bile duct.

Cytoplasmic maturation (of gametes) Cytoplasmic changes occurring during the process of gametogenesis within the male and female germ cell line, converting them into mature gametes.

Cytotrophoblast Cells of the trophoblast that retain their cell membranes and enclose the blastocyst cavity.

D

Decidua basalis Zone of decidual tissue in the wall of the uterus underlying the embedded embryonic pole of the embryo.

Decidua capsularis Zone of decidua overlying the part of the embryo that protrudes into the lumen of the uterus.

Decidual cells Formed as cells of the endometrial stroma within the wall of the uterus differentiate in response to the implanting embryo by accumulating lipid and glycogen.

Decidual parietalis Does not directly cover the embryo (like the decidua basalis and capsularis).

Decidual reaction In response to implantation endometrial stromal cells accumulate lipid and glycogen; the endometrium thickens, endometrial glands enlarge, and endometrial veins and spiral arteries make connections with trophoblastic lacunae.

Decidual (placental) septa Wedge-like walls of decidual tissue that grow into the intervillous spaces to separate the villi into 15 to 25 cotyledons.

Decision-making point Nerve fibers leave nerve trunk to innervate end organs at a specific point; divergence of the nerve may occur in response to a chemoattractant or tropic substance or result from the growth cone's unique capacity to follow structural or molecular cues present in the substrate.

Deep ring (of inguinal canal) Site of weakening and evagination of the transversalis fascia produced by the evagination of the processus vaginalis.

Definitive (secondary) endoderm Germ layer of the trilaminar embryo arising from the epiblast during gastrulation; forms the gastrointestinal tract and its derivatives.

Definitive left atrium Heart chamber formed by incorporation of pulmonary veins into the posterior wall of the primitive atrium.

Definitive left ventricle Heart chamber primarily derived from the primitive ventricle; in part formed by left wall of the conus cordis.

Definitive oocyte or definitive spermatocyte (spermatid) The definitive haploid (IN); spermatocyte and oocyte have completed both meiotic divisions.

Definitive pericardial cavity An anterior cavity containing the heart that forms, along with the pleural cavities, as the primitive pericardial cavity (in which developing heart is suspended) is divided by two coronal pleuropericardial folds in the fifth week; folds fuse at the midline, and, with esophageal mesoderm, form the pericardial sac.

Definitive right atrium Heart chamber formed by incorporation of the sinus venosus into the posterior wall of the primitive atrium.

Definitive right ventricle Heart chamber primarily derived from the inferior end of the bulbus cordis; also incorporates part of the right wall of the conus cordis and primitive ventricle.

Definitive urogenital sinus Lower expanded region of the primitive urogenital sinus; gives rise to the vestibule of the vagina in the female and the penile urethra in the male.

Dendrite Short neuronal processes, often highly branched; usually conduct impulses toward the neuronal cell body and its axon and form synapses with the axons of other neurons.

Dental laminae U-shaped ridges of surface ectoderm that appear on the upper and lower jaws in the seventh week; each forms the ectodermal component of ten primary tooth buds.

Dental papilla Concentrations of mesenchyme, derived from migrating neural crest cells, form under the surface ectoderm of the upper and lower jaw, respectively, stimulating ten centers of ingrowth from each dental lamina; together with each ingrowth, forms a primary tooth bud.

Dental pulp A canal within the core of the mature tooth that transports nerves and blood vessels into the tooth.

Dental sac Mesenchymal investment that encloses the tooth bud at the end of the second month; forms cementoblasts and the periodontal ligament and contributes to the alveolus.

Dermal papilla of dermis Evaginations of the papillary layer of the dermis that interdigitate with overlying epidermal ridges to form the pattern of external ridges and grooves of the skin.

Dermal papilla of hair follicle Mesenchyme that invaginates into the tips of hair pegs, converting them to bulbous hair pegs; layer of proliferating ectoderm overlying it forms the germinal matrix that forms the hair shaft.

Dermatome Formed as a dermomyotome splits; contributes to development of the dermis.

Dermis (corium) Derived from both lateral plate mesoderm and the dermatomes of the somites; consists of two layers: a papillary layer just underlying the epidermis and a deeper, dense, irregular layer (reticular layer).

Dermomyotome Portion of the somite that remains in place after the sclerotome migrates medially; quickly splits into a myotome and a dermatome.

Dextrocardia Condition resulting from an opposite "dextral" looping of the primary heart tube displacing the apex of the left ventricle to the right.

Diaphragm Chief respiratory muscle of humans; derivative of four embryological structures: septum transversum, pleuroperitoneal membranes, paraxial mesoderm of the body wall, and lateral plate mesoderm.

Diaphysis Shaft of the long bone.

Diarthroidal (synovial) joint See **Synovial joint.**

Diencephalon (between-brain) One of two secondary brain vesicles formed by the prosencephalon (forebrain); gives rise to the epithalamus and its derivatives and to the thalamus and the hypothalamus.

Dihydrotestosterone Androgen that is produced by conversion of testosterone by the enzyme 5-α-reductase; responsible for male development of the prostate, bulbourethral glands, seminal vesicles, and male differentiation of the external genitalia during embryonic and fetal life.

Distal tongue buds (lateral lingual swellings) Overgrow the median tongue bud to give rise to most of the anterior two-thirds of the tongue.

Dizygotic (fraternal) twins Arise from two separate oocytes; do not share any fetal membranes.

Doppler ultrasonography Ultrasound mode that allows visualization and analysis of blood flow within the fetal heart and blood vessels.

Dorsal mesentery Thin peritoneal membrane that suspends abdominal viscera in the coelomic cavity; forms mesentery of the abdominal esophagus, mesogastrium, greater omentum, small intestines, and transverse and sigmoid colons.

Dorsal mesocardium Dorsal mesentery of the primitive heart tube that ruptures in the fourth week to form the transverse pericardial sinus.

Dorsal nucleus of the vagus Contains preganglionic parasympathetic neurons that innervate the viscera via the vagus nerve.

Dorsal pancreatic bud Sprouts from the dorsal duodenal wall to form the head, body, and tail of the pancreas after fusion with the ventral pancreatic bud.

Dorsal primary ramus Dorsal branch of any spinal nerve that innervates skin and deep muscles of the back; contains motor, sensory, and sympathetic fibers.

Dorsal root Comprised of the dorsal root ganglion and its centripetal and centrifugal fibers.

Dorsal root ganglion Formed from concentrations of neural crest cells that collect just lateral to the second cervical to first coccygeal segments of the spinal cord.

E

Ectoderm Descends from epiblast cells following completion of gastrulation; differentiates into surface ectoderm (forms the epidermis) and neural epithelium (forms neurons, supporting cells, neural crest cells, and ependyma of the central nervous system).

Ectodermal placodes Ectodermal thickenings including the nasal and otic placodes, trigeminal placode, and four epibranchial (epipharyngeal) placodes; all play major roles in producing neurons within several of the sensory ganglia associated with the cranial nerves.

Ectodactyly Absence of any number of fingers or toes.

Edinger-Westphal nucleus Contains preganglionic parasympathetic neurons that innervate postganglionic neurons within the ciliary ganglia that innervate the sphincter pupillae muscle of the iris and the smooth muscle cells of the ciliary body.

Efferent ductules (ductuli efferentes) Formed as epigenital mesonephric tubules unite with the presumptive rete testis; provide pathway for sperm from seminiferous and rete testis tubules to the vas deferens.

Embryoblast Arises from inner cell mass of the morula during first week of development and gives rise to the embryo proper.

Embryonic period Typically described as the period when most of the organ systems are developing, between the late third week and the eighth week.

Embryonic stem cells Arise from the inner cell mass during in vitro culture of blastocysts removed from a fertilized genital tract; totipotent; produce injection chimeras when introduced into a normal blastocyst.

Enamel Mineralized secretion of the ameloblasts (derived from the inner enamel epithelium of the enamel organ) that covers the dentin of the crown of the mature tooth.

Enamel organ Differentiates from the dental lamina; consists of an inner and outer enamel epithelium with a middle enamel or stellate reticulum of star-shaped cells embedded in an extracellular matrix; inner enamel epithelium secretes enamel.

Endocardial cushions Thickenings in the atrioventricular canal are regions of thickened cardiac jelly.

Endocardium Lining of the heart tube derived from the lateral endocardial tubes; consists of endothelium and thin subendothelial connective tissue.

Endochondral ossification Ossification of a cartilaginous precursor.

Endometrial stroma Fleshy part of the uterine wall immediately underlying the endometrial epithelium.

Endometrium Consists of an epithelial lining of the uterine lumen and a mesodermal stroma (lamina propria) containing vasculature and endometrial glands.

Endosonography Miniature ultrasound probe is inserted into a body orifice to visualize internal structures.

Endothelial cells Arise from angioblasts to form initial vascular network; provide endothelial lining for the entire cardiovascular system.

Enteric ganglia Ganglia embedded within the walls of the gastrointestinal tract derived from vagal and sacral neural crest cells.

Ependyma Cellular membrane lining the ventricles of the brain and the central canal of the spinal cord; arises directly from the ventricular layer; may participate in the development of the choroid plexuses and specialized circumventricular organs that produce cerebrospinal fluid.

Ependymal cell Last cells to differentiate from the ventricular layer of the brain and spinal cord; form an ependymal lining of the neural canal.

Epiblast Sheet of cells that appears with the hypoblast as the embryoblast differentiates to form the bilaminar embryo; eventually gives rise to all cells and tissues of the amnion and the embryo proper.

Epibranchial (epipharyngeal) placodes Four regions of ectoderm located just dorsal to the pharyngeal arches; produce neurons that form more distal sensory ganglia of the cranial nerves.

Epicardium (visceral pericardium) Outer tunic of thin serous membrane that covers the myocardium; derived from splanchnopleuric mesoderm; forms the coronary vessels.

Epidemiologic studies Examination of the spread and prevalence of diseases in communities.

Epidermal ridges Invaginations of epidermis that interdigitate with the dermal papillae to produce the distinctive ridges and grooves of the skin.

Epididymis Convoluted region of the vas deferens attached to the posterior side of the testis that serves as a reservoir for spermatozoa.

Epigenital mesonephric tubules Degenerates in females to form a remnant called the epoophoron; in males, 5 to 12 of these give rise to the efferent ductules.

Epiglottis Covers the opening of the trachea during swallowing; formed within the region of the fourth arch.

Epimere Formed from splitting of myotomes; gives rise to the deep epaxial muscles of the back, including the erector spinae and transversospinalis groups.

Epiphyseal plate Cartilaginous segments at the base of the epiphysis at both ends of long bones; provide a mechanism for the elongation of the long bones until about the 20th year.

Epiphysis Part of a long bone that develops from a site of secondary ossification, usually at the end of a bone.

Epiploic foramen of Winslow Narrow canal just posterior to the lesser omentum formed from reduction of the communication of the lesser and greater sacs of the peritoneal cavity as the stomach, liver, and lesser omentum are repositioned during the sixth week.

Epithalamus Forms the pineal gland; also forms the trigonum habenulae, including the habenular nucleus and the posterior and habenular commissures.

Epithelial root sheath (of the tooth) Epithelium immediately overlying the dentin of the tooth root; formed by the confluence of inner and outer enamel epithelium.

Eponychium Thin layer of epidermis initially covering the nail plate.

Epoophoron Vestiges of the epigenital mesonephric tubules scattered in the mesovarium.

Erythroblastosis fetalis If a mother who lacks Rh factors bears an Rh+ baby and fetal blood leaks across the placenta into the maternal circulation (usually at birth), the mother may make antibodies against these factors; if she bears a second Rh+ fetus, the anti-Rh antibodies cross into the fetal circulation and destroy the fetus' red blood cells; the fetus then overproduces red blood cells; the number of immature nucleated erythroblasts increases within the fetal circulation.

Ethmoid sinuses Paranasal air sinuses; begin to form within the ethmoid bone, communicating with the nasal passages through the middle meatus; complete their growth during puberty.

Exocoelomic cavity (primary yolk sac) Formed as cells at the periphery of the hypoblast proliferate and migrate out onto the cytotrophoblast to line the blastocyst cavity.

Exocoelomic membrane (Heuser's membrane) Arises from hypoblast cells that line the primary yolk sac (exocoelomic cavity).

Exocoelomic vesicles Collection of vesicles at the abembryonic pole arising from disintegration of the primary yolk sac, which also ultimately disintegrate.

External auditory meatus Derivative of the first pharyngeal cleft consisting of a channel from the pinna to the tympanic membrane.

External germinal (granular) layer (of the cerebellum) Forms superficial to the marginal layer during the third month; beginning in the fourth month its neuroblasts successively give rise to basket neuroblasts, granule neuroblasts, and stellate neuroblasts.

Extraembryonic coelom See **Chorionic cavity.**

Extraembryonic endoderm Cells arising from the periphery of the hypoblast (primary endoderm) that form the exocoelomic membrane and secrete the extraembryonic reticulum; a second wave of hypoblast proliferation forms the extraembryonic endoderm that lines the secondary yolk sac.

Extraembryonic mesoderm Lines the primary and secondary yolk sacs during the second week and is said to arise from the epiblast at the caudal end of the bilaminar germ disc; migrates out to form two layers that gradually separate the amnion from the cytotrophoblast.

Extraembryonic reticulum Acellular matrix secreted between exocoelomic membrane and cytotrophoblast by the exocoelomic membrane; vacuoles form within it during the second week that coalesce to form the chorionic cavity.

F

Facial nerve (VII) Contains branchial efferent, sensory, and visceral efferent fibers; grows into the second pharyngeal arch where it innervates muscles of facial expression and provides sensory innervation to the soft palate.

Facial skeleton (viscerocranium) Supports pharyngeal arches and their derivatives; evolved from skeletal elements of the branchial arches; in humans, much of the original branchial arch skeleton of the upper jaw has been replaced by dermal bones.

False ribs Includes ribs 8 to 12, which do not articulate directly with the sternum ventrally (see **True ribs**).

Fate map Diagram of the differentiation of epiblast cells showing developmental fate of each of its regions constructed using cell tracing and lineage studies.

Fertilization A spermatozoon penetrates the cumulus mass and zona pellucida, causing fusion of spermatozoon and secondary oocyte membranes; fusion of male and female pronuclei form a diploid, 2N zygote.

Fetal liver transplant   Fetal liver cells, suspended in a culture medium, are injected into the umbilical vein of a fetus to colonize the fetal liver, providing stem cells for hemopoiesis.

Fetal period   From end of the 8th through 38th week of gestation; characterized by growth and maturation of the organ systems.

Fibrocartilage   Type of cartilage usually occurring between bones, ligaments, or tendons; composes structures such as the menisci of the knee or shoulder joint.

Filopodia   Cellular extensions thought to be responsible for motility of axonal growth cones.

First meiotic division   Involves DNA replication and recombination and yields two haploid 2N daughter cells; produces two secondary spermatocytes in the male and a secondary oocyte and the first polar body in the female.

First trimester   First 3 months of gestation.

Fissuration   Process (along with the process of foliation) producing fissures within the cerebellar cortex.

Flocculonodular lobes   Most posterior (and primitive) lobes of the cerebellum; separated from the more cranial vermis and cerebellar hemispheres by a posterolateral fissure.

Floor plate   Formed as the ventral midline of the neural plate thins; becomes a hinge allowing the lateral lips of the developing neural folds to rise and meet in the dorsal midline during neurulation.

Foliation   See **Fissuration.**

Follicle cells   Nurse cells of the oocyte that develop from secondary cortical sex cords; form the cumulus oophorus and membrana granulosa cells.

Follicular canal   Canal lined by the inner and outer epidermal root sheath of the hair follicle; contains the outgrowing hair shaft.

Foramen cecum   Endodermal pit lying in the midline of the tongue within the terminal sulcus; gives rise to the thyroglossal duct (transient) and thyroid gland.

Foramen ovale   Inferior opening in the septum secundum that allows blood to flow from the right to left atrium during embryonic and fetal life.

Foregut   Develops from the cranial end of the primitive gut tube to form the pharyngeal foregut, thoracic esophagus, and abdominal foregut (abdominal esophagus, stomach, and superior half of duodenum).

Formative zone (root; of nail plate)   Arises from the stratum germinative of the proximal nail fold; produces the horny nail plate.

Fossa ovalis   Formed as foramen ovalis closes as septum primum and septum secundum fuse following birth.

Fourth ventricle   Forms by expansion of the neural canal in the region of the rhombencephalon.

Fraternal (dizygotic) twins   Arise from two separate oocytes and therefore do not share any of the fetal membranes.

Frontal lobes   Large superoventral lobes of the cerebral hemispheres separated from the more posterior parietal lobes by a groove called the central sulcus; each consists of two major regions, the prefrontal (largely "association" cortex) and precentral (sensorimotor) regions.

Frontal sinuses   Paranasal air sinuses: appear at fifth or sixth postnatal year; comprised of two separate cavities within the frontal bone—an extension of the ethmoid sinus and an independent invagination of the middle meatus.

Frontonasal prominence   One of five processes that give rise to the face (with two maxillary swellings and two mandibular swellings); forms the skull and forehead; gives rise to the nasal placodes that form the medial and lateral nasal processes.

Fundus   Superoposterior expansion of the stomach that is superior to a horizontal plane drawn through the apex of the cardiac incisure.

G

Ganglion   A discrete cell body composed of a concentration of neurons of the peripheral nervous system.

Gartner's cysts   Vestiges of the inferior end of the mesonephric duct located in the wall of the vagina.

Gastrulation   Process of epiblast ingress through the primitive streak forming the primary germ layers, namely, the definitive endoderm and mesoderm.

Gene therapy   Genetically defective stem cells are removed and then "cured" at the genetic level by gene targeting techniques and reintroduced into the individual.

General afferent   Refers to that part of the nervous system involved in the reception of impulses of general sensation: served by the trigeminal (V) and facial (VII) nerves and pharyngeal and laryngeal cavities (V, IX, X).

Genetic screening (of polar bodies)   Polar bodies contain DNA that can be screened to obtain genetic information about a female's germ cell line.

Genital ridge   Primordial gonad formed by germ cell migration just medial to the mesonephroi (embryonic kidneys).

Germ line   Cells originating within primary ectoderm that migrate into the yolk sac and differentiate into primordial germ cells during early weeks of embryonic development; cells then migrate to genital ridge, where they differentiate into gametes.

Germinal matrix   See **Dermal papilla of hair follicle.**

Germinal vesicle   Large, watery nucleus formed during the dictyotene stage of the first meiotic prophase in the primary oocyte that may protect genetic material within the primary oocyte from destructive effects of teratogens or irradiation.

Germinal vesicle breakdown   Reinitiation of nuclear maturation in primary oocytes resulting in disintegration of germinal vesicle membrane.

Germinative layer (stratum germinativum) Layer of the mature epidermis derived from the basal proliferating layer of surface ectoderm; contains stem cells that differentiate into the keratinized cells of overlying layers that proliferate to replenish its own stem cell population.

GIFT (Gamete intrafallopian transfer) Technique often employed for anovulatory syndrome or suboptimal spermatozoa motility; male and female gametes are collected and then separately reintroduced through a catheter into oviduct for fertilization (see also **ZIFT**).

Glans (of clitoris; of penis) Distal end of the clitoris and penis demarcated from the shaft by the coronary sulcus.

Glioblast Produced after the formation of neuroblasts ceases by the ventricular neuroectoderm of the neural tube; differentiate into glial cells.

Glomerulus Small bundle of capillaries surrounded by the Bowman's capsule of the metanephric tubule; form the renal corpuscle.

Glossopharyngeal nerve (IX) Innervates structures that develop from tissues within the third pharyngeal arch; contains branchial and visceral efferent fibers; provides general sensory innervation to most of the posterior one third of the tongue, pharyngeal cavity, and superior esophagus; also contains special (taste) fibers that conduct impulses from the vallate papillae; innervates the stylopharyngeus muscle.

Gonocyte Cells of the germ line of males or females during meiosis, including primary, secondary, and definitive oocytes or spermatocytes.

Granular layer Stratum of the cerebellum composed of granule cells and some stellate and basket cells that arise within and migrate from the external germinal layer.

Granule neuroblasts Formed during the second wave of neuroblasts formation by the external germinal layer of the cerebellar cortex; migrate inward to establish the granular layer.

Gray matter Regions of the central nervous system containing neuronal cell bodies; initially organized into a marginal layer, then into ventral and dorsal columns that may further differentiate into motor and associational nuclei, respectively.

Gray ramus communicans Diminutive bundle of neuronal fibers connecting the sympathetic chain ganglion to the spinal nerve; contain postganglionic sympathetic fibers only.

Greater omentum Fold of the dorsal mesogastrium that encloses the lower recess of the lesser sac; forms a repository of fat in the adult.

Greater sac Remainder of the peritoneal cavity after formation of the lesser sac.

Greater splanchnic nerve Comprised of preganglionic fibers originating from central neurons located in the intermediolateral columns at spinal cord levels T5 to T12; collect into a single nerve that innervates the celiac ganglia.

Growth cone Develops at the advancing end of elongating axons and is thought to provide locomotory force required for axonal growth; capable of sensing chemical and physical characteristics of the extracellular matrix and mesenchyma.

Gubernaculum Ligamentous cord that condenses in the seventh week to effect descent of the testes in males; forms the round ligaments of the uterus and ovarian ligaments in females.

H

Hair follicles Formed from the epidermis and dermis; form the hair shafts and sebaceous glands; first evident as concentrations of epidermal cells (hair germs) in the basal layer of the primitive two-layered epidermis that elongate to form hair pegs.

Hair germ Ectodermal concentrations arising in the basal layer of the primitive epidermis; form hair follicles.

Hair peg Rod-like structure formed from elongation of the hair germ.

Hair shaft Specialized aggregations of keratinocyte generated by the germinal matrix of the hair follicle and pushed outward through the follicular canal.

Hard palate Formed subsequent to fusion of the palatine shelves when mesenchyme within the anterior region ossifies.

Harlequin fetus Results from defect of the mechanism that bundles the keratin fibers in the stratum granulosum; keratinocytes cannot be sloughed; these babies usually die shortly after birth.

Hematopoietic stem cell Arise in primary ectoderm; migrate to yolk sac, liver, and (possibly) to aorta-gonad-mesonephros (AGM) region to form blood cells that ultimately seed adult hematopoietic organs (spleen, thymus, and bone marrow).

Hemimelia Reduction or stunting of distal limb segments.

Hemivertebra Lopsided vertebra produced when the notochord fails to induce the ventral sclerotome on one side; may result in lateral curvature of the spinal column (scoliosis).

Hepatic diverticulum Endodermal outgrowth of the duodenum; forms on day 22 on the ventral wall of the descending segment of the duodenum; grows into the ventral mesentery, where it forms liver parenchyma (hepatocytes), bile canaliculi, and hepatic ducts.

Higher centers More complex structures of the brain (cerebellum, diencephalon, and cerebral hemispheres); retain very few traces of spinal cord organization.

Hindgut Segment formed from the caudal end of the primitive gut tube; vascularized by the inferior mesenteric artery; forms left one third of the transverse colon, the descending colon, and rectum.

Hippocampal (fornix) commissure Fiber tract that develops within the lamina terminalis; connects left and right hippocampi of the cerebral hemispheres.

Horny layer (stratum corneum)   Outermost layer of the mature epidermis produced as lytic enzymes are released; metabolic activity ceases in cells of the outer layer of the stratum granulosum, producing flattened, scale-like, terminally differentiated keratinocytes.

Horny nail plate   Compressed keratinocytes produced by the formative zone or root of the nail plate.

Horseshoe kidney   Fusion of the inferior poles of the metanephroi during their ascent from the sacral region may result in formation of a horseshoe-shaped kidney that may be caught under the inferior mesenteric artery.

Hydramnios (oligohydramnios)   Insufficient amounts of amniotic fluid within the amnion; may be caused by renal agenesis or an obstructive uropathy that prevents fetus from urinating into the amnion.

Hydrops   Accumulation of water in the fetus.

Hymen   Endodermal membrane that initially partitions the lumen of the inferior vagina from the vestibule; usually partially ruptured after the fifth fetal month but remnants may persist.

Hyoid bone   Ossifies from cartilage of the second pharyngeal arch (Reinchert's cartilage) and the third pharygeal arch; stabilizes the tongue and the larynx.

Hypoblast (primary endoderm)   Sheet of cells that appears with the epiblast as the embryoblast laminates; it eventually forms the extraembryonic endoderm.

Hypodermis (subcorium)   Subcutaneous fatty connective tissue underlying the dermis.

Hypoglossal nerve (XII)   Develops in association with occipital somites and innervates all of the intrinsic muscles of the tongue except the palatoglossus; exclusively motor in function.

Hypomere   Formed from splitting of myotomes; gives rise to the deep hypaxial muscles of the lateral and ventral body wall in the thorax and abdomen.

Hypopharyngeal (hypobranchial) eminence   Swelling on the floor of the pharynx in the region of the third and fourth pharyngeal arches; gives rise to the posterior one third of the tongue.

Hypophyseal cartilages   Forms the body of the sphenoid bone of the chondrocranium.

Hypothalamic sulcus   Groove that demarcates the boundary between the thalamus and the hypothalamus.

Hypothalamus   Inferoventral swelling of the diencephalon; regulates endocrine activity of the pituitary and many autonomic responses; also functions in the limbic system, which controls/regulates emotion and sleep/waking mechanisms.

I

Identical (monozygotic) twins   Arise from the same oocyte, which may split at the two-cell stage or at later stages of development; possess the same genetic makeup; may or may not share fetal membranes.

Immature intermediate villi   Extensions of the stem villi formed during the first and second trimester by development of trophoblastic and villous sprouts; contain a core of connective tissue and blood vessels, within an incomplete jacket of cytotrophoblast, covered by a complete layer of syncytiotrophoblast; do not possess terminal villous branches.

In situ vesicle formation and fusion   See **Vasculogenesis.**

Incus bone   Auditory ossicle arising from the palatopterygoquadrate bar.

Indifferent phase   See **ambisexual stage.**

Inferior colliculi   Develop from alar plate neuroblasts that migrate into the mesencephalic roof plate; relay information from the cochlea to auditory areas of the cerebral cortex.

Inferior (geniculate) ganglion of cranial nerve VII   Formed by neural crest cells and cells of the first epibranchial (epipharyngeal) placode; relays impulses of general sensation to the brain stem from the skin of the auricular concha, small patch of skin behind the ear, and external tympanic membrane; also conveys sensation of taste from the anterior two thirds of the tongue and from the hard and soft palates to the nucleus of the tractus solitarius.

Inferior (nodose) ganglion of cranial nerve X (vagus)   Neurons within this ganglion arise from third and fourth epibranchial placodes; relay general and special (taste) sensations to the general afferent column and the nucleus of the tractus solitarius, respectively.

Inferior (petrosal) ganglion of cranial nerve IX (glossopharyngeal)   Neurons within this ganglion are derived from the second epibranchial placode; relay general and special (taste) sensations to the general afferent column and the nucleus of the tractus solitarius, respectively.

Inferior vena cava   Vessel that returns systemic blood from the trunk and lower extremities to the right atrium; formed from the right vitelline, subcardinal, supracardinal, and posterior cardinal veins.

Infundibulum   Evagination of the floor of the diencephalon formed in the third week; forms the posterior pituitary gland (neurohypophysis).

Inguinal canal   Defect occurring in both males and females formed in the anterior abdominal wall by the processus vaginalis as it forces thin sock-like extensions of transversalis fascia, internal oblique muscle, and external oblique muscle into the labioscrotal swelling.

Inner cell mass (embryoblast)   Blastomeres arising from first cells to divide during early cleavages that segregate within the center of the morula and differentiate into the embryo (outer cells differentiate into placental membranes).

Inner enamel epithelium Derived from the ectoderm of the dental lamina; differentiates into the ameloblasts that secrete the enamel of the root crown.

Inner epidermal root sheath (of the hair follicle) Directly lines the follicular canal.

Insemination Deposition of seminal fluid within the vagina, during coitus, or with a catheter as in "artificial" insemination.

Insula Portion of the cerebral cortex forming the floor of the lateral cerebral fossa; eventually covered by the temporal lobe.

Intermaxillary process Formed by the growth and fusion of the inferior regions of the left and right medial nasal processes; forms the philtrum of the upper lip and the primary palate.

Intermediate layer (of the dermis) Produced in the 11th week by the basal layer of the epidermis; gives rise to outer layers of the mature epidermis.

Intermediate mesoderm Lies between paraxial mesoderm and lateral plate mesoderm from the cervical to sacral regions; forms embryonic and definitive kidneys and part of the male genital system.

Intermediate zone Formed between the ventricular and marginal zone; neuroblasts within it and the ventricular zone migrate outward to form the cortical plate; eventually forms white matter of the cerebral hemispheres.

Intermediolateral cell columns Collections of gray matter containing central (preganglionic) neurons of the sympathetic nervous system (T1 to L2).

Internal capsule Massive fiber bundle that carries fibers from the thalamus to the cerebral cortex and from the cerebral cortex to lower regions of the brain and spinal cord.

Internal germinal layer Neuroblast-producing layer of the cerebellum; arises from the ventricular layer to form primitive nuclear neuroblasts (form the cerebellar nuclei), primitive Purkinje neuroblasts, and Golgi neuroblasts.

Intersegmental artery Paired intersegmental arteries that sprout from the dorsal aorta; vascularize all of the derivatives of the somites and the extremities (see **Axis artery**).

Interthalamic adhesions May form as the thalami expand into the third ventricle.

Interventricular foramen of Munro Openings that allow passage of cerebrospinal fluid between the third ventricle and lateral ventricles.

Intervillous space Blood-filled cavities within the placenta arising from the trophoblastic lacunae.

Interzone Region of fibroblastic tissue, within the rod-like bone precursor, that will form the joint.

Intraembryonic coelomic cavity Formed as cavities between splanchnopleuric and somatopleuric lateral plate mesoderm on the left and right sides coalesce during embryonic folding; forms the definitive pericardial, left and right pleural, and peritoneal cavities.

Intraperitoneal (organ) Suspended within the peritoneal cavity by a mesentery.

Intrauterine growth retardation (IUGR) Effects of some toxins, teratogens, or disease states of the mother may lead to an inhibition of fetal growth.

Intrinsic muscles of the larynx Move laryngeal parts; change the length and tension of the vocal folds and the space between the vocal folds; except for the cricothyroid muscle, innervated by the recurrent laryngeal branch of the vagus nerve.

K

Karyotype Description of the composition of the genome with respect to the number and condition of autosomes and sex chromosomes or a preparation of condensed chromosomes that may be viewed with a microscope.

Keratinocytes Cells of the epidermis produced by the stratum germinative forming three additional superficial layers: the stratum spinosum, the stratum granulosum, and the stratum corneum (in order of maturation); contain keratin proteins.

L

Labia minora Medial swellings of the female external genitalia that border the vestibule of the vagina and arise from the urethral folds; homologous to the corpus spongiosum (spongy or penile urethra) of the penis.

Labioscrotal swellings Develop lateral to the urethral (urogenital) folds in both males and females; form the labia majora in females and the scrotum in males.

Lamellar ichthyosis Excessive keratinization of the skin; skin may scale off in flakes; babies are usually viable.

Lamina terminalis Point of final closure of the cranial neuropore; extends from the dorsal region of the optic chiasm to rostrum of the corpus callosum; includes the anterior and hippocampal commissures.

Langerhans cells Formed within the bone marrow; migrate to the epidermis (initially in the seventh week) to form the macrophage immune cells of the skin.

Larynx Formed from cartilage arising from lateral plate mesoderm of the fourth and sixth pharyngeal arches; musculature formed from cranial paraxial mesoderm of these arches.

Lateral apertures (foramina of Luschka) Facilitate transfer of cerebrospinal fluid from the fourth ventricle to the subarachnoid space of the brain stem and spinal cord.

Lateral cerebral fossa See **Lateral cerebral sulcus.**

Lateral cerebral sulcus Formed as the lateral cerebral fossa becomes a deeper, elongated cleft.

Lateral cervical sinuses See **Cervical cysts.**

Lateral endocardial tubes Paired tubes that form within the lateral regions of the cardiogenic area by vasculogenesis; fuse to form the primitive heart tube.

Lateral folding Results in fusion of the lateral edges of the ectoderm, somatopleuric mesoderm, presumptive coelomic cavities, splanchnopleuric mesoderm, and endoderm in the 4- to 5-week embryo; cylindrical vertebrate body is formed with its integument, musculature, and gut tube.

Lateral nasal process Form from the lateral regions of the nasal placodes of the frontonasal prominence; give rise to the lateral regions of the nose.

Lateral plate mesoderm Mesodermal sheet lateral to the intermediate mesoderm; splits into somatopleuric mesoderm (forms parietal serous lining of body cavities) and splanchnopleuric mesoderm (forms serous membrane ensheathing visceral organs).

Lateral ventricles Two cavities within the cerebral hemispheres arising from expansion of the neural canal within the telencephalon; initially occupy most of the volume of the cerebral hemispheres, but are gradually constricted by growth and thickening of the cerebral cortex; communicate with the third ventricle through the interventricular foramina of Munro.

Least splanchnic nerve Composed of preganglionic sympathetic axons originating from central sympathetic neurons at spinal cord level T12; innervates peripheral neurons within ganglia associated with the superior mesenteric artery.

Left brachiocephalic vein Develops from thymic and thymus veins to connect the distal end of the left anterior cardinal vein with the right; drains blood from the left side of the head and neck to the superior vena cava.

Lesser omentum Mesentery between the liver and lesser curvature of the stomach derived from the ventral mesentery; includes the hepatogastric and hepatoduodenal ligaments.

Lesser sac Portion of the peritoneal cavity posterior to the stomach; partially segregated by rotation of the stomach and secondary fixation of the duodenum to the posterior body wall.

Lesser splanchnic nerve Composed of sympathetic preganglionic fibers originating from central sympathetic neurons located within the intermediolateral columns at spinal cord levels T10 and T11; innervates peripheral neurons located within the aorticorenal ganglia.

Leydig (interstitial) cells Differentiate in response to the protein encoded by the sex-determining region of the Y chromosome from mesenchymal stroma in the genital ridge; secrete male steroid hormones.

Limb bud Formed as somites in the limb regions (C5 to C8, L3 to L5) induce somatopleuric lateral plate mesoderm within the flank to proliferate; upper extremity limb buds appear at about 24 days; lower extremity limb buds appear at about 28 days.

Lobes (of the cerebellum) Initial subdivisions of the cerebellum; consist of the anterior, middle, and flocculonodular.

Lumbar splanchnic nerve Composed of sympathetic preganglionic axons originating from central neurons located within the intermediolateral columns at spinal cord levels L1 to L2; innervates peripheral neurons located in the diffuse inferior mesenteric ganglia or plexus.

Lung bud Endodermal foregut diverticulum that bifurcates into primary bronchiole buds; forms the bronchioles and alveoli of the lungs; also called respiratory diverticulum and pulmonary diverticulum.

M

Major calyces Calyces of the metanephric collecting system formed after formation of the renal pelvis as the next four generations of ureteric bud bifurcations coalesce.

Malleus bone Auditory ossicle arising from Meckel's cartilage.

Mammary glands Modified apocrine glands; develop within a pair of epidermal thickenings (mammary ridges) that extend from the axilla to the inguinal region; two primary buds of the mammary glands appear by the seventh week; numerous secondary buds appear by the fourth month that become canalized to form lactiferous ducts by the sixth month; each mammary gland consists of 15 to 25 lactiferous ducts by birth.

Mammary pit Depression that is the opening to the lactiferous ducts of the mammary gland that form in the sixth month.

Mammary ridges See **Mammary glands.**

Mandible bone Formed largely of dermal elements that have invested the Meckel's cartilage within the mandibular swelling of the first pharyngeal arch.

Mandibular swellings Inferior divisions of the first pharyngeal arch that give rise to the lower jaw and lip; contain Meckel's cartilage.

Mantle layer Layer of gray matter peripheral to the ventricular layer formed by differentiating neuroblasts of the neural tube.

Marginal layer Most peripheral layer of white matter of the developing neural tube composed of nerve cell fibers that emanate from the neuronal cell bodies of the mantle layer.

Maternal sinusoids Expanded maternal capillaries within the endometrium that become connected to trophoblastic lacunae to establish uteroplacental circulation.

Mature alveoli Differentiate from branches of respiratory bronchioles (immature alveoli or terminal sacs); first appear at about week 28, produced through year 8; differentiation involves thinning of squamous epithelial lining of terminal sacs and production of surfactant.

Mature intermediate villi Slender side branches of

the tertiary stem villi that begin to form near the end of the second trimester; produce small nodular secondary branches called terminal villi.

Maxilla bone   In primitive jawed fishes, formed largely from cartilage within the palatopterygoquadrate bar; in humans, formed largely of dermal bone.

Maxillary sinuses   Paranasal air sinuses that form within the maxilla during the third fetal month; grow larger during childhood.

Maxillary swellings   Superior divisions of the first pharyngeal arch that give rise to the upper jaw and lip.

Meckel's cartilage   Cartilaginous element that forms from neural crest cells within the mandibular swelling of the first pharyngeal arch; forms the malleus in humans; a remnant of this cartilage may be evident within the core of the mandible.

Medial nasal processes   Formed from the medial regions of the nasal placodes; from the medial region of the nose and the intermaxillary process.

Median aperture (foramen of Magendie)   Single median opening in the roof plate of the fourth ventricle allows cerebrospinal fluid to flow from the fourth ventricle to the subarachnoid space of the brain stem and spinal cord.

Median sulcus   Groove that demarcates the medial line of fusion of the distal tongue buds.

Median tongue bud (tuberculum impar)   Medial swelling of the first pharyngeal arch that is largely overgrown by distal tongue buds; forms a small part of the posterior region of the anterior two thirds of the tongue.

Medulla oblongata   Most caudal region of the rhombencephalon; arises from the myelencephalon and is most like the spinal cord in organization; most of the cranial nerve nuclei are formed within this part of the brain; acts as a relay between higher centers and the spinal cord; regulates respiration, heartbeat, reflex movements, and several other functions.

Medullary sex cords   Primitive sex cords in the medullary region of the genital ridge that differentiate into pre-Sertoli cells to form testis cords; at puberty these cords become canalized to form the seminiferous tubules; also form the rete testis tubules that connect the seminiferous tubules to the efferent ductules.

Meiotic arrest in the female germ line, first stage   Cells of the female germ line initiate meiosis during late embryonic or early fetal life, synthesize DNA, and enter the prophase stage of the first meiotic division; chromosomes condense during the dictyotene stage, meiotic progress is suspended, and the nucleus swells with fluid, producing the germinal vesicle.

Meiotic arrest in the female germ line, second stage   Meiotic arrest of the primary oocyte at the first meiotic prophase is overcome following an ovulatory stimulus producing a secondary oocyte arrested at the second meiotic metaphase; second-ary oocyte does not resume meiotic progress unless fertilized.

Meiotic maturation   Changes in the chromosomes and DNA that occur during both meiotic divisions.

Melanocytes   Neural crest-derived cells that migrate from the neural tube into the epidermis by the sixth to seventh week; are the pigment cells of the integument.

Membrane bones (of skull)   Arise from the dermal armor of the armored fishes; form the cranial vault, including frontal, parietal, and superior regions of the occipital squamata; have also overgrown cartilages of the facial skeleton to form most of the maxilla, zygomatic bone, squamata of the temporal bone, and mandible.

Membranous ossification   Bony tissue that develops within mesenchymal tissue in the absence of a cartilaginous precursor.

Membranous urethra   Arises from the pelvic urethra of the primitive urogenital sinus in the region of the developing sphincter urethra muscle.

Membranous ventricular septum   Develops from migrating neural crest cells; failure of neural crest cell migration into the heart may result in ventricular septal defects.

Meningocele   Type of spina bifida in which the meninges evaginate through a dorsal defect of the vertebral canal.

Meningohydroencephalocele   Anomaly of the occipital region in which part of the brain (ventricle and meninges) evaginate through a defect resulting from inadequate ossification of the cranial vault.

Meningomyelocele   Severe example of spina bifida in which a sac or cele (including meninges and a segment of spinal cord) protrude through a defect in the vertebral canal.

Meniscus (of joint)   Crescent-shaped fibrocartilaginous structure serving to increase the concavity of the joint.

Merkel cells   Contain keratin and form desmosomes with adjacent keratinocytes; lie at the base of the epidermis and are associated with nerve endings where they function as pressure-sensing mechanoreceptors; found only in palmar or plantar regions.

Mesencephalic (cranial) flexure   Initial flexure of the brain that develops at the level of the future mesencephalon on day 22.

Mesencephalon (midbrain)   One of the three primary brain vesicles; also one of the five secondary brain vesicles; primarily a relay center but also contains cranial nerve nuclei, visual and auditory centers, and other structures.

Mesoderm   "Middle" layer of trilaminar embryo arising from the epiblast by gastrulation during the third week; classified as paraxial, intermediate, or lateral plate mesoderm.

Mesodermal core   Precursor of the limb buds; lateral plate mesoderm (the mesodermal core) and a cap of ectoderm.

Mesonephric (wolfian) ducts   First function in elimination of urine; sprout ureteric buds that form the collecting system of the metanephroi; exstrophy into the posterior wall of the bladder to form trigone of the bladder; degenerate in females; form the spermatic ducts (vasa deferentia) in males.

Mesonephric excretory unit Renal corpuscle and its connection to the mesonephric duct.

Mesonephric tubules First function to form the urine of the mesonephros and transport it to mesonephric ducts; degenerate in females to form the epoophoron and paroophoron; 5 to 12 of these persist in males to form efferent ductules.

Mesonephroi "Middle" kidneys that develop from intermediate mesoderm in the thoracic and lumbar regions; functional from the 6th to the 10th week.

Metanephric excretory unit Includes the renal corpuscle (Bowman's capsule enclosing a glomerulus), proximal convoluted tubule, loops of Henle, and distal convoluted tubule.

Metanephroi Definitive kidneys that arise through inductive interactions between the ureteric bud and metanephric blastema in the sacral region; ascend to superior lumbar levels.

Metaphysis Growing region of the long bone located between the epiphyseal plate (physis) and the shaft (diaphysis).

Metencephalon (behind-brain) Cranial region of the rhombencephalon; gives rise to the pons and the cerebellum.

Midgut Region of the primitive gut tube vascularized by the superior mesenteric artery; communicates directly with the cavity of the yolk sac via the vitelline duct; gives rise to portions of the duodenum, jejunum, ileum, ascending colon, and transverse colon.

Minor calyces Formed after formation of the major calyces as an additional four generations of ureteric bud bifurcations coalesce; each drains a tree of collecting ducts (renal pyramid) that converge to form a renal papilla.

Molecular layer Layer of the cerebellar cortex formed primarily by Purkinje and basket neuroblasts and the dendritic trees of the Golgi and granule cells in the underlying granular layer.

Monosomy Absence of one chromosome of a single pair of chromosomes in an otherwise genotypically normal embryo.

Monozygotic (identical) twins See **Identical twins.**

Mosaic (embryo) Composed of a mixture of cells with different karyotypes; chromosome 21 nondisjunction may occur in a single embryonic cell during cleavage; resulting fetus develops as a mosaic of normal and trisomy 21 cells.

Motor neurons Develop within the gray matter of the ventral gray columns of the spinal cord and brain stem; innervated by axons of association neurons and in turn sprout axons that exit the spinal cord via the ventral roots.

Müllerian-inhibiting substance (MIS) See **Anti-müllerian hormone.**

Müllerian tubercle Remnant of the inferior end of the paramesonephric duct in males.

Muscles of facial expression Formed from the paraxial mesoderm (from somitomere 6) in the second pharyngeal arch.

Muscles of mastication Formed from the paraxial mesoderm (from somitomere 4) in the first pharyngeal arch.

Muscular ventricular septum Septation of the ventricles is initiated by growth of this thickened ridge of musculature; anterior trabeculated region is the primary ventricular fold (septum); smooth posterior region is the inlet septum; demarcated by the septomarginal trabecula or moderator band.

Myelencephalon (medulla brain) Caudal region (secondary brain vesicle) of the rhombencephalon; gives rise to the medulla oblongata and is most like the spinal cord in organization.

Myelin sheath Lamellar covering of nerve axons of the peripheral nervous system produced by Schwann cells; those investing axons of the central nervous system are formed by oligodendrocytes.

Myocardium Cardiac muscle arising from splanchnopleuric mesoderm that invests the primary heart tube; secretes cardiac jelly and gives rise to the conduction system.

Myoepithelial cells Muscle cells of epidermal origin form the outer layer of the sweat glands; innervated by sympathetic fibers that stimulate contractions to expel sweat from the gland.

Myotome Formed as the dermomyotome splits; further splits into epimeres and hypomeres and also gives rise to myoblasts that form upper and lower extremity musculature.

N

N number Applied to descriptions of meiotic or mitotic cells; the number of copies of each unique DNA strand within the cell.

Nail folds Two lateral ectodermal folds and a single proximal ectodermal fold surround the nail field; proximal nail fold produces the formative zone or root of the nail plate.

Nasal fin Thickened floor of the nasal sac; vacuolates and thins to form the oronasal membrane, which breaks down to form an opening between the nasal sac and oral cavity (primitive choana).

Nasal pits Shallow depressions that form within the central regions of the nasal placodes in the sixth week; posterior regions fuse together to form a single nasal sac.

Nasal placodes Ectodermal thickenings on the ventral surface of the frontonasal prominence that appear in the fourth week; form medial and lateral nasal processes.

Nasal sac See **Nasal pits.**

Nasolacrimal duct Ectodermal duct that forms through the invagination of the nasolacrimal groove; invested by bone during ossification of maxilla; drains lacrimal secretions from the conjunctival sac into the nasal cavity.

Nasolacrimal groove   See **Nasolacrimal duct.**

Nephric (renal) vesicle (nephrotome)   Derived from intermediate mesoderm of the mesonephroi and metanephroi; form nephric tubules.

Nephric tubules   General term denoting the mesonephric and metanephric tubules derived from intermediate mesoderm; form the nephrons of the mesonephroi and metanephroi, respectively.

Neural canal   A lumen formed within the neural tube during neurulation that becomes the central canal of the spinal cord and the ventricles of the brain.

Neural cord   Solid midline structure formed from the caudal eminence during secondary neurulation; fuses with the caudal end of the neural tube; neural canal develops within it; forms the caudal end of the spinal cord and pia and dura of the filum terminale.

Neural crest   Population of cells arising from the lateral lips of the neural plate that detach during formation of the neural tube and migrate to form a variety of structures.

Neural groove   Thin longitudinal midline groove that bisects the neural plate into presumptive right and left neural folds.

Neural plate   Begins to form on day 18 in epiblast along the midsagittal axis cranial to the primitive pit; undergoes neurulation in the fourth week to form the neural tube (precursor of the central nervous system).

Neurenteric canal   Formed as ventral floor of hollow notochordal process degenerates; facilitates communication between amniotic cavity and yolk sac through the primitive pit.

Neuroblasts   Formed as neuroepithelial cells within the central nervous system divide and differentiate; subsequently elongate and migrate to form the mantle layer of the neural tube.

Neuroectoderm   Neural epithelium arising from the ectoderm within the neural plate.

Neurohypophysis (posterior pituitary)   Region of the pituitary gland formed by the infundibulum of the diencephalon.

Neuromere   Transitory subdivisions of the brain first evident on day 20 as transverse sulci separate the presumptive brain into small segments; nine such segments (rhombomeres) may form in the presumptive rhombencephalon.

Neuronal fibers   Nerve cell axons and their accompanying glial investment.

Neurosensory cells of the olfactory epithelium   Produced by cells of the nasal placode; cell bodies located within the olfactory epithelium of the nasal cavity; axons penetrate the cribriform plate of the ethmoid bone to synapse with secondary neurosensory cells within the olfactory bulb.

Neurulation   Process of folding of the neural plate and closure of the cranial and caudal neuropores to form the neural tube.

Notochord   A solid cylinder formed as the notochordal plate detaches from the endoderm; later induces the spinal cord and vertebral bodies.

Notochordal plate   Flattened midventral bar of mesoderm formed from the hollow notochordal process.

Notochordal process   One of the first mesodermal structures to arise by gastrulation as cells surround the primitive pit, forming hollow tube extending cranially in the axial midline; elongates as cells are added at its caudal end.

Nuclear maturation (of gamete)   Process of nuclear remodeling and changes in DNA content and chromosome number occurring during meiosis without regard to cytoplasmic changes.

Nucleus ambiguus   Located in the caudal hindbrain; provides branchial efferent fibers for cranial nerves IX, X, and XI.

Nucleus habenulae   Formed within the epithalamus; may function as a relay for olfactory, somatic, and visceral afferent pathways.

Nucleus pulposus   Central region of the intervertebral disc arising directly from the notochord; original tissue may be replaced by cells of the annulus fibrosis in early childhood.

Nutrient artery   Single dominant artery that supplies the medullary cavity of a long bone.

O

Oblique vein of the left atrium   Drains the wall of the left atrium; arises from the distal end of the left sinus horn and is directly connected to the coronary sinus.

Occipital lobes   Posterior lobes of the cerebral hemispheres demarcated from the parietal lobes by the occipital sulcus; contains visuosensory areas that interpret visual information passed from the lateral geniculate bodies.

Occipital sulcus   See **Occipital lobes.**

Oculomotor nerve (III)   Supplies motor innervation to the following extrinsic muscles of the eye: levator palpebrae superioris, superior rectus, medial rectus, inferior rectus, and inferior oblique and parasympathetic innervation to the sphincter pupillae and ciliary muscles.

Odontoblast   Neural crest-derived cells arising from the dental papilla; secrete the nonmineralized matrix of the dentin (predentin) in the seventh month; predentin calcifies to form the dentin.

Olfactory bulb   Outgrowth of the telencephalon that appears in the sixth week as axons of primary sensory neurons differentiating within the nasal placodes begin to synapse with neurons; neurons become secondary sensory neurons of the olfactory system; axons of the secondary olfactory neurosensory cells elongate forming a stalk-like olfactory tract; these synapse within olfactory centers of the cerebral hemispheres; olfactory bulbs and tracts are also called the olfactory nerve (I).

Olfactory epithelium   Arises from the nasal placode to form the primary olfactory neurosensory cells.

Olfactory nerve (I)   See **Olfactory bulb.**

Olfactory tract   See **Olfactory bulb.**

Oligodendrocytes   Supporting cells within the central nervous system; arise from glioblasts that arise from the ventricular layer; form sheet-like processes that wrap around axons to form myelin sheaths within the central nervous system.

Oligohydramnios   See **Hydramnios.**

Olivary nuclei   Rhombencephalic nuclei formed by alar column gray matter that migrate into ventral regions of the rhombencephalon, reeling their axons out behind them.

Oogonium   Differentiates directly from a primordial germ cell; constitutes the stem cells of the female germ line.

Optic nerve (II)   Composed of the axons of ganglion cells in the anterior layer of the neural retina that pass from the eyeball at the optic disc as the optic nerve; convey visual sensation from the retina to the lateral geniculate bodies.

Oronasal membrane   See **Nasal fin.**

Ostium primum   Opening in the septum primum that closes as the septum primum fuses with the septum intermedium.

Ostium secundum   Develops by programmed cell death (apoptosis) within the superior region of the septum primum as the ostium primum closes.

Otic ganglion   Parasympathetic ganglion of the glossopharyngeal nerve; houses peripheral neurons whose postganglionic fibers innervate the parotid gland.

Outer cell mass (trophoblast)   Formed by "late-dividing" cells of the morula that remain at the periphery and serve as the primary source for placental membranes.

Outer enamel epithelium   Derived from the ectoderm of the dental lamina.

Outer epidermal root sheath   Constitutes the outer epidermal wall of the root canal of the hair follicle.

P

Palatine shelves   Medial growths of the maxillary processes that form the secondary palate.

Palatine tonsils   Lymphoid structures that form from endoderm of the second pharyngeal pouch and mesoderm of the second pharyngeal membrane.

Palatopterygoquadrate bar (maxillary process)   Forms from neural crest cells within the maxillary swellings of the first pharyngeal arch; gives rise to the alisphenoid bone of the orbit and the incus bone of the middle ear.

Papillary muscles   Muscular specializations of the ventricular walls that anchor the chordae tendineae of the atrioventricular valves.

Papillary region (of the dermis)   Superficial layer elaborated into ridge-like dermal papillae that interdigitate with the epidermal ridges.

Parachordal cartilages   Gives rise to the base of the occipital bone.

Paradidymis   Remnants of the degenerate paragenital mesonephric tubules in the male genital system (see **Paragenital mesonephric tubules**).

Parafollicular (C) cells   Calcitonin-secreting cells of the thyroid that arise from the telopharyngeal (ultimobranchial) body of the fifth pouch.

Paragenital mesonephric tubules   Adjacent to the developing gonad; degenerate to form the paradidymis; degenerate in females to form the paraoophoron.

Paramesonephric (müllerian) ducts   Paired ducts that develop in the early seventh week; degenerate in males, leaving the appendix, testis, and müllerian tubercle; form superior end of the vagina, the uterus, and fallopian tubes (oviducts) in females.

Parasympathetic ganglia   Peripheral neurons of the parasympathetic nervous system are housed in one of four cranial ganglia (ciliary [III], sphenopalatine and submandibular [VII], and otic [IX]) or numerous small ganglia embedded within the walls of the viscera of the thorax, abdomen, and pelvis (vagus [X]).

Parasympathetic nervous system   Two-neuron subdivision of the autonomic nervous system that includes central motor neurons within nuclei of the brain stem and intermediolateral columns of the spinal cord (S2 to S4); sprouts preganglionic fibers that synapse with motor neurons of peripheral ganglia in the head and in the walls of trunk viscera that in turn sprout postganglionic fibers that innervate end organs; termed a craniosacral system and is involuntarily active during periods of peace and relaxation.

Parietal lobes   Lobes of the cerebral hemispheres bounded anteriorly by the central sulcus from the frontal lobe and posteriorly by the occipital sulcus from the occipital lobe; contain motor and somatosensory areas and a speech area; function largely in discrimination and interpretation.

Paroophoron   Remnants of the paragenital mesonephric tubules in females; scattered in the mesovarium.

Parotid (salivary) glands   Develop from ectoderm within the groove formed by fusion of the maxillary and mandibular swellings.

Pelvic kidney   Metanephric kidney that fails to ascend between the sixth and ninth weeks; remains within the pelvis.

Pelvic splanchnic nerves   Formed by parasympathetic preganglionic fibers emerging from the ventral surface of the sacral cord (S2 to S4); innervates ganglia of target viscera.

Pelvic urethra   Constricted region of the primitive urogenital sinus at the base of the presumptive bladder; gives rise to the membranous urethra in females and the membranous and prostatic urethras in males.

Penile urethra   Part of the urethra in males enclosed within the corpora spongiosum of the penis; derived from the definitive urogenital sinus.

Penis   Male phallus derived from the genital tubercle and the fusion of urethral folds.

Pericardioperitoneal canals   Facilitate communication between the superior primitive pericardial cavity and inferior peritoneal cavity through the septum transversum.

Periderm   During the fourth week the surface ectoderm proliferates to produce this superficial epidermal cell layer; usually sloughed by the 21st week; with sebaceous gland secretions, produces a waterproof covering called the vernix caseosa.

Periodontal ligaments   Derivatives of the inner layer of the dental sac that anchor the root of the tooth to the alveolus.

Periotic (petromastoid) bones   Arise from mesenchyme of the otic capsule to form the bony labyrinth enclosing the inner ear.

Peritoneal cavity   Derived from the region of the intraembryonic coelomic cavity inferior to the diaphragm; forms the abdominal and pelvic cavities.

Permissive pathways   Pathways for growth cones of elongating nerves; most notably devoid of dense mesenchyme or glycosaminoglycans.

Phallus (indifferent stage)   Gives rise to the clitoris in the female and the penis in the male.

Pharyngeal arches   Paired structures in human embryos evolved from branchial arches 1, 2, 3, 4, and 6 of primitive fishes to form facial and pharyngeal structures.

Pharyngeal clefts   Outer grooves between the pharyngeal arches.

Pharyngeal membranes   Thin, three-layered membranes consisting of ectoderm, mesoderm, and endoderm; separate the pharyngeal pouches from the pharyngeal clefts; first pharyngeal membrane forms the tympanic membrane or eardrum.

Pharyngeal pouches   Inner grooves within the pharynx; separate the pharyngeal arches but also give rise to important cavities and glands.

Philtrum   Medial groove of the upper lip; formed from the inferior region of the intermaxillary process.

Phocomelia   Shortened limbs may lack several intermediary segments, taking the form of seal-like appendages.

Pineal gland   Small pine-cone-shaped gland; develops from an evagination of the epithalamus.

Pioneer axon   Provides pathway along which other axons may grow.

Pituitary   Formed from the roof of the stomodeum (Rathke's pouch) and the infundibulum (floor of the diencephalon); Rathke's pouch gives rise to the anterior lobe and pars intermedia and the infundibulum forms the posterior pituitary (neurohypophysis).

Placenta   Derived from the maternal decidua basalis and the fetal chorion; provides a mechanism to exchange oxygen, nutrients, carbon dioxide, and wastes between the fetal and the maternal circulations.

Pleural cavities   Formed along with the definitive pericardial cavity by division of the primitive pericardial cavity by the pleuropericardial folds.

Pleuropericardial folds   Coronal folds of the lateral body wall that grow into the primitive pericardial cavity during the fifth week; folds fuse together in the midline and, with esophageal mesoderm, form the left and right pleural cavities and an anterior definitive pericardial cavity; forms the parietal pericardium, mediastinal pleura, and fibrous pericardium.

Pleuroperitoneal membranes   Grow from the posterolateral body walls in the plane of the septum transversum to seal off the pericardioperitoneal canals.

Ploidy   Number of copies of distinct chromosomes within a cell nucleus; haploid cell nucleus contains 23 chromosomes; diploid cell nucleus contains a pair of 23 chromosomes (46 chromosomes).

Polar body   Three minute, nonfunctional products of unequal meiotic divisions in the female germ line.

Polydactyly   Existence of extra fingers or toes.

Polyhydramnios   An excess of amniotic fluid; may occur if the fetus is not able to swallow amniotic fluid as in cases of esophageal atresia or anencephaly.

Pons   Functions to relay signals between the spinal cord and the cerebral and cerebellar cortices; composed largely of white matter; also contains pontine nuclei that relay input from the cerebrum to the cerebellum.

Pontine flexure   Third flexure of the brain; begins bending the cerebellum back upon the myelencephalon in the fifth week of development at the level of the metencephalon.

Pontine nuclei   Formed by alar column gray matter that migrates into the ventral region of the brain stem.

Portal system   Specialized system of veins that drains the gastrointestinal tract into the liver for processing of nutrients; arises from right and left vitelline veins and their median anastomoses.

Posterior and habenular commissures   Fiber tracts that connect the left and right epithalami and, with the nucleus habenulae, form the trigonum habenulae.

Posterior cardinal veins   Bilateral paired vessels that drain the trunk and lower extremities between the fourth and eighth weeks; superseded by the subcardinal and supracardinal systems.

Posterior lobe (of pituitary)   See **Neurohypophysis.**

Postganglionic fibers   See **Preganglionic fibers** and **Parasympathetic nervous system.**

Pre-Sertoli cell   Formed by medullary sex cord cells that differentiate during the sixth or seventh week of development and then give rise to Sertoli cells.

Prechordal cartilages   Form the ethmoid bone of the chondrocranium.

Prechordal plate   Small block of mesoderm that forms

just cranial to the tip of the notochordal process; induces cranial midline structures such as the brain.

Predentin Nonmineralized matrix of the dentin; first secreted by the odontoblasts in the seventh month.

Preganglionic fibers Sympathetic or parasympathetic autonomic fibers emanating from central neurons that innervate neurons in peripheral ganglia.

Prevention of polyspermy Contents of cortical granules are released into the perivitelline space (between oocyte membrane and zona pellucida) as the first spermatozoon fuses with the oocyte membrane, preventing further binding of additional sperm.

Prevertebral (preaortic) ganglion Peripheral sympathetic ganglia that house the second neuron of the two-neuron sympathetic pathway innervating the abdominal viscera; associated with major abdominal branches of the descending aorta.

Primary brain vesicles Form upon complete closure of the cranial neuropore; expansions that form each vesicle are apparent within the neural tube.

Primary buds (of mammary glands) Paired ingrowths of mammary ridge epidermis; precursors of the mammary glands.

Primary endoderm See **Hypoblast.**

Primary intestinal loop During the fifth week the midgut forms this hairpin loop that herniates into the umbilicus.

Primary oocyte or **spermatocyte** During preparatory stage of the first meiotic division oogonium and spermatogonium are converted to the primary oocyte or primary spermatocyte respectively.

Primary palate Short dorsal extension of the intermaxillary process; fuses with the palatine shelves (secondary palate) in the region of the incisive foramen.

Primary sensory cells of the olfactory system See **Olfactory epithelium** and **Olfactory bulb.**

Primary (deciduous) teeth Ten are formed within both upper and lower dental laminae; in each half-jaw will form two incisors, one canine, and two premolars; begin to erupt in the sixth month; fully erupted by 2 years of age; replaced by secondary or permanent teeth.

Primary yolk sac Formed by transformation of the blastocyst cavity; is later pushed toward abembryonic pole and degenerates to form exocoelomic vesicles and cysts.

Primitive atrium Appears as a small expansion of the primitive heart tube early in the fourth week; forms right auricle as it is displaced on the right side by incorporation of the right sinus venosus and left auricle as it is displaced on the left side by intussusception of the pulmonary veins.

Primitive groove Shallow groove running from the primitive pit to the caudal end of the primitive streak.

Primitive (primary) heart tube Formed by fusion of the lateral endocardial tubes.

Primitive node Lip of ectoderm around the primitive pit at the cranial end of the primitive streak forming the notochordal process.

Primitive nuclear neuroblasts Formed by the inner germinal layer of the cerebellum in the fourth month; migrate and give rise to the deep cerebellar nuclei.

Primitive pericardial cavity See **Definitive pericardial cavity.**

Primitive pit Depression surrounded by the primitive node at the cranial end of the primitive streak.

Primitive sex cords Form within the presumptive gonads (genital ridges) in response to arrival of the primordial germ cell; arise from cells of the coelomic epithelium and possibly cells of the mesonephros.

Primitive streak Composed of the primitive node, primitive pit, and primitive groove; forms at beginning of third week and provides the mechanism for gastrulation.

Primitive urogenital sinus Formed from the ventral region of the cloaca as it is divided by the urorectal septum; gives rise to the bladder, pelvic urethra, and definitive urogenital sinus.

Primitive ventricle Expansion of the primitive heart tube apparent early in the fourth week; mainly forms the definitive left ventricle; small portion contributes to formation of the definitive right ventricle.

Processus vaginalis Evagination of the peritoneum that plays an active role in formation of the inguinal canal; normally obliterated in females; distal remnant in the male is the tunica vaginalis; in both sexes, may remain intact and give rise to a congenital indirect hernia.

Pronucleus Chromosomes and nucleoplasm of definitive oocyte and definitive spermatocyte become separately enclosed within their own nuclear envelopes during fertilization to form female and male pronuclei, respectively.

Prosencephalon (forebrain) Region of neural plate forming this primary brain vesicle is apparent even prior to closure of the cranial neuropore; will form two secondary brain vesicles: the cranial telencephalon and diencephalon.

Prostate Male gland formed from five endodermal lobes that sprout from the pelvic urethra at the base of the bladder in the 10th week; smooth muscle and connective tissue components are derived from the splanchnopleuric mesoderm that initially covers the hindgut; formed under influence of dihydrotestosterone.

Prostatic urethra Segment of the pelvic urethra that becomes enclosed within the developing prostate gland.

Proximal nail fold See **Nail folds.**

Psoriasis Hyperproliferative skin disease; may be caused by overproduction of transforming growth factor-α.

Pulmonary diverticulum See **Lung bud.**

Pulmonary trunk Outflow tract of the right ventricle that develops from the truncus arteriosus.

Pulmonary valve   See **Semilunar valves**.

Purkinje neuroblasts   Formed by the internal germinal layer of the cerebellum and, with the basket neuroblasts formed by the external germinal layer, contribute to formation of the molecular layer of the cerebellum.

Q

Quail-chick chimera system   Experimental model (originally developed by Le Douarin) in which small pieces of chick embryo tissue are removed and replaced with tissue obtained from a quail embryo; the quail cells may differentiate and/or migrate and, due to their distinctive nucleoli, may be followed throughout their subsequent development.

R

Rachischisis   Synonym for spina bifida; craniorachischisis may refer to anencephaly.

Rathke's pouch   Ectodermal evagination of the roof of the stomodeum; forms the anterior lobe of the pituitary and the pars intermedia.

Recurrent laryngeal branch of the vagus nerve   Provides motor innervation to the intrinsic muscles of the larynx and also includes sensory fibers that innervate the mucous membrane of the larynx below the vocal cords; also possesses general visceral efferent fibers innervating the mucous membrane of the trachea.

Reichert's cartilage   Cartilage of the second pharyngeal arch formed by neural crest cells.

Renal (Malpighian) corpuscle   Comprised of the Bowman's capsule and glomerulus.

Renal papilla   Convergence of collecting ducts from a single renal pyramid at the minor calyx.

Renal pelvis   Large expansion of the hilus of the developing kidney formed from the initial bifurcation of the ureteric bud.

Renal pyramid   Pyramidal grouping of collecting ducts extending from the tip of each minor calyx (from the renal papilla) to connect with metanephric excretory units within the renal cortex.

Respiratory bronchial   Sprout from terminal bronchials between 16 and 28 weeks; branch to form terminal sacs.

Respiratory diverticulum   See **Lung bud**.

Rete testis   Thin-walled tubules that connect the seminiferous tubules with the efferent ductules formed as the deepest medullary sex cords differentiate.

Reticular layer   Thick layer of dense irregular connective tissue; deep layer of the dermis.

Retroperitoneal (organ)   Embedded within the subserous fascia of the peritoneum lining the body wall and located behind the parietal peritoneum from a point of view within a body cavity.

Rh factor   Genetically determined surface molecules present on the plasma membranes of red blood cells in most but not all individuals (see **Erythroblastosis fetalis**).

Rhombencephalon (hindbrain)   Region of the neural plate forming this primary brain vesicle is evident prior to closure of the cranial neuropore; will form two secondary brain vesicles: the metencephalon and myelencephalon.

Rhombic lips (of the hindbrain)   Arise as thickenings of the alar columns; form the cerebellar primordia that in turn give rise to the cerebellum; some of the gray matter within it migrates into the ventral floor of the hindbrain to form the pontine and olivary nuclei.

Rhombomere   Neuromeres of the rhombencephalon (see **Neuromere**).

Roof plate   Thin dorsal wall of the spinal cord and brain stem.

Root of nail plate   See **Formative zone (root; of nail plate)**.

Root of the tooth   Region deep to the boundary of the cementoenamel junction; embedded within the alveolus and covered with cementum.

S

Sacral plexus   Large plexus of nerves (anterior to the pyriformis muscle and the sacrum) composed of ventral primary rami of the lumbosacral trunk (L4, L5) and S1 to S4.

Salivatory nuclei   Innervate the salivary and lacrimal glands via nerves VII and IX.

Schwann cells   See **Myelin sheath**.

Sclerotome   Results from differentiation of somites; ventromedial and loose core cells migrate and surround the notochord and neural tube to eventually form the vertebrae.

Scoliosis   Curvature of the spine often caused by unequal development or growth of the left and right halves of a vertebral body (see **Hemivertebra**).

Scrotum   Contains the testes in the male; homologous to the labia majora of the female; arises from the labioscrotal swellings.

Sebaceous glands   Usually form as diverticula of the hair follicles within 4 weeks after the hair germ begins to elongate; formed in most regions of the body; branch into a small system of ducts that expand into small terminal acini that secrete sebum through a holocrine mechanism.

Second meiotic division   Double-stranded chromosomes divide within secondary gonocyte yielding two haploid 1N daughter cells; two definitive spermatocytes or spermatids in males and a definitive oocyte and polar body in females.

Second trimester   Fourth through sixth months of gestation.

Secondarily retroperitoneal (organ)   Appears to be retroperitoneal; initially an intraperitoneal organ that became secondarily fused to the body wall.

Secondary buds (of mammary glands) See **Mammary glands.**

Secondary endoderm See **Definitive (secondary) endoderm.**

Secondary neurosensory cells of the olfactory system See **Olfactory bulb.**

Secondary neurulation Process resulting in formation of the caudal spinal cord and filum terminale by the caudal eminence.

Secondary oocyte or **Secondary spermatocyte** Products of the first meiotic division that are haploid and 2N.

Secondary teeth See **Primary (deciduous) teeth.**

Secondary yolk sac Forms first blood vessels and blood cells; typically disappears, but may form anomalous Meckel's diverticulum.

Semilunar (trigeminal) ganglion of cranial nerve V Sensory ganglion of the fifth cranial nerve; comprised of neurons arising from the neural crest as well as from the trigeminal placode; serves general afferent functions of the trigeminal nerve.

Semilunar valves Valves of the aortic and pulmonary outflow tracts that arise as cell death foci sculpt cusps from the left and right truncoconal septa, a minor anterior truncus swelling (a cusp of the pulmonary valve), and a minor posterior swelling (a cusp of the aortic valve).

Seminal vesicles Diverticula of the mesonephric ducts; form convoluted glands that contribute secretions to the seminal fluid that nourish and protect sperm following ejaculation.

Seminiferous tubules Derived from the cells of the primitive medullary sex cords; form pre-Sertoli cells and then Sertoli cells that differentiate at puberty.

Sensitive period Period in which an organ or organ system is sensitive to effects of teratogens.

Sensory capsules Evolved from primitive ossification centers to protect the nasal epithelium, eyeball, and ear.

Sensory neurons Arise from neural crest cells that then collect lateral to the spinal cord within dorsal root ganglia; form both axons and dendritic processes that innervate the association neurons of the dorsal gray columns and target organs, respectively; may also be applied to neurons within the cranial sensory ganglia associated with cranial nerves V, VII, IX, and X and to the special sensory neurons of the retina, the nose, and the ears; may also be loosely applied to the association neurons within the dorsal (sensory) gray columns of the spinal cord and brain stem.

Septum intermedium Divides the single atrioventricular canal into right and left atrioventricular canals as the superior and inferior endocardial cushions meet and fuse during the sixth week.

Septum primum Membranous interatrial septum that forms adjacent to the left atrium; first contains an **Ostium primum,** which closes when the septum fuses with the **Septum intermedium; Ostium secundum** then forms in its superior region.

Septum secundum Grows from the atrial roof just to the right of the septum primum; forms the foramen ovale.

Septum transversum Cranial block of mesoderm apparent at the leading edge of the trilaminar germ disc on about day 22; translocated inferiorly and ventrally to the region of the presumptive diaphragm during embryonic folding; becomes innervated by cervical nerves C3, C4, and C5 and gives rise to the central tendon of the diaphragm.

Sertoli cells Arise through differentiation of medullary sex cord cells in male embryos and actively participate in nuclear and cytoplasmic maturation of male germ cells; differentiation is not complete until puberty, when they form seminiferous tubules.

Sex determination The male sex is determined by presence of a Y sex chromosome (XY), and female sex is determined by absence of a Y sex chromosome (XX).

Sex-determining region of the Y chromosome (SRY) Gene in the 1A1 region of the Y chromosome that encodes a transcription factor (the SRY protein) with a pivotal role in male sex determination and development.

Shaft (of the clitoris; of the penis) Short shaft of the female clitoris arises from the proximal end of the genital tubercle; longer shaft of the male penis is derived from the proximal end of the genital tubercle and the fusing urethral folds.

Sinus venarum Smooth-walled region of the definitive right atrium formed by intussusception of the right horn of the sinus venosus.

Sinus venosus Chamber at the inferior end of the primitive heart tube; site of confluence of the left and right common cardinal, vitelline, and umbilical veins prior to remodeling of the inflow region of the heart; left sinus horn forms the coronary sinus, and right horn forms the sinus venarum and thus the definitive right atrium.

Sinusal tubercle Endodermal thickening at the posterior wall of the pelvic urethra in the region of contact of the paramesonephric ducts; expands to form the sinuvaginal bulbs, which later form the inferior segment of the vagina.

Soft palate Most posterior region of the secondary palate; contains muscle that differentiates from its enclosed mesenchyme.

Somatic efferent Characterizes cranial nerves III, IV, VI, and XII, which provide motor innervation to striated muscles that do not develop within the pharyngeal arches.

Somatic nervous system Subdivision of the peripheral nervous system responsible for carrying conscious sensations and for innervating the voluntary (striated) muscles of the body.

Somites Appear at about day 20 as blocks of segmental mesoderm developed from somitomeres; cervical, thoracic, lumbar, and sacral somites establish segmental organization of the body by giving rise to most of the axial skeleton (including vertebral column), part of the dermis, and the voluntary musculature.

Somitomeres Segmental whorls produced prior to segmentation of paraxial mesoderm into somites; all but the first seven cranial pairs differentiate into somites.

Special somatic afferent Neuronal function served by the olfactory (I: smell), optic (II: vision), and vestibulocochlear (VIII: hearing and balance) nerves.

Special visceral afferent Characterizes sensory pathways that serve the sense of taste (gustatory function) provided by cranial nerves VII, IX, and X.

Spermatic duct (vas deferens) Arises from the mesonephric ducts in the male (see **Vas deferens**).

Spermatic fascia Processus vaginalis elongates and pushes this inguinal "sock," composed of internal (from transversalis fascia), cremasteric (from internal oblique muscle), and external (from the external oblique muscle) spermatic fascia, into the scrotal swelling.

Spermatogenesis The nuclear and cytoplasmic changes that transform primordial germ cells of the male germ line into mature spermatocytes.

Spermiation The release of the spermatozoon from the seminal epithelium into the lumen of the seminiferous tubule.

Spermiogenesis Process of cytoplasmic maturation that converts a spermatid to a spermatozoon.

Sphenoid bone Arises from the hypophyseal cartilages; greater and lesser wings have evolved from the optic capsule.

Sphenoid sinuses Extensions of the ethmoid sinuses into the sphenoid bone; first appear during the fifth fetal month and enlarge during infancy and childhood.

Sphenopalatine ganglion Parasympathetic ganglion of the facial nerve (VII); houses the peripheral neurons of the pathway that provides parasympathetic motor innervation to the lacrimal glands and mucous glands within the nasal cavity.

Spina bifida Spectrum of anomalies including spina bifida occulta, meningocele, meningomyelocele, rachischisis, and cranioschisis arising from failure of complete development and closure of the vertebral arches in one or more segments.

Spinal accessory nerve (XI) Classified as branchial efferent since it is located within the same plane of the brain stem as motor columns serving the trigeminal (V), facial (VII), glossopharyngeal (IX), and vagus (X) nerves.

Spinal nerves Originate at the point where dorsal and ventral roots join to form bundles of nerve fibers containing sensory, motor, and, in most cases, postganglionic sympathetic fibers.

Stapes bone Auditory ossicle arising from Reichert's cartilage of the second pharyngeal arch.

Stellate neuroblasts Final population of neuroblasts produced by the external germinal layer of the developing cerebellum; found in both the molecular and granular layers of the definitive cerebellar cortex.

Stem villus At 11 days, proliferation of syncytiotrophoblast and cytotrophoblast produce primary stem villi that evaginate into the trophoblastic lacunae; by day 16, an innermost core of extraembryonic somatopleuric mesoderm transforms these into secondary stem villi; by day 21, extraembryonic mesoderm differentiates into blood vessels and blood cells, converting these into tertiary stem villi.

Stratum corneum See **Horny layer.**

Stratum germinativum See **Germinative layer.**

Stratum granulosum Production of keratin and envelope proteins ceases as cells move from the stratum spinosum into this layer; produce filagrin, which helps to bundle keratin filaments within the cell.

Stratum spinosum Layer of keratinocytes overlying the stratum germinativum; as cells move into this layer they produce large amounts of keratin and envelope proteins that cover the inner surface of the plasma membranes.

Stylohyoid ligament Connects the tip of the styloid process to the lesser horn (cornua) of the hyoid; formed by Reichert's cartilage within the second pharyngeal arch.

Styloid process Inferior extension of the temporal bone; formed by Reichert's cartilage within the second pharyngeal arch.

Subarachnoid space Space between the arachnoid and pia layers of the brain and spinal cord; filled with cerebrospinal fluid.

Sublingual (salivary) glands Form from endodermal invaginations in the paralingual sulci of the oral cavity.

Submandibular ganglion Parasympathetic ganglion of the facial nerve (VII); houses peripheral neurons that provide parasympathetic postganglionic fibers to the submandibular and sublingual salivary glands.

Submandibular (salivary) glands Arise from endodermal invaginations in the floor of the oral cavity.

Subplate See **Cerebral cortex.**

Subventricular zone Layer of proliferating cells between the ventricular and intermediate layers of the cerebellum that supersedes the ventricular zone.

Sulcus dorsalis Shallow groove that appears in the sixth week to demarcate the epithalamus from the thalamus; obliterated by enlargement of the thalamus.

Sulcus limitans Narrow groove running longitudinally along the inner surface of the lateral wall of the neural tube that divides the dorsal (alar) columns from the ventral (basal) columns.

Superficial ring (of inguinal canal) Inferior medial boundary of the inguinal canal; deficiency of the external oblique muscle from which the external spermatic fascia evaginates into the scrotum.

Superior colliculi Paired swellings within the roof plate of the mesencephalon formed by proliferation of alar column neuroblasts; receive fibers from the retinas and mediate ocular reflexes.

Superior ganglion of cranial nerve IX (glossopharyngeal) Relays general sensory and special sensory (taste) impulses from the glossopharyngeal nerve to the visceral afferent nuclei; serves cranial nerve IX and the nucleus of the tractus solitarius, respectively.

Superior ganglion of the vagus (X) Relays general sensory, interoceptive, and special sensory (taste) impulses from the vagus nerve to the general afferent, visceral afferent nuclei, and nucleus of the tractus solitarius, respectively; serves cranial nerve X.

Superior laryngeal branch of the vagus nerve Innervates the musculature that develops in association with the fourth pharyngeal arch, including the cricothyroid, levator veli palatini, and pharyngeal constrictors; provides general and special (taste) sensory innervation to the very posterior region of the tongue and general sensory fibers to the epiglottis and mucous membrane of the larynx.

Superior parathyroid glands Named for their final position superior to the inferior parathyroids in the dorsal wall of the thyroid gland.

Superior vena cava Vessel arising from the proximal end of the right anterior cardinal vein.

Sweat glands First appear at about 20 weeks as buds of the stratum germinativum grow into the dermis to form unbranched highly coiled glands; secrete fluid by an eccrine mechanism; found in virtually all regions of the body except the nipples.

Sympathetic chain ganglion Paired ganglia formed at almost every segment from the cervical region to the first coccygeal level.

Sympathetic nervous system Two-neuron subdivision of the autonomic nervous system composed of central motor neurons within intermediolateral columns of the spinal cord (T1 to L2) and peripheral neurons within sympathetic chain ganglia or prevertebral ganglia; central neurons sprout preganglionic fibers that synapse with neurons in peripheral ganglia; neurons within peripheral ganglia produce postganglionic fibers that innervate target organs; termed a thoracolumbar system and is active during periods of "fight and flight."

Sympathetic trunk Composed of chain ganglia and the preganglionic fiber tract that interconnects them on either side of the vertebral column; paired sympathetic trunks run from the first cervical to the first coccygeal vertebral segment.

Synchondroidal joint Union of two bones comprised of hyaline cartilage or fibrocartilage.

Syncytiotrophoblast Expanding peripheral syncytial layer produced by mitoses within cells of the cytotrophoblast at the embryonic pole of the blastocyst beginning at day 6; secretes human chorionic gonadotropin maintaining thickened endometrium of uterus until placental membranes later usurp this function.

Syndactyly Insufficient cell death within the radial necrotic zones between digital rays results in fusion of the digits; may be manifested in webbing of the skin; bony elements of the digits may be fused.

Synovial (diarthroidal) joint Contains a cavity lined by a synovial membrane that in turn contains a slippery, lubricating fluid permitting unfettered movement between joined bones.

T

Tela choroidea Thin membrane covering the roof of the fourth ventricle; formed by ependyma and a well-vascularized layer of pia mater.

Telencephalon (end-brain) Secondary brain vesicle arising from the prosencephalon; forms the cerebral vesicles and the rhinencephalon (nose-brain).

Telopharyngeal (ultimobranchial) body Formed from a controversial fifth pharyngeal pouch; migrates into the thyroid gland to form the calcitonin-secreting parafollicular (C) cells.

Temporal lobes First appear as a forward growth of the caudal end of the lengthening cerebral hemisphere in the fourth month; involved in hearing, language, and perception.

Temporal squamosa Dermal bone that forms in association with the maxillary process of the first pharyngeal arch.

Temporomandibular joint Arose in evolution with the emergence of mammals; replaces the incus and malleus, which served as the jaw joint of vertebrates other than mammals.

Teratogen Agent that acts on the developing embryo, causing abnormal development.

Terminal bronchial Bronchial branches formed after about 17 generations of branchings of the lung bud by the 16th week; between weeks 16 and 28 they each subdivide into two or more respiratory bronchioles.

Terminal sac See **Mature alveoli.**

Terminal sulcus Transverse groove that demarcates the boundary between the anterior two thirds and posterior one third of the tongue.

Terminal villi Lateral branches of the mature intermediate villi; contain folded, coiled capillaries.

Thalamus Region of the diencephalon initially separated superiorly from the epithalamus by the sulcus dorsalis and from the inferior hypothalamus by the hypothalamic sulcus; relays information to the cerebral cortex and nuclei within the thalamus; functions in sight (lateral geniculate body) and hearing (medial geniculate body).

Third trimester Seventh through the ninth month of gestation.

Third ventricle Expansion of the neural canal enclosed within the diencephalon.

Thymus gland Arises from endoderm within the third pharyngeal pouch; descends to a position just dorsal to the sternum, where it grows to a maximum size at puberty and then regresses.

Thyroglossal cyst (sinus)   Formed when the normally degenerating thyroglossal duct persists.

Thyroglossal duct   See **Thyroid gland** and **Thyroglossal cyst.**

Thyroid gland   Forms at the apex of the thyroglossal duct as it elongates from the foramen cecum of the tongue; elongation of the thyroglossal duct places the thyroid just ventral and inferior to the developing larynx by the seventh week of development.

Tooth bud   Specialization of the dental lamina that may give rise to a primary or secondary tooth in collaboration with a dental papilla; derived from neural crest cells and an investing layer of dermal mesenchyme called the dental sac; forms the enamel organ of the growing tooth and the epithelial root sheath.

Transgenic animal   Produced by introducing foreign DNA into its genome by direct injection of the DNA into the male or the female pronucleus or by using DNA targeting techniques.

Tricuspid valve   See **Atrioventricular valves.**

Trigeminal nerve (V)   Innervates the maxillary process and mandibular process; contains branchial efferent and general sensory fibers; general sensory innervation provided by the mandibular division to the anterior two thirds of the tongue and by the maxillary division to the nasal passages and primary and hard palates.

Trigeminal placode   Ectodermal placode that gives rise to the neurons within the distal part of the semilunar ganglion.

Trigone (of the bladder)   Smooth-walled region of the posterior bladder wall (between the orifices of the two ureters and the opening into the pelvic urethra); formed by the intussusception of the inferior ends of the mesonephric ducts.

Trilaminar germ disc   Three-layered (trilaminar) embryo consisting of ectoderm, mesoderm, and definitive endoderm.

Triploid   Nucleus contains three copies of all 23 chromosomes (69 chromosomes).

Trisomy   Results from the presence of two of the same kind of chromosome in one of the gametes forming a zygote containing three copies of the same kind of chromosome.

Trochlear nerve (IV)   Somatic efferent fibers within this cranial nerve innervate the superior oblique muscle of the eyeball.

Trophic substance   Supports the growth or viability of a cellular subpopulation such as brain-derived neural growth factor (BDNF).

Trophoblast   Arises from the outer cell mass during the morula stage and initially lines blastocyst cavity but then forms the syncytiotrophoblast and cytotrophoblast of the chorionic plate; development is largely under control of the male genome.

Trophoblastic lacunae   Cavities formed within the syncytiotrophoblast in the second week that then join with maternal sinusoids to establish uteroplacental circulation.

Tropic substance   Attracts cells or growth cones to the target structures that secrete them such as netrin.

True ribs   First seven ribs that articulate with the sternum via costal cartilages.

Truncoconal septa   Septa of the outflow tracts formed from neural crest cells migrating to the truncus arteriosus through the third, fourth, and sixth aortic arches; fusion simultaneously separates the right and left ventricular chambers along with their respective outflow tracts the pulmonary trunk and aorta.

Truncus arteriosus   Distal segment of the bulbus cordis, which is divided into the ascending aorta and pulmonary trunk by formation and fusion of the truncoconal septa between weeks 5 and 9.

Tuberculum impar   See **Median tongue bud.**

Tubotympanic recess   Develops from the first pharyngeal pouch; further differentiates into the eustachian (auditory) tube and the tympanic cavity.

Tubulobulbar complexes   Formed by Sertoli cells to siphon cytoplasm from spermatids, reducing the cytoplasmic-nuclear ratio during maturation of the spermatozoon.

Tunica vaginalis   Inferior remnant of the processus vaginalis in males; enwraps the testis but is also enclosed (like the spermatic cord) in three layers of spermatic fascia; potential lumen may become filled with serous fluid following injury or disease of the serosal membrane.

U

Ultimobranchial body   See **Telopharyngeal (ultimobranchial) body.**

Ultrasonography   Body is scanned with an ultrasound beam (3 to 10 MHz); computer analyzes returning echoes imaging internal structures.

Umbilical cord   Formed by association of the connecting stalk and neck of the yolk sac (vitelline duct) as they become invested in amniotic membrane at the conclusion of embryonic folding in week 8.

Uncinate process   Hook-like region of the pancreas; derived from the ventral pancreatic bud; contains the main pancreatic duct.

Urachus (median umbilical ligament)   Vestige arising from obliteration of the allantois; may rarely remain patent.

Ureter   Duct that drains the kidneys into the bladder; derived from the ureteric bud.

Ureteric buds   Sprout from the mesonephric ducts; lengthen to penetrate the metanephric blastema; undergo a prescribed series of bifurcations to form the renal pelvis, major and minor calyces, and collecting tubules of the metanephros; tips (ampullae) induce development of the metanephric excretory units.

Urethral (urogenital) folds   Arise from the cloacal folds; give rise to the labia minora (females) and shaft (spongy urethra) of the penis (males).

Urogenital membrane   Arises from the anterior end of

the cloacal membrane in the seventh week as the urorectal septum fuses with the cloacal membrane.

Urorectal septum Mesenchymal septum that divides the cloaca composed of a Tourneaux fold, which grows inferiorly to the presumptive pelvic urethra, and left and right inferolateral Rathke folds that subdivide the inferior cloaca.

Uterovaginal (genital) canal Single cavity formed within the developing vagina and uterus by fusion of the paramesonephric ducts; produces the inferior end of the vaginal lumen.

Uterus Formed by fusion of the paramesonephric (müllerian) ducts.

V

Vagina Composite structure primarily arising from fusion of the paramesonephric ducts; smaller inferior segment is formed by growth of the sinusal tubercle.

Vaginal (sinuvaginal) bulbs Hollow expansions of the sinusal tubercle; give rise to the inferior segment of the vagina.

Vaginal plate Endodermal proliferation that occludes the inferior end of the genital canal; later canalized by desquamation to form the lower end of the vaginal canal.

Vagus nerve (X) Relays interoceptive information from the trachea, larynx, esophagus, and thoracic and abdominal viscera and stretch and chemoreceptors within the aortic arch and aortic bodies, respectively; transmits impulses from the skin behind the ear, external acoustic meatus, external surface of the tympanic membrane, and pharynx; innervates striated muscles of the fourth and sixth pharyngeal arches, glands, and smooth muscle of the pharynx, larynx, and thoracic and abdominal viscera.

Vas deferens (pl. **vasa deferentia;** also **Spermatic duct**) Male genital ducts that arise from the mesonephric ducts; differentiate in response to testosterone.

Vasculogenesis Blood vessels form throughout the entire embryo as endoderm induces overlying splanchnopleuric mesoderm to form networks of vasculature characteristic of each specific region; angioblasts form angiocysts that coalesce to form angioblastic cords and then angioblastic plexuses.

Ventral mesentery Fold of peritoneum derived from the inferior septum transversum; initially suspends the abdominal esophagus and stomach from the anterior abdominal wall; forms the falciform ligament, the visceral peritoneum of the liver and coronary ligament, and the lesser omentum.

Ventral pancreatic bud Endodermal diverticulum that sprouts just inferior to the cystic diverticulum on the ventral duodenal wall at the end of the fourth week; forms the uncinate process and main pancreatic duct.

Ventral primary ramus Ventral branch of any spinal nerve that innervates muscles of the lateral and anterior trunk and muscles of the upper and lower extremities; contains motor, sensory, and sympathetic fibers.

Ventral roots Paired bundles of nerve fibers emanating from the left and right ventrolateral wall of the spinal cord at every segmental level from the first cervical to first coccygeal level; contain motor axons of the ventral (basal) columns and preganglionic sympathetic fibers of the intermediolateral cell columns from T1 to L2.

Ventricular layer Layer of neuroepithelium located adjacent to the neural canal; gives rise to neurons, supporting cells, and ependyma of the central nervous system.

Vermis Median region of the cerebellum bounded laterally by the cerebellar hemispheres and caudally by the posterolateral fissure that separates it from the flocculonodular lobe.

Vernix caseosa See **Periderm.**

Vestibular ganglion of cranial nerve VIII Serves the special sensory function of balance; neurons arise from the otic placode (mainly) along with the neural crest.

Vestibule of the vagina Entrance to the vagina between the labia minora; derived directly from definitive urogenital sinus.

Vestibulocochlear nerve (VIII) Serves the special senses of hearing and balance.

Visceral afferent Part of the nervous system receiving interoceptive impulses via the glossopharyngeal (IX) and vagus (X) nerves from thoracic, abdominal, and pelvic viscera.

Visceral efferent Function served by cranial nerves III, VII, IX, and X; preganglionic fibers innervate parasympathetic ganglia that emit postganglionic fibers that innervate smooth muscles and glands of viscera from the head to the left colic flexure.

Vitelline arteries Initially vascularize the yolk sac; become the chief arteries of the gastrointestinal tract.

Vitelline duct Formed as growth of the embryo overtakes the stagnating yolk sac; connection between the yolk sac and midgut of the developing gastrointestinal tract narrows into this slim duct.

W

White matter Contains myelinated nerve fibers that arise from neuronal cell bodies within ventral gray column, nuclei, and specialized cortical layers of the higher centers.

White ramus communicans Connection between spinal nerves and chain ganglia at spinal cord levels T1 to L3 containing preganglionic sympathetic fibers originating from neurons within the intermediolateral column at each respective level.

Z

ZIFT (Zygote intrafallopian transfer) Male and female gametes are collected and combined in a culture dish for fertilization and subsequently introduced into the oviduct where they develop during transport to the uterus (see also **GIFT**).

Zona pellucida Protective shell around the oocyte initially formed during early stages of folliculogenesis.

Zygomatic bone Bone of the upper jaw that develops within the maxillary process; composed of dermal bone that has superseded the function of the palatopterygoquadrate bar in this location.

Index

Note: Page numbers in *italic* indicate illustrations; those followed by t refer to tables.